Biosensor Technology i
Materials into Practical

Vinay Patel • Rajendra Prasad Meena
Rohit Srivastava • Pranjal Chandra
Editors

Biosensor Technology in Translating Novel Materials into Practical Devices

Springer

Editors
Vinay Patel
Bioscience and Biotechnology
Indian Institute of Technology Kharagpur
Kharagpur, West Bengal, India

Rajendra Prasad Meena
Biochemical Engineering
Indian Institute of Technology (BHU)
Varanasi, Uttar Pradesh, India

Rohit Srivastava
Biosciences and Bioengineering
Indian Institute of Technology Bombay
Mumbai, Maharashtra, India

Pranjal Chandra
Biochemical Engineering
Indian Institute of Technology (BHU)
Varanasi, Uttar Pradesh, India

ISBN 978-981-95-5518-5 ISBN 978-981-95-5519-2 (eBook)
https://doi.org/10.1007/978-981-95-5519-2

This Springer imprint is published by the registered company Springer Nature Singapore Pte Ltd.
The registered company address is: 152 Beach Road, #21-01/04 Gateway East, Singapore 189721, Singapore

Preface

For the last 50 years, biosensing devices have evolved due to rapid development in sensor technologies, miniaturized electronics, flexible substrates, material development, and a push toward better patient management. Multiple biosensing devices have been developed and commercialized as point-of-care devices. The success of commercialized biosensing devices is owed to the development of stable biorecognition elements, nanomaterials, stable sensor substrates, immobilization methods, and various scalable fabrication methods. The emergence of mass fabrication methods has brought down the cost of these devices and their consumables making them available for the masses.

Moreover, recent advances in the miniaturization of analytical systems and newly emerging technologies also offer platforms with greater automation and multiplexing capabilities than traditional biological binding assays. Multiplexed commercial assay cartridges like i-STAT, and EPOC, have paved the way for bedside testing of multiple parameters with a sample volume of less than 100 μl. Numerous studies have proposed further development based on these multiplexed sensor arrays. Also, multiple AI/ML-based sensors are proposed to further improve these sensing systems. Further developments in flexible substrates have helped the growth of self-monitoring wearable sensors for healthcare and sports monitoring. These sensors can be used to measure common biochemical parameters such as lactate, glucose, and electrolytes.

Additionally, recent developments in materials especially nanomaterials with high surface area, tunable electrochemical and optical properties, potential surface modifications, and dynamic catalytic properties have helped the translation of different biosensors. Different nanomaterials like graphene, carbon nanotube, MXenes, and others have opened the doors for the development of multiple high-performance rapid biosensing devices with high selectivity and sensitivity. Further, these numerous composite materials with high stability and improved performance have emerged to assist the development of next-generation devices.

This book focuses on translating the biosensing devices from research to the masses. This book discusses in details about the material development, miniaturization of biosensing devices, on-chip sensors, scalable sensor fabrication methods, multiplexed sensing arrays, wearable sensors, and use of artificial intelligence and machine learning in current biosensing devices. This book also covers the use of smartphones to further miniaturize these devices and incorporates various biosensing technologies which are translated over the years will be discussed thoroughly.

The primary audience for this will be newcomers in the field of biomedical engineering, biotechnology, medical technology, and biochemistry and other related engineering professionals. Biomedical engineers, sensor technologists, biochemists, and nanobiotechnologists will find this book useful, as well as graduate students working in biomedical devices and sensor technologies. It might also serve as a reference book for schools offering graduate and postgraduate courses in biomedical engineering and their commercial fabrication. With the help of leading scientists, we are most pleased to bring this book to the readership.

Kharagpur, West Bengal, India — Vinay Patel
Varanasi, Uttar Pradesh, India — Rajendra Prasad Meena
Mumbai, Maharashtra, India — Rohit Srivastava
Varanasi, Uttar Pradesh, India — Pranjal Chandra

Contents

Editors and Contributors

About the Editors

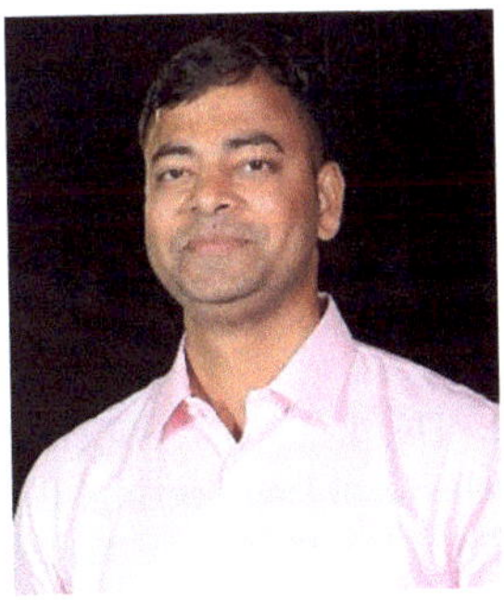

Vinay Patel is an Assistant Professor at Department of Bioscience and Biotechnology, IIT Kharagpur, India. He has 8+ years of combined experience in industrial end-to-end product development. He is leading One Health Technologies Laboratory at IIT Kharagpur. He earned his PhD from McMaster University, Canada, focusing on sensor technologies. He held postdoctoral position at IIT Bombay. His research areas include electrochemical sensing and medical diagnostics. He has published over 20+ papers and filed multiple international and national patents (one granted). He has been recognized for his outstanding work, including an outstanding graduate student award at McMaster University, Canada, and Institute Silver Medal at IIT Kharagpur.

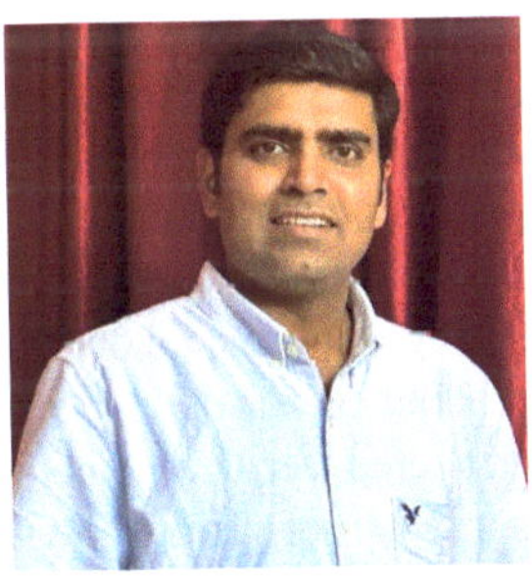

Rajendra Prasad Meena is an Assistant Professor at the School of Biochemical Engineering, IIT (BHU) Varanasi, India. He is leading the Bright NanoGhost group for early-stage CANCER diagnosis and therapeutics. Before joining the faculty position, he has done postdoctoral trainings from Tufts University, Medford, Boston, MA, USA; Technion-Israel Institute of Technology, Haifa, Israel; NOVA Medical School, Faculdade de Ciências Médicas Campo Mártires da Pátria, Lisboa, Portugal; and Indian Institute of Technology, Bombay, India. He received his PhD degree in 2017 from CSIR-NCL, Pune, India. He holds membership for World Molecular Imaging Society, American Association for Cancer Research, Royal Society of Chemistry, and American Chemical Society. He is also serving as an Associate Editor at various journals.

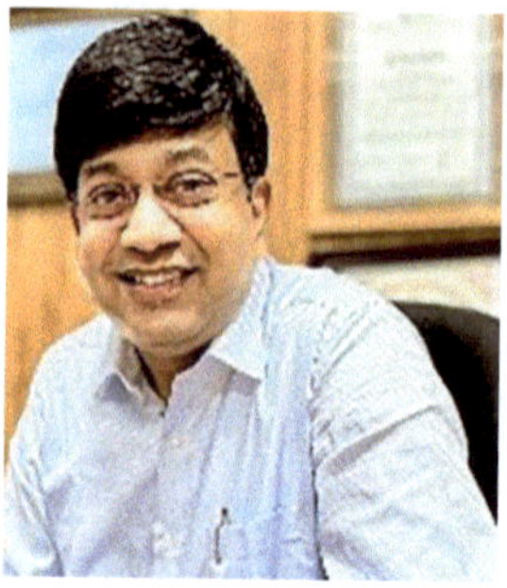

Rohit Srivastava is the Himanshu Patel Chair Professor at the Department of Biosciences and Bioengineering, IIT Bombay, India. He completed his PhD in biomedical engineering from Louisiana Tech University, USA, and has been with IIT Bombay since 2005. He specializes in point-of-care devices and cancer nanomedicine. Among his numerous awards, he received the multiple prestigious awards including Shanti Swarup Bhatnagar Prize, Vigyan Shri in Technology and Innovation, TATA innovation fellowship, and Shri Om Prakash Bhasin Award 2018 for excellence in Health and Medical Sciences. He is honored to be part of the compendium featuring "75 under 50 Scientists Shaping Today's India" published by Vigyan Prasar, Department of Science and Technology, 2022. More than 150 of his current ideas have been submitted as patents and design applications to the US and Indian Patent Office with 25+ granted patents. He has already published in more than 230+ international journals, books and books chapters, and 100+ conference proceedings.

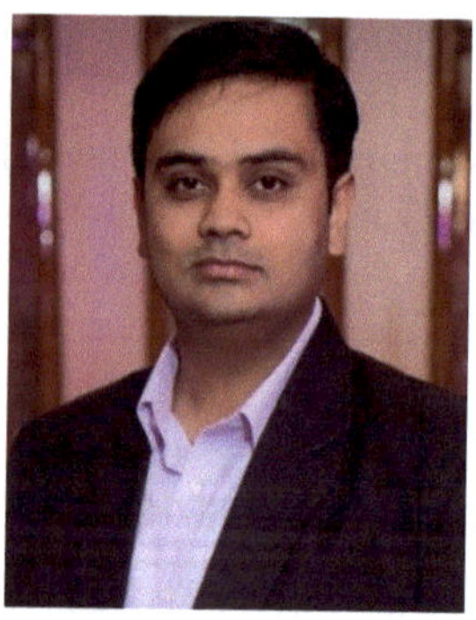

Pranjal Chandra is currently Head and an Associate Professor at the School of Biochemical Engineering, IIT (BHU) Varanasi, India. He earned his PhD from Pusan National University, South Korea, and did postdoctoral training at Technion-Israel Institute of Technology, Israel. With 15+ years of professional experience, he focuses on interdisciplinary research in biotechnology, nanobiosensors, and biochemical diagnostics. His group has designed several commercially viable prototypes that can be operated for onsite analysis. He has two international (South Korea), and four national patents granted. His work is published in 200+ journal articles/invited chapters in top-tier journals/books and has been greatly highlighted/featured in over 450 news agencies/media outlets globally. He has published 20+ books on various aspects of biosensors/diagnostics/material engineering. He is an associate editor/editorial board member of various international journals. He is the recipient of many prestigious awards, honors, and fellowships, including Fellow of National Academy of Sciences, India (FNASc); Fellow of Royal Society of Biology, London (FRSB); Associate fellow of Indian National Science Academy (INSA); Fellow of Indian Chemical Society (FICS); etc. He is also listed among the world's top 2% scientists from last 5 years by Stanford University, USA.

Contributors

Mangilal Agarwal Integrated Nanosystems Development Institute, Indiana University Indianapolis, Indianapolis, IN, USA

Department of Chemistry & Chemical Biology, Indiana University Indianapolis, Indianapolis, IN, USA

Department of Biomedical Engineering & Informatics, Indiana University Indianapolis, Indianapolis, IN, USA

Kaifi Ali Department of Biosciences and Bioengineering, Indian Institute of Technology Jammu, Jagti, Jammu, Jammu and Kashmir, India

Dilnawaz Ansari MGM University, Aurangabad, Maharashtra, India

Krishna Prasad Aryal Department of Biomedical Engineering, University of Calgary, Calgary, AB, Canada

Gizem Baysan Department of Biomechanics, Institute of Health Science, Dokuz Eylul University, Izmir, Turkey

Volkan Cecen Department of Biomedical Engineering, Newark College of Engineering, New Jersey Institute of Technology, Newark, NJ, USA

Chandhana J. P. Department of Chemistry, Amrita School of Physical Sciences Coimbatore, Coimbatore, India

Biosensor Research Lab, Amrita School of Engineering Coimbatore, Coimbatore, India

Moshfiq-Us-Saleheen Chowdhury Department of Electrical and Software Engineering, University of Calgary, Calgary, AB, Canada

Johnson Dalmieda Department of Chemistry, Columbia University, New York, NY, USA

Sreekant Damodara Verv Technologies, Sudbury, ON, Canada

Kishor Deshmukh MGM University, Aurangabad, Maharashtra, India

Sudhaunsh Deshpande David Price Evans Global Health and Infectious Diseases Group, Pharmacology & Therapeutics, Institute of Systems, Institute of Systems, Molecular and Integrative Biology, University of Liverpool, Liverpool, UK

Alev Erdi Department of Biomedical Engineering, Newark College of Engineering, New Jersey Institute of Technology, Newark, NJ, USA

Shivaum Heranjal Integrated Nanosystems Development Institute, Indiana University Indianapolis, Indianapolis, IN, USA

Department of Electrical & Computer Engineering, Purdue University Indianapolis, Indianapolis, IN, USA

Krishna Jangid Volta Labs Inc., Boston, MA, USA

Archita Jha MKSSS's Cummins College of Engineering for Women, Pune, Maharashtra, India

Wei Jiang Microelectronic Thrust, Hong Kong University of Science and Technology (Guangzhou), Guangzhou, China

Dhruvi Kakadiya Department of Biomedical Engineering, University of Calgary, Calgary, AB, Canada

Yeshwant Kasa Integrated Nanosystems Development Institute, Indiana University Indianapolis, Indianapolis, IN, USA

Department of Computer Science, Purdue University Indianapolis, Indianapolis, IN, USA

Paras J. Keyravan Department of Biosciences and Bioengineering, Indian Institute of Technology Bombay, Powai, Mumbai, India

Amey Khatavkar MIT-ADT University, Pune, Maharashtra, India

Priya Kumari CL203E Core Laboratory, Department of Chemistry, Indian Institute of Technology Kanpur, Kanpur, Uttar Pradesh, India

Sumit Majumder Department of Biomedical Engineering, Chittagong University of Engineering and Technology, Chattogram, Bangladesh

Akshay Mane Integrated Nanosystems Development Institute, Indiana University Indianapolis, Indianapolis, IN, USA

Department of Electrical & Computer Engineering, Purdue University Indianapolis, Indianapolis, IN, USA

Rohit Mohite Department of Biosciences and Bioengineering, Indian Institute of Technology Bombay, Powai, Mumbai, India

Aditya Shekhar Nittala Department of Computer Science, University of Calgary, Calgary, AB, Canada

Richa Pandey Department of Biomedical Engineering, University of Calgary, Calgary, AB, Canada

Hotchkiss Brain Institute, University of Calgary, Calgary, AB, Canada

Rajan Patyal Department of Biosciences and Bioengineering, Indian Institute of Technology Jammu, Jagti, Jammu, Jammu and Kashmir, India

Sasha Cai Lesher Perez Department of Chemical Engineering, University of Michigan, Ann Arbor, MI, USA

Buddhadev Purohit Department of Biosciences and Bioengineering, Indian Institute of Technology Bombay, Powai, Mumbai, India

Sutirtha Roy Department of Electrical and Software Engineering, University of Calgary, Calgary, AB, Canada

Sudip Saha Xzom Inc., San Diego, CA, USA

T. G. Satheesh Babu Department of Chemistry, Amrita School of Physical Sciences Coimbatore, Coimbatore, India

Biosensor Research Lab, Amrita School of Engineering Coimbatore, Coimbatore, India

Amrita Biomedical Engineering Centre, Amrita School of Engineering Coimbatore, Coimbatore, India

Eray Schulz Integrated Nanosystems Development Institute, Indiana University Indianapolis, Indianapolis, IN, USA

Department of Chemistry & Chemical Biology, Indiana University Indianapolis, Indianapolis, IN, USA

Manish S. Sengar Laboratory for Life, Sciences and Technology (LiST), Department of Chemistry, Danube Private University (DPU), Austria, Wiener Neustadt, Austria

Fatemeh Sharifi Department of Chemical Engineering, University of Michigan, Ann Arbor, MI, USA

Amit Kumar Sharma Department of Materials Science and Engineering, National Cheng Kung University, Tainan, Taiwan

Sanjiv Sharma David Price Evans Global Health and Infectious Diseases Group, Pharmacology & Therapeutics, Institute of Systems, Institute of Systems, Molecular and Integrative Biology, University of Liverpool, Liverpool, UK

Sushant Sharma Department of Biosciences and Bioengineering, Indian Institute of Technology Bombay, Powai, Mumbai, India

Vinay Sharma Department of Biosciences and Bioengineering, Indian Institute of Technology Jammu, Jagti, Jammu, Jammu and Kashmir, India

Vikas Kumar Shukla Department of Chemistry and Biochemistry, Worcester Polytechnic Institute, Worcester, MA, USA

Rohit Srivastava Biosciences and Bioengineering, Indian Institute of Technology Bombay, Mumbai, Maharashtra, India

Tanushri Department of Mathematics and Computing Technology, National Institute of Technology Patna, Patna, India

Akanksha Tipparti Integrated Nanosystems Development Institute, Indiana University Indianapolis, Indianapolis, IN, USA

Department of Biomedical Engineering & Informatics, Indiana University Indianapolis, Indianapolis, IN, USA

Cihangir Turemis Department of Orthopedics and Traumatology, Dokuz Eylul University, Faculty of Medicine, Izmir, Turkey

Hussain Valikarimwala MIT-ADT University, Pune, Maharashtra, India

Geetha Satya Sainaga Jyothi Vaskuri Department of Pharmaceutical Sciences, University of Tennessee Health Science Center (UTHSC), Memphis, TN, USA

Lalitkumar K. Vora School of Pharmacy, Queen's University Belfast, Belfast, UK

Mark Woollam Integrated Nanosystems Development Institute, Indiana University Indianapolis, Indianapolis, IN, USA

Department of Chemistry & Chemical Biology, Indiana University Indianapolis, Indianapolis, IN, USA

Introduction to Biosensing Devices 1

Amit Kumar Sharma

Abstract

Biosensing device (BioDe) technology has rapidly evolved, driven by breakthroughs in materials science, nanotechnology, and data analytics. These innovations have led to the development of highly sensitive, selective, and portable biosensors. Miniaturization of biosensors has enables high-throughput screening and precise analyte detection, while advancements in electrochemical transduction mechanisms—such as piezoelectric and triboelectric nanogenerators—allow biochemical interactions to be converted into electrical signals, facilitating real-time healthcare monitoring and p aving the way for self-powered sensors. This chapter introduces the concepts of BioDe, tracing its progression across generations to modern sensor platforms. It outlines the key structural components of biosensing devices and their evolution over time. Furthermore, this chapter briefly discusses the ongoing integration of machine learning (ML) and artificial intelligence (AI) into BioDe, enabling robust data analysis, pattern recognition, and predictive capabilities, ultimately improving sensor specificity and sensitivity. This chapter concludes with an outlook on upcoming BioDe and its impact on precision medicine and diagnostics.

Keywords

Biosensors · Wearable technology · Machine learning · Artificial intelligence · Signal transducers

A. K. Sharma (✉)
Department of Materials Science and Engineering, National Cheng Kung University, East District, Tainan, Taiwan

V. Patel et al. (eds.), *Biosensor Technology in Translating Novel Materials into Practical Devices*, https://doi.org/10.1007/978-981-95-5519-2_1

1.1 Biosensors to Biosensing Device: Introduction

Much like Beethoven's Ninth Symphony, which celebrates the joy of life, the human body is an excellent marvel of nature's finest creations, a symphony of biological processes that constantly communicates with itself and the world around it. From heartbeat to electrical stimulus in neurons, a symphony of molecular interactions orchestrates every movement and every thought in the human body. Through rigorous and unrelenting efforts, scientists have been able to eavesdrop on these molecular whisperings to better understand the language of life. For centuries, we could only listen to this symphony from a distance, through invasive procedures, predictions, and scepticism, or until it turned terminal, inferring the underlying patterns based on indirect signals. The complex nature of the human body, with its intricate biomolecular interactions, creates an environment that is suitable for a plethora of microorganisms to attack and cause disease. Due to the cell cycle and constant multiplication of human cells, genetic mutations and environmental factors often lead to cancerous growth in organs and tissues, making it one of the leading causes of human death. From cardiac arrest, neurological ailments, diabetes, and obesity, the human body is in continuous battle against internal and external threats.

The ability to detect and identify a disease for its root cause is among the fundamental challenges in medicine. The accurate pathophysiology of a disease is often hindered and becomes strenuous due to overlapping symptoms and interfering biomolecular composition, contributing to unnatural deaths. For instance, persistent fatigue can be associated with anaemia, hypothyroidism, or even chronic illness (Goërtz et al. 2021). Without identifying the responsible biomolecule accurately, treatment would be ineffective, or in some cases, even harmful. This is specifically evident in patients suffering from autoimmune diseases (Fugger et al. 2020; Fatani et al. 2021), where the immune system begins attacking the body's own tissues (Cojocaru et al. 2011). Biomolecules, including proteins, nucleic acids, lipids, carbohydrates, and metabolites, play a fundamental role in cellular function, physiological regulation, and disease pathogenesis. Despite their abundance and diversity in the human body, concentrations of certain biomolecules are highly specific to physiological ailments. These critical biomolecules are termed biomarkers (Steckl and Ray 2018). Biomarkers can be defined as the measurable biomolecular or biochemical indicators to detect, diagnose, and monitor diseases (Füzéry et al. 2013; Strimbu and Tavel 2010). Their structural modifications or presence in minute to elevated concentrations in blood (Angioni et al. 2022; Henry and Hayes 2012; Rajan et al. 2019), cerebrospinal fluid (Robey and Panegyres 2019; Blennow et al. 2010), salivary mucous (Yoshizawa et al. 2013; Dongiovanni et al. 2023), sweat (Gao et al. 2023; Zhang et al. 2024a), urine (Zhang et al. 2024b; Jordaens et al. 2023), or breath (Chan et al. 2020; Moura et al. 2024) are a testimony to disease onset, progression, and response to prescribed therapeutics.

In an era defined by rapid technological advancements, growing demands for precision medicine, and patient-driven healthcare monitoring, biosensors are transformative tools at the intersection of biology, chemistry, and engineering that are undergoing continuous refinement. Biosensors can be defined as analytical tools and processes composed of a biological or non-biological recognition element—such as enzymes, antibodies, nucleic acids, chemical or physical entities—that convert a biochemical reaction with target analytes into a quantifiable response. These tiny translators bridge the gap between biology and technology, aimed at detecting minute changes in the human body, whether it is a spike in blood sugar, the presence of a pathogen, or stress hormones. The unique selectivity of the sensing component towards the analyte/biomolecule is central to the lock-and-key principle, enabling high sensitivity and precise determination of the physiological state. Additionally, ensuring long-term biocompatibility is crucial to prevent adverse reactions and probe degradation within biological systems, especially as ongoing efforts aim not only for accurate diagnosis and treatment but also to predict and prevent the onset of diseases in the distant future. Achieving ultra-low detection limits is another significant challenge, necessary for identifying minute concentrations of target analytes. Furthermore, developing scalable fabrication methods is essential for the cost-effective and widespread deployment of advanced biosensors, ultimately supporting their role in proactive healthcare. For example, coronary heart disease is the leading cause of human death globally takes several years to progress in patients who suffer from myocardial infarction (Klein and Gheorghiade 2004; Papafaklis et al. 2016; Shah et al. 2015; Sharma et al. 2018).

Conventional biosensors typically rely on invasive sampling of biological fluids—commonly blood—to quantify specific biomarker concentrations for diagnostic assessment. Even today, most of the clinical biosensors are based on enzymes (Fan et al. 2023), immunoglobulins (Malhotra and Chaubey 2003), and nucleic acids (Piunno and Krull 2005) for disease determination (Lino et al. 2022). However, with technological advancements, non-invasive methodologies are gaining popularity among users and patients (Backiyalakshmi et al. 2024).

The biochemical reaction between the biosensor and target analyte molecule is outdated, as we wish to foresee the ongoing physiological changes and predict the user's health in real-time. This is where the second component, the transducer, comes into play. Transducers assist in translating the biological interactions into electrical or optical signals that can be quantified and translated to a real-time monitoring device. The choice of the transducer depends on the nature of the biological interaction and the analyte target. The seamless integration of biosensor and transducer components culminates in a user-centric platform known as the Biosensing Device (BioDe), enabling precise monitoring of biomarkers with exceptional sensitivity. BioDe has evolved from paper-based lateral flow assay (Toubanaki et al. 2020; Borse and Srivastava 2019), lab on a chip (Weng and Neethirajan 2016), and transdermal patch (Dervisevic et al. 2024), to on-body wearable sensors (Smith et al. 2023), wearable smartwatch (Marchianò et al. 2024), smart rings (Sempionatto et al. 2017a), offering an advanced route to disease detection. These systems function through integrated transducers, signal processors, and increasingly, AI-driven analytics (Qureshi et al. 2023). For example, wearable BioDe, including fabric (Fu et al. 2024) and eyewear (Shetty et al. 2024) can connect to a user's smartphone providing continuous real-time monitoring of physiological and biochemical parameters such as lactate (Chen et al. 2024), glucose (Sunstrum et al. 2025), and

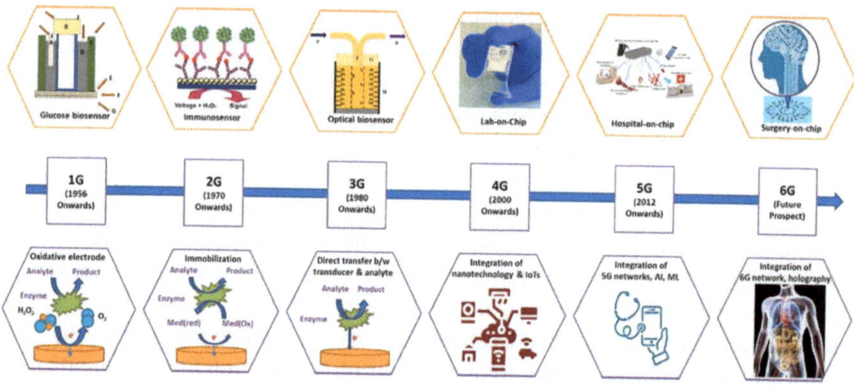

Fig. 1.1 Representative timeline showing the evolution of biosensors and biosensing devices from first generation to fourth generation and projected future prediction to six generation. (Adapted from Chaudhary et al. (2023))

hydration status (Rodin et al. 2022; Sempionatto et al. 2017b). Recent advancements in material science, device miniaturization, and wireless communication have greatly improved the functionality, comfort, and accessibility of wearable BioDe. Through its non-invasive approach and ease of usage, BioDe can play a crucial role in managing chronic diseases such as diabetes (Cappon et al. 2019) and cardiovascular conditions (Barrett et al. 2014) through continuous monitoring feature and reducing the need for frequent doctor visits. Moreover, integration of nanotechnology and development of flexible biocompatible materials are enhancing the performance and comfort of these BioDe (Hu et al. 2023). Current research on BioDe is aimed at integrating AI and digital health platforms, enabling personalized health management, early disease prediction, and secure data tracking. These advancements have supplemented preventive medicine and reduced the burden of terminal and chronic diseases. The evolution of biosensors developed over time is broadly illustrated in Fig. 1.1 (Chaudhary et al. 2023).

1.2 The Rise of BioDe—Empowering Detection and Monitoring

The modern iteration of BioDe has created a revolution in healthcare monitoring through the integration of real-time, precise, and non-invasive tracking of physiological parameters and the consequence of environmental factors on the human body (Shetty et al. 2023). Advanced BioDe are analytical tools that combine biological components with physicochemical and optoelectronic detectors to measure specific or multi-analyte biomarkers in biological fluids and tissue samples (Nagamine and Tokito 2021; Elgazar et al. 2024). For example, to facilitate point-of-care diagnostic and real-time monitoring, the reporters/probes are usually selected from organic (Sun et al. 2021; Hopkins et al. 2019), inorganic (Sokolov et al. 2023; Tang et al. 2025a) or hybrid (Park et al. 2020; Yilmaz et al. 2020) materials depending on the desired output response from the biochemical interactions. High specificity towards the target biomarker is a primary requisite in the efficient functioning of the BioDe, while the reporter/probe should be able to convert the biochemical interaction into an optical or electrical signal. As per the current research trends, BioDe can be classified into three generations.

1.2.1 First-Generation BioDe

First-generation BioDe are classified based on the use of enzymes (Sharpes et al. 2021) or organic (Norvaiša et al. 2020) molecules with high affinity against the target biomarker in a lock-and-key model, and could be detected using spectrophotometers (Khumngern and Jeerapan 2024). Enzymes are remarkable proteins that act as biocatalysts in biochemical interactions, with high specificity against their substrates, making them an ideal probe. Through their substrate-binding active sites, enzymes undergo a complex transformation upon interaction with biomarkers to produce reaction products. These products then detach from the enzyme, validating the presence of the biomarker. Glucose oxidase-based glucose sensor is a hallmark detection methodology (Brown et al. 2005). The catalytic product of glucose oxidase-based reaction, hydrogen peroxide, is exploited to quantify glucose through colorimetric and electrochemical response (Ahmed et al. 2022) using reporter materials like gold nanoparticles (Chi et al. 2020), α-MoO_{3-x} (Nerthigan et al. 2018), carbon 60-carboxyfullerenes (Li et al. 2013). This reaction is further exploited meticulously to design several wearable glucose-sensing technologies, such as in contact lens (Jeon et al. 2021) (that will be discussed later). Owing to this high specificity, enzymes are also used in enzyme-linked immunosorbent assays (ELISA)-based detection kits for cancers (Saadi et al. 2013; Chen et al. 2022) and viral zoonotic outbreaks like COVID-19 (Yadegari et al. 2023; Liu et al. 2023).

Nucleic acids have been instrumental in targeting biomarkers and identifying diseases through their complementary base pairing property leading to the development of DNA array sensors (Sassolas et al. 2008; Park et al. 2023). Nucleic acid driven sensors based on single-stranded DNA probes have played a key role in genomics and recently for COVID-19 detection (Vindeirinho et al. 2022). Its unparalleled specificity plays a critical role in identifying genetic mutations (Yeong Lee et al. 2024; Zhao et al. 2023), viral infections (Feng et al. 2024), and bacteria (Tang et al. 2025b). These biosensors exploit the specific hybridization property of nucleic acids to its complementary sequences forming double-stranded structure and triggers a measurable signal in a BioDe. For example, Guardant360 CDx and FoundationOne Liquid CDx are FDA-approved liquid biopsy tests for detecting genetic mutations in EGFR, BRCA, L858R, and T790M mutations for determining circulating tumour cells (Takai and Yachida 2016; Gupta et al. 2020). Abbott ID NOW™, developed for detecting viral genetic material for SARS-CoV-19, proved a vital alternative to conventional RT-PCR tests during the pandemic (Burnes et al. 2021). Similarly, point-of-care nucleic acid BioDe, like the Cepheid GeneXpert System (Ioannidis et al. 2011) and loop-mediated isothermal amplification (LAMP)

(Choopara et al. 2021) biosensor is developed for tuberculosis and methicillin-resistant *Staphylococcus aureus* (MRSA), respectively. Gene editing capabilities of clustered regularly interspaced short palindromic repeats (CRISPR) are used to design CRISPR-Cas biosensors to detect specific genetic sequences, enabling ultra-fast diagnostics (Masi et al. 2023).

The first-generation BioDe relied on the direct use of natural biological elements, primarily, enzymes and nucleic acids, to detect specific biomarkers. The signal generated by enzymatic reaction was typically electrochemical, such as differential pulse voltammetry, square wave voltammetry, chronoamperometry, and fluorescence spectroscopy, measuring oxidation products or hydrogen peroxide. However, a major limiting factor for these first-generation BioDe was its limited stability and lifespan of enzymes, susceptibility to environmental conditions like temperature or pH, potential interference from competitive inhibitors, loss of enzyme activity over time, reproducibility, and reliability of measurements.

1.2.2 Second-Generation BioDe

The peculiar challenges of the first-generation BioDe were overcome by the second-generation BioDe, which involved electron transfer as the vital communication medium between the analyte target biomarker and the biosensor probe (Monošík et al. 2012). The incorporation of appropriate biosensor probes facilitated a more robust signal while adhering to sensitivity and reduced susceptibility to environmental factors.

The concurrent rise of nanotechnology, in the form of metallic sub-atomic nanomaterials with functional properties (Anker et al. 2008), boosted the research toward the development of the second-generation BioDe and laid the foundation for present-day advanced monitoring systems. In contrast to first-generation BioDe, second-generation BioDe relied heavily on the specific interactions between the nanomaterial probe and the target biomarker to generate a colorimetric, electrochemical, or electrical signal. For example, the use of gold nanoparticles in developing a lateral flow assay for quick determination of nodavirus (as shown in Fig. 1.2a) (Toubanaki et al. 2020), and a peanut allergen Ara h1 detection device using quantum dots-aptamer-graphene oxide conjugates (Fig. 1.2b). These biosensors eliminated the need for detecting reaction byproducts, instead utilizing electron transfer mediators to improve sensitivity, accuracy, and response time (Li et al. 2022). Additionally, artificial redox mediators facilitating electron transfer and reducing response time with high reproducibility, enabled miniaturization of the BioDe towards the era of point-of-care diagnostics (Kaur et al. 2021). Noble metal nanoparticles (Sharma et al. 2025), metal oxide nanomaterials (Solanki et al. 2011), and carbon-based nanomaterials (Khan et al. 2023) were on the font-line as reporters owing to their high sensitivity for single electron transfers and quick optoelectronic response (Sharma et al. 2021). This further enabled us to reach lower detection limits and set new standards for BioDe. Ferrocene-based glucose biosensors (Guven et al. 2021), Biosen C-Line for lactate (EKF Global n.d.), and hydrogen

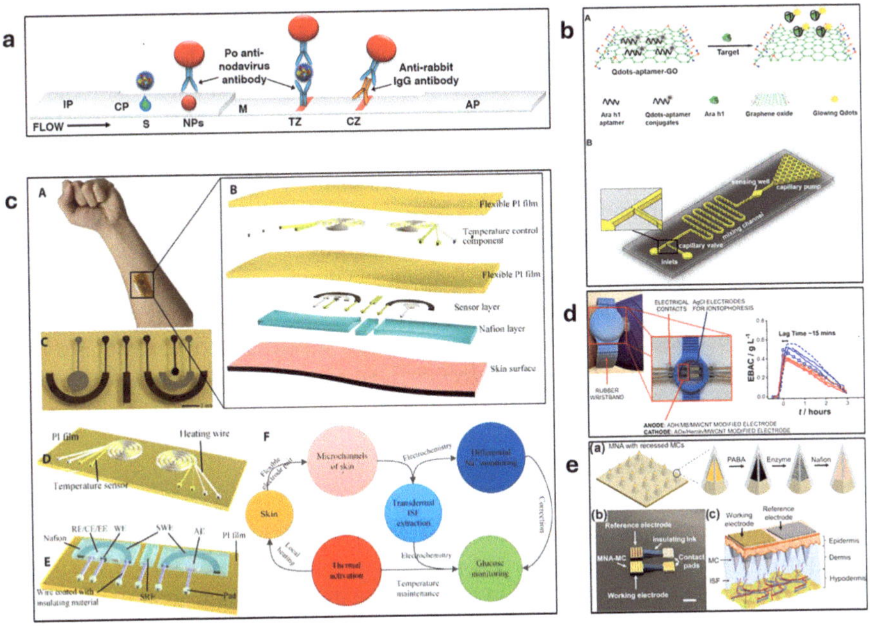

Fig. 1.2 (**a**) Nanoparticle-based lateral flow assay for detecting nodavirus. (Adapted from Toubanaki et al. (2020)). (**b**) Working principle (A) and device design (B) of Quantum dots-aptamer-Graphene oxide based lateral flow assay design for allergen detection. (Adapted from Weng and Neethirajan (2016)). (**c**) Pictorial representation of skin-adhering non-invasive continuous blood glucose monitor, showing the proposed design (A), integrated structure (B), detection components (C), temperature regulator (D), device structure (E), and working mechanism. (Adapted from Smith et al. (2023)). (**d**) Self-powered wearable wrist band biosensor incorporating iontophoretic electrodes developed for non-invasive blood alcohol detection. Adapted from Marchianò et al. (2024)). (**e**) Wearable microneedle patch architecture for blood urea detection through interstitial fluid. (Adapted from Dervisevic et al. (2024))

peroxide-mediated oxidative stress biomarkers (Giaretta et al. 2022) are a few examples of the second-generation BioDe. Notably, second-generation BioDe suffered from limited biocompatibility, signal drift due to prolonged exposure to biomarkers, single-molecule specificity, cost of production, and interference from biological fluids hinders its long-life success.

1.2.3 Third-Generation BioDe

The prerequisite of mediators for electron transfers between biomarkers and biosensor probes was a major challenge for second-generation BioDe, which was resolved simply through eliminating these mediators. The direct electron transfer between biomarkers and transducers is an obvious choice for advanced BioDe to achieve a higher accuracy, eliminate competitive inhibition and interference due to biological fluids (Das et al. 2016). For instance, the direct electron transfer between the biomarker and electrode, in an electrochemical biosensing device, improved the response time and stability. Nanomaterials, such as graphene (Mehmeti et al. 2017; Zhao et al. 2016), carbon nanotubes (Gomes et al. 2019), and phenyl boronic acid (Elsherif et al. 2018a), enhance sensitivity and selectivity by improving conductivity and enzyme stability. The use of biocompatible polymers ensures controlled interaction between the probe and biomarkers in biological fluids, leading to the development of implantable and long-term monitoring BioDe (Ghazizadeh et al. 2024; Tomioka et al. 2022). Thus, the third-generation BioDe are capable of detecting multiple biomarkers simultaneously owing to their selective response, i.e. electrochemical signals (Yokus et al. 2020; Cheng et al. 2023; Wang et al. 2022), enabling their integration in flexible polymers for a skin-adherent sensor for non-invasive analyte detection through sweat analysis (Gao et al. 2023).

1.2.4 Fourth-Generation BioDe

The integration of reporter/probes into wearable devices, in the form of biocompatible polymers, or smart gadgets, led to the rise of the fourth-generation BioDe. These BioDe are primarily focused on multi-analyte detection while being non-invasive and on-body wearable units in operation. For example, Fig. 1.2c shows the skin-adhering glucose BioDe that functions on the direct interaction between electrodes and analytes in sweat (Smith et al. 2023), while rapid blood alcohol detection through non-invasive BioDe (Fig. 1.2d) exploits iontophoresis to extract sweat to measure blood alcohol levels (Marchianò et al. 2024). Partially invasive microneedle patch-based BioDe gained popularity in theranostics applications for their ability to integrate with a smartphone and execute controlled release and simultaneous detection of analytes through interstitial fluids (Dervisevic et al. 2024) (Fig. 1.2e).

1.2.5 Fifth-Generation BioDe

The forthcoming advancements in AI and machine learning (ML) (Han et al. 2025) are anticipated to enhance predictive capabilities for early disease detection, personalized medication, remote health monitoring through 5G and 6G connectivity, and designing sustainable implantable biosensors (Zhang et al. 2023; Bhaiyya et al. 2024). As a subset of AI, ML algorithms can assist in handling large datasets acquired over a period of days and weeks from on-body continuous monitoring sensors (Kadian et al. 2023). Additionally, ML algorithms facilitate categorization of the measured signals, differentiate and interpret signals as a consequence of interfering factors, reduce noise, and determine a pattern appropriate for interpretation of the collected data (Cui et al. 2020). ML algorithms like (i) κ-nearest neighbour—a supervised learning model functions based on classifying new data by finding the "κ" most similar past measurements and assigning new point based on the majority class or average value of those neighbours (Florimbi et al. 2018); (ii) support vector machine—operates by finding an optimal hyperplane that separates different classes of the acquired data, maximizing the margin between the closest data points from each class; (iii) decision tree—that uses a flowchart-like structure to classify or predict outcomes. It splits biosensor data based on a series of "if-then-else" rules derived from features such as biomarker concentration thresholds until it reaches a final decision or prediction; (iv) random forest—an ensemble learning model that combines predictions from multiple individual decision trees. Each tree is built using a random subset of the acquired data and a random subset of features, leading to a more robust and accurate model that reduces overfitting compared to a single decision tree; it has been applicable in third and fifth-generation BioDe predicting disease progression (Elsherif et al. 2018b; van de Goor et al. 2018; Alfian et al. 2018; Zhang et al. 2021; Mondal et al. 2023; Flynn and Chang 2024).

Furthermore, AI-driven bioinformatics tools have now begun to analyse and interpret biosensor-generated nucleic acid data, improving diagnostic accuracy (Kamya et al. 2024). Coupled with electrochemical transducers, the biochemical response is amplified through current, voltage, or impedance signal. Optical transducers, on the other hand, complement the development of cholesterol (Yunianto et al. 2017; Li et al. 2022), cortisol (Arcadio et al. 2024) and lactate (Ignatov et al. 2001) biosensors to detect obesity and other physiological diseases.

1.3 Components in BioDe

BioDe functions by detecting biological interactions and converting them into measurable signals. The fundamental principle of BioDe lies in the specific recognition of a target analyte by a recognition element and the subsequent conversion of this biochemical interaction into an electrical, optical, thermal, magnetic, or mechanical signal is termed signal transduction. This signal can be analysed to determine the presence, concentration, or activity of the target analyte. The choice of the transduction mechanism dictates the sensitivity, specificity, and reliability of the biosensing device.

1.3.1 Electrochemical Transduction

Electrochemical transduction method primarily involves measuring changes in current, voltage, or impedance resulting from the biochemical interaction between analyte and probe (Yang et al. 2021). Such BioDe are highly popular due to their high sensitivity, rapid response time, and compatibility with miniaturized devices. Owing to its facile integration with electrochemical detectors, these BioDe are increasingly integrated into smartphones for convenient access to biomarker concentration and ease of monitoring (Su et al. 2022). Voltammetry/potentiometry-based BioDe involves measuring current as a function of applied voltage to analyse the redox reaction at the interface of the probe and target analyte. This technique is largely explored in developing continuous glucose monitoring devices, such as in Dexcomm CGM (Kumar Das et al. 2022) and pathogen sensing (Lopez-Tellez et al. 2022;

Vidic and Manzano 2021). Chronoamperometry-based BioDe, on the other hand, measures the steady-state current in response to a fixed voltage over time. This technique is suitable and employed in elastomers and flexible polymer-based wearable BioDe for monitoring lactate (Rasitanon et al. 2023), levodopa (Goud et al. 2019), and dopamine (Domingo-Roca et al. 2022) levels. Impedimetric BioDe are based on changes in electrical resistance or capacitance caused by biochemical interactions between the analyte and probe. These are considered relatively robust and employed in skin-based wearable devices owing to its specificity for the biological impedance of the skin (Siboro et al. 2024). Piezoelectric BioDe operates by detecting mechanical vibrations generated when a biological molecule binds to the sensor surface. The change in frequency is proportional to the mass of the bound analyte. For example, quartz crystal microbalance sensors are used in virus detection and biomolecular interaction analysis (Lim et al. 2020). Piezoelectric BioDe provides the highest accuracy among electrochemical transduction techniques, prominently in wearable continuous blood pressure monitoring devices (Yi et al. 2022a; Yi et al. 2022b).

1.3.2 Optical Transduction

The optical signal transduction method relies largely on the light absorption, fluorescence, or luminescence caused by biochemical interactions between biomarkers and the reporter entity. Also termed colorimetric sensors, these BioDe operate on visible colour changes caused by chemical reactions. This method, although a simple operating mechanism, suffers from low sensitivity, interference from sample components, and subjectivity in colour interpretation. Despite these drawbacks, colorimetric sensors have stood the test of time as it provide a quick verification of the analyte (Li et al. 2022; Seo et al. 2023).

1.3.3 Signal Processing

Signal processing plays a crucial role in converting the raw data from the BioDe into meaningful information for decision-making. This process involves multiple stages, including amplification, filtering, noise reduction, analogue-to-digital conversion, and microcontroller-based data processing. The raw data obtained after biochemical interactions are transformed using the signal transduction mechanisms. However, these signals are often too weak (in the range of microvolts to millivolts), low signal-to-noise ratio, or in an analogue format that needs further amplification. Operational amplifiers (op-amps) are a primary choice for signal enhancement without introducing distortions. For example, the microcurrent generated in a glucose wearable patch is amplified to accurately determine its levels (Croce et al. 2013). The second step is to eliminate the interfering signals from external electrical sources, environmental factors, or physiological variations through noise reduction and filtering to avoid false positives and inaccuracies. Various filtering techniques, such as low-pass, high-pass, and band-pass filters, help remove unwanted signal components. Low-pass filtering eliminates high-frequency noise, while high-pass filtering removes slow signal drift. Additionally, adaptive filtering techniques such as wavelet transform and Kalman filtering are also employed in wearable BioDe (Ward et al. 2021).

1.3.4 Analogue-to-Digital Conversion

The next step is to convert the analogue signal to a digital format for further processing. Analog-to-digital conversion (ADC) is an essential step in modern BioDe as most biological signals exist in continuous analogue form. ADC transforms these signals into discrete numerical values that can be processed, analysed, and stored by digital systems. The accuracy of the ADC system depends on its bit resolution and sampling rate. Higher bit ADC provides precise signal representations while a higher sampling rate ensures rapid changes in biosensor readings are accurately captured. For example, ADC assists in converting enzymatic-dependent output current into blood glucose values, and nucleic acid hybridization-dependent electrical signal into interpretable data. The final stage of biosensor signal processing involves microcontroller-based data handling and processing. Microcontroller serves as the computational core of BioDe, executing algorithms for real-time analysis, calibration, and decision-making. They enable the device to perform operations such as drift comparison, pattern recognition, and ML-based diagnostics. Microcontrollers also facilitate wireless connectivity or near-field communications (NFC) for smartphone connectivity and cloud-based data sharing with healthcare professionals.

1.3.5 Output Device and Power Supply

BioDe is designed not only to detect biochemical interaction signals but also to provide meaningful and accessible information to users. The user interface and data output mechanisms play a crucial role in ensuring that sensor-generated data is effectively displayed, transmitted, and analysed. The key components of this system include display technology, wireless connectivity, and software-driven analysis tools. A major challenge in the choice of display technology is associated directly with power consumption, which becomes more crucial in case of battery-operated BioDe, such as a smart watch. Energy consumption, energy efficiency, readability, and compact size are the associated parameters governing this aspect of BioDe (Arya et al. 2024). Organic Light Emitting Diodes (OLED) screens are now replacing conventional liquid crystal displays (LCD) owing to the high contrast, flexibility, and low power consumption (Kim 2017). Power supply is another critical component of BioDe, directly impacting its portability, longevity, and efficiency (Sun et al. 2023a). Most modern BioDe rely on lithium ion (Li-ion), lithium polymer (Li-Po), and coin-cell batteries due to their high energy density, stability, and compact size. Wearable devices use ultrathin batteries that provide sustained power while maintaining the flexibility and comfort for the user. However, low battery usability and limited lifespan present challenges that lead to the exploration of alternative power solutions. Ongoing research indicates piezoelectric (Xu et al. 2021) and triboelectric nanogenerators (Munirathinam and Chandrasekhar 2023; Tao et al. 2025) as potential replacements for wearable BioDe. The future of BioDe lies in self-powered and energy-efficient systems where innovative power solutions will enable long-term, continuous monitoring without frequent charging and battery replacements.

1.4 Transformations of BioDe—From Bench to Bedside

1.4.1 Chemical Sensors

The first-generation BioDe, primarily chemical sensors, emerged in the mid-twentieth century, primarily driven by the need for rapid and accurate detection of biological analytes. These devices used a continuous flow analysis technique to process multiple samples simultaneously, significantly increasing the throughput of chemical testing laboratories. The advent of functional nanomaterials in the late twentieth century further advanced the detection capabilities of the BioDe. Reported literature has shown that plasmonic metals such as gold, silver, copper, iron, and cobalt have been exploited for detecting biomarkers in biological fluids with remarkable sensitivities in solutions (Jain et al. 2008). Owing to the surface plasmon effect, the quantum confined nanostructures exhibit excellent optical properties that are varied upon interaction with biomarkers. These biochemical interactions laid the foundation for the development of second-generation BioDe, such as paper strip lateral flow assays (LFA). LFA is deemed an advanced technique for qualitative assessment of the biological fluid (Zhao et al. 2018). It uses an adsorbing nitrocellulose membrane paper as a medium for the biological fluid to flow through the pre-adsorbed biosensors on cellulose paper (usually plasmonic materials bound to the complementary molecule) and generate a colorimetric response post-interaction. Biochemical entities like enzymes, selective proteins, nucleic acids have been used for devising a plethora of qualitative sensors for several acute diseases. Pregnancy test kits are the most popular example of LFA, where gold nanoparticles are bound to human chorionic gonadotropin (hCG)-antibodies and conjugated on the substrate pad (Zhang et al. 2020). The hCG protein in the urine sample is dropped on the nitrocellulose membrane and reaches the conjugate pad to bind to the specific antibodies. The presence of the hCG is confirmed by the test line and control line appearing on the test strip, indicating a positive result. Similar strategies are employed in the detection of glucose (using glucose oxidase) (Huang et al. 2022), malaria (using lactate dehydrogenase) (Mthembu et al. 2017), human immunodeficiency virus (HIV) (Chen et al. 2023), and cardiac troponin (Omidfar et al. 2023). Recently, lateral flow immunoassay (LFIA) was exploited to design COVID-19 rapid detection kits (Huang et al. 2020). Despite the remarkable success of LFA and LFIA, this technique suffers from low clinical sensitivity and specificity to low analyte concentration, lack of quantifiable data, and a lack of multiplex detection.

1.4.2 Complex Sensors for Multiplex Analysis

Lab-on-a-Chip (LOC) BioDe are unique technology addressing the limitation of LFA and facilitating multiplex analysis of analytes. LOC BioDe aims for robust detection strategies, facile scalability, real-time detection capabilities, miniaturization, and incorporation of electrochemical principles as sensors (Cinti et al. 2023). LOC builds upon the core principles of LFA while incorporating sophisticated microfluidic channels, automated sample processing, and real-time detection mechanisms (Economou et al. 2018). Unlike LFAs, which rely on the capillary action of the nitrocellulose membrane substrate for fluid transport and use colorimetric readouts, LOC BioDe uses active fluid manipulation, electrochemical, optical, or piezoelectric sensing, and integrates nucleic acids amplifiers technology for improved sensitivity and specificity. This allows for the detection of multiple biomarkers simultaneously, providing more accurate and quantitative diagnostic (Guan et al. 2022). A notable example is the development of an aptamer-based LOC system for prostate-specific antigen (PSA) biomarker detection. This device utilizes aptamers—short, single-stranded nucleic acid molecules—that specifically bind to PSA biomarkers in patient samples, demonstrating its potential as an indispensable tool for point-of-care cancer biomarker detection (Uludag et al. 2016). Another example of LOC for nucleic acid testing is shown by Tong et al., where the authors demonstrate an integrated 3D-printed biosensing device incorporating CRISPR/Cas12a-based dual-enzymatic mechanism. This device eliminates the need for amplification of the nucleic acid sequence, achieving a limit of detection as low as 10 pM. Furthermore, the biosensing device can be patched with a smartphone for quantitative analysis, thus, a promising tool for rapid nucleic acid screening in clinical diagnostics (Tong et al. 2025).

1.4.3 Smartphone Integrated BioDe

Building upon LOC advancements, smartphone-integrated BioDe leverage the widespread use and technological capabilities of smartphones to further democratize healthcare. This enables continuous health monitoring and personalized healthcare, serving as storage and data sharing units with healthcare professionals, providing adequate computational prowess for accurately predicting and projecting patients' physiological state. The foundations laid by second-generation BioDe, like LOC, are a benchmark for introducing innovative methodologies such as piezoelectric and triboelectric nanogenerators (TENG) for disease diagnosis. These advanced sensors, coupled with smartphones' computational capabilities, offer enhanced sensitivity and selectivity against biomarkers. Piezoelectric nanogenerators are known to convert mechanical energy into electrical energy (Yeo 2023), on the other hand, TENG generates electrical energy through contact electrification and electrostatic induction (Bulathsinghala et al. 2023). These technologies have enabled the development of wearable and implantable sensors that continuously monitor physiological parameters (Xu et al. 2024).

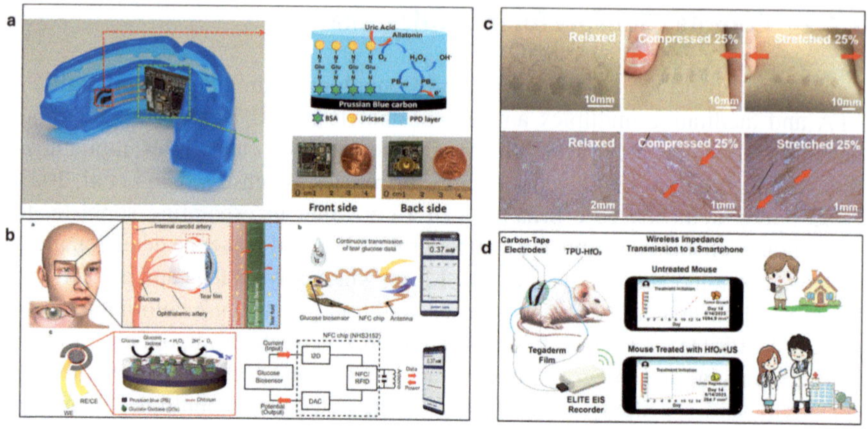

Fig. 1.3 (**a**) Uricase-based salivary uric acid detection through mouthguard BioDe. (Adapted from Kim et al. (2015)). (**b**) Smart Contact lens enabled with glucose sensing capabilities and a wireless module for data transfer. Adapted from Park et al. (2024a)). (**c**) Characterizations of Graphene electronic tattoo mounted on skin that serve as functional electrodes for biosensing analytes in sweat. (Adapted from Kabiri Ameri et al. (2017)). (**d**) HfO_2 embedded thermoplastic polyurethane elastomer sensor integrated with a smartphone for continuous monitoring of tumour progression. (Adapted from Siboro et al. (2024))

Wearable and implantable sensors represent the next frontier in BioDe technology. These devices are often integrated with clothing, accessories, or even directly attached to the skin (Alberto et al. 2020; Shang et al. 2023) allowing for non-invasive health monitoring. Implantable sensors, on the other hand, are embedded within the body, offering more accurate and comprehensive data collection. Figure 1.3a shows uricase-based uric acid detection using a mouthguard that is also enabled with wireless modalities for data collection (Kim et al. 2015). Park et al. demonstrate a robust glucose monitoring contact lens, meticulously excluding the tears from reflex (Fig. 1.3b) (Park et al. 2024a). Graphene electronic tattoo (Kabiri Ameri et al. 2017) (Fig. 1.3c) is exemplary as BioDe, which harvests the capabilities of graphene's electrical conductivity to develop an on-body sensor, housing electrochemical interactions between biomarkers in the sweat. This device registers the movement of the user through piezoelectric signals and time-dependent change in voltage. The sensitivity of the tattoo is adequate in detecting electrocardiogram signals and skin hydration. Similarly, Yetisen et al. have developed dermal tattoos for glucose, albumin, and pH detection over the skin using sweat as a biofluid (Yetisen et al. 2019). Kim et al. have demonstrated a colorimetric approach integrated with an on-body skin sensor that qualitatively detects micronutrients and vitamins in sweat (Kim et al. 2022). Intriguingly, thermoelastic polymers entrapping metal oxide nanomaterials, such as HfO_2, have shown promising results in monitoring cancer tumour progression over the skin (Siboro et al. 2024) (Fig. 1.3d). Bioelectronic Tongues (BETs) and Bioelectronic Noses (BENs) emerge as non-invasive BioDe to detect biomarkers associated with Alzheimer's disease (Park et al. 2024b). Seo et al. have reviewed the fabrication of wearable contact lenses as a point-of-care diagnostic and disease management platform in detail; interested readers may seek (Seo et al. 2023) for further reading. Zhang et al. have integrated an image optimization algorithm for quantitation of hCG in a LFA BioDe (Zhang et al. 2020); such an approach opens a new platform for upgrading earlier second-generation BioDe while retaining its simplicity.

1.4.4 Artificial Intelligence Enabled Fourth-Generation BioDe

The innovation of AI and facile availability in smartphones has further boosted the advancements in BioDe. With machine learning approaches, advanced BioDe can predict oncoming diseases like cardiac myopathy, obesity, and diabetes that usually take several years to develop (Bhaiyya et al. 2024). One notable application of machine learning in BioDe is the detection and classification of cells. Machine learning algorithms can differentiate between healthy and diseased cells, enabling early diagnosis and monitoring of various medical conditions. This capability is particularly valuable in oncology, where early detection of cancer cells can significantly improve patient outcomes. AI enables BioDe to analyse data from electrochemical sensors for different biomarkers in biological fluids. AI algorithms can process this data, identify relevant biomarkers and provide insight into patient health status (Wang et al. 2024). This capability is particularly valuable in managing chronic conditions, such as diabetes, where continuous monitoring and personalized treatment plans are essential. Table 1.1 shows the successive generation of BioDe (Fig. 1.4).

1.5 Outlook and Conclusion

Recent years have witnessed remarkable advancements in BioDe driven by innovations in materials science, nanotechnology, and data analytics. These advancements have led to the development of highly sensitive, selective, and portable biosensors, transforming various fields, including healthcare, environmental monitoring, and food safety. One of the key aspects is the miniaturization of devices. Lab-on-chip technology has enabled the integration of multiple laboratory functions onto a single chip, allowing for high-throughput screening and precise detection of analytes. These miniaturized devices are not only portable but also offer rapid and accurate results, making them ideal for point-of-care diagnostics. Another significant trend is the incorporation of advanced methodologies such as piezoelectric and triboelectric nanogenerators. These technologies enhance the performance of biosensors by converting mechanical energy into electrical signals, enabling real-time biomarker analysis. Wearable and implantable sensors, leveraging these technologies, provide continuous health monitoring and early diagnosis. The integration of ML and AI has also revolutionized BioDe. ML and AI algorithms can analyse complex datasets, identify patterns, and make accurate predictions, enhancing the sensitivity and specificity of biosensors. These algorithms can also optimize sensor design, reduce false positives and provide personalized recommendations. Moreover, the development

Table 1.1 Tabular representation of various generations of BioDe

BioDe generations	Target biomolecule	Reporter/probe	Biochemical/physical interaction	Transduction method	Limit of detection	Reference
Generation 1	Glucose	H_2O_2	Glucose oxidase/glucose	Electrochemical	0.06—10 mM	Adeloju and Moline (2001)
	Cholesterol	Cholesterol oxidase	Electrode interaction	Microneedle-Pt	0.5 μM	Uchayash et al. (2025)
	Lactate	Lactate dehydrogenase	Gold nanopillar electrode	Square wave voltammetry	1.0 U/L	Li et al. (2023)
	H_2O_2 released from cells	Gold nanowires	Electrode interaction	Chronoamperometry	3.2 μM	Patella et al. (2024)
	Phosphate	Ce–UiO–66-NO_2	Free oxygen radical generation	Fluorometry and colorimetry	7.60 μM	Qin et al. (2024)
Generation 2	Tyrosinase	$NaYF_4$:Yb,tm	Dopamine-controlled photoinduced energy transfer	Upconversion fluorescence spectroscopy	0.3 U/ml	Li et al. (2019)
	Alkaline phosphatase	p-Nitrophenol	Phenyl phosphate/p-nitrophenol	Square wave voltammetry	0.29 μM	Sappia et al. (2019)
	Glucose	Glucose-6-phosphate	Glucose/hexacyanoferrate	Field effect transistor	50 μM	Anan et al. (2013)
	D-2-hydroxyglutaric acid	d-2-hydroxyglutarate dehydrogenase regulator	Chemiluminescent signal due to energy transfer between reporter and target molecule	AlphaScreen technology	2—50 μM	Xiao et al. (2021)
	Thrombin	Amine reactive phenazine ethosulphate	Aptamer-antibody sandwich	Electrochemical	1.5 pM	Kim and Yang (2024)

Generation 3	CA-15-3	MIL-156/gold nanoparticles	Antibody binding gold nanoparticle	Differential pulse voltammetry	2.6 nU/ml	Dezhakam et al. (2024)
	BRCA1	Carbon electrode	Polyethylene glycol/gold nanoparticles	Electrochemical impedance spectroscopy	1.72 fM	Wang et al. (2015)
	Beta-amyloid	Graphene electrode	Poly(1,5-diaminonaphthalene)/beta amyloid	Differential pulse voltammetry	1.4 pg/ml	Abbasi Hina et al. (2021)
	Cholesterol	Pencil graphite electrode	Cholesterol oxidase/cholesterol	Electrochemical impedance spectroscopy	62 μM	Eksin et al. (2024)
	Cardiac troponin I	Gold nanoparticles on graphene electrode	Physical interaction	Differential pulse voltammetry	11.2 pg/ml	Sun et al. (2023b)
Generation 4	Glucose	Cerium oxide nanoparticles on contact lens	Glucose oxidase/glucose	Colorimetry	0.1—0.6 mM	Jeon et al. (2021)
	Multi-analyte	Contact lens	Physical interaction	Electrochemical		Moreddu et al. (2020)
	Cortisol	Poly(glycidylmethacrylate-coethylene glycol dimethacrylate)	On-body sweat absorption	Conductivity	2 ng/ml	Mugo and Alberkant (2020)
	Metabolic biomarkers	Prussian blue working electrode	On-body sweat absorption	Amperometry		Sempionatto et al. (2021)
	Multi-analyte	Tear-eyeglasses	On-body tear absorption	Square-wave voltammetry		Sempionatto et al. (2019)

(continued)

Table 1.1 (continued)

BioDe generations	Target biomolecule	Reporter/probe	Biochemical/physical interaction	Transduction method	Limit of detection	Reference
Generation 5—Real-time monitoring wearable sensors	Uric acid and tyrosine	Contact lens sensor	On-body tear absorption	Amperometry		Yang et al. (2020)
	Cortisol	Skin patch sensor	On-body sweat absorption	Amperometry		Singh et al. (2023)
	Metabolites	Molecular imprinted polymer—Graphene	On-body sweat absorption	Amperometry		Wang et al. (2022)
	Cancer tumour progression	Stretchable elastomer	On-body wearable	Amperometry		Abramson et al. (2022)
	Alzheimer's disease	Wireless body area network	Multiple wearable platforms	Internet of things		Zheng et al. (2025)
	Cerebral blood flow	Transcranial doppler ultrasonography	On-body conformal ultrasound patch	Doppler imaging		Zhou et al. (2024)

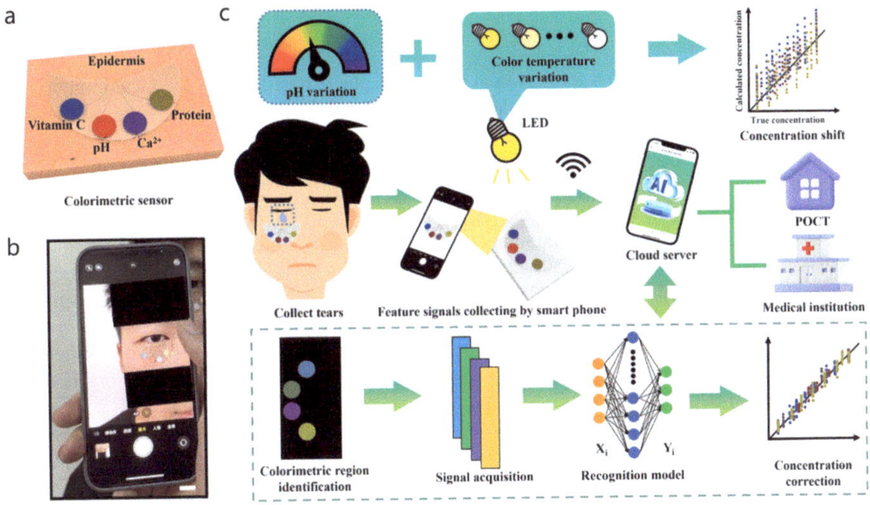

Fig. 1.4 (**a**) AI-assisted wearable microfluidic colorimetric sensor (AI-WMCS) developed using polydimethyl siloxane (PDMS) for multiplex detection of vitamin C, pH, Ca^{2+}, and proteins from tears. (**b**) Image acquisition after tears interact with the sensor. (**c**) The sensor platform is integrated with a cloud-based data analysis system to train the neural network model for improving sensitivity. (Adapted from Wang et al. (2024))

of smartphone-integrated BioDe has brought healthcare diagnostics to user fingertips. These devices can connect to smartphones, enabling real-time data analysis and visualization. The integration with cloud platforms further expands data analytics and sharing, allowing healthcare professionals to monitor patients remotely and provide timely interventions.

The future of BioDe looks promising, with several exciting directions and challenges on the horizon. One of the key areas of focus is the development of multi-analyte sensors that can detect multiple biomarkers simultaneously. This capability can provide a comprehensive understanding of complex diseases and improve diagnostic accuracy. Another important direction is the enhancement of sensor sensitivity and specificity. Researchers are exploring novel materials, such as graphene and carbon nanotubes, to improve the performance of biosensors. Additionally, the integration of ML and AI algorithms can further enhance sensor accuracy and provide personalized health insights. However, there are several challenges that need to be addressed to fully realize the potential of BioDe. Data privacy and security still remain a major concern, especially with the increasing use of cloud platforms and data-sharing technologies. Ensuring the confidentiality and integrity of patient data is crucial for building trust among users. Scalability and production costs are also significantly challenging. While advanced biosensors offer numerous benefits, their widespread adoption requires scalable manufacturing processes and cost-effective production methods. We should expect appropriate regulations for academic research and manufacturers in near future to develop strategies for large-scale production and commercialization of BioDe.

References

Abbasi Hina Y, Tehrani Z, Devadoss A et al (2021) Graphene based electrochemical immunosensor for the ultra-sensitive label free detection of Alzheimer's beta amyloid peptides Aβ(1–42). Nanoscale Adv 3:2295–2304. https://doi.org/10.1039/D0NA00801J

Abramson A, Chan CT, Khan Y et al (2022) A flexible electronic strain sensor for the real-time monitoring of tumor regression. Sci Adv 8. https://doi.org/10.1126/sciadv.abn6550

Adeloju SB, Moline AN (2001) Fabrication of ultra-thin polypyrrole–glucose oxidase film from supporting electrolyte-free monomer solution for potentiometric biosensing of glucose. Biosens Bioelectron 16:133–139. https://doi.org/10.1016/S0956-5663(00)00117-2

Ahmed I, Jiang N, Shao X et al (2022) Recent advances in optical sensors for continuous glucose monitoring. Sens Diagn 1:1098–1125. https://doi.org/10.1039/D1SD00030F

Alberto J, Leal C, Fernandes C et al (2020) Fully untethered battery-free biomonitoring electronic tattoo with wireless energy harvesting. Sci Rep 10:5539. https://doi.org/10.1038/s41598-020-62097-6

Alfian G, Syafrudin M, Ijaz MF et al (2018) A personalized healthcare monitoring system for diabetic patients by utilizing BLE-based sensors and real-time data processing. Sensors 18:2183. https://doi.org/10.3390/s18072183

Anan H, Kamahori M, Ishige Y, Nakazato K (2013) Redox-potential sensor array based on extended-gate field-effect transistors with ω-ferrocenylalkanethiol-modified gold electrodes. Sens Actuators B Chem 187:254–261. https://doi.org/10.1016/j.snb.2012.11.016

Angioni D, Delrieu J, Hansson O et al (2022) Blood biomarkers from research use to clinical practice: what must be done? A report from the EU/US CTAD task force. J Prev Alzheimers Dis 9:569–579. https://doi.org/10.14283/jpad.2022.85

Anker JN, Hall WP, Lyandres O et al (2008) Biosensing with plasmonic nanosensors. Nat Mater 7:442–453. https://doi.org/10.1038/nmat2162

Arcadio F, Soares S, Nedoma J et al (2024) POF-based biosensors for cortisol detection in seawater as a tool for aquaculture systems. Sci Rep 14:13117. https://doi.org/10.1038/s41598-024-63870-7

Arya S, Sharma A, Singh A et al (2024) Review—energy and power requirements for wearable sensors. ECS Sensors Plus 3:022601. https://doi.org/10.1149/2754-2726/ad54d2

Backiyalakshmi G, Snekhalatha U, Salvador AL (2024) Recent advancements in non-invasive wearable electrochemical biosensors for biomarker analysis—a review. Anal Biochem 692:115578. https://doi.org/10.1016/j.ab.2024.115578

Barrett PM, Komatireddy R, Haaser S et al (2014) Comparison of 24-hour Holter monitoring with 14-day novel adhesive patch electrocardiographic monitoring. Am J Med 127:95.e11–95.e17. https://doi.org/10.1016/j.amjmed.2013.10.003

Bhaiyya M, Panigrahi D, Rewatkar P, Haick H (2024) Role of machine learning assisted biosensors in point-of-care-testing for clinical decisions. ACS Sens 9:4495–4519. https://doi.org/10.1021/acssensors.4c01582

Blennow K, Hampel H, Weiner M, Zetterberg H (2010) Cerebrospinal fluid and plasma biomarkers in Alzheimer disease. Nat Rev Neurol 6:131–144. https://doi.org/10.1038/nrneurol.2010.4

Borse V, Srivastava R (2019) Fluorescence lateral flow immunoassay based point-of-care nanodiagnostics for orthopedic implant-associated infection. Sens Actuators B Chem 280:24–33. https://doi.org/10.1016/j.snb.2018.10.034

Brown JQ, Srivastava R, McShane MJ (2005) Encapsulation of glucose oxidase and an oxygen-quenched fluorophore in polyelectrolyte-coated calcium alginate microspheres as optical glucose sensor systems. Biosens Bioelectron 21:212–216. https://doi.org/10.1016/j.bios.2004.08.020

Bulathsinghala RL, Ding W, Dharmasena RDIG (2023) Triboelectric nanogenerators for wearable sensing applications: a system level analysis. Nano Energy 116:108792. https://doi.org/10.1016/j.nanoen.2023.108792

Burnes LE, Clark ST, Sheldrake E et al (2021) One swab, two tests: validation of dual SARS-CoV-2 testing on the Abbott ID NOW™. J Clin Virol 141:104896. https://doi.org/10.1016/j.jcv.2021.104896
Cappon G, Vettoretti M, Sparacino G, Facchinetti A (2019) Continuous glucose monitoring sensors for diabetes management: a review of technologies and applications. Diabetes Metab J 43:383. https://doi.org/10.4093/dmj.2019.0121
Chan LW, Anahtar MN, Ong T-H et al (2020) Engineering synthetic breath biomarkers for respiratory disease. Nat Nanotechnol 15:792–800. https://doi.org/10.1038/s41565-020-0723-4
Chaudhary V, Khanna V, Ahmed Awan HT et al (2023) Towards hospital-on-chip supported by 2D MXenes-based 5th generation intelligent biosensors. Biosens Bioelectron 220:114847. https://doi.org/10.1016/j.bios.2022.114847
Chen L-Y, Schirmer U, Widder M et al (2022) Breast cancer cell-based ELISA: a potential material for better detection of heparin-induced thrombocytopenia antibodies. J Mater Chem B 10:7708–7716. https://doi.org/10.1039/D2TB01228F
Chen X, Du C, Zhao Q et al (2023) Rapid and visual identification of HIV-1 using reverse transcription loop-mediated isothermal amplification integrated with a gold nanoparticle-based lateral flow assay platform. Front Microbiol 14. https://doi.org/10.3389/fmicb.2023.1230533
Chen Y, Hu X, Liang Q et al (2024) Large-scale flexible fabric biosensor for long-term monitoring of sweat lactate. Adv Funct Mater 34. https://doi.org/10.1002/adfm.202401270
Cheng Y, Feng S, Ning Q et al (2023) Dual-signal readout paper-based wearable biosensor with a 3D origami structure for multiplexed analyte detection in sweat. Microsyst Nanoeng 9:36. https://doi.org/10.1038/s41378-023-00514-2
Chi J, Guo M, Zhang C et al (2020) Glucose oxidase and au nanocluster co-encapsulated metal–organic frameworks as a sensitive colorimetric sensor for glucose based on a cascade reaction. New J Chem 44:13344–13349. https://doi.org/10.1039/C9NJ06339K
Choopara I, Suea-Ngam A, Teethaisong Y et al (2021) Fluorometric paper-based, loop-mediated isothermal amplification devices for quantitative point-of-care detection of methicillin-resistant *Staphylococcus aureus* (MRSA). ACS Sens 6:742–751. https://doi.org/10.1021/acssensors.0c01405
Cinti S, Singh S, Covone G et al (2023) Reviewing the state of biosensors and lab-on-a- chip technologies: opportunities for extreme environments and space exploration. Front Microbiol 14. https://doi.org/10.3389/fmicb.2023.1215529
Cojocaru M, Cojocaru IM, Silosi I, Vrabie CD (2011) Manifestations of systemic lupus erythematosus. Maedica (Bucur) 6:330–336
Croce RA, Vaddiraju S, Kondo J et al (2013) A miniaturized transcutaneous system for continuous glucose monitoring. Biomed Microdevices 15:151–160. https://doi.org/10.1007/s10544-012-9708-x
Cui F, Yue Y, Zhang Y et al (2020) Advancing biosensors with machine learning. ACS Sens 5:3346–3364. https://doi.org/10.1021/acssensors.0c01424
Das P, Das M, Chinnadayyala SR et al (2016) Recent advances on developing 3rd generation enzyme electrode for biosensor applications. Biosens Bioelectron 79:386–397. https://doi.org/10.1016/j.bios.2015.12.055
Dervisevic M, Jara Fornerod MJ, Harberts J et al (2024) Wearable microneedle patch for transdermal electrochemical monitoring of urea in interstitial fluid. ACS Sens 9:932–941. https://doi.org/10.1021/acssensors.3c02386
Dezhakam E, Vayghan RF, Dehghani S et al (2024) Highly efficient electrochemical biosensing platform in breast cancer detection based on MOF-COF@Au core-shell like nanostructure. Sci Rep 14:29850. https://doi.org/10.1038/s41598-024-78836-y
Domingo-Roca R, Macdonald AR, Hannah S, Corrigan DK (2022) Integrated multi-material portable 3D-printed platform for electrochemical detection of dopamine and glucose. Analyst 147:4598–4606. https://doi.org/10.1039/D2AN00862A
Dongiovanni P, Meroni M, Casati S et al (2023) Salivary biomarkers: novel noninvasive tools to diagnose chronic inflammation. Int J Oral Sci 15:27. https://doi.org/10.1038/s41368-023-00231-6

Economou A, Kokkinos C, Prodromidis M (2018) Flexible plastic, paper and textile lab-on-a chip platforms for electrochemical biosensing. Lab Chip 18:1812–1830. https://doi.org/10.1039/C8LC00025E

EKF Global. launch of new Biosen C-Line glucose and lactate analyzer

Eksin E, Senturk H, Erdem A (2024) Cost-effective cholesterol monitoring by enzyme-based electrochemical assay. ChemistrySelect 9. https://doi.org/10.1002/slct.202304593

Elgazar A, Sabouni R, Ghommem M, Majdalawieh AF (2024) Novel metal–organic framework biosensing platform for detection of COVID-19 RNA. Sci Rep 14:25437. https://doi.org/10.1038/s41598-024-75668-8

Elsherif M, Hassan MU, Yetisen AK, Butt H (2018a) Glucose sensing with Phenylboronic acid functionalized hydrogel-based optical diffusers. ACS Nano 12:2283–2291. https://doi.org/10.1021/acsnano.7b07082

Elsherif M, Hassan MU, Yetisen AK, Butt H (2018b) Wearable contact lens biosensors for continuous glucose monitoring using smartphones. ACS Nano 12:5452–5462. https://doi.org/10.1021/acsnano.8b00829

Fan Y-F, Guo Z-B, Ge G-B (2023) Enzyme-based biosensors and their applications. Biosensors (Basel) 13:476. https://doi.org/10.3390/bios13040476

Fatani AZ, Bugshan NA, AlSayyad HM et al (2021) Causes of the failure of biological therapy at a tertiary center: a cross-sectional retrospective study. Cureus. https://doi.org/10.7759/cureus.18253

Feng R-M, Liu Y, Liu Z-Q et al (2024) Advances in nucleic acid aptamer-based detection of respiratory virus and bacteria: a mini review. Virol J 21:237. https://doi.org/10.1186/s12985-024-02513-9

Florimbi G, Fabelo H, Torti E et al (2018) Accelerating the K-nearest neighbors filtering algorithm to optimize the real-time classification of human brain tumor in hyperspectral images. Sensors 18:2314. https://doi.org/10.3390/s18072314

Flynn CD, Chang D (2024) Artificial intelligence in point-of-care biosensing: challenges and opportunities. Diagnostics 14:1100. https://doi.org/10.3390/diagnostics14111100

Fu W, Yu B, Ji D et al (2024) Intelligent fibers and textiles for wearable biosensors. Respons Mater 2. https://doi.org/10.1002/rpm.20240018

Fugger L, Jensen LT, Rossjohn J (2020) Challenges, progress, and prospects of developing therapies to treat autoimmune diseases. Cell 181:63–80. https://doi.org/10.1016/j.cell.2020.03.007

Füzéry AK, Levin J, Chan MM, Chan DW (2013) Translation of proteomic biomarkers into FDA approved cancer diagnostics: issues and challenges. Clin Proteomics 10:13. https://doi.org/10.1186/1559-0275-10-13

Gao F, Liu C, Zhang L et al (2023) Wearable and flexible electrochemical sensors for sweat analysis: a review. Microsyst Nanoeng 9:1. https://doi.org/10.1038/s41378-022-00443-6

Ghazizadeh E, Naseri Z, Deigner H-P et al (2024) Approaches of wearable and implantable biosensor towards of developing in precision medicine. Front Med (Lausanne) 11. https://doi.org/10.3389/fmed.2024.1390634

Giaretta JE, Duan H, Oveissi F et al (2022) Flexible sensors for hydrogen peroxide detection: a critical review. ACS Appl Mater Interfaces 14:20491–20505. https://doi.org/10.1021/acsami.1c24727

Goërtz YMJ, Braamse AMJ, Spruit MA et al (2021) Fatigue in patients with chronic disease: results from the population-based Lifelines Cohort Study. Sci Rep 11:20977. https://doi.org/10.1038/s41598-021-00337-z

Gomes FO, Maia LB, Delerue-Matos C et al (2019) Third-generation electrochemical biosensor based on nitric oxide reductase immobilized in a multiwalled carbon nanotubes/1-n-butyl-3-methylimidazolium tetrafluoroborate nanocomposite for nitric oxide detection. Sens Actuators B Chem 285:445–452. https://doi.org/10.1016/j.snb.2019.01.074

Goud KY, Moonla C, Mishra RK et al (2019) Wearable electrochemical microneedle sensor for continuous monitoring of levodopa: toward Parkinson management. ACS Sens 4:2196–2204. https://doi.org/10.1021/acssensors.9b01127

Guan T, Shen Y, Jiang Z et al (2022) An ultrasensitive microfluidic chip-based immunoassay for multiplex determination of 11 PDE-5 inhibitors in adulterated health foods. Sens Actuators B Chem 358:131450. https://doi.org/10.1016/j.snb.2022.131450

Gupta R, Othman T, Chen C et al (2020) Guardant360 circulating tumor DNA assay is concordant with FoundationOne next-generation sequencing in detecting actionable driver mutations in anti-EGFR naive metastatic colorectal cancer. Oncologist 25:235–243. https://doi.org/10.1634/theoncologist.2019-0441

Guven N, Apetrei R-M, Camurlu P (2021) Next step in 2nd generation glucose biosensors: Ferrocene-loaded electrospun nanofibers. Mater Sci Eng C 128:112270. https://doi.org/10.1016/j.msec.2021.112270

Han G-R, Goncharov A, Eryilmaz M et al (2025) Machine learning in point-of-care testing: innovations, challenges, and opportunities. Nat Commun 16:3165. https://doi.org/10.1038/s41467-025-58527-6

Henry NL, Hayes DF (2012) Cancer biomarkers. Mol Oncol 6:140–146. https://doi.org/10.1016/j.molonc.2012.01.010

Hopkins J, Fidanovski K, Lauto A, Mawad D (2019) All-organic semiconductors for electrochemical biosensors: an overview of recent progress in material design. Front Bioeng Biotechnol 7. https://doi.org/10.3389/fbioe.2019.00237

Hu H, Huang H, Li M et al (2023) A wearable cardiac ultrasound imager. Nature 613:667–675. https://doi.org/10.1038/s41586-022-05498-z

Huang C, Wen T, Shi F-J et al (2020) Rapid detection of IgM antibodies against the SARS-CoV-2 virus via colloidal gold nanoparticle-based lateral-flow assay. ACS Omega 5:12550–12556. https://doi.org/10.1021/acsomega.0c01554

Huang H-J, Lin Y-T, Chung M-C et al (2022) Glucose and ethanol detection with an affinity-switchable lateral flow assay. Anal Chem 94:5084–5090. https://doi.org/10.1021/acs.analchem.1c05316

Ignatov SG, Ferguson JA, Walt DR (2001) A fiber-optic lactate sensor based on bacterial cytoplasmic membranes. Biosens Bioelectron 16:109–113. https://doi.org/10.1016/S0956-5663(00)00144-5

Ioannidis P, Papaventsis D, Karabela S et al (2011) Cepheid GeneXpert MTB/RIF assay for mycobacterium tuberculosis detection and rifampin resistance identification in patients with substantial clinical indications of tuberculosis and smear-negative microscopy results. J Clin Microbiol 49:3068–3070. https://doi.org/10.1128/JCM.00718-11

Jain PK, Huang X, El-Sayed IH, El-Sayed MA (2008) Noble metals on the nanoscale: optical and Photothermal properties and some applications in imaging, sensing, biology, and medicine. Acc Chem Res 41:1578–1586. https://doi.org/10.1021/ar7002804

Jeon H-J, Kim S, Park S et al (2021) Optical assessment of tear glucose by smart biosensor based on nanoparticle embedded contact lens. Nano Lett 21:8933–8940. https://doi.org/10.1021/acs.nanolett.1c01880

Jordaens S, Zwaenepoel K, Tjalma W et al (2023) Urine biomarkers in cancer detection: a systematic review of preanalytical parameters and applied methods. Int J Cancer 152:2186–2205. https://doi.org/10.1002/ijc.34434

Kabiri Ameri S, Ho R, Jang H et al (2017) Graphene electronic tattoo sensors. ACS Nano 11:7634–7641. https://doi.org/10.1021/acsnano.7b02182

Kadian S, Kumari P, Shukla S, Narayan R (2023) Recent advancements in machine learning enabled portable and wearable biosensors. Talanta Open 8:100267. https://doi.org/10.1016/j.talo.2023.100267

Kamya P, Ozerov IV, Pun FW et al (2024) PandaOmics: an AI-driven platform for therapeutic target and biomarker discovery. J Chem Inf Model 64:3961–3969. https://doi.org/10.1021/acs.jcim.3c01619

Kaur J, Srivastava R, Borse V (2021) Recent advances in point-of-care diagnostics for oral cancer. Biosens Bioelectron 178:112995. https://doi.org/10.1016/j.bios.2021.112995

Khan A, DeVoe E, Andreescu S (2023) Carbon-based electrochemical biosensors as diagnostic platforms for connected decentralized healthcare. Sens Diagn 2:529–558. https://doi.org/10.1039/D2SD00226D

Khumngern S, Jeerapan I (2024) Synergistic convergence of materials and enzymes for biosensing and self-sustaining energy devices towards on-body health monitoring. Commun Mater 5:135. https://doi.org/10.1038/s43246-024-00557-6

Kim KJ (2017) Shape and size matter for smartwatches: effects of screen shape, screen size, and presentation mode in wearable communication. J Comput-Mediat Commun 22:124–140. https://doi.org/10.1111/jcc4.12186

Kim G, Yang H (2024) Electrochemical biosensor using direct electron transfer and an antibody–aptamer hybrid sandwich for target detection in complex biological samples. Biosens Bioelectron 253:116184. https://doi.org/10.1016/j.bios.2024.116184

Kim J, Imani S, de Araujo WR et al (2015) Wearable salivary uric acid mouthguard biosensor with integrated wireless electronics. Biosens Bioelectron 74:1061–1068. https://doi.org/10.1016/j.bios.2015.07.039

Kim J, Wu Y, Luan H et al (2022) A skin-interfaced, miniaturized microfluidic analysis and delivery system for colorimetric measurements of nutrients in sweat and supply of vitamins through the skin. Adv Sci 9. https://doi.org/10.1002/advs.202103331

Klein L, Gheorghiade M (2004) Coronary artery disease and prevention of heart failure. Med Clin North Am 88:1209–1235. https://doi.org/10.1016/j.mcna.2004.03.002

Kumar Das S, Nayak KK, Krishnaswamy PR et al (2022) Review—electrochemistry and other emerging technologies for continuous glucose monitoring devices. ECS Sensors Plus 1:031601. https://doi.org/10.1149/2754-2726/ac7abb

Li R, Zhen M, Guan M et al (2013) A novel glucose colorimetric sensor based on intrinsic peroxidase-like activity of C60-carboxyfullerenes. Biosens Bioelectron 47:502–507. https://doi.org/10.1016/j.bios.2013.03.057

Li Y, Jia D, Ren W et al (2019) A versatile Photoinduced electron transfer-based Upconversion fluorescent biosensing platform for the detection of disease biomarkers and nerve agent. Adv Funct Mater 29. https://doi.org/10.1002/adfm.201903191

Li S, Zhu Y, Haghniaz R et al (2022) A microchambers containing contact lens for the noninvasive detection of tear exosomes. Adv Funct Mater 32. https://doi.org/10.1002/adfm.202206620

Li Q, Ding L, Zhang Y, Wu T (2022b) A cholesterol optical fiber sensor based on CQDs-COD/CA composite. IEEE Sensors J 22:6247–6255. https://doi.org/10.1109/JSEN.2022.3146150

Li Z, Kadian S, Mishra RK et al (2023) Electrochemical detection of cholesterol in human biofluid using microneedle sensor. J Mater Chem B 11:6075–6081. https://doi.org/10.1039/D2TB02142K

Lim HJ, Saha T, Tey BT et al (2020) Quartz crystal microbalance-based biosensors as rapid diagnostic devices for infectious diseases. Biosens Bioelectron 168:112513. https://doi.org/10.1016/j.bios.2020.112513

Lino C, Barrias S, Chaves R et al (2022) Biosensors as diagnostic tools in clinical applications. Biochimica et Biophysica Acta (BBA) Rev Cancer 1877:188726. https://doi.org/10.1016/j.bbcan.2022.188726

Liu J, Pang S, Wang M et al (2023) An ultrasensitive ELISA to assay femtomolar level SARS-CoV-2 antigen based on specific peptide and tyramine signal amplification. Sens Actuators B Chem 387:133746. https://doi.org/10.1016/j.snb.2023.133746

Lopez-Tellez J, Ramirez-Montes S, Ferreira TA et al (2022) Application of Voltammetric sensors for pathogen bacteria detection: a review. Chemosensors 10:424. https://doi.org/10.3390/chemosensors10100424

Malhotra BD, Chaubey A (2003) Biosensors for clinical diagnostics industry. Sens Actuators B Chem 91:117–127. https://doi.org/10.1016/S0925-4005(03)00075-3

Marchianò V, Tricase A, Macchia E et al (2024) Self-powered wearable biosensor based on stencil-printed carbon nanotube electrodes for ethanol detection in sweat. Anal Bioanal Chem 416:5303–5316. https://doi.org/10.1007/s00216-024-05467-7

Masi A, Antonacci A, Moccia M et al (2023) CRISPR-Cas assisted diagnostics: a broad application biosensing approach. TrAC Trends Anal Chem 162:117028. https://doi.org/10.1016/j.trac.2023.117028

Mehmeti E, Stanković DM, Chaiyo S et al (2017) Wiring of glucose oxidase with graphene nanoribbons: an electrochemical third generation glucose biosensor. Microchim Acta 184:1127–1134. https://doi.org/10.1007/s00604-017-2115-5

Mondal HS, Ahmed KA, Birbilis N, Hossain MZ (2023) Machine learning for detecting DNA attachment on SPR biosensor. Sci Rep 13:3742. https://doi.org/10.1038/s41598-023-29395-1

Monošík R, Stred'anský M, Šturdík E (2012) Application of electrochemical biosensors in clinical diagnosis. J Clin Lab Anal 26:22–34. https://doi.org/10.1002/jcla.20500

Moreddu R, Elsherif M, Adams H et al (2020) Integration of paper microfluidic sensors into contact lenses for tear fluid analysis. Lab Chip 20:3970–3979. https://doi.org/10.1039/D0LC00438C

Moura PC, Raposo M, Vassilenko V (2024) Breath biomarkers in non-carcinogenic diseases. Clin Chim Acta 552:117692. https://doi.org/10.1016/j.cca.2023.117692

Mthembu CL, Sabela MI, Mlambo M et al (2017) Google Analytics and quick response for advancement of gold nanoparticle-based dual lateral flow immunoassay for malaria—Plasmodium lactate dehydrogenase (pLDH). Anal Methods 9:5943–5951. https://doi.org/10.1039/C7AY01645J

Mugo SM, Alberkant J (2020) Flexible molecularly imprinted electrochemical sensor for cortisol monitoring in sweat. Anal Bioanal Chem 412:1825–1833. https://doi.org/10.1007/s00216-020-02430-0

Munirathinam P, Chandrasekhar A (2023) Wearable triboelectric nanogenerator for real-time IoT-supported security applications. Sustain Mater Technol 37:e00700. https://doi.org/10.1016/j.susmat.2023.e00700

Nagamine K, Tokito S (2021) Organic-transistor-based biosensors interfaced with human skin for non-invasive perspiration analysis. Sens Actuators B Chem 349:130778. https://doi.org/10.1016/j.snb.2021.130778

Nerthigan Y, Sharma AK, Pandey S et al (2018) Glucose oxidase assisted visual detection of glucose using oxygen deficient α-MoO3-x nanoflakes. Microchim Acta 185:65. https://doi.org/10.1007/s00604-017-2612-6

Norvaiša K, Kielmann M, Senge MO (2020) Porphyrins as colorimetric and photometric biosensors in modern bioanalytical systems. Chembiochem 21:1793–1807. https://doi.org/10.1002/cbic.202000067

Omidfar K, Riahi F, Kashanian S (2023) Lateral flow assay: a summary of recent Progress for improving assay performance. Biosensors (Basel) 13:837. https://doi.org/10.3390/bios13090837

Papafaklis MI, Mavrogiannis MC, Stone PH (2016) Identifying the progression of coronary artery disease: prediction of cardiac events. Contin Cardiol Educ 2:105–114. https://doi.org/10.1002/cce2.25

Park W, Shin H, Choi B et al (2020) Advanced hybrid nanomaterials for biomedical applications. Prog Mater Sci 114:100686. https://doi.org/10.1016/j.pmatsci.2020.100686

Park G, Lee H, Jang M et al (2023) Rapid electrical biosensor consisting of DNA aptamer/carbon nanonetwork on microelectrode array for cardiac troponin I in human serum. Sens Actuators B Chem 393:134295. https://doi.org/10.1016/j.snb.2023.134295

Park W, Seo H, Kim J et al (2024a) In-depth correlation analysis between tear glucose and blood glucose using a wireless smart contact lens. Nat Commun 15:2828. https://doi.org/10.1038/s41467-024-47123-9

Park JS, Ahmad W, Choe K et al (2024b) Biosensors and biomarkers: a dynamic duo towards Alzheimer's disease detection. Sens Biosensing Res 46:100704. https://doi.org/10.1016/j.sbsr.2024.100704

Patella B, Di Vincenzo S, Moukri N et al (2024) Gold nanowires-based sensor for quantification of H2O2 released by human airway epithelial cells. Talanta 272:125772. https://doi.org/10.1016/j.talanta.2024.125772

Piunno PAE, Krull UJ (2005) Trends in the development of nucleic acid biosensors for medical diagnostics. Anal Bioanal Chem 381:1004–1011. https://doi.org/10.1007/s00216-004-3024-0

Qin Y, Li S, Liang L et al (2024) Regulating the redox and non-redox enzyme-mimicking activities of Ce-UiO-66-NO2 nanozyme for dual-mode sensing of phosphate. Sens Actuators B Chem 412:135782. https://doi.org/10.1016/j.snb.2024.135782

Qureshi R, Irfan M, Ali H et al (2023) Artificial intelligence and biosensors in healthcare and its clinical relevance: a review. IEEE Access 11:61600–61620. https://doi.org/10.1109/ACCESS.2023.3285596

Rajan MR, Sotak M, Barrenäs F et al (2019) Comparative analysis of obesity-related cardiometabolic and renal biomarkers in human plasma and serum. Sci Rep 9:15385. https://doi.org/10.1038/s41598-019-51673-0

Rasitanon N, Ittisoponpisan S, Kaewpradub K, Jeerapan I (2023) Wearable electrodes for lactate: applications in enzyme-based sensors and energy biodevices. Anal Sens 3. https://doi.org/10.1002/anse.202200066

Robey TT, Panegyres PK (2019) Cerebrospinal fluid biomarkers in neurodegenerative disorders. Future Neurol 14. https://doi.org/10.2217/fnl-2018-0029

Rodin D, Shapiro Y, Pinhasov A et al (2022) An accurate wearable hydration sensor: real-world evaluation of practical use. PLoS One 17:e0272646. https://doi.org/10.1371/journal.pone.0272646

Saadi H, Seillier M, Sandi MJ et al (2013) Development of an ELISA detecting tumor protein 53-induced nuclear protein 1 in serum of prostate cancer patients. Results Immunol 3:51–56. https://doi.org/10.1016/j.rinim.2013.05.002

Sappia L, Felice B, Sanchez MA et al (2019) Electrochemical sensor for alkaline phosphatase as biomarker for clinical and in vitro applications. Sens Actuators B Chem 281:221–228. https://doi.org/10.1016/j.snb.2018.10.105

Sassolas A, Leca-Bouvier BD, Blum LJ (2008) DNA biosensors and microarrays. Chem Rev 108:109–139. https://doi.org/10.1021/cr0684467

Sempionatto JR, Mishra RK, Martín A et al (2017a) Wearable ring-based sensing platform for detecting chemical threats. ACS Sens 2:1531–1538. https://doi.org/10.1021/acssensors.7b00603

Sempionatto JR, Nakagawa T, Pavinatto A et al (2017b) Eyeglasses based wireless electrolyte and metabolite sensor platform. Lab Chip 17:1834–1842. https://doi.org/10.1039/C7LC00192D

Sempionatto JR, Brazaca LC, García-Carmona L et al (2019) Eyeglasses-based tear biosensing system: non-invasive detection of alcohol, vitamins and glucose. Biosens Bioelectron 137:161–170. https://doi.org/10.1016/j.bios.2019.04.058

Sempionatto JR, Lin M, Yin L et al (2021) An epidermal patch for the simultaneous monitoring of haemodynamic and metabolic biomarkers. Nat Biomed Eng 5:737–748. https://doi.org/10.1038/s41551-021-00685-1

Seo H, Chung WG, Kwon YW et al (2023) Smart contact lenses as wearable ophthalmic devices for disease monitoring and health management. Chem Rev 123:11488–11558. https://doi.org/10.1021/acs.chemrev.3c00290

Shah P, Bajaj S, Virk H et al (2015) Rapid progression of coronary atherosclerosis: a review. Thrombosis 2015:1–6. https://doi.org/10.1155/2015/634983

Shang C, Xu Q, Liang N et al (2023) Multi-parameter e-skin based on biomimetic mechanoreceptors and stress field sensing. NPJ Flex Electron 7:19. https://doi.org/10.1038/s41528-023-00252-5

Sharma AK, Pandey S, Nerthigan Y et al (2018) Aggregation of cysteamine-capped gold nanoparticles in presence of ATP as an analytical tool for rapid detection of creatine kinase (CK-MM). Anal Chim Acta 1024:161–168. https://doi.org/10.1016/j.aca.2018.03.027

Sharma AK, Huang W-S, Pandey S, Wu H-F (2021) Solvent-free low-temperature annealing method for aqueous stable perovskite nanofibers and its role in peroxide catalysis. ACS Sustain Chem Eng 9:7678–7686. https://doi.org/10.1021/acssuschemeng.1c02676

Sharma M, Mahajan P, Alsubaie AS et al (2025) Next-generation nanomaterials-based biosensors: real-time biosensing devices for detecting emerging environmental pollutants. Mater Today Sustain 29:101068. https://doi.org/10.1016/j.mtsust.2024.101068

Sharpes CE, McManus JB, Blum SM et al (2021) Assessment of colorimetric reporter enzymes in the PURE system. ACS Synth Biol 10:3205–3208. https://doi.org/10.1021/acssynbio.1c00360
Shetty SS, Deepthi D, Harshitha S et al (2023) Environmental pollutants and their effects on human health. Heliyon 9:e19496. https://doi.org/10.1016/j.heliyon.2023.e19496
Shetty KH, Desai DT, Patel HP et al (2024) Contact lens as an emerging platform for non-invasive bio-sensing: a review. Sens Actuators A Phys 376:115617. https://doi.org/10.1016/j.sna.2024.115617
Siboro PY, Sharma AK, Lai P-J et al (2024) Harnessing HfO_2 nanoparticles for wearable tumor monitoring and Sonodynamic therapy in advancing cancer care. ACS Nano 18:2485–2499. https://doi.org/10.1021/acsnano.3c11346
Singh NK, Chung S, Chang A-Y et al (2023) A non-invasive wearable stress patch for real-time cortisol monitoring using a pseudoknot-assisted aptamer. Biosens Bioelectron 227:115097. https://doi.org/10.1016/j.bios.2023.115097
Smith AA, Li R, Tse ZTH (2023) Reshaping healthcare with wearable biosensors. Sci Rep 13:4998. https://doi.org/10.1038/s41598-022-26951-z
Sokolov P, Samokhvalov P, Sukhanova A, Nabiev I (2023) Biosensors based on inorganic composite fluorescent hydrogels. Nano 13:1748. https://doi.org/10.3390/nano13111748
Solanki PR, Kaushik A, Agrawal VV, Malhotra BD (2011) Nanostructured metal oxide-based biosensors. NPG Asia Mater 3:17–24. https://doi.org/10.1038/asiamat.2010.137
Steckl AJ, Ray P (2018) Stress biomarkers in biological fluids and their point-of-use detection. ACS Sens 3:2025–2044. https://doi.org/10.1021/acssensors.8b00726
Strimbu K, Tavel JA (2010) What are biomarkers? Curr Opin HIV AIDS 5:463–466. https://doi.org/10.1097/COH.0b013e32833ed177
Su J, Chen S, Dou Y et al (2022) Smartphone-based electrochemical biosensors for directly detecting serum-derived exosomes and monitoring their secretion. Anal Chem 94:3235–3244. https://doi.org/10.1021/acs.analchem.1c04910
Sun C, Wang X, Auwalu MA et al (2021) Organic thin film transistors-based biosensors. EcoMat 3. https://doi.org/10.1002/eom2.12094
Sun Y, Li Y-Z, Yuan M (2023a) Requirements, challenges, and novel ideas for wearables on power supply and energy harvesting. Nano Energy 115:108715. https://doi.org/10.1016/j.nanoen.2023.108715
Sun B, Kan L, Liu Y et al (2023b) An electrochemical Immunosensor based on GO@CS for highly sensitive and accurate detection of cardiovascular markers-cTn- I. J Electrochem Soc 170:117502. https://doi.org/10.1149/1945-7111/ad066a
Sunstrum FN, Khan JU, Li N-W, Welsh AW (2025) Wearable textile sensors for continuous glucose monitoring. Biosens Bioelectron 273:117133. https://doi.org/10.1016/j.bios.2025.117133
Takai E, Yachida S (2016) Circulating tumor DNA as a liquid biopsy target for detection of pancreatic cancer. World J Gastroenterol 22:8480. https://doi.org/10.3748/wjg.v22.i38.8480
Tang Y, Zhang Q, Yuan H et al (2025a) Recent applications and challenges of inorganic nanomaterial-based biosensing devices for detecting nucleic acid biomarkers. Adv Sensor Energy Mater:100136. https://doi.org/10.1016/j.asems.2025.100136
Tang Y, Li Y, Chen P et al (2025b) Nucleic acid Aptamer-based sensors for bacteria detection: a review. BioEssays. https://doi.org/10.1002/bies.202400111
Tao D, Su P, Chen A et al (2025) Electro-spun nanofibers-based triboelectric nanogenerators in wearable electronics: status and perspectives. NPJ Flex Electron 9:4. https://doi.org/10.1038/s41528-024-00357-5
Tomioka Y, Sekino M, Gu J et al (2022) Wearable, wireless, multi-sensor device for monitoring tissue circulation after free-tissue transplantation: a multicentre clinical trial. Sci Rep 12:16532. https://doi.org/10.1038/s41598-022-21007-8
Tong G, Nath P, Hiruta Y, Citterio D (2025) Amplification-free CRISPR/Cas based dual-enzymatic colorimetric nucleic acid biosensing device. Lab Chip. https://doi.org/10.1039/D4LC01039F
Toubanaki DK, Margaroni M, Prapas A, Karagouni E (2020) Development of a nanoparticle-based lateral flow strip biosensor for visual detection of whole nervous necrosis virus particles. Sci Rep 10:6529. https://doi.org/10.1038/s41598-020-63553-z

Uchayash S, Que SS, Rubby MF et al (2025) Lactate dehydrogenase electrochemical sensing using electrodes with 3D gold nanostructures. ACS Appl Nano Mater 8:11404–11414. https://doi.org/10.1021/acsanm.5c01308
Uludag Y, Narter F, Sağlam E et al (2016) An integrated lab-on-a-chip-based electrochemical biosensor for rapid and sensitive detection of cancer biomarkers. Anal Bioanal Chem 408:7775–7783. https://doi.org/10.1007/s00216-016-9879-z
van de Goor R, van Hooren M, Dingemans A-M et al (2018) Training and validating a portable electronic nose for lung cancer screening. J Thorac Oncol 13:676–681. https://doi.org/10.1016/j.jtho.2018.01.024
Vidic J, Manzano M (2021) Electrochemical biosensors for rapid pathogen detection. Curr Opin Electrochem 29:100750. https://doi.org/10.1016/j.coelec.2021.100750
Vindeirinho JM, Pinho E, Azevedo NF, Almeida C (2022) SARS-CoV-2 diagnostics based on nucleic acids amplification: from fundamental concepts to applications and beyond. Front Cell Infect Microbiol 12. https://doi.org/10.3389/fcimb.2022.799678
Wang W, Fan X, Xu S et al (2015) Low fouling label-free DNA sensor based on polyethylene glycols decorated with gold nanoparticles for the detection of breast cancer biomarkers. Biosens Bioelectron 71:51–56. https://doi.org/10.1016/j.bios.2015.04.018
Wang M, Yang Y, Min J et al (2022) A wearable electrochemical biosensor for the monitoring of metabolites and nutrients. Nat Biomed Eng 6:1225–1235. https://doi.org/10.1038/s41551-022-00916-z
Wang Z, Dong Y, Sui X et al (2024) An artificial intelligence-assisted microfluidic colorimetric wearable sensor system for monitoring of key tear biomarkers. NPJ Flex Electron 8:35. https://doi.org/10.1038/s41528-024-00321-3
Ward SJ, Layouni R, Arshavsky-Graham S et al (2021) Morlet wavelet filtering and phase analysis to reduce the limit of detection for thin film optical biosensors. ACS Sens 6:2967–2978. https://doi.org/10.1021/acssensors.1c00787
Weng X, Neethirajan S (2016) A microfluidic biosensor using graphene oxide and aptamer-functionalized quantum dots for peanut allergen detection. Biosens Bioelectron 85:649–656. https://doi.org/10.1016/j.bios.2016.05.072
Xiao D, Zhang W, Guo X et al (2021) A d-2-hydroxyglutarate biosensor based on specific transcriptional regulator DhdR. Nat Commun 12:7108. https://doi.org/10.1038/s41467-021-27357-7
Xu C, Song Y, Han M, Zhang H (2021) Portable and wearable self-powered systems based on emerging energy harvesting technology. Microsyst Nanoeng 7:25. https://doi.org/10.1038/s41378-021-00248-z
Xu K, Ko SH, Chen J (2024) Advances in wearable and implantable bioelectronics for precision medicine. Biodes Manuf 7:383–387. https://doi.org/10.1007/s42242-024-00302-5
Yadegari H, Mohammadi M, Maghsood F et al (2023) Diagnostic performance of a novel antigen-capture ELISA for the detection of SARS-CoV-2. Anal Biochem 666:115079. https://doi.org/10.1016/j.ab.2023.115079
Yang Y, Song Y, Bo X et al (2020) A laser-engraved wearable sensor for sensitive detection of uric acid and tyrosine in sweat. Nat Biotechnol 38:217–224. https://doi.org/10.1038/s41587-019-0321-x
Yang B, Jiang X, Fang X, Kong J (2021) Wearable chem-biosensing devices: from basic research to commercial market. Lab Chip 21:4285–4310. https://doi.org/10.1039/D1LC00438G
Yeo HG (2023) Piezoelectric energy-harvesting devices for wearable self-powering system. JMST Adv 5:37–43. https://doi.org/10.1007/s42791-023-00053-x
Yeong Lee E, Gyu Kim M, Joo Lee H et al (2024) Programmable DNA-based nanostructure sensors for mutation detection coupled with asymmetric amplification in precision genome profiling. Chem Eng J 500:157436. https://doi.org/10.1016/j.cej.2024.157436
Yetisen AK, Moreddu R, Seifi S et al (2019) Dermal tattoo biosensors for colorimetric metabolite detection. Angew Chem Int Ed 58:10506–10513. https://doi.org/10.1002/anie.201904416
Yi Z, Zhang W, Yang B (2022a) Piezoelectric approaches for wearable continuous blood pressure monitoring: a review. J Micromech Microeng 32:103003. https://doi.org/10.1088/1361-6439/ac87ba

Yi Z, Liu Z, Li W et al (2022b) Piezoelectric dynamics of arterial pulse for wearable continuous blood pressure monitoring. Adv Mater 34. https://doi.org/10.1002/adma.202110291

Yilmaz YY, Yalcinkaya EE, Demirkol DO, Timur S (2020) 4-aminothiophenol-intercalated montmorillonite: organic-inorganic hybrid material as an immobilization support for biosensors. Sens Actuators B Chem 307:127665. https://doi.org/10.1016/j.snb.2020.127665

Yokus MA, Songkakul T, Pozdin VA et al (2020) Wearable multiplexed biosensor system toward continuous monitoring of metabolites. Biosens Bioelectron 153:112038. https://doi.org/10.1016/j.bios.2020.112038

Yoshizawa JM, Schafer CA, Schafer JJ et al (2013) Salivary biomarkers: toward future clinical and diagnostic utilities. Clin Microbiol Rev 26:781–791. https://doi.org/10.1128/CMR.00021-13

Yunianto M, Permata AN, Eka D et al (2017) Design of a fiber optic biosensor for cholesterol detection in human blood. IOP Conf Ser Mater Sci Eng 176:012014. https://doi.org/10.1088/1757-899X/176/1/012014

Zhang T, Wang H-B, Zhong Z-T et al (2020) A smartphone-based rapid quantitative detection platform for lateral flow strip of human chorionic gonadotropin with optimized image algorithm. Microchem J 157:105038. https://doi.org/10.1016/j.microc.2020.105038

Zhang K, Wang J, Liu T et al (2021) Machine learning-reinforced noninvasive biosensors for healthcare. Adv Healthc Mater 10. https://doi.org/10.1002/adhm.202100734

Zhang Y, Hu Y, Jiang N, Yetisen AK (2023) Wearable artificial intelligence biosensor networks. Biosens Bioelectron 219:114825. https://doi.org/10.1016/j.bios.2022.114825

Zhang Z, Li Z, Wei K et al (2024a) Sweat as a source of non-invasive biomarkers for clinical diagnosis: an overview. Talanta 273:125865. https://doi.org/10.1016/j.talanta.2024.125865

Zhang C, Liu T, Wang X et al (2024b) Urine biomarkers in type 2 diabetes mellitus with or without microvascular complications. Nutr Diabetes 14:51. https://doi.org/10.1038/s41387-024-00310-5

Zhao Y, Li W, Pan L et al (2016) ZnO-nanorods/graphene heterostructure: a direct electron transfer glucose biosensor. Sci Rep 6:32327. https://doi.org/10.1038/srep32327

Zhao S, Wang S, Zhang S et al (2018) State of the art: lateral flow assay (LFA) biosensor for on-site rapid detection. Chin Chem Lett 29:1567–1577. https://doi.org/10.1016/j.cclet.2017.12.008

Zhao J, Xia K, He P et al (2023) Recent advances of nucleic acid-based cancer biomarkers and biosensors. Coord Chem Rev 497:215456. https://doi.org/10.1016/j.ccr.2023.215456

Zheng M, Wu Y, Weng C (2025) A digital intelligence visualization health monitoring device for Alzheimer's disease patients based on WBAN technology. Sci Rep 15:15997. https://doi.org/10.1038/s41598-025-99637-x

Zhou S, Gao X, Park G et al (2024) Transcranial volumetric imaging using a conformal ultrasound patch. Nature 629:810–818. https://doi.org/10.1038/s41586-024-07381-5

Small-Scale Biomedical Devices for Healthcare Applications

2

Sumit Majumder, Wei Jiang, and Sudip Saha

Abstract

The increase in global life expectancy has led to a growing elderly population, creating an urgent need for efficient, long-term healthcare solutions. Significant advancements in material sciences and fabrication technologies, along with progress in low-power, high-speed electronics, computing, and communications, have enabled the development of high-performance, small-scale biomedical devices. These devices, including wearable, implantable, and ingestible systems, facilitate continuous monitoring of physiological parameters and support closed-loop therapeutic interventions through the integration of the Internet of Things (IoT), artificial intelligence, and data analytics. However, design considerations, such as size, safety, biocompatibility, and user comfort, must be carefully addressed, particularly for long-term monitoring applications. Furthermore, ensuring reliable, secure, and energy-efficient operation, while addressing scalability and integration complexities owing to their compact form factors, is crucial for widespread adoption. With advances in flexible electronics, material sciences, and ultra-low-power computing and communication systems, these miniaturized biomedical devices have the potential to transform healthcare delivery.

S. Majumder (✉)
Department of Biomedical Engineering, Chittagong University of Engineering and Technology, Chattogram, Bangladesh
e-mail: s.majumder@cuet.ac.bd

W. Jiang
Microelectronic Thrust, Hong Kong University of Science and Technology (Guangzhou), Guangzhou, China
e-mail: weijiang2@hkust-gz.edu.cn

S. Saha
Xzom Inc., San Diego, CA, USA
e-mail: ssaha@xzom.com

V. Patel et al. (eds.), *Biosensor Technology in Translating Novel Materials into Practical Devices*, https://doi.org/10.1007/978-981-95-5519-2_2

Keywords

Wearable · Implantable · Ingestible · AI · Biomedical devices · Biosensors · Bio-MEMs · Biochips · Smart sensors · Telehealth · Remote monitoring

2.1 Introduction

Across the globe, the elderly demographic is growing rapidly due to increased life expectancy and declining birth rates. In fact, the worldwide population aged 60 years and older is projected to reach 1.4 billion by 2030 (Ageing and Health 2025). Aging is commonly associated with chronic conditions such as cardiovascular diseases, diabetes, hypertension, arthritis, hearing loss, cataracts, and dementia. For instance, in the United States (US), nearly 95% of adults over 60 live with at least one chronic illness (The top 10 most common chronic conditions in older adults 2025). These chronic diseases not only affect the quality of life of older adults but also raise healthcare expenditures. In 2023, US healthcare spending rose by 7.5% from the previous year, outpacing its 6.6% growth rate of the gross domestic product (GDP) and accounting for 17.6% of the nation's GDP (Trends in health care spending 2025).

Therefore, there is a growing interest in developing efficient and cost-effective healthcare solutions. Significant advances in materials science and fabrication methods; Complementary Metal-Oxide-Semiconductor (CMOS)-based low-power electronics, computing, and communication technologies; energy harvesting techniques; and microelectromechanical systems (MEMS) have collectively enabled the development of high-performance miniature biomedical systems such as wearable, implantable, and ingestible devices. These miniature devices enable continuous monitoring of physiological parameters, such as heart rate, blood pressure, respiratory rate, body temperature, and biochemical markers, and may even incorporate therapeutic functions such as regulating heart rhythm and restoring hearing. However, continuous and long-term monitoring requires these devices to remain in close contact with the human body for extended periods, making factors such as size, safety, unobtrusiveness, and comfort key concerns for users. This has led to an increasing demand for miniature biomedical devices to enable long-term physiological monitoring, especially for chronic disease management and therapeutic interventions (Majumder et al. 2017a).

In fact, the market for small-scale medical systems, including wearable and implantable devices, is expanding rapidly. The wearable device market is projected to grow from USD 81.15 billion in 2024 to USD 324.7 billion by 2032 at a compounded annual growth rate (CAGR) of 17.2%. Besides, the implantable device market is expected to rise from USD 122.63 billion in 2023 to USD 266.33 billion by 2032 (CAGR 9.0%) (Wearable medical devices market in-depth insights and analysis 2024–2032 2025). Several wearable and implantable biomedical devices, such as pacemakers, glucose monitoring systems, neural stimulators, and cochlear implants, are currently commercially available. Nevertheless, there remains significant potential for developing miniaturized biomedical systems that enable unobtrusive, continuous, and remote monitoring of a broader range of health indicators.

Although the market projections for miniature biomedical devices are highly promising, critical challenges, including manufacturing scalability, integration complexity within compact form factors, energy requirements, and operational safety within the human body, must be addressed for their widespread adoption. Moreover, concerns regarding long-term reliability, biocompatibility, and stability, as well as data security and privacy, and energy-efficient communication are pivotal for clinical acceptance and regulatory approval.

In this chapter, we explore emerging technologies that contribute to the development of low-power, miniaturized biomedical systems, which can potentially transform healthcare by enabling continuous and real-time physiological monitoring. These technologies, altogether, enable designing small-scale biomedical devices under stringent size, power, and biocompatibility constraints without compromising performance and reliability. In order to systematically investigate the evolution of miniature biomedical devices, we first introduce the key components of these devices (Sect. 2.2), followed by an in-depth discussion of the core technologies driving their miniaturization (Sect. 2.3). Then, a brief overview of recent advancements in miniature biomedical devices is presented in Sect. 2.4. In Sect. 2.5, we discuss critical challenges, ranging from energy requirements and safety to data security and device interoperability, that must be addressed to enable broader clinical adoption. Finally, the chapter concludes by highlighting the research and innovation required to address current limitations, along with the potential of integrating technologies such as the Internet of Things (IoT), Artificial Intelligence (AI), and big data analytics to realize the full potential of small-scale biomedical systems in modern healthcare.

2.2 Key Components of Modern Biomedical Devices

A typical biomedical measurement device consists of several key components, as shown in Fig. 2.1. The front end of the device comprises a sensing unit and a signal conditioning unit (Majumder et al. 2018).

2.2.1 Sensing Unit

The sensing unit detects electrical (e.g., biopotentials such as electrocardiogram (ECG), electroencephalogram (EEG), and electromyography (EMG)), chemical (e.g., pH, glucose, lactate, and ionic concentrations), mechanical (e.g., pulse pressure, movement), acoustic (e.g., heart sound and lung sound) and optical signals (e.g., photoplethysmogram (PPG)) from the human body and converts them into electrical signals for further processing.

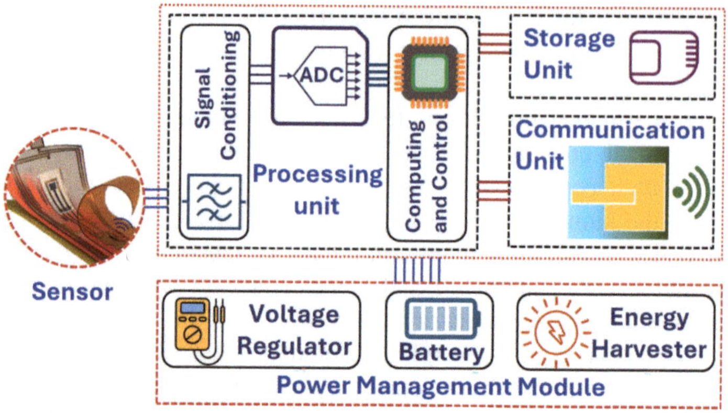

Fig. 2.1 Key components of a modern biomedical device

Since these sensors remain in close contact with the human body, it is critical for the materials to be biocompatible and safe for prolonged use. In addition, these sensors need to be unobtrusive to enable continuous monitoring without compromising user comfort. Flexible substrates not only enhance user comfort but also improve skin contact, thereby enhancing signal quality by reducing motion artifacts. Proper design considerations, including electrode geometry (Majumder et al. 2018) and materials with high surface-to-volume ratios, such as carbon nanotubes (CNTs), Graphene, and MXenes (Majumder et al. 2025), can further enhance signal quality. Material composition plays a crucial role in achieving desired sensing performance, including response time, sensitivity, selectivity, and long-term stability. However, periodic calibration of the sensors may be required to ensure measurement accuracy and long-term stability.

2.2.2 Signal Conditioning

The signal conditioning unit includes critical components such as filters, instrumentation amplifiers, and protective circuitry. Filters are designed to remove unwanted signals, including DC offset, low-frequency motion artifacts, high-frequency noise, and powerline interference (50/60 Hz). Instrumentation amplifiers amplify weak differential biosignals while effectively eliminating common-mode noise such as motion artifacts or power-line interference. To enhance signal quality, it is essential for the amplifier to have a high (>80 dB) common-mode rejection ratio (CMRR) along with high input impedance, low output impedance, and high linearity (Malekzadeh-Arasteh et al. 2021).

Miniature biomedical devices facilitate continuous physiological monitoring, typically through direct contact with the human body. Therefore, these devices must limit patient leakage currents to specified levels, for instance, below 100 μA in normal conditions for Body Floating (BF)-rated devices, as directed by the IEC 60601-1 (Sutanto et al. 2017). Additionally, they must also be protected against electrostatic discharge (ESD) and overheating to ensure patient safety. Leakage currents can be minimized by reducing input-to-output capacitance and employing isolation amplifiers (e.g., optocouplers) and unity-gain buffers. The high input impedance of the buffer effectively isolates the sensor from the rest of the signal conditioning circuit, thus ensuring minimal current draw from the sensor. Furthermore, the buffer amplifier offers a low output impedance, thus efficiently transmitting signals to subsequent circuitry, thus maintaining signal integrity.

2.2.3 Computing and Control

The conditioned analog signal is fed to an analog-to-digital converter (ADC) for digitization, which is then passed on to the computing and control unit. In small devices, components like microcontrollers, digital signal processors (DSPs), and application-specific integrated circuits (ASICs) are typically used for on-board signal processing and control (Yazicioglu et al. 2010; Yan et al. 2014). These devices are programmed to perform application-specific processing tasks such as digital filtering, artifact or drift removal, fast Fourier transform (FFT), and wavelet transforms (Yazicioglu et al. 2010; Chen et al. 2015) as well as preliminary data analysis to extract physiological parameters like heart rate, body temperature, and glucose concentration (Deepu et al. 2016). This unit manages device operation, including settings such as sampling rates and sleep modes. Additionally, it may incorporate a closed-loop feedback system to enable adaptive therapy, as realized in modern continuous glucose monitoring (CGM) systems with integrated insulin pumps (MiniMed™ 780G System | Medtronic 2025). The unit also manages on-board storage and ensures secure communication through encrypted channels.

2.2.4 Data Storage and Communication

The digitized and processed data can be stored in an on-board storage device. However, small biomedical devices typically have limited on-board storage capacity. Recent devices incorporate low-power communication modules such as Bluetooth® Low Energy (BLE), ZigBee, Near-Field Communication (NFC), Low Range (LoRa), and Narrowband IoT (NB-IoT) (Majumder et al. 2017b). The processing and control unit drives the communication module to transmit encrypted data securely to a nearby computing device such as a smartphone. The computing device can relay the data to a distant server over the internet, where large volumes of data can be stored and analyzed for real-time physiological monitoring and clinical assessment. Advanced encryption protocols like advanced encryption standard (AES) and secure sockets layer/transport layer security (SSL/TLS) ensure secure bidirectional communication for tasks including firmware updates, data retrieval, and device control through user interaction.

Nevertheless, each technology offers distinct performance characteristics in terms of data transmission speed, range, and power efficiency, making its selection highly specific to application requirements. For instance, fast-varying physiological signals like ECG, EMG, and PPG require higher bandwidth and lower latency for real-time transmission and monitoring compared to body temperature or glucose concentration measurements. Additionally, coverage area and power consumption must be considered when selecting these technologies. In general, BLE is widely used in consumer-grade wearable devices owing to its balanced power requirements, transmission range, and data throughput.

2.2.5 Power Management

Another key component of medical devices is the power management module, which ensures a stable power supply for device operation. Wearable devices typically use rechargeable batteries like lithium-ion (Li-ion) or lithium polymer (Li-polymer) batteries, which require periodic charging. However, charging may interrupt the measurement and monitoring operations of the wearables. Inductive power transfer technologies enable wireless battery charging without interrupting device operation, making them particularly valuable for implantable and ingestible devices where conventional cable-based charging is not feasible (Ben Amar et al. 2015; Campi et al. 2021). Moreover, energy harvesting techniques can be integrated into such devices to scavenge energy from the surroundings by exploiting the photovoltaic, piezoelectric, and thermoelectric properties of materials (Zhang et al. 2013; Nagaveni et al. 2024; Zeng et al. 2022).

Regardless, efficient power management is critical for small devices to achieve prolonged operation without frequent charging. Typically, wireless communication and data processing are the most power-intensive functions in these devices. Effective energy management strategies, including duty cycling, different power modes (such as sleep, standby, and wakeup modes), and dynamic voltage scaling (DVS), along with low power electronics, are employed to minimize power consumption, thereby extending the operational time of devices (Singh et al. 2020).

2.2.6 Enclosure

Since biomedical devices remain in close contact with the human body, they must be safely and securely housed in robust enclosures made of bio-compatible, non-irritant, and hypoallergenic materials such as medical-grade silicone, polyimide, and PDMS (Majumder et al. 2023, 2025). These enclosures must effectively shield the internal electronic circuitry to safeguard against leakage currents, electric shock, and thermal hazards. It is critical for these devices to comply with ISO 10993 and IEC 60601-1 standards to ensure bio- and electrical safety for human use (Proposed changes to the medical devices directorate's draft guidance document – list of recognized standards for medical devices 2025). Additionally, enclosures with Ingress Protection (IP) ratings (e.g., IP67 or IP68) are required to protect the devices from dust, moisture, and sweat ingress (IP Ratings 2025). Nonetheless, the enclosures must be ergonomically designed to ensure user comfort while maintaining robust mechanical integrity against the stresses and wear of daily use.

2.2.7 User Interface

Furthermore, wearable devices typically incorporate simple and minimalistic user interfaces with a few buttons or touch-sensitive intuitive controls. These devices are often paired with supporting smartphone applications for enhanced monitoring and user interaction. However, direct physical interaction is infeasible for implantable or ingestible devices. Nevertheless, integrated wireless communication capabilities of these devices enable users to interact via smartphone apps.

2.3 Technologies Enabling Miniaturization

In recent years, there has been growing interest in developing miniature biomedical systems for long-term, unobtrusive health monitoring and therapeutic interventions via wearable, implantable, and ingestible devices. Advances in material science and nanotechnology, microfabrication processes, MEMS technology, and CMOS-based low-power systems, including microelectronic, computing, and communication devices, have collectively contributed to integrating multiple functionalities seamlessly to create standalone and miniature biomedical devices.

2.3.1 Advanced Materials and Nanotechnology

Materials are the key enablers of flexible, biocompatible, and high-precision sensors. Nanomaterials offer a high surface-to-volume ratio and exhibit excellent electrical, mechanical, and thermal properties. These properties render them highly sensitive to various stimuli, making them excellent candidates for biosensing applications. A variety of 2D nanomaterials (Fig. 2.2), such as graphene and graphene oxide (GO), MXenes, hexagonal boron nitride (h-BN), transition metal

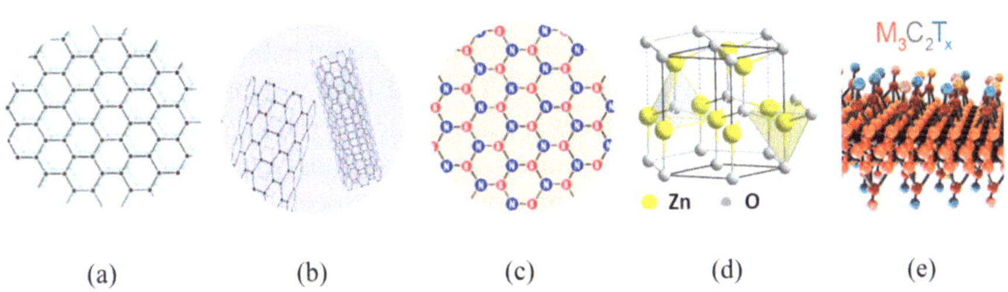

Fig. 2.2 Some widely used nanomaterials in biomedical sensors: (**a**) graphene, (**b**) carbon nanotube, (**c**) h-BN, (**d**) ZnO wurtzite cell (File:Wurtzite_polyhedra.png), public domain, (**e**) MXene. (Reproduced from Babar et al. (2025) with permission from the Royal Society of Chemistry)

dichalcogenides (TMD), and metal oxides (ZnO, TiO_2, SnO_2), are widely used in biosensors (Majumder et al. 2025). In addition, carbon nanotubes (CNTs) and metallic nanoparticles (NPs), such as Au-NPs, Ag-NPs, and Pt-NPs, are extensively used in sensor fabrication.

These nanomaterials are often incorporated into conductive polymers, such as poly(3,4-ethylenedioxythiophene) polystyrene sulfonate (PEDOT: PSS), polyaniline (PANI), and polypyrrole (PPy) or their derivatives, to enhance sensor sensitivity (Majumder et al. 2025). These conductive biocompatible polymers, as well as conductive polymer hydrogels, exhibit high mechanical flexibility and tunable electrical properties, thereby making them good candidates for fabricating flexible sensors. These flexible sensors can be designed to detect a wide range of physiological signals, including strain, biopotentials, temperature, humidity, pH, and biochemicals such as glucose, lactate, and electrolytes.

By leveraging flexible and stretchable polymer substrates, wearable sensors can achieve good conformity to irregular body surfaces, thus enhancing signal quality and user comfort. However, these substrates must be resistant to sweat and heat, insulating in nature, and mechanically durable to withstand daily wear and tear. Polymers, such as polyimide (PI), polyethylene terephthalate (PET), polyvinylidene fluoride (PVDF), polyvinyl alcohol (PVA), and polyethylene naphthalate (PEN), are extensively used as substrate materials in flexible sensors due to their good mechanical strength, thermal stability, and corrosion resistance (Majumder et al. 2023, 2025). Nevertheless, these polymers can often be brittle, particularly after prolonged use and exposure to heat and sweat.

Elastomers such as polydimethylsiloxane (PDMS) and polyurethane (PU) are highly elastic and biocompatible, making them good candidates as substrates for flexible medical devices and skin-worn sensors. In recent years, textile- and paper-based substrates have gained attention for biosensor fabrication (Majumder et al. 2023). Paper as well as most textile materials, including cotton, wool, and silk, are derived from eco-friendly sources and extensively used in daily life. These substrates are typically functionalized with conductive nanomaterials, conductive polymers, or nanomaterial-polymer composites to enhance sensor strength, flexibility, stability, and sensing performance. Moreover, the inherent biocompatibility, flexibility, and softness of paper and textile materials, coupled with their low cost and abundance, render them excellent candidates for developing skin-friendly, disposable sensors.

In addition, carbonized materials are increasingly used in biosensors due to their high electrical conductivity, thermal stability, and light weight. Highly sensitive, stretchable strain sensors with excellent gauge factors (GFs) and wide detection ranges were developed using carbonized fabrics such as cotton and silk (Zhang et al. 2017; Wang et al. 2016). Capacitive pressure sensors based on carbonized cotton fabric and porous Ecoflex® have also demonstrated high sensitivity and broad detection ranges, demonstrating the potential of carbonized materials for wearable sensor applications (Ko et al. 2021).

Recently, hydrogels have emerged as a promising class of materials for flexible sensors due to their unique combination of flexibility, stretchability, biocompatibility, and water-retention capabilities (Yu et al. 2022; Li et al. 2020). Beyond electrical conductivity, conductive hydrogel-based fibers and composites exhibit multifunctional properties, including self-healing, strain sensitivity, and responsiveness to external stimuli (Yu et al. 2022; Li et al. 2020). Functional additives such as CNTs, cellulose nanofibers, and metal nanoparticles can significantly enhance the electrochemical performance of hydrogels, enabling applications in sensing, energy harvesting, and drug delivery. However, achieving an optimal balance between sensitivity, conductivity, mechanical robustness, and self-healing efficiency remains a key challenge (Han et al. 2019).

Furthermore, small biomedical devices require uninterrupted energy supplies for continuous operation. Advanced material compositions have been explored to develop small-scale energy solutions, including nanobatteries, nanogenerators, and energy-harvesting technologies (Tiwari and Singh 2023; Lu et al. 2020). For instance, high-energy-density nanobatteries can be fabricated using nanostructured conducting polymer electrolytes (e.g., PANI, PPy, and polythiophene), with $LiMn_2O_4$ and $LiCoO_2$ nanoparticles serving as cathodes and Si, SnO, Sb, and graphene nanoparticles forming the anodes (Tiwari and Singh 2023). Additionally, carbonized silk integrated with vertically aligned molybdenum disulfide (MoS_2) nanosheets has demonstrated high energy-storage capacity (Lu et al. 2020).

Moreover, a wide variety of nanomaterial–conductive polymer composites have been explored to achieve piezoelectric, photovoltaic, thermoelectric, and triboelectric properties (Fakhri et al. 2019; Veeralingam et al. 2022; Wang et al. 2021). These composites can be integrated into biosensors to harvest electrical energy from the ambient environment. Nevertheless, ensuring a stable, reliable, and continuous energy supply to drive all components of the miniature device, including signal conditioning, processing, and communication systems, remains an engineering challenge.

2.3.2 Synthesis and Fabrication Techniques

While materials play key roles in enhancing the sensing properties in biomedical devices, synthesis of highly pure materials and their precise deposition are crucial for achieving desired performance metrices, including sensitivity, dynamic range, stability, and mechanical strength. Advanced fabrication techniques (Fig. 2.3) have enabled the synthesis of high-purity nanomaterials and thin-film deposition.

Physical vapor deposition (PVD) is such technique that enables high precision thin-film deposition of nanomaterials onto flexible substrates such as Kapton and PDMS. PVD methods, including RF/DC sputtering, pulsed laser deposition, thermal evaporation, and e-beam evaporation, are used to fabricate highly flexible, skin-conformable resistive strain sensors for applications such as motion detection, voice recognition and electronic skin, and soft robotics (Ben Amar et al. 2015; Majumder et al. 2023).

Chemical vapor deposition (CVD) techniques allow for uniform and precise deposition of conductive materials onto flexible substrates, thus facilitating

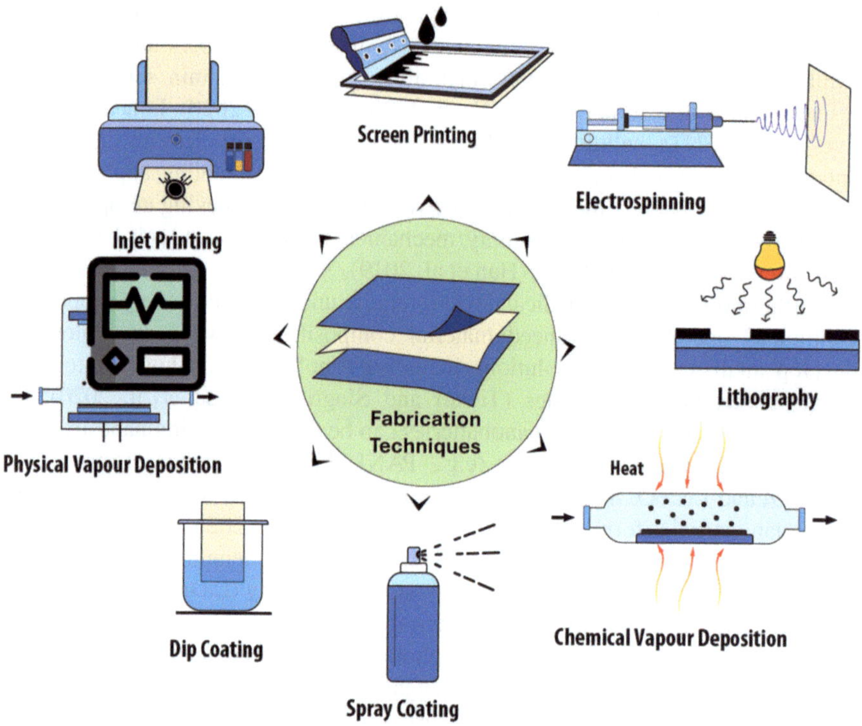

Fig. 2.3 Modern fabrication techniques

fabrication of lightweight and biocompatible flexible devices. For instance, CVD was used in (Conti et al. 2020) to grow MoS_2 layers for fabricating field-effect transistors on paper substrates. In addition, flexible PDMS-based temperature sensors were developed by incorporating CVD-grown graphene nanowalls (GNWs) (Yang et al. 2015) and CNTs (Ben-Shimon and Ya'akobovitz 2021) for small-scale health monitoring applications.

Screen printing and inkjet printing are cost-effective, scalable techniques for fabricating flexible wearable sensors. These methods enable precise patterning of functional inks onto substrates such as paper, textiles, or flexible polymers. These ubiquitous methods make them ideal for the mass production of lightweight, flexible wearable sensors, including skin-conformable sensors for strain (Thiyagarajan et al. 2021; Yoshida et al. 2024; Liao et al. 2016), temperature, and humidity detection (Vuorinen et al. 2016; Bouhamed et al. 2021).

Another cost-effective and scalable technique is spray coating, which is used to deposit thin layers of conductive or composite materials in complex, irregular patterns onto a wide range of substrates, including PDMS, cotton fabric, and silicone rubber (Majumder et al. 2023). While spray coating preserves substrate flexibility, achieving uniform and precise coating thickness remains challenging. Additionally, this method often requires surface treatments or binders to ensure strong adhesion between the coating material and substrate.

The dip coating technique deposits uniform thin films onto substrates by immersing and withdrawing them from a coating solution at a controlled speed (Majumder et al. 2023). This method enables multilayer deposition of conductive polymers and nanomaterials onto various substrates, including spandex, polyurethane (PU), and paper. However, dip coating requires large volumes of coating solution and precise process control to achieve the desired adhesion and film thickness.

Functional nanofibers are extensively used in flexible and stretchable sensors. These fibers can be produced using the electrospinning technique, which exploits a high-voltage power supply to create Taylor cones from charged polymer solutions or molten materials. The Taylor cones are stretched into fine nanofibers and collected as nonwoven meshes on a grounded collector. A conductive coating is then applied to the polymer core to form composites, such as PANI/PU, PVDF/CNT, and PVA/MXene, with enhanced sensing capabilities (Majumder et al. 2025).

Furthermore, micromachining techniques, including lithography, etching, and bonding, are widely used to fabricate MEMS and microfluidic devices, flexible biochips, microelectrode arrays (MEAs), and biosensors such as multifunctional e-skin sensors and microfluidic pressure sensors (Xu et al. 2018). Methods like photolithography, electron-beam lithography, and nanoimprint lithography enable high-resolution patterning of metal films on flexible substrates, thus providing sensor stretchability and skin-conformability while allowing microchannel integration (Gao et al. 2017) for enhanced sensing performance.

Additionally, techniques such as sol–gel processing, dry–wet spinning, and chemical cross-linking are extensively employed to incorporate nanomaterials, conductive polymers (Wang et al. 2025a), and reinforcing materials such as cellulose nanofibrils or protein-based fibers (Lin et al. 2022) into hydrogel matrices, thus yielding material composites with enhanced mechanical strength, conductivity, and durability.

2.3.3 CMOS IC, MEMS, and SoC Technologies

Semiconductor process technologies have advanced remarkably in the last three decades. Metal-oxide-semiconductor field-effect transistors (MOSFETs) have evolved from 130-nm CMOS planar technology in the early 2000s to 3-nm non-planar FinFET technology in 2022 (Bohr and Young 2017), keeping pace with the pace of transistor scaling predicted by Moore's law. Recently, a 2-nm process using gate-all-around (GAA) nanosheet transistors was introduced, offering a ~1.15-fold increase in transistor density, along with a 15% improvement in transistor speed or a 30% reduction in power consumption compared to its 3-nm counterpart (Vaughan 2024). These advances enable the fabrication of high-speed, low-power miniature multi-modal system-on-chip (SoC) devices that integrate multiple functionalities such as sensing, signal conditioning, processing, storage, and communication on a single chip.

A key design consideration for biomedical SoCs is minimizing power consumption to enable prolonged monitoring. Various architectural and circuit-level design strategies, including subthreshold digital signal processing and duty-cycled radio frequency (RF) operation, help minimize power consumption (Zhang et al. 2013; Khayatzadeh et al. 2012). Furthermore, automatic gain control (AGC) techniques can enhance signal quality by dynamically adjusting the input level of low-power sigma-delta ADCs (Vemishetty et al. 2016). Moreover, an independent AGC coupled with ADC triggering after gain adjustment can reduce overall power requirements. By employing energy-efficient analog front end (AFE) designs, including ac-coupled amplifiers (Deepu et al. 2016; Harpe et al. 2016), complementary differential input amplifiers (Zhang et al. 2012; Wang et al. 2014), and chopper-stabilized amplifiers (Yazicioglu et al. 2010; Chen et al. 2015; Tseng et al. 2012), power consumption can be reduced to hundreds of nanowatts.

To avoid amplifier saturation, AFEs must effectively eliminate large DC electrode offsets (DEO), typically up to ±300 mV in ECG systems (Becchetti and Neri 2013). Various techniques, including AC-coupled amplifiers, capacitive feedback amplifiers (Yan et al. 2014; Khayatzadeh et al. 2012; Wang et al. 2014) and DC-servo loops (DSLs) (Harpe et al. 2016; Yoo et al. 2012), are used to eliminate DEO. Although these techniques are effective in eliminating DEO, each comes with inherent limitations. For example, AC-coupled amplifiers exhibit poor input impedance and suffer from capacitor mismatch issues, thus affecting the common-mode rejection ratio (CMRR). Capacitive feedback amplifiers use MOS-based capacitors and resistors (e.g., PMOS pseudoresistors or floating-gate transistors) to implement high-pass filters that, however, potentially introduce nonlinearity and process-dependent variations (Wang et al. 2014). Therefore, application-specific optimization is required for the AFEs to trade off performance, cost, and reliability.

SoCs may further incorporate on-chip noise reduction techniques, such as switched-capacitor high-pass filters (Yan et al. 2014) and baseline stabilization circuits (Zhang et al. 2015), to enhance signal quality by eliminating high-frequency noise and baseline shifts, albeit at the cost of increased chip area. Furthermore, on-chip signal processing like the 1-D discrete wavelet transform (Vemishetty et al. 2016) and fast Fourier transform (FFT) (Chen et al. 2015) enable real-time denoising and feature extraction, for example, QRS peak detection for real-time heart rate monitoring (Zhang et al. 2013; Yang et al. 2015; Wang et al. 2025a).

On-chip integration of wireless communication technologies facilitates real-time data transmission, which is particularly critical for implantable and ingestible devices. Biomedical SoCs with integrated transceivers supporting ZigBee (Wang et al. 2015), Medical Implant Communication Service (MICS) (Zhang et al. 2013; Khayatzadeh et al. 2012), and ultra-wideband (UWB) (Ren et al. 2016; Lee et al. 2018; Mahfuz et al. 2022) communications, occasionally integrated with energy harvesting technologies, have been widely demonstrated (Zhang et al. 2013).

CMOS technology also enables the fabrication of high-density microelectrode arrays (MEAs) for diverse applications, including electrochemical sensing, implantable biopotential recording, electrical brain stimulation (EBS), brain–computer interfaces (BCIs), and retinal prostheses, with the number of electrodes ranging

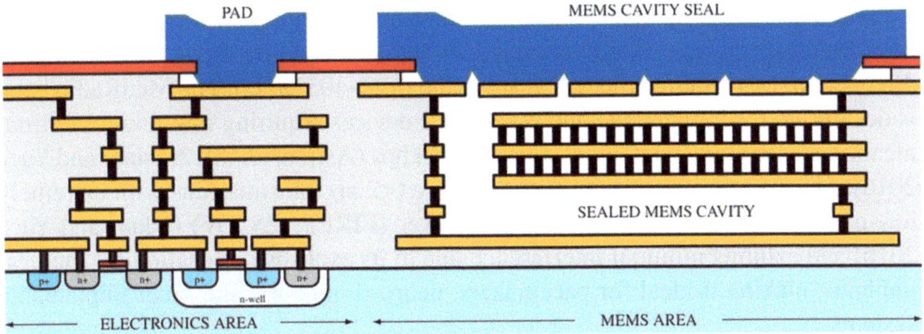

Fig. 2.4 CMOS–MEMS process cross-section. (Adapted from Valle et al. (2021), CC BY-NC-ND 4.0)

from hundreds to thousands (Liu et al. 2023). These MEAs can be monolithically integrated into biochip and biosensor SoCs using submicron lithography, thereby significantly reducing device footprint while achieving robust interconnections and enhanced noise performance.

MEMS technologies enable the integration of electrical and mechanical functionalities at a highly miniaturized scale. The CMOS-compatible micromachining processes allow for the fabrication of robust, high-performance biomedical SoCs with integrated MEMS-based sensors and actuators, and energy harvesters (Fig. 2.4). These technologies facilitate the fabrication of self-powered biosensors and implantable devices, including cochlear implants, ocular implants, micropumps, and pacemakers, for diagnostic and therapeutic purposes (Li 2012).

In addition, MEMS technologies are used to fabricate precise microfluidic components, including pumps, valves, and channels, which are integrated into biosensors to precisely control fluid flow, mixing, and chemical reactions at microliter to nanoliter scale volumes. Such precise and microscale manipulation of liquids facilitates diverse applications, including cell sorting, in vitro cell culture, droplet microfluidics, targeted drug delivery, and real-time biochemical analysis of biofluids (e.g., sweat, saliva, interstitial fluid). These capabilities of precise fluid manipulation further lead to the emergence of modern BioMEMS systems such as point-of-care, lab-on-a-chip and organ-on-a-chip devices (Azizipour et al. 2020). Systems like organ-on-a-chip provide controlled microenvironments that mimic human organ functions to study diseases, test drugs, and understand organ physiology, thus eliminating the need for traditional cell cultures or animal models.

2.3.4 Low-Power Communication Technologies

Small biomedical devices, including wearables, implantables, and ingestibles, require energy-efficient, miniaturized communication systems to reduce power consumption, extend operational lifetime, and meet stringent size constraints. Moreover, reliable and secure data transmission is critical to ensure data integrity, patient privacy, and protection against unauthorized access.

Two license-free frequency bands are allocated for biomedical communications. The Medical Device Radiocommunications (MedRadio) Service band spans 401–406 MHz, including the MICS sub-band (402–405 MHz). The MedRadio band is designated for implantable and body-worn devices requiring low-power communication at a moderate data rate of up to 800 kbps (Asili et al. 2012; Islam and Yuce 2016). This band is optimized for short-range (<2 m) transmissions with extremely low-power (effective isotropic radiated power (EIRP) ≤25 μW) (Islam and Yuce 2016) and exhibits minimal interference due to its exclusive allocation for medical implants, making it ideal for pacemakers, neurostimulators, and other implantable systems.

Additionally, the 433–434.8 MHz Industrial, Scientific, and Medical (ISM) band is utilized for short-range transmissions due to its moderate penetration depth and lower absorption in body tissues compared to higher frequencies. The ISM band also encompasses the 902–928 MHz, 2.4–2.5 GHz, and 5.725–5.875 GHz bands. However, the 2.4–2.5 GHz band is predominantly employed in wearable devices, including smartwatches, fitness trackers, health monitoring devices, and Wireless Body Area Networks (WBANs), owing to its high data rates and compact antenna design (Marasco et al. 2023; Lee et al. 2020a). The 5 GHz band offers higher bandwidth, reduced interference, and smaller antennas than lower-frequency bands, thus enabling faster data transmission with low latency (<5 ms) for WBAN-connected sensors (Preethichandra et al. 2023). Nevertheless, these high-frequency bands are more susceptible to absorption and scattering in biological tissues, limiting their range and reliability in WBAN applications.

To enable energy-efficient short-range wireless communication, compact biomedical devices utilize low-power technologies including BLE, ZigBee, MICS, NFC, UWB, LoRa, and NB-IoT (Majumder et al. 2017a, b). Most of these can be integrated into biomedical SoCs to support real-time physiological monitoring (Khayatzadeh et al. 2012; Wang et al. 2015; Lee et al. 2020b). Furthermore, energy harvesting methods, such as RF energy harvesting, piezoelectric, and thermoelectric generators, can be integrated to achieve self-sustaining operation for these systems (Zhang et al. 2013; Nagaveni et al. 2024). A summary of key short-range communication technologies is presented in Table 2.1.

Antennas are essential components of wireless systems that facilitate bidirectional conversion between electrical signals and propagating electromagnetic waves. With the growing demand for portable and wearable devices, the design of flexible, conformal, and small-scale antennas has become increasingly important. These compact antennas are particularly critical for small biomedical applications, including implantable and ingestible systems, which must meet stringent spatial, mechanical, and biocompatibility requirements.

Microstrip patch antennas operating in the 2.4 GHz ISM band are extensively used in biomedical applications due to their compact size, ease of circuit integration, and low cost, thus making them well-suited for miniature medical devices. These antennas can be designed for short-range biomedical communication through careful selection of biocompatible substrate materials (e.g., ceramic composites, PDMS, parylene) and conductive layers (e.g., silver nanoparticles, graphene inks).

Table 2.1 Short-range communication technologies for biomedical devices (Majumder et al. 2017a, b)

Technology	Frequency band(s)	Typical data rate	Range	Power/current consumption
Bluetooth®	2.4 GHz ISM	~1–3 Mbps	~10–100 m	upto100 mW
BLE	2.4 GHz ISM	~125 kbps–2 Mbps	~10–100 m	10–100 mW
ZigBee	2.4 GHz, 868 MHz, 915 MHz	~250 kbps (2.4 GHz)	~10–100 m	~1 mW RF power, 9.5–30 mA during transmission
MICS	402–405 MHz	Up to 800 kbps	~2 m (implants)	25 μW–2.5 mW
NFC	13.56 MHz	~106–424 kbps	<10 cm	<15 mA during active reading
UWB	3.1–10.6 GHz	~110 Mbps–1 Gbps	~1–10 m	~39 μW–10 mW
LoRa	433 MHz, 868 MHz, 915 MHz	~0.3–50 kbps	~2–15 km	7.66 μA–34 mA (sleep mode) 38.9 mA–117 mA (active)
NB-IoT	LTE bands (700–2100 MHz)	~20–250 kbps	~1–10 km	~8 μA (sleep), up to 130 mA during transmission

Additionally, bio-based polymers are being investigated to develop conformal, flexible antennas optimized for ISM band operation (Zahedi et al. 2024; Sid et al. 2023). Furthermore, textile-based antennas using cotton, silk, and polyester substrates are gaining traction in wearable health monitoring applications and WBAN connectivity (Mahfuz et al. 2022). The inherently low dielectric constants of these substrate materials reduce surface wave propagation, thereby enhancing impedance bandwidth and radiation efficiency.

In addition, miniaturized nanoantennas (Tiwari and Sharma 2025) and normal-mode helical antennas (Karnaushenko et al. 2015) operating in ISM bands are particularly suitable for compact implantable biomedical systems, including pacemakers (Feng et al. 2022), neural stimulators (Mohan and Kumar 2024), and drug delivery systems (Mirvakili and Langer 2021). In drug-releasing implants, these nanoantennas enable wireless triggering of drug carriers for targeted release (Mirvakili and Langer 2021). Furthermore, brain implants incorporating such antennas facilitate precise neural stimulation, offering therapeutic potential for neurological disorder treatment (Mohan and Kumar 2024).

Unlike conventional RF antennas, the human body itself can serve as a transmission medium for intra-body communication in body area network (BAN)-connected sensors. This mode of communication, known as human body communication (HBC), exploits the conductive and dielectric properties of body tissues to propagate electrical signals (Maity et al. 2020; Kodama and Muramatsu 2024). HBC offers significant advantages over traditional RF methods owing to its ultra-low power requirement and enhanced data security resulting from the signal confinement within the body's vicinity. HBC enables signal transmission via displacement currents induced in the body's electric field (capacitive coupling) or via low-amplitude current injection through tissues (galvanic coupling) (Maity et al. 2020). These mechanisms offer reliable, secure, and energy-efficient short-range communication, making HBC particularly suitable for implantable and wearable medical devices (Kodama and Muramatsu 2024).

2.4 Recent Trends

2.4.1 Monitoring and Therapeutic Devices

Wearable devices have gained significant popularity in recent years. Small-scale devices like smartwatches and fitness trackers, such as the Apple Watch Series 9 (Apple Watch Series 9 – technical specifications – Apple support 2025) and the Fitbit Sense 2 (Fitbit Sense 2 technical specs 2025), integrate multiple sensors with wireless connectivity to track health parameters such as heart rate, oxygen levels, body temperature, and activity patterns. Some FDA-cleared wearable devices, such as the BioSticker™ (BioIntelliSense announces FDA clearance of the BioSticker™, the first single-use medical device enabling 30 days of continuous vital signs monitoring 2025) and BioButton® (BioIntelliSense launches new BioButton® rechargeable wearable device for continuous medical grade monitoring of 20+ vital signs and biometrics 2025) from BioIntelliSense and the ScanWatch (Withings announces the FDA clearance of ScanWatch – its most advanced hybrid smartwatch 2025) from Withings, are currently available on the market that enable continuous multi-parameter monitoring remotely. These systems leverage cloud-based data storage and AI-driven analytics to provide users with personalized health insights, including activity patterns, sleep quality, and atrial fibrillation detection. Such smart biosensors are increasingly used in telemedicine, allowing physicians to remotely assess patient conditions and provide timely recommendations (Faham et al. 2023), thus enhancing patient care and accessibility to medical diagnostics.

In addition to wearable devices, there are other miniature biomedical instruments that are used for diagnostic purposes. One such instrument is capsule endoscopy, which enables non-invasive imaging of the gastrointestinal (GI) tract to diagnose digestive diseases such as obscure GI bleeding, celiac disease, and inflammatory bowel disease (IBD). These miniature ingestible capsules, including PillCam™ SB 3 (PillCam™ SB 3 Capsule | Medtronic 2025), and PillCam™ COLON 2 (PillCam™ COLON 2 System | Medtronic 2025) from Medtronic, CapsoCam Plus® SV-3 (Product Specifications – Capsovision 2025) from CapsoVision, and NaviCam® SB (NaviCam® SB System – AnX Robotics 2025) from AnX Robotica, are equipped with cameras, LEDs, and batteries, and support wireless communication (PillCam™ SB 3 Capsule | Medtronic 2025; PillCam™ COLON 2 System | Medtronic 2025) to capture and transmit images of the gastrointestinal tract.

While wearable and ingestible devices are non-invasive and typically used for health monitoring and diagnostic purposes, implantable devices are generally therapeutic and may require surgical procedures. Advances in CMOS–MEMS fabrication processes and low-power wireless technologies have significantly contributed to the development of a new generation of miniaturized, highly sensitive, and low-power implantable devices for a wide range of clinical applications. Currently, several FDA-cleared/CE-marked implantable medical devices, including insertable cardiac monitors, pacemakers, cochlear implants, deep brain stimulation (DBS) systems, spinal cord stimulation (SCS) devices, continuous glucose monitoring (CGM) systems, and intraocular pressure (IOP) monitoring devices, are available on the market.

Insertable cardiac monitors, such as Medtronic's LINQ II™ (LINQ IITM Insertable Cardiac Monitor | Medtronic 2025), are implanted beneath the skin to continuously record the electrical activity associated with cardiac rhythms and detect arrhythmias. For glaucoma management, devices like the Sensimed Triggerfish® (Sensimed Triggerfish – Sensimed S.A. 2025) use smart contact lenses embedded with strain gauges to track ocular shape changes, enabling wireless monitoring of intraocular pressure for 24 hours. Continuous glucose monitoring (CGM) systems, such as the Eversense E3® (Eversense Diabetes Eversense E3® CGM SYSTEM 2005) and MiniMed™ 780G (MiniMed™ 780G System | Medtronic 2025), use subcutaneous electrochemical sensors to provide real-time glucose measurements.

Therapeutic implants such as pacemakers, like the Micra™ AV and VR (Micra AV and VR – Pacing Systems | Medtronic Diabetes 2025), deliver electrical pulses directly to the heart to maintain proper rhythm in patients with bradycardia. Cochlear implants like Cochlear™ Nucleus® (Cochlear Americas | Hear Now and Always | Cochlear Implants 2025) converts sound into electrical signals that bypass damaged cochlear hair cells to stimulate the auditory nerve and thereby restore partial hearing. Deep brain stimulation (DBS) systems, such as the Percept™ PC (Percept™ PC Neurostimulator | Medtronic 2025), target specific brain regions with controlled electrical impulses to alleviate symptoms of neurological disorders like Parkinson's disease. Similarly, spinal cord stimulation (SCS) devices like Abbott's Proclaim™ Plus and Proclaim™ XR (SCS Therapies | Abbott 2025) deliver electrical pulses to the spinal cord to disrupt pain signaling and relieve chronic pain.

These wireless commercial devices generally come with proprietary mobile applications and data analytics tools for real-time patient health monitoring and assessment, thus potentially enabling remote healthcare delivery. Some advanced systems, such as CGM devices with integrated insulin pumps like the MiniMed™ 780G (MiniMed™ 780G System | Medtronic 2025), may even support the automatic adjustment of therapies, e.g., insulin dosing via a closed-loop system.

2.4.2 AI-Based Data Analytics

AI and big data analytics hold immense potential in transforming healthcare. These technologies can process large datasets generated by biomedical sensors and diagnostic tools to uncover subtle patterns and anomalies, which otherwise may not be detectable through conventional methods. AI-driven data analytics enhances diagnostic accuracy and enables early interventions, facilitating the development of intelligent healthcare applications for predictive diagnostics, personalized treatment, and real-time physiological monitoring (Esteva et al. 2019).

Most manufacturers of the smart biomedical devices mentioned above offer cloud-based, AI-driven proprietary data analytics platforms for their users. For example, Medtronic's LINQ II™ ICM utilizes a deep learning-based AccuRhythm™ AI algorithm to analyze cardiac data for abnormalities such as atrial fibrillation (AF) and pauses in heart rhythm (LINQ IITM Insertable Cardiac Monitor | Medtronic 2025). Additionally, Medtronic recently received FDA clearance for its adaptive deep brain stimulation (aDBS) technology, BrainSense™, which can be incorporated with the Percept™ neurostimulator to automatically adjusts therapy in real time based on a patient's brain activity (Medtronic earns U.S. FDA approval for the world's first adaptive deep brain stimulation system for people with Parkinson's 2025). Furthermore, their MiniMed™ 780G system incorporates the SmartGuard™ adaptive technology to automatically predict and correct glucose level on a regular basis by adjusting insulin delivery (MiniMed™ 780G System | Medtronic 2025).

Some recent devices incorporate onboard AI accelerators for faster, more efficient local data processing. For example, the Apple Watch Series 9 includes a 4-core Neural Engine in its S9 SiP processor to facilitate onboard AI tasks that enable features like fall detection and irregular heart rhythm detection (Apple Watch Series 9 – technical specifications – Apple support 2025). Similarly, Starkey's Genesis AI (Genesis AI – Hearing Aids | Starkey 2025) hearing aids employ a sound processor with an embedded Deep Neural Network (DNN) accelerator to dynamically enhance sound clarity.

Nevertheless, on-device AI presents several critical challenges stemming from energy requirements, limited computational resources, privacy and security concerns, and algorithmic bias. Computational resource and energy constraints are inherent to small-scale smart devices such as smartphones, wearables, and implantables, and edge computing platforms. Careful design of model architectures, encompassing compression and optimization strategies, is required to balance among inference accuracy, latency, and resource efficiency (Wang et al. 2025b). Additionally, on-device AI systems often rely on large volumes of medical data for training, thereby raising concerns about data breaches, compromised privacy, and unauthorized data usage (Murdoch 2021). Moreover, imbalanced or non-representative datasets and flawed model architectures can cause algorithmic bias, potentially leading to diagnostic inaccuracies and poor treatment outcomes (Mittermaier et al. 2023). Therefore, it is critical to implement comprehensive strategies for efficient model development, robust data governance, and regulatory oversight to ensure the responsible and ethical deployment of on-device AI in clinical practice. Table 2.2 summarizes key healthcare applications incorporating AI technologies.

Table 2.2 Healthcare applications areas incorporating AI technologies

Application Area	Techniques used	Data sources	Functionality	Example systems/ devices	Reference
Predictive analytics	Machine learning, deep learning	EHRs, wearable sensor data, historical records	Predict disease progression, hospital readmissions, or patient deterioration	Epic Systems, Google Health Predictive AI	Ristevski and Chen (2018)
Real-time decision support	Deep learning, rule-based AI	Biomedical sensors, diagnostic devices	Supports clinicians via alerts and diagnostic suggestions	Medtronic LINQ II™ with AccuRhythm™ AI	LINQ IITM Insertable Cardiac Monitor I Medtronic (2025)
Personalized medicine	Reinforcement learning, genomic AI	Genomic data, longitudinal medical records	Tailored treatment plans and drug dosages to individual profiles	IBM Watson for Oncology, Tempus AI	Ristevski and Chen (2018)
Anomaly detection	CNNs, Autoencoders	ECG, EEG, glucose monitors, motion sensors	Detects irregular heartbeats, seizure precursors, and metabolic anomalies	Apple Watch Series 9, MiniMed™ 780G with SmartGuard™	MiniMed™ 780G System I Medtronic (2025) and Apple Watch Series 9 – technical specifications – Apple support (2025)
Adaptive neuromodulation	Embedded AI, real-time feedback algorithms	Brain activity signals (LFPs, EEG)	Dynamically adjusts neurostimulation parameters based on patient-specific brain responses	Medtronic Percept™ PC with BrainSense™ technology	Percept™ PC Neurostimulator I Medtronic (2025)
On-device AI processing	Neural Engines, TinyML, DNN accelerators	Local wearable and hearable sensor data	Facilitates low-latency processing, reduces reliance on cloud infrastructure	Apple S9 SiP Neural Engine, Starkey Genesis AI hearing aids	Apple Watch Series 9 – technical specifications – Apple support (2025) and Genesis AI – Hearing Aids I Starkey (2025)
Automated insulin delivery	Predictive modeling, adaptive control algorithms	CGM, insulin pumps	Predicts and adjusts insulin dosing to maintain euglycemia	Medtronic MiniMed™ 780G with SmartGuard™	MiniMed™ 780G System I Medtronic (2025)

2.4.3 Internet of Things (IoT) in Medical Devices

Advances in computing technologies, such as edge computing platforms and processors with integrated AI accelerators, along with developments in low-power wireless communication systems and miniaturized sensor technologies, have paved the way for realizing the Internet of Things (IoT) (Majumder et al. 2017b). The Internet of Things connects diverse smart devices, including sensors, actuators, appliances, and mobile systems, to create intelligent, distributed ecosystems that enable both machine-to-machine and human-machine interactions.

In healthcare, IoT enables the seamless integration of biomedical sensors and devices for continuous monitoring of physiological parameters, patient safety, and overall well-being (Majumder et al. 2017b). When augmented with AI and big data analytics, IoT systems automate data collection from multiple sources and provide real-time clinical insights. This not only facilitates data-driven decision-making, precision medicine, and effective chronic disease management but also enhances healthcare efficiency through remote care capabilities.

Smart biomedical devices can potentially be integrated with IoT platforms to enable seamless data transmission and real-time remote monitoring. Devices such as Medtronic's LINQ II™ ICM (LINQ IITM Insertable Cardiac Monitor | Medtronic 2025) and Micra™ AV/VR pacemakers (Micra AV and VR – Pacing Systems | Medtronic Diabetes 2025) use BLE to communicate with proprietary smartphone apps, which then transmit data via the internet to cloud platforms for clinician access and assessment. Systems like MiniMed™ 780G insulin pump (MiniMed™ 780G System | Medtronic 2025) and Eversense E3® CGM (Eversense Diabetes Eversense E3® CGM SYSTEM 2005) stream interstitial glucose levels to smartphones to facilitate continuous monitoring. The MiniMed™ 780G further connects wirelessly to its insulin pump to realize an automated closed-loop delivery system.

Sensimed Triggerfish® smart contact lenses support glaucoma management by transmitting hourly intraocular pressure readings to a wearable recorder (Sensimed Triggerfish – Sensimed S.A. 2025). Similarly, wearable patches such as BioIntelliSense's BioSticker™ (BioIntelliSense announces FDA clearance of the BioSticker™, the first single-use medical device enabling 30 days of continuous vital signs monitoring 2025) and Philips Healthdot™ (Philips Healthdot | Philips 2025) collect vital signs (e.g., heart and respiratory rate, temperature) via Bluetooth® and upload data to cloud platforms to enable continuous health tracking. The Hailie® solution incorporates a Bluetooth®-connected sensor attached to the patient's inhaler, which transmits inhalation data to a smartphone app and cloud platform to monitor medication usage and receive clinician support (The Hailie™ solution helps patients track their inhaler usage 2025).

Beyond patient monitoring, IoT plays a vital role in hospital operations and patient logistics (Akkaş et al. 2020). RFID and BLE-enabled wearables enable real-time patient tracking, bed occupancy monitoring, and contact tracing, which became critical during the COVID-19 pandemic (Ye et al. 2023). Furthermore, smart ambulances equipped with IoT-enabled devices can transmit real-time vital signs and medical imaging data to emergency departments, allowing for care preparedness and faster interventions upon arrival (Fong et al. 2018).

2.5 Challenges and Concerns

Miniaturized biomedical devices hold significant potential for real-time and long-term physiological monitoring. However, there remain several challenges and concerns (Fig. 2.5) that must be addressed to achieve their widespread adoption in clinical practice.

First, miniaturized biomedical devices, such as wearables and implantables, require a continuous and reliable energy supply for long-term operation. However, the onboard battery capacity is constrained by the stringent size limitations of these devices. Although energy harvesting techniques can be integrated into the device, they often yield low power densities (μW to mW/cm^2), which may be insufficient to support active RF transmission and real-time on-board signal processing.

Second, sub-wavelength ($<\lambda/10$) antennas typically exhibit reduced radiation resistance owing to their small size and are prone to higher internal losses due to factors including conductor, dielectric, and structural losses, resulting in lower radiation efficiency.

Third, the heterogeneous integration of sensing, processing, memory, communication, and energy harvesting components into compact SoC platforms presents significant challenges stemming from thermal management issues in highly compact devices, high fabrication costs and complexities, and the need for reliable hermetic sealing and biocompatible encapsulation, particularly for implantable devices.

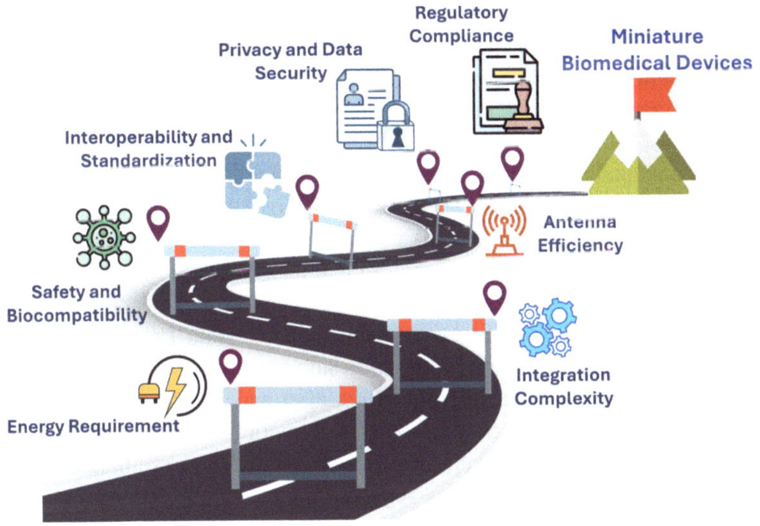

Fig. 2.5 Challenges and concerns associated with miniature biomedical devices

Fourth, safety and biocompatibility remain critical concerns for biomedical devices. Hydrolysis of polymers and metal ion leaching can degrade the structural integrity of implants over long-term use, thus potentially inducing local toxicity or immune responses. Implants may also trigger foreign body responses (FBR), leading to inflammation, fibrotic encapsulation, and device failure. Additionally, nanomaterials, which are extensively used to enhance sensor performance, have long-term health implications that are still not fully understood. Reports of cytotoxicity, oxidative stress, apoptosis, platelet aggregation, and inflammatory cytokine release associated with various nanomaterials raise concerns about their long-term use. Furthermore, high-density SoCs in wearables and implants can generate excessive heat and leakage currents, posing thermal and electrical hazards to surrounding tissues.

Fifth, the connectivity of smart medical devices makes them highly susceptible to data privacy and cybersecurity threats. Unauthorized access to sensitive health data can lead to serious consequences like identity theft, financial fraud, and clinical errors. Ensuring end-to-end security, including secure data, encrypted transmission, and protected storage, is therefore critical for such medical devices. It is essential to comply with standards like IEEE 2621 and IEEE 2933 to ensure the cybersecurity of medical devices (Palombini 2025). However, implementing robust encryption and secure communication in small-scale devices like implantable devices remains a major challenge due to strict power and size constraints.

Sixth, ensuring interoperability among biomedical devices from different manufacturers and their integration into existing healthcare systems is essential for seamless data exchange. However, proprietary legacy systems, data integrity issues, and data security measures can pose significant challenges to achieving interoperability. The IEEE 11073 family of standards provides a comprehensive framework for the secure exchange of physiological data and control commands, as well as effective integration across heterogeneous systems. Nevertheless, implementing IEEE 11073 in miniaturized biomedical devices may be constrained by the limited memory, processing power, and energy resources of the wearable and implantable devices.

Seventh, medical devices must comply with stringent regulatory standards established by authorities such as the US Food and Drug Administration (FDA) and the European Medicines Agency (EMA) to ensure their safety, clinical efficacy, and quality prior to commercialization and clinical use. In addition, adherence to data protection regulations, such as the Health Insurance Portability and Accountability Act (HIPAA) in the United States and the General Data Protection Regulation (GDPR) in the European Union, is critical to safeguarding sensitive personal health information. However, securing regulatory approval is a time-consuming and resource-intensive process that typically involves comprehensive preclinical studies, multi-phase clinical trials, and rigorous post-market surveillance. Moreover, navigating the diverse and complex regulatory landscapes and legal frameworks across different jurisdictions presents substantial challenges for manufacturers seeking timely and successful market access.

2.6 Conclusions and Future Perspectives

Advances in materials science, microfabrication techniques, MEMS, and SoC technologies, combined with low-power, small-scale electronic, computing, and communication systems, have collectively contributed to the miniaturization of biomedical devices. These technologies allow for the development of reliable, safe, and energy-efficient wearable and implantable devices to enable long-term health monitoring, and thereby facilitating early diagnosis, personalized healthcare, and enhanced health management through remote monitoring, while ensuring patient comfort and mobility.

However, biomedical devices must meet stringent safety, performance, and security standards established by regulatory bodies, such as the FDA and EMA, before commercialization to guarantee patient safety and clinical efficacy. Advanced materials based on nanoparticles, flexible and conductive polymers, and composites can be tailored to specific applications using precise material synthesis and fabrication techniques. These materials enhance signal quality and sensing performance while ensuring biocompatibility as well as user safety and comfort. In addition, significant progress in semiconductor process technologies has led to the emergence of low-power, and high-speed electronic, computing, and communication devices. CMOS technology, coupled with advances in micromachining processes, has enabled the integration of diverse components, including MEMS, sensing, signal processing, and communication systems, into a single SoC, thus leading to the development of low-power and miniature biomedical devices.

Nevertheless, the progress of small-scale biomedical devices can be hindered by several factors, including the energy requirements for supporting on-board signal processing and communication, safety and biocompatibility concerns, and the complexity of integrating diverse functional units within a compact form factor.

These challenges need to be addressed to realize high-performance miniaturized biomedical devices. Innovations in material science will be pivotal in driving the development of ultra-high-sensitivity biosensors, high-energy-density micro-batteries, and efficient energy harvesters for prolonged, autonomous operation. In addition, effective encapsulation techniques using advanced biocompatible materials, such as ALD-grown nanolaminates or multinetwork zwitterionic hydrogels, with tailored surfaces can enhance the mechanical resilience and long-term stability of the device, as well as improve its acceptance by, or integration into, the human body, potentially reducing allergic and foreign body responses. Such materials are especially important for implantable systems, where mitigating foreign body responses and ensuring long-term biostability is critical.

Moreover, electromagnetic metamaterials tailored to specific electric permittivity and magnetic permeability, coupled with advanced antenna architectures, such as high-Q cavity structures and sub-wavelength resonators, offer significant potential for enhancing antenna radiation efficiency while reducing antenna size. Nonetheless, challenges such as fabrication complexity, especially in achieving nanoscale geometric precision, as well as concerns related to manufacturing

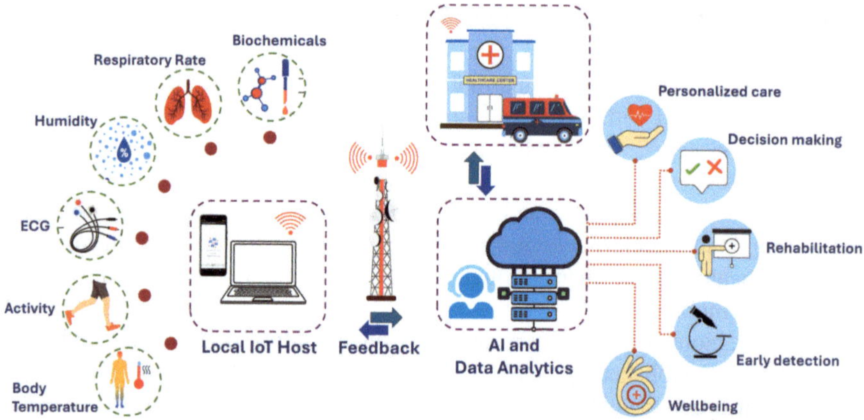

Fig. 2.6 A complete framework for physiological monitoring to enable predictive, preventive, and personalized care

scalability and cost-effectiveness must be carefully addressed. In addition, advanced thermal management strategies, such as integrated microfluidic cooling channels for localized heat dissipation, phase-change materials with high latent heat capacity for passive thermal buffering, and diamond-based ultra-high thermal heat dissipators, should be further investigated to ensure reliable device performance and patient safety during prolonged operation.

IoT technology can potentially facilitate the continuous acquisition of physiological data using these miniature low-power biomedical devices and transmit them securely to edge or cloud computing platforms. With the aid of AI algorithms and big data analytics, the large volume of data generated by the IoT-enabled medical devices can be processed in real time to support predictive, preventive, and personalized care (Fig. 2.6). However, the exchange and handling of sensitive medical data raises critical concerns regarding data security and patient privacy. Therefore, energy-efficient and light-weight data encryption algorithms and privacy-preserving protocols are essential, particularly for resource-constrained wearable and implantable devices.

Moreover, continued research should focus on developing efficient methods to implement complex interoperability standards within resource-constrained devices, without compromising their core functionalities or performance.

References

Ageing and Health (2025) [Online]. Available: https://www.who.int/news-room/fact-sheets/detail/ageing-and-health. Accessed 09 June 2025

Akkaş MA, Sokullu R, Ertürk Çetin H (2020) Healthcare and patient monitoring using IoT. Internet of Things (Netherlands) 11. https://doi.org/10.1016/j.iot.2020.100173

Apple Watch Series 9 – technical specifications – Apple support (2025) [Online]. Available: https://support.apple.com/en-us/111833. Accessed11 June 2025

Asili M, Green R, Seran S, Topsakal E (2012) A small implantable antenna for medradio and ISM bands. IEEE Antennas Wirel Propag Lett 11:1683–1685. https://doi.org/10.1109/LAWP.2013.2241723

Azizipour N, Avazpour R, Rosenzweig DH, Sawan M, Ajji A (2020) Evolution of biochip technology: a review from lab-on-a-chip to organ-on-a-chip. Micromachines 11(6):1–15. https://doi.org/10.3390/mi11060599

Babar ZUD et al (2025) MXenes in healthcare: synthesis, fundamentals and applications. Chem Soc Rev. https://doi.org/10.1039/d3cs01024d

Becchetti C, Neri A (2013) Medical instrument design and development: from requirements to market placements. [Online]. Available: https://books.google.com/books?id=P3VeLRVMdQ8C&pgis=1

Ben Amar A, Kouki AB, Cao H (2015) Power approaches for implantable medical devices. Sensors (Switzerland) 15(11):28889–28914. https://doi.org/10.3390/s151128889

Ben-Shimon Y, Ya'akobovitz A (2021) Flexible and bio-compatible temperature sensors based on carbon nanotube composites. Meas J Int Meas Confed 172. https://doi.org/10.1016/j.measurement.2020.108889

BioIntelliSense announces FDA clearance of the BioSticker™, the first single-use medical device enabling 30 days of continuous vital signs monitoring (2025) [Online]. Available: https://www.biointellisense.com/wp-content/uploads/2023/02/biointellisense-announces-fda-clearance-of-the-biosticker.pdf. Accessed 10 June 2025

BioIntelliSense launches new BioButton® rechargeable wearable device for continuous medical grade monitoring of 20+ vital signs and biometrics (2025) [Online]. Available: https://www.biointellisense.com/wp-content/uploads/2023/02/biobutton-rechargeable-press-release.pdf. Accessed 10 June 2025

Bohr MT, Young IA (2017) CMOS scaling trends and beyond. IEEE Micro 37(6):20–29. https://doi.org/10.1109/MM.2017.4241347

Bouhamed A et al (2021) Customizing hydrothermal properties of inkjet printed sensitive films by functionalization of carbon nanotubes. Nanotechnology 32(10). https://doi.org/10.1088/1361-6528/abcc95

Campi T, Cruciani S, Maradei F, Feliziani M (2021) Innovative wireless charging system for implantable capsule robots. IEEE Trans Electromagn Compat 63(5):1726–1734. https://doi.org/10.1109/TEMC.2021.3078846

Chen YP et al (2015) An injectable 64 nW ECG mixed-signal SoC in 65 nm for arrhythmia monitoring. IEEE J Solid State Circuits 50(1):375–390. https://doi.org/10.1109/JSSC.2014.2364036

Cochlear Americas | Hear Now and Always | Cochlear Implants (2025) [Online]. Available: https://www.cochlear.com/us/en/home. Accessed 11 June 2025

Conti S et al (2020) Low-voltage 2D materials-based printed field-effect transistors for integrated digital and analog electronics on paper. Nat Commun 11(1). https://doi.org/10.1038/s41467-020-17297-z

Deepu CJ, Zhang X, Heng CH, Lian Y (2016) A 3-Lead ECG on-chip with QRS detection and lossless compression for wireless sensors. IEEE Trans Circuits Syst II Express Briefs 63(12):1151–1155. https://doi.org/10.1109/TCSII.2016.2613564

Esteva A et al (2019) A guide to deep learning in healthcare. Nat Med 25(1):24–29. https://doi.org/10.1038/s41591-018-0316-z

Eversense Diabetes Eversense E3® CGM SYSTEM (2005) [Online]. Available: https://global.eversensediabetes.com/. Accessed 11 June 2025

Faham S, Salimi A, Ghavami R (2023) Electrochemical-based remote biomarker monitoring: toward Internet of Wearable Things in telemedicine. Talanta 253. https://doi.org/10.1016/j.talanta.2022.123892

Fakhri P et al (2019) Flexible hybrid structure piezoelectric nanogenerator based on ZnO nanorod/PVDF nanofibers with improved output. RSC Adv 9(18):10117–10123. https://doi.org/10.1039/c8ra10315a

Feng Y, Li Z, Qi L, Shen W, Li G (2022) A compact and miniaturized implantable antenna for ISM band in wireless cardiac pacemaker system. Sci Rep 12(1). https://doi.org/10.1038/s41598-021-04404-3

File:Wurtzite_polyhedra.png [Online]. Available: https://commons.wikimedia.org/wiki/File:Wurtzite_polyhedra.png

Fitbit Sense 2 technical specs (2025) [Online]. Available: https://store.google.com/ie/product/fitbit_sense_2_specs?hl=en-GB. Accessed11 June 2025

Fong B, Fong ACM, Li CK (2018) Internet of Things in smart ambulance and emergency medicine. In: Internet Things A to Z, pp 475–506. https://doi.org/10.1002/9781119456735.ch17

Gao Y et al (2017) Wearable microfluidic diaphragm pressure sensor for health and tactile touch monitoring. Adv Mater 29(39). https://doi.org/10.1002/adma.201701985

Genesis AI – Hearing Aids | Starkey (2025) [Online]. Available: https://www.starkey.com/hearing-aids/genesis-artificial-intelligence-hearing-aids. Accessed 11 June 2025

Han J et al (2019) A self-healable and highly flexible supercapacitor integrated by dynamically cross-linked electro-conductive hydrogels based on nanocellulose-templated carbon nanotubes embedded in a viscoelastic polymer network. Carbon NY 149:1–18. https://doi.org/10.1016/j.carbon.2019.04.029

Harpe P, Gao H, Van Dommele R, Cantatore E, Van Roermund AHM (2016) A 0.20 mm2 3 nW signal acquisition IC for miniature sensor nodes in 65 nm CMOS. IEEE J Solid State Circuits 51(1):240–248. https://doi.org/10.1109/JSSC.2015.2487270

IP Ratings (2025) [Online]. Available: https://www.iec.ch/ip-ratings. Accessed 09 June 2025

Islam MN, Yuce MR (2016) Review of medical implant communication system (MICS) band and network. ICT Express 2(4):188–194. https://doi.org/10.1016/j.icte.2016.08.010

Karnaushenko DD, Karnaushenko D, Makarov D, Schmidt OG (2015) Compact helical antenna for smart implant applications. NPG Asia Mater 7(6). https://doi.org/10.1038/am.2015.53

Khayatzadeh M, Zhang X, Tan J, Liew WS, Lian Y (2012) A 0.7-V 17.4-μW 3-lead wireless ECG SoC. 2012 IEEE Biomed Circuits Syst Conf Intell Biomed Electron Syst Better Life Better Environ BioCAS 2012 Conf Publ:344–347. https://doi.org/10.1109/BioCAS.2012.6418426

Ko Y, Vu CC, Kim J (2021) Carbonized cotton fabric-based flexible capacitive pressure sensor using a porous dielectric layer with tilted air gaps. Sensors 21(11). https://doi.org/10.3390/s21113895

Kodama M, Muramatsu D (2024) Determining carrier frequency for implantable human body communication based on transmission efficiency-electromagnetic interference trade-off. AIP Adv 14(7). https://doi.org/10.1063/5.0210654

Lee Y et al (2018) A novel non-contact heart rate monitor using impulse-radio ultra-wideband (IR-UWB) radar technology. Sci Rep 8(1). https://doi.org/10.1038/s41598-018-31411-8

Lee SY, Cheng PH, Tsou CF, Lin CC, Shieh GS (2020a) A 2.4 GHz ISM band OOK transceiver with high energy efficiency for biomedical implantable applications. IEEE Trans Biomed Circuits Syst 14(1):113–124. https://doi.org/10.1109/TBCAS.2019.2963202

Lee J et al (2020b) NB-IoT and GNSS all-in-one system-on-chip integrating RF transceiver, 23-dBm CMOS power amplifier, power management unit, and clock management system for low cost solution. IEEE J Solid State Circuits 55(12):3400–3413. https://doi.org/10.1109/JSSC.2020.3012742

Li W (2012) MEMS as ocular implants. MEMS Biomed Appl:396–431. https://doi.org/10.1533/9780857096272.4.396

Li S, Zhou X, Dong Y, Li J (2020) Flexible self-repairing materials for wearable sensing applications: elastomers and hydrogels. Macromol Rapid Commun 41(23). https://doi.org/10.1002/marc.202000444

Liao X et al (2016) Flexible and printable paper-based strain sensors for wearable and large-area green electronics. Nanoscale 8(26):13025–13032. https://doi.org/10.1039/c6nr02172g

Lin X, Zhao X, Xu C, Wang L, Xia Y (2022) Progress in the mechanical enhancement of hydrogels: fabrication strategies and underlying mechanisms. J Polym Sci 60(17):2525–2542. https://doi.org/10.1002/pol.20220154

LINQ II™ Insertable Cardiac Monitor | Medtronic (2025) [Online]. Available: https://www.medtronic.com/en-us/healthcare-professionals/products/cardiac-rhythm/cardiac-monitoring/insertable-cardiac-monitors/linq-ii-icm.html. Accessed 10 June 2025

Liu Y et al (2023) Nanomaterial-based microelectrode arrays for in vitro bidirectional brain–computer interfaces: a review. Microsyst Nanoeng 9(1). https://doi.org/10.1038/s41378-022-00479-8

Lu W et al (2020) Molybdenum disulfide nanosheets aligned vertically on carbonized silk fabric as smart textile for wearable pressure-sensing and energy devices. ACS Appl Mater Interfaces 12(10):11825–11832. https://doi.org/10.1021/acsami.9b21068

Mahfuz MMH et al (2022) Wearable textile patch antenna: challenges and future directions. IEEE Access 10:38406–38427. https://doi.org/10.1109/ACCESS.2022.3161564

Maity S, Nath M, Bhattacharya G, Chatterjee B, Sen S (2020) On the safety of human body communication. IEEE Trans Biomed Eng 67(12):3392–3402. https://doi.org/10.1109/TBME.2020.2986464

Majumder S, Mondal T, Deen MJ (2017a) Wearable sensors for remote health monitoring. Sensors (Switzerland) 17(1). https://doi.org/10.3390/s17010130

Majumder S et al (2017b) Smart homes for elderly healthcare—recent advances and research challenges. Sensors (Switzerland) 17(11):2496. https://doi.org/10.3390/s17112496

Majumder S, Chen L, Marinov O, Chen CH, Mondal T, Jamal Deen M (2018) Noncontact wearable wireless ECG systems for long-term monitoring. IEEE Rev Biomed Eng 11:306–321. https://doi.org/10.1109/RBME.2018.2840336

Majumder S, Roy AK, Jiang W, Mondal T, Deen MJ (2023) Smart textiles to enable in-home health care: state of the art, challenges, and future perspectives. IEEE J Flex Electron 3(4):120–150. https://doi.org/10.1109/jflex.2023.3339587

Majumder S, Roy AK, Mondal T, Jamal Deen M (2025) Flexible sensors for IoT-based health monitoring. IEEE J Flex Electron. https://doi.org/10.1109/JFLEX.2025.3538808

Malekzadeh-Arasteh O, Danesh AR, Do AH, Nenadic Z, Heydari P (2021) An analysis of CMRR degradation in multi-channel biosignal recording systems. IEEE Trans Circuits Syst II Express Briefs 68(1):151–155. https://doi.org/10.1109/TCSII.2020.3011180

Marasco I et al (2023) Wearable heart rate monitoring device communicating in 5G ISM band for IoHT. Bioengineering 10(1). https://doi.org/10.3390/bioengineering10010113

Medtronic earns U.S. FDA approval for the world's first adaptive deep brain stimulation system for people with Parkinson's (2025) [Online]. Available: https://news.medtronic.com/2025-02-24-Medtronic-earns-U-S-FDA-approval-for-the-worlds-first-Adaptive-deep-brain-stimulation-system-for-people-with-Parkinsons. Accessed 11 June 2025

Micra AV & VR – Pacing Systems | Medtronic Diabetes (2025) [Online]. Available: https://www.medtronic.com/in-en/healthcare-professionals/products/cardiac-rhythm/pacemakers/micra-pacing-system.html. Accessed 11 June 2025

MiniMed™ 780G System | Medtronic (2025) [Online]. Available: https://www.medtronic-diabetes.com/en-gb/insulin-pump-therapy/minimed 780g-system. Accessed 11 June 2025

Mirvakili SM, Langer R (2021) Wireless on-demand drug delivery. Nat Electron 4(7):464–477. https://doi.org/10.1038/s41928-021-00614-9

Mittermaier M, Raza MM, Kvedar JC (2023) Bias in AI-based models for medical applications: challenges and mitigation strategies. NPJ Digit Med 6(1). https://doi.org/10.1038/s41746-023-00858-z

Mohan A, Kumar N (2024) Implantable antennas for biomedical applications: a systematic review. Biomed Eng Online 23(1). https://doi.org/10.1186/s12938-024-01277-1

Murdoch B (2021) Privacy and artificial intelligence: challenges for protecting health information in a new era. BMC Med Ethics 22(1). https://doi.org/10.1186/s12910-021-00687-3

Nagaveni S, Hunasigidad P, Pathak D, Dutta A (2024) On-chip configurable RF energy harvester for biomedical implantable devices. IEEE Trans Circuits Syst I Regul Pap:1–10. https://doi.org/10.1109/tcsi.2024.3416252

NaviCam® SB System – AnX Robotics (2025) [Online]. Available: https://www.anxrobotics.com/products/navicam-sb-capsule-system/. Accessed 10 June 2025

Palombini M (2025) Bolstering cybersecurity for connected medical devices. [Online]. Available: https://standards.ieee.org/beyond-standards/medical-devices-cybersecurity/. Accessed 09 June 2025

Percept™ PC Neurostimulator | Medtronic (2025) [Online]. Available: https://www.medtronic.com/en-us/healthcare-professionals/products/neurological/deep-brain-stimulation/electrical-stimulation-systems/percept-pc-neurostimulator.html. Accessed 11 June 2025

Philips Healthdot | Philips (2025) [Online]. Available: https://www.philips.com.tr/healthcare/e/healthdot. Accessed 10 June 2025

PillCam™ COLON 2 System | Medtronic (2025) [Online]. Available: https://www.medtronic.com/en-us/healthcare-professionals/products/digestive-gastrointestinal/capsule-endoscopy/endoscopy-systems/pillcam-colon-2-system.html. Accessed 10 June 2025

PillCam™ SB 3 Capsule | Medtronic (2025) [Online]. Available: https://www.medtronic.com/en-us/healthcare-professionals/products/digestive-gastrointestinal/capsule-endoscopy/capsules/pillcam-sb-3-capsule.html. Accessed 10 June 2025

Preethichandra DMG, Piyathilaka L, Izhar U, Samarasinghe R, De Silva LC (2023) Wireless body area networks and their applications – a review. IEEE Access 11:9202–9220. https://doi.org/10.1109/ACCESS.2023.3239008

Product Specifications – Capsovision (2025) [Online]. Available: https://capsovision.com/physicians/product-specifications/. Accessed 10 June 2025

Proposed changes to the medical devices directorate's draft guidance document – list of recognized standards for medical devices (2025) [Online]. Available: https://www.canada.ca/en/health-canada/programs/consultation-draft-guidance-list-recognized-standards-medical-devices/document.html. Accessed 09 June 2025

Ren L, Wang H, Naishadham K, Kilic O, Fathy AE (2016) Phase-based methods for heart rate detection using UWB impulse Doppler radar. IEEE Trans Microw Theory Tech 64(10):3319–3331. https://doi.org/10.1109/TMTT.2016.2597824

Ristevski B, Chen M (2018) Big data analytics in medicine and healthcare. J Integr Bioinform 15(3). https://doi.org/10.1515/jib-2017-0030

SCS Therapies | Abbott (2025) [Online]. Available: https://www.neuromodulation.abbott/us/en/chronic-pain/how-neurostimulation-treats/proclaim-xr-scs-system.html. Accessed 11 June 2025

Sensimed Triggerfish – Sensimed S.A. (2025) [Online]. Available: https://www.sensimed.ch/sensimed-triggerfish/. Accessed 11 June 2025

Sid A, Cresson PY, Joly N, Braud F, Lasri T (2023) Bio-based substrate for flexible electronics – application to a 2.45 GHz wearable patch antenna. Mater Today Electron 5. https://doi.org/10.1016/j.mtelec.2023.100049

Singh J, Kaur R, Singh D (2020) A survey and taxonomy on energy management schemes in wireless sensor networks. J Syst Archit 111. https://doi.org/10.1016/j.sysarc.2020.101782

Sutanto E, Chandra F, Dinata R (2017) Simulation of leakage current measurement on medical devices using helmholtz coil configuration with different current flow. J Phys Conf Ser 853(1). https://doi.org/10.1088/1742-6596/853/1/012004

The Hailie™ solution helps patients track their inhaler usage (2025) [Online]. Available: https://www.hailie.com/. Accessed 13 June 2025

The top 10 most common chronic conditions in older adults (2025) [Online]. Available: https://www.ncoa.org/article/the-top-10-most-common-chronic-conditions-in-older-adults/. Accessed 09 June 2025

Thiyagarajan K, Rajini GK, Maji D (2021) Flexible, highly sensitive paper-based screen printed MWCNT/PDMS composite breath sensor for human respiration monitoring. IEEE Sensors J 21(13):13985–13995. https://doi.org/10.1109/JSEN.2020.3040995

Tiwari P, Sharma N (2025) The potential of Nanoantennas. In: Choudhury B, Tewary VK, Kanth VK (eds) Handbook of nano-metamaterials. Springer Nature Singapore, Singapore, pp 1–48. https://doi.org/10.1007/978-981-13-0261-9_56-1

Tiwari A, Singh RK (2023) Polymeric materials for nanobatteries, pp 419–432. https://doi.org/10.1007/978-981-99-4193-3_24

Trends in health care spending (2025) [Online]. Available: https://www.ama-assn.org/about/ama-research/trends-health-care-spending. Accessed 09 June 2025

Tseng Y, Ho Y, Kao S, Su C (2012) A 0.09 μ W low power front-end biopotential amplifier for biosignal recording. IEEE Trans Biomed Circuits Syst 6(5):508–516. https://doi.org/10.1109/TBCAS.2012.2188029

Valle J, Fernandez D, Gibrat O, Madrenas J (2021) Manufacturing issues of BEOL CMOS-MEMS devices. IEEE Access 9:83149–83162. https://doi.org/10.1109/ACCESS.2021.3086867

Vaughan O (2024) Two nanometre CMOS technology: semiconductor manufacturing. Nat Electron. https://doi.org/10.1038/s41928-024-01320-y

Veeralingam S, Bharti DK, Badhulika S (2022) Lead-free PDMS/PPy based low-cost wearable piezoelectric nanogenerator for self-powered pulse pressure sensor application. Mater Res Bull 151. https://doi.org/10.1016/j.materresbull.2022.111815

Vemishetty N et al (2016) Low power personalized ECG based system design methodology for remote cardiac health monitoring. IEEE Access 4:8407–8417. https://doi.org/10.1109/ACCESS.2016.2629486

Vuorinen T, Niittynen J, Kankkunen T, Kraft TM, Mäntysalo M (2016) Inkjet-printed graphene/PEDOT:PSS temperature sensors on a skin-conformable polyurethane substrate. Sci Rep 6. https://doi.org/10.1038/srep35289

Wang TY, Lai MR, Twigg CM, Peng SY (2014) A fully reconfigurable low-noise biopotential sensing amplifier with 1.96 noise efficiency factor. IEEE Trans Biomed Circuits Syst 8(3):411–422. https://doi.org/10.1109/TBCAS.2013.2278659

Wang LH, Chen TY, Lin KH, Fang Q, Lee SY (2015) Implementation of a wireless ECG acquisition SoC for IEEE 802.15.4 (ZigBee) applications. IEEE J Biomed Health Inform 19(1):247–255. https://doi.org/10.1109/JBHI.2014.2311232

Wang C et al (2016) Carbonized silk fabric for ultrastretchable, highly sensitive, and wearable strain sensors. Adv Mater 28(31):6640–6648. https://doi.org/10.1002/adma.201601572

Wang D, Zhang D, Li P, Yang Z, Mi Q, Yu L (2021) Electrospinning of flexible poly(vinyl alcohol)/MXene nanofiber-based humidity sensor self-powered by monolayer molybdenum diselenide piezoelectric nanogenerator. Nano Micro Lett 13(1). https://doi.org/10.1007/s40820-020-00580-5

Wang Y et al (2025a) Graphene-doped hydrogels with enhanced conductivity and stretchability for all-weather wearable devices. Adv Funct Mater. https://doi.org/10.1002/adfm.202425014

Wang X et al (2025b) Empowering edge intelligence: a comprehensive survey on on-device AI models. ACM Comput Surv 57(9):1–39. https://doi.org/10.1145/3724420

Wearable medical devices market in-depth insights and analysis 2024–2032 (2025) [Online]. Available: https://www.introspectivemarketresearch.com/reports/wearable-medical-devices-market/. Accessed 09 June 2025

Withings announces the FDA clearance of ScanWatch – its most advanced hybrid smartwatch (2025) [Online]. Available: https://media.withings.com/press/press-releases/scan-watch/20211012_US_EN_FDA_Clearance_ScanWatch.pdf. Accessed 10 June 2025

Xu F et al (2018) Recent developments for flexible pressure sensors: a review. Micromachines 9(11). https://doi.org/10.3390/mi9110580

Yan L et al (2014) A 680 nA ECG acquisition IC for leadless pacemaker applications. IEEE Trans Biomed Circuits Syst 8(6):779–786. https://doi.org/10.1109/TBCAS.2014.2377073

Yang J et al (2015) Wearable temperature sensor based on graphene nanowalls. RSC Adv 5(32):25609–25615. https://doi.org/10.1039/c5ra00871a

Yazicioglu RF, Kim S, Torfs T, Merken P, Van Hoof C (2010) A 30μW analog signal processor ASIC for biomedical signal monitoring. Dig Tech Pap IEEE Int Solid-State Circuits Conf 53:124–125. https://doi.org/10.1109/ISSCC.2010.5434026

Ye F et al (2023) A framework for infectious disease monitoring with automated contact tracing – a case study of COVID-19. IEEE Internet Things J 10(1):144–165. https://doi.org/10.1109/JIOT.2022.3199216

Yoo J et al (2012) An 8-channel scalable EEG acquisition SoC with fully integrated patient-specific seizure classification and recording processor. Dig Tech Pap IEEE Int Solid-State Circuits Conf 55:292–293. https://doi.org/10.1109/ISSCC.2012.6177019

Yoshida A, Méhes G, Okuyama Y, Murakata M, Shiba T, Tokito S (2024) Blood oxygen and heart rate monitoring by a flexible hybrid electronics device fabricated by multilayer screen-printing. Adv Electron Mater 10(5). https://doi.org/10.1002/aelm.202300615

Yu X et al (2022) Highly stretchable, ultra-soft, and fast self-healable conductive hydrogels based on polyaniline nanoparticles for sensitive flexible sensors. Adv Funct Mater 32(33). https://doi.org/10.1002/adfm.202204366

Zahedi A, Liyanapathirana R, Thiyagarajan K (2024) Biodegradable and renewable antennas for green IoT sensors: a review. IEEE Access. https://doi.org/10.1109/ACCESS.2024.3515274

Zeng X, Peng R, Fan Z, Lin Y (2022) Self-powered and wearable biosensors for healthcare. Mater Today Energy 23. https://doi.org/10.1016/j.mtener.2021.100900

Zhang F, Holleman J, Otis BP (2012) Design of ultra-low power biopotential amplifiers for biosignal acquisition applications. IEEE Trans Biomed Circuits Syst 6(4):344–355. https://doi.org/10.1109/TBCAS.2011.2177089

Zhang Y et al (2013) A batteryless 19 μw MICS/ISM-band energy harvesting body sensor node SoC for ExG applications. IEEE J Solid-State Circuits 48(1):199–213. https://doi.org/10.1109/JSSC.2012.2221217

Zhang X, Zhang Z, Li Y, Liu C, Guo YX, Lian Y (2015) A 2.89-μW clockless wireless dry-electrode ECG SoC for wearable sensors. In: 2015 IEEE Asian solid-state circuits conference, A-SSCC 2015 – proceedings, pp 1–4. https://doi.org/10.1109/ASSCC.2015.7387498

Zhang M, Wang C, Wang H, Jian M, Hao X, Zhang Y (2017) Carbonized cotton fabric for high-performance wearable strain sensors. Adv Funct Mater 27(2). https://doi.org/10.1002/adfm.201604795

Nanostructured Nanomaterials for High-Performance Biosensing

3

Sudhaunsh Deshpande, Sanjiv Sharma, and Lalitkumar K. Vora

Abstract

Electrochemical biosensors represent a rapidly growing field, offering sensitive and cost-effective detection of diverse biomarkers. However, achieving optimal performance often requires advanced materials engineering. Nanostructured materials (1–100 nm) have become integral to high-performance electrochemical biosensors due to their unique physicochemical properties. Their high surface-area-to-volume ratio enhances bioreceptor loading, while materials like carbon nanotubes and metallic nanoparticles facilitate rapid electron transfer, boosting sensitivity. Nanomaterials serve multiple crucial functions: signal amplification (e.g., AuNPs, carbon nanotubes, nanoporous metals, MXenes, dendrimers), improving stability and activity of bioreceptors, enhancing resistance to biofouling through surface modifications (e.g., PEGylation, zwitterionic polymers, hPG coatings), facilitating advanced synthetic bioreceptors, and acting as direct sensing elements. Notably, nanozymes (e.g., CeO_2, Fe_3O_4 NPs) mimic enzyme activity, while electrocatalytic nanomaterials (e.g., CuNPs, PtNPs, NiO) enable enzyme-free detection of analytes like glucose, creatinine, urea, and insulin. Despite challenges in reproducibility, long-term stability, biocompatibility, and device integration, ongoing research into rational design, hybrid nanomaterials, multiplexed detection, wearable/implantable sensors, and AI integration promises continued advancements. Nanomaterials have fundamentally

S. Deshpande · S. Sharma
David Price Evans Global Health and Infectious Diseases Group, Pharmacology & Therapeutics, Institute of Systems, Institute of Systems, Molecular and Integrative Biology, University of Liverpool, Liverpool, UK

L. K. Vora (✉)
School of Pharmacy, Queen's University Belfast, Belfast, UK
e-mail: l.vora@qub.ac.uk

V. Patel et al. (eds.), *Biosensor Technology in Translating Novel Materials into Practical Devices*, https://doi.org/10.1007/978-981-95-5519-2_3

transformed electrochemical biosensing, paving the way for next-generation diagnostic and monitoring tools with significant potential impacts.

Keywords

Electrochemical biosensors · Optical sensing · Signal amplification · Biofouling resistance · Nanozymes · Electrocatalysis

3.1 Introduction

The demand for rapid, sensitive, and cost-effective analytical tools for healthcare, environmental surveillance, and food safety has driven significant innovation in biosensor technology (Mehrotra 2016; Nath 2024). Among the various transduction methods, electrochemical biosensors have garnered substantial attention due to their inherent advantages, including high sensitivity, portability, low power requirements, and compatibility with modern microfabrication techniques, making them ideal for point-of-care diagnostics and in-field applications (Jannath and Saputra 2025; Che et al. 2022). These devices translate the biochemical interaction between a biorecognition element and a target analyte into a measurable electrical signal, offering a powerful platform for detecting a vast and ever-expanding library of biomarkers, from small molecules like glucose and creatinine to complex proteins and nucleic acids (Huang et al. 2017).

The performance of any electrochemical biosensor is fundamentally dictated by the efficacy of its biorecognition layer. Historically, the field has been dominated by enzyme-based sensors, which capitalize on the high specificity and catalytic efficiency of natural enzymes. The archetypal glucose biosensor, which employs glucose oxidase (GOx) (Yang et al. 2025; Navarro-Nateras et al. 2023; Zhang et al. 2021; Lucisano et al. 2017; Tang et al. 2014), stands as a testament to the success of this approach, having revolutionized diabetes management. However, the reliance on natural enzymes presents inherent limitations, including sensitivity to environmental factors such as temperature and pH, potential denaturation, and the challenge of immobilizing them onto an electrode surface without compromising their activity. Furthermore, this strategy is confined to analytes that have a corresponding and readily available enzyme partner.

To overcome these constraints and broaden the scope of detectable analytes, the field has pivoted toward the development of synthetic bioreceptors. Advanced synthetic recognition elements, such as molecularly imprinted polymers (MIPs) (Deshpande et al. 2025; Arjun et al. 2025, 2024; Liu et al. 2021) and nucleic acid aptamers (Manuel et al. 2022), offer compelling alternatives. MIPs are robust, custom-made polymer networks that possess bespoke cavities complementary to the target analyte in shape, size, and functionality, earning them the moniker "plastic antibodies" (Deshpande et al. 2025; Arjun et al. 2025; Liu et al. 2021; Amarh et al. 2024; Canfarotta et al. 2016). Similarly, aptamers, single-stranded DNA or RNA molecules identified through an in vitro selection process (SELEX), can be engineered to bind to virtually any target—from small ions to whole cells—with high affinity and specificity comparable to monoclonal antibodies (Manuel et al. 2022). These synthetic receptors provide significant advantages in terms of stability, cost-effectiveness, and the ability to be rationally designed for targets that lack natural biological receptors.

Regardless of the chosen recognition element—be it enzymatic or synthetic—achieving the analytical performance required for real-world applications often necessitates sophisticated materials engineering at the nanoscale. Nanomaterials, defined as materials with at least one dimension between 1 and 100 nanometers (Agraja et al. 2025; Karuppaiah et al. 2025; Liu et al. 2025), have emerged as a cornerstone of modern high-performance biosensors. Their unique physicochemical properties, including exceptionally high surface-area-to-volume ratios, quantum effects, and highly tunable surface chemistries, make them ideal for enhancing the interface between biological recognition and electronic signal transduction. Nanomaterials serve a multitude of critical functions: they act as signal amplifiers, provide a stable and biocompatible scaffold for bioreceptor immobilization, improve conductivity, and enhance catalytic activity. Materials such as gold nanoparticles, carbon nanotubes, graphene, and quantum dots have been instrumental in pushing the detection limits of electrochemical biosensors to unprecedented levels (Table 3.1). These materials are used to enhance the performance in biosensing at the analyte recognition, signal amplification, and/or biofouling (Fig. 3.1). This chapter will comprehensively explore the diverse roles of these nanostructured materials, detailing their mechanisms of action and their transformative impact on the design and performance of next-generation electrochemical biosensors.

3.2 Why Nanomaterials for Biosensing?

The integration of nanomaterials into biosensor design is driven by several key advantages over traditional bulk materials. Firstly, nanomaterials possess exceptionally high surface-area-to-volume ratios (Agraja et al. 2025; Karuppaiah et al. 2025). This allows for significantly higher loading of biorecognition elements (enzymes, antibodies, DNA probes, etc.) per unit area of the electrode, leading to a stronger signal response and increasing the available sites for interaction with the target analyte. Secondly, many nanomaterials, particularly carbon-based structures like graphene and carbon nanotubes, alongside metallic nanoparticles, exhibit enhanced electron transfer kinetics (Fig. 3.2). Their excellent electrical conductivity facilitates faster electron transfer between the bioreceptor/analyte complex and the electrode surface, which is crucial for improving sensitivity and lowering detection limits in amperometric and voltammetric sensors.

Furthermore, nanomaterials offer unique optical and catalytic properties. For instance, quantum dots provide size-tunable fluorescence valuable for optical biosensing, while metallic nanoparticles like gold (Au), silver (Ag), and platinum (Pt) display localized surface plasmon resonance (LSPR) effects sensitive to analyte binding. Many nanomaterials, including metal oxides and nanoparticles like PtNPs

Table 3.1 A comprehensive literature survey on the use of nanomaterials for detection of analytes using electrochemical biosensor

Title	Nanomaterial	Dynamic range	Limit of detection	Sample matrix	Reference
Development of a biosensor for phosphorylated Tau 181 protein detection in early-stage Alzheimer's disease	Multi-walled carbon nanotubes (MWCNTs) and platinum nanoparticles (PtNPs)	8.6 to 1100 pg/mL	0.24 pg/mL	Human serum	Eduarda Schneider et al. (2022)
Novel biomimetic Prussian blue nanocubes-based biosensor for Tau-441 protein detection	Graphene oxide/Prussian Blue nanocubes (GO/PBNCs)	74.12 to 148.24 ng/mL	0.680 pg/mL	PBS	Ben Hassine et al. (2023)
Alzheimer's diagnosis beyond cerebrospinal fluid: Probe-free detection of tau proteins using MXene-based redox systems and molecularly imprinted polymers	Vanadium MXene (V_x)	74.12 to 148.24 pg/mL	0.680 pg/mL	Artificial ISF and serum	Arjun et al. (2024)
Electrochemical tau protein immunosensor based on MnS/GO/PANI and magnetite-incorporated gold nanoparticles	MnS/GO/PANI and AuNPs@Fe3O4	6.8 to pg/mL to 68 μg/mL	0.68 pg/mL	PBS	Yola et al. (2022)
High-performance plasma biomarker panel for Alzheimer's disease screening using a femtomolar-level label-free biosensing system	Graphene-based field-effect transistor (gFET)	1 fg/mL to 1 ng/mL	Not specified	Human plasma	Wang et al. (2024)
Electrochemical impedance-based biosensor for label-free determination of plasma P-tau181 levels for clinically accurate diagnosis of mild cognitive impairment and Alzheimer's disease	Reduced graphene oxide/β--cyclodextrin (rGO/β-CD) nanocomposite	10^{-3} to 10^{3} pg/mL	0.92 fg/mL	Human plasma	Tieu et al. (2023)

(continued)

Table 3.1 (continued)

Title	Nanomaterial	Dynamic range	Limit of detection	Sample matrix	Reference
Vertical graphene-based printed electrochemical biosensor for simultaneous detection of four Alzheimer's disease blood biomarkers	Vertical graphene (VG) modified with gold nanoparticles (AuNPs).	0.1 pg/mL to 1 ng/mL	0.051 pg/mL	1:3 dilute human serum	Li et al. (2023)
Novel designed electrochemical sensor for simultaneous determination of linezolid and meropenem pneumonia drugs	Graphene + CNT-hydroquinone + Fe-Ni alloy nanoparticles	0.01–12 μM	1.3 nM	Human Serum	Atta et al. (2021)
Voltammetric monitoring of linezolid, meropenem and theophylline in plasma	Multi-walled carbon nanotubes	0.08–90 μM	Not specified	Human plasma	Attia et al. (2018)

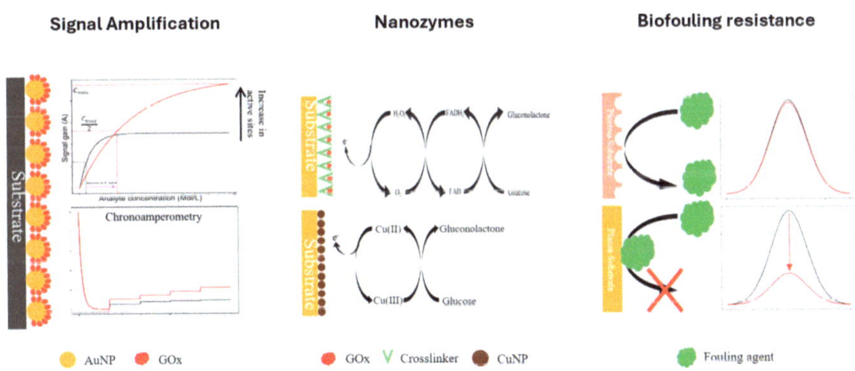

Fig. 3.1 An illustration of the functions of nanoparticle systems and nanomaterials in high-performance electrochemical biosensors

or CuNPs, also possess intrinsic catalytic or electrocatalytic activity. They can act as enzyme mimics (nanozymes) or directly catalyze electrochemical reactions relevant to detection, such as H_2O_2 turnover or glucose oxidation. The tunable surface chemistry of nanomaterials is another significant benefit, allowing for ready functionalization with various chemical groups (e.g., –COOH, $–NH_2$, –SH). This enables stable covalent attachment of bioreceptors, often improving their orientation and stability compared to simple physical adsorption, and can also be exploited to

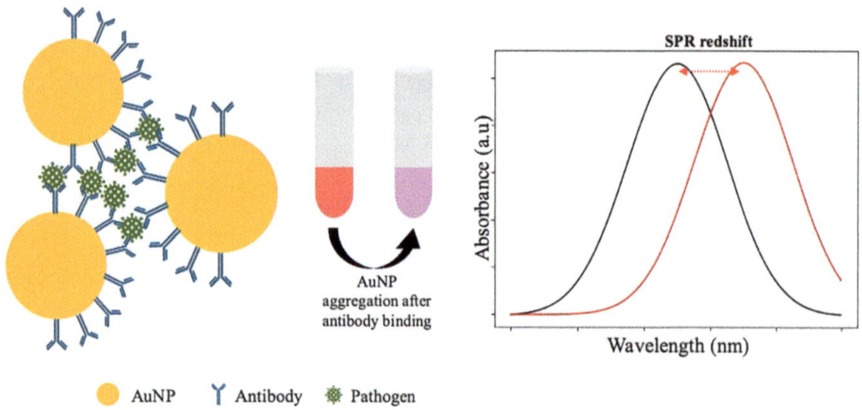

Fig. 3.2 An illustration of nanoparticles in optical sensing. Gold nanoparticles are functionalized with antibodies specific to a target antigen. When the antigen is present, it cross-links the nanoparticles, causing them to aggregate. This aggregation changes the solution's optical properties, leading to a color change from red to purple/blue, which can be visually detected. The graph illustrates the corresponding shift in the localized surface plasmon resonance (LSPR) peak to a longer wavelength (a "redshift"), which can be quantified spectrophotometrically to determine the analyte concentration (Ghasemi et al. 2018)

enhance biocompatibility or reduce biofouling. Finally, while toxicity requires careful evaluation, many nanomaterials can be engineered or surface-modified to exhibit good biocompatibility, providing a favorable microenvironment that helps preserve the activity of immobilized biomolecules.

3.3 Nanomaterials for Signal Amplification

One of the primary roles of nanomaterials in biosensing is to amplify the signal generated upon analyte recognition, thereby lowering detection limits and enhancing sensitivity (Table 3.2). Nanomaterials are mainly used for signal amplification as they are known for their high surface area to volume ratio (Arjun et al. 2025). Nanomaterials have a small size, which can be concentrated in a smaller geometric area to provide a high surface area. In comparison to planar materials, having a nanostructured surface can dramatically improve the active surface area to provide more active sites for the bioreceptor (Deshpande et al. 2025; Arjun et al. 2025).

Metal nanoparticles, such as those made of gold (AuNPs), silver (AgNPs), and platinum (PtNPs), are widely utilized *for signal amplification* (Bezuneh et al. 2022). AuNPs are particularly popular due to their excellent conductivity, stability, biocompatibility, and the ease with which they can be synthesized and functionalized, often via thiol chemistry, providing a large surface area for immobilizing bioreceptors. PtNPs serve as excellent electrocatalysts, frequently used in sensors detecting hydrogen peroxide (H_2O_2), a common byproduct of oxidase enzyme activity (Huang et al. 2025). AuNPs can also function as detectable labels in electrochemical

Table 3.2 Overview of nanostructured materials for high-performance biosensing

Nanomaterial type	Examples	Applications in biosensing	Unique properties and advantages	References
Metal nanoparticles	AuNPs, AgNPs, PtNPs	Signal amplification, immunoassays, glucose detection	High conductivity, biocompatibility, catalytic activity	Kim et al. (2019), Baruch-Shpigler and Avnir (2021)
Carbon-based nanomaterials	Graphene, SWCNTs, MWCNTs, rGO	Enhanced electron transfer, glucose sensing, immunoassays	High conductivity, large surface area, easy functionalization	Zhu et al. (2023); Jia et al. (2014)
Nanoporous metals	NPG, NPPt	High bioreceptor loading, glucose sensing	Extremely high surface area, catalytic properties	Bollella et al. (2019), McCormick and McCrudden (2020)
2D materials (TMDs, MXenes)	MoS_2, $Ti_3C_2T_x$	Alzheimer's biomarker detection, catalysis	High conductivity, electrocatalytic activity, tunable surface chemistry	Arjun et al. (2024)
Dendrimers and hyperbranched polymers	PAMAM dendrimers, hPG	Enzyme immobilization, antifouling coatings	High density of functional groups, enhanced loading capacity	Abbina et al. (2017), Li et al. (2014)
Nanozymes	CeO_2 NPs, Fe_3O_4 NPs	Enzyme mimicry, peroxide sensing	Intrinsic catalytic activity, robustness compared to enzymes	Zhang et al. (2021)
Electrocatalytic nanomaterials	CuNPs, PtNPs, NiO	Non-enzymatic glucose, creatinine, insulin detection	Direct catalytic activity, robustness, reduced sensor complexity	Zhang et al. (2020), Yu et al. (2016)
Antifouling nanomaterials	PEGylated surfaces, zwitterionic polymers	Reducing biofouling in biosensors	Strong hydration, resistance to nonspecific adsorption	Karuppaiah et al. (2025), Saxena et al. (2024)

immunoassays or DNA sensors, where their presence, often quantified after dissolution and voltammetric measurement of released metal ions, indicates analyte binding. A common example is the use of AuNPs in enzymatic glucose sensors, where decorating an electrode surface with AuNPs increases the loading of Glucose Oxidase (GOx), providing more active sites for the enzymatic reaction, and facilitates electron transfer, boosting the amperometric signal corresponding to glucose concentration (Kim et al. 2019). Furthermore, techniques like entrapping Glucose Oxidase within AuNP structures, or co-entrapping enzymes with surfactants like CTAB within nanomaterial matrices to create general saccharide oxidase activity, extend these applications (Baruch-Shpigler and Avnir 2021). Such approaches are valuable not only for specific glucose monitoring but also for total sugar sensing relevant to metabolic diseases and quality control in the food and beverage industry.

Carbon nanomaterials, including single-walled (SWCNTs) and multi-walled carbon nanotubes (MWCNTs), graphene, and reduced graphene oxide (rGO), offer exceptional electrical conductivity, large surface areas, and high mechanical strength. Their sp^2-hybridized carbon structure promotes rapid electron transfer, making them excellent base materials or modifiers for enhancing biosensor performance (Ashwini et al. 2021; Velický et al. 2014). Their surfaces can also be functionalized (e.g., carboxylated) to allow covalent linking of biomolecules. As an example, rGO provides a highly conductive, high-surface-area platform often used in composites with metal nanoparticles or enzymes as a common strategy for signal amplification in sensors for various analytes (Zhu et al. 2023; Jia et al. 2014).

Nanoporous metals, such as nanoporous gold (NPG) and nanoporous platinum (NPPt), represent another morphology providing extremely high surface areas (Fig. 3.3). These materials consist of interconnected ligaments and pores on the nanoscale, typically formed by dealloying processes. The significantly increased surface area of NPG directly translates to a higher Electrochemically Active Surface Area (ECSA), which enhances signal amplification by allowing for greater loading of biorecognition molecules or providing more sites for electrochemical reactions (Bollella et al. 2019). Similarly, the high surface area of NPPt contributes to signal amplification (Tang et al. 2024) alongside its notable catalytic properties discussed later.

2D transition metal dichalcogenides (TMDs) and MXenes represent another important class. Materials like Molybdenum disulfide (MoS_2) and MXenes (e.g., $Ti_3C_2T_x$, where T_x represents surface terminations) possess layered structures with unique electronic properties, high surface areas, and good conductivity (especially MXenes). Some TMDs and MXenes also exhibit electrocatalytic activity toward specific analytes or reaction intermediates like H_2O_2. Their surfaces naturally

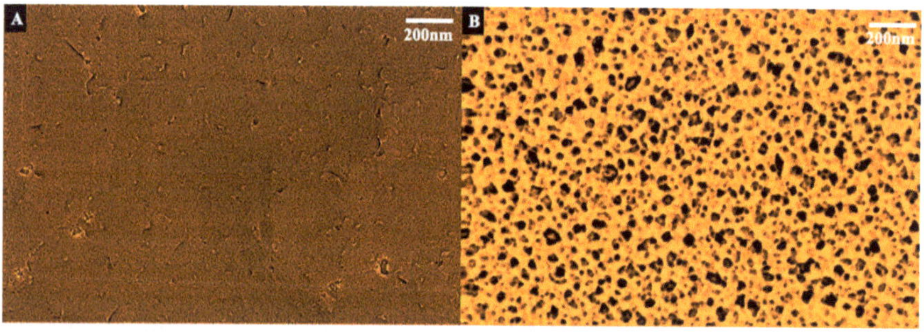

Fig. 3.3 Surface morphology of planar versus nanoporous gold electrodes. Coloured SEM images comparing the topography of different electrode surfaces. (**a**) A planar gold electrode, showing a smooth surface with minor irregularities from the manufacturing process. (**b**) A highly porous gold electrode, revealing a feature-rich, sponge-like structure. This three-dimensional architecture of interconnected pores and ligaments dramatically increases the electrochemically active surface area (ECSA) compared to the planar electrode, which is critical for enhancing signal amplification in biosensors. (Scale bars = 200 nm)

contain functional groups (e.g., –O, –OH, –F for MXenes, depending on synthesis routes) that aid in biomolecule immobilization. A specific example involves using a vanadium MXene polydopamine (VxPDA) composite combined with a molecularly imprinted polymer (MIP) specific for the Alzheimer's disease biomarker Tau-441. This electrochemical sensor demonstrated highly sensitive, mediator-free detection of Tau-441 down to femtogram per milliliter levels, where the nanomaterial composite structure likely contributes to signal enhancement by providing a high surface area for increased active sites within the MIP recognition layer (Arjun et al. 2024).

Dendrimers and hyperbranched polymers (hPG) offer a different approach through their unique architecture. Materials like hyperbranched polyglycerol (hPG) or poly(amidoamine) (PAMAM) dendrimers possess well-defined, three-dimensional structures with a high density of functional groups concentrated on their periphery. This architecture allows for extremely high loading capacity for enzymes, antibodies, or nanoparticles, resulting in increased active sites per unit area and leading to significant signal amplification. For example, hPG can be employed as a scaffold to immobilize large quantities of enzymes, thereby enhancing the sensitivity of enzymatic biosensors (Abbina et al. 2017; Dahlgren et al. 2025; Li et al. 2014).

3.4 Nanomaterials for Biofouling Resistance

Biofouling, the non-specific adsorption of biomolecules such as proteins and cells onto a sensor surface, is a primary obstacle in the development of reliable biosensors for complex biological media like blood or serum (Abbina et al. 2017; Flemming 2002). This undesirable accumulation can passivate the sensing interface, obstruct analyte transport, and generate significant background noise, ultimately compromising sensor sensitivity, accuracy, and operational lifetime. Nanomaterials offer a versatile platform to engineer anti-biofouling surfaces through two principal strategies: surface modification with anti-fouling molecules and the utilization of intrinsic material properties, including surface chemistry and topography.

The most common approach involves functionalizing nanomaterials to create a physical and energetic barrier that resists protein adsorption. This is primarily achieved by forming a tightly bound hydration layer at the sensor-solution interface, which prevents proteins from making direct contact with the surface.

Steric Repulsion via PEGylation The grafting of polyethylene glycol (PEG) chains, a process known as PEGylation, is a widely adopted technique (Chen et al. 2019). PEG is a hydrophilic, flexible, and uncharged polymer. When tethered to a nanomaterial surface, the chains extend into the aqueous solution, trapping a significant number of water molecules and creating a dense hydration layer. This layer serves two functions: (1) It presents an energetically unfavorable barrier, as a protein would need to displace this stable water layer to adsorb, a process with a high energetic cost. (2) The flexible PEG chains are in constant thermal motion, creating a dynamic, fluctuating volume that sterically repels approaching biomolecules, effectively forming a soft, repulsive shield (Chen et al. 2019).

Strong Hydration via Zwitterionic Materials Zwitterionic materials, which contain an equal number of positive and negative charges on their polymer chains (e.g., poly(sulfobetaine methacrylate)), represent a highly effective class of anti-fouling agents (Luc et al. 2023). Their efficacy stems from the strong electrostatic interactions between the charged moieties and surrounding water molecules. This creates an exceptionally stable and tightly bound hydration layer that is even more resistant to displacement than that formed by PEG. The near-neutral overall charge also minimizes non-specific electrostatic interactions with charged proteins, further enhancing its anti-fouling performance (Luc et al. 2023).

The schematic above illustrates how both steric repulsion from PEG chains and the robust hydration layer formed by zwitterionic polymers prevent proteins from adsorbing onto a functionalized nanomaterial surface. Alternatively, the inherent chemical or physical characteristics of certain nanomaterials can be leveraged to resist biofouling.

Surface Chemistry Control The surface chemistry of a nanomaterial is a critical determinant of its interaction with proteins. For instance, while pristine graphene is susceptible to biofouling due to strong hydrophobic and $\pi - \pi$ stacking interactions with proteins, its anti-fouling properties can be dramatically improved. Covalent functionalization with hydrophilic groups (e.g., –OH, –COOH) or the creation of composites with polymers like hPG transforms the surface from hydrophobic to hydrophilic, establishing the repulsive hydration layer discussed previously (Saxena et al. 2024).

Topographical Effects of Nanoporous Gold (NPG) NPG exhibits enhanced resistance to biofouling compared to its atomically flat gold counterpart, a phenomenon attributed primarily to its unique surface topography (Deshpande et al. 2025; Arjun et al. 2025). The anti-fouling mechanism of NPG is multifaceted:

Reduced Protein Contact Area Proteins are large molecules, typically several nanometers in size. On a flat surface, a protein can maximize its contact points, leading to a large adsorption footprint and strong, multi-point binding (high adsorption enthalpy). In contrast, the high curvature of the ligaments and pores within NPG restricts the available contact area for an incoming protein. This limitation reduces the overall binding energy, making adsorption weaker and more reversible (Noguchi et al. 2024; Lee et al. 2024).

Conformational Restriction For a protein to adsorb onto the highly curved or confined surfaces within the nanopores, it may be forced to adopt an energetically unfavorable conformation. This conformational penalty adds to the energy barrier for stable adsorption, discouraging irreversible binding (Noguchi et al. 2024; Lee et al. 2024).

Increased Surface Hydrophilicity The electrochemical or chemical dealloying process used to create NPG can result in a surface that is more hydrophilic than a flat gold film, which can further contribute to the formation of a repulsive hydration layer and reduce hydrophobic-driven protein adsorption (Noguchi et al. 2024; Lee et al. 2024).

By understanding and applying these mechanisms—from creating hydrated barriers with polymers to exploiting the intrinsic topography of materials like NPG—nanotechnology provides a powerful toolkit to overcome the persistent challenge of biofouling in modern biosensor design.

3.5 Nanomaterials as Direct Sensing Elements (Nanozymes and Electrocatalysts)

In certain biosensor designs, nanomaterials themselves possess intrinsic properties that allow them to participate directly in the sensing mechanism, reducing or even eliminating the need for potentially fragile biological recognition elements like enzymes. This often leads to more robust and stable sensors.

One category involves *nanozymes*, which are nanomaterials exhibiting enzyme-like catalytic activity. Peroxidase mimics, such as cerium oxide nanoparticles (CeO_2 NPs), iron oxide nanoparticles (Fe_3O_4 NPs), and even some forms of AuNPs, can catalyze the oxidation of chromogenic or electroactive substrates in the presence of H_2O_2, similar to horseradish peroxidase (HRP). This activity can be exploited in various colorimetric or electrochemical assays. Similarly, oxidase mimics, like PtNPs and other noble metal nanoparticles, can catalyze oxidation reactions analogous to those performed by oxidase enzymes.

Another major application is in direct electrocatalysis, where nanomaterials catalyze the oxidation or reduction of target analytes directly at the electrode surface, often at lower overpotentials and/or with higher sensitivity compared to conventional electrode materials. A prominent example involves copper nanoparticle (CuNP)-based non-enzymatic sensors. CuNPs and copper oxide nanoparticles (CuO NPs, Cu_2O NPs) exhibit excellent electrocatalytic activity toward the direct oxidation of glucose (Zhang et al. 2020) and creatinine (Boobphahom et al. 2019), enabling the development of enzyme-free sensors for these important metabolites. Composites incorporating CuNPs, such as copper oxide nanoparticles combined with cobalt (II,III) oxide (Co_3O_4) and multi-walled carbon nanotubes (CuO/Co_3O_4-MWCNTs) nanocomposite, have also been developed for the direct electrochemical detection of urea (Magar et al. 2023).

Platinum-based nanomaterials are also highly effective electrocatalysts; nanoporous platinum (NPPt), leveraging its high surface area and intrinsic catalytic activity, is particularly noted for its efficiency in direct glucose oxidation, making it a key material for non-enzymatic glucose sensors (McCormick and McCrudden 2020). Furthermore, other nanomaterials show promise for direct sensing; for instance, nickel oxide (NiO) nanoparticles (Yu et al. 2016) have been explored for the electrochemical detection of insulin. Extending beyond metabolites and proteins, nanomaterial composites like carbon nanotubes functionalized with polyethylenimine (CNT-PEI) have been utilized for the sensitive detection of dissolved gases such as carbon dioxide (CO_2) (Han et al. 2021; Liu et al. 2023). Other metal oxides like Co_3O_4 and MnO_2 are also widely investigated for non-enzymatic sensing applications.

3.6 Challenges and Future Perspectives

Despite the tremendous progress and demonstrated potential, several challenges remain in the development and practical application of nanomaterial-based biosensors. Ensuring the reproducibility and scalability of nanomaterial synthesis to achieve consistent size, shape, and properties is critical for reliable sensor performance and commercial viability. The long-term stability of both the nanomaterials and any immobilized bioreceptors, especially when operating in complex biological media over extended periods, needs further improvement for applications like continuous monitoring. Toxicity and biocompatibility also require thorough assessment, particularly for nanomaterials intended for in vivo or frequent ex vivo use. Significant hurdles also exist in the integration and miniaturization required to incorporate these advanced materials into practical, robust, and user-friendly devices suitable for point-of-care testing or wearable applications. Finally, while offering high performance, the cost-effectiveness of certain nanomaterial synthesis and sophisticated surface modification processes can be a barrier to widespread adoption compared to established technologies.

Furthermore, the fabrication and functionalization processes themselves contribute to the challenges of reproducibility and scalability, varying significantly in complexity. Relatively straightforward methods exist, such as preparing reduced graphene oxide (rGO) electrodes by simply drop-casting water-soluble graphene oxide (GO) onto an electrode surface followed by in situ electrochemical reduction using techniques like cyclic voltammetry (CV) in phosphate-buffered saline (PBS) (Chen et al. 2023). Synthesizing gold nanoparticles (AuNPs) often involves the well-established Turkevich method or similar approaches, where a gold salt (e.g., $HAuCl_4$) is reduced by an agent like sodium citrate under controlled heating and stirring, followed by purification steps like centrifugation (Kimling et al. 2006). Creating more intricate structures like highly porous gold involves more steps, potentially including the electrochemical deposition of "soft" gold layers from a solution containing gold salts (like $HAuCl_4$) and ammonium chloride (NH_4Cl), followed by an electroporation step using chronoamperometry to create the porous structure through the electrolysis of the ammonium salt (Bollella 2020).

Moving to more advanced materials like MXenes introduces significantly greater complexity and potential hazards. Their synthesis typically involves selectively etching the "A" layer (often aluminum) from a precursor MAX phase material (e.g., Ti_3AlC_2) using highly corrosive and hazardous etchants, most commonly concentrated hydrofluoric (HF) acid. This etching step is followed by processes like sonication or intercalation to exfoliate the resulting multilayered MXene into few-layer or single-layer sheets (e.g., $Ti_3C_2T_x$) (Bollella 2020). The reliance on extremely dangerous chemicals like HF not only poses significant safety risks requiring specialized handling protocols and facilities but also complicates waste disposal and raises environmental concerns, adding another layer to the challenges of scalable and sustainable production for widespread biosensor application. Significant hurdles also exist in the integration and miniaturization required to incorporate these advanced materials into practical, robust, and user-friendly devices suitable for point-of-care testing or wearable applications. Finally, while offering high performance, the cost-effectiveness of certain nanomaterial synthesis and sophisticated surface modification processes can be a barrier to widespread adoption compared to established technologies.

Nevertheless, the field is rapidly evolving, with several exciting future research directions. Rational design, potentially aided by computational modeling, aims to create nanomaterials with precisely tailored properties optimized for specific sensing tasks. The development of hybrid nanomaterials, which combine different types of nanomaterials (e.g., AuNP-decorated CNTs, MXene-graphene composites), seeks to leverage synergistic effects for enhanced performance. There is a strong interest in multiplexed detection, developing sensor arrays capable of measuring multiple biomarkers simultaneously using different nanomaterial-based sensing elements on a single platform. Significant effort is focused on creating wearable and implantable sensors by improving miniaturization, stability, and biocompatibility for continuous health monitoring. Lastly, the integration with artificial intelligence (AI) and machine learning offers powerful tools to analyze complex sensor data, potentially improving accuracy, extracting subtle diagnostic patterns, and managing sensor drift or calibration.

A particularly promising area within this drive toward minimally invasive and continuous monitoring involves accessing alternative biofluids and adapting microneedle (MN) technology. Extracellular tissue fluids, such as interstitial fluid (ISF), contain significant biomarkers, and measuring them directly can offer greater clinical value for localized diseases compared to systemic measurements (Himawan et al. 2022). However, accessing these abundant fluids is a major challenge, as current methods are often invasive and costly. This is where MN technology presents a significant opportunity. Traditionally used for drug delivery, there is a notable paradigm shift toward employing MNs for biosensing purposes (Vora et al. 2024), leveraging their ability to minimally invasively access tissue fluids like ISF (Himawan et al. 2022). MN-based biosensors, therefore, have the potential to serve as a powerful platform for high-throughput, rapid diagnosis and monitoring, particularly for localized conditions, offering significant benefits for patients needing convenient, continuous health surveillance. Continued development of novel sensing modalities integrated with MNs aims to enhance the accuracy, precision, and sensitivity of these devices. However, despite their potential, multiple translational hurdles related to large-scale manufacturing, regulatory approval, and ensuring long-term reliability must be overcome before MN-based biosensors become widely available in the market (Vora et al. 2024). Lastly, the integration with artificial intelligence (AI) and machine learning offers powerful tools to analyze complex sensor data, potentially improving accuracy, extracting subtle diagnostic patterns, and managing sensor drift or calibration across all these advanced sensing platforms. The work was recently published by Arjun. A.M and Deshpande. S et al. (Deshpande et al. 2025; Arjun et al. 2025), has shown how machine learning (ML) can be integrated into biosensing to improve the sensing performance and ultimately patient outcomes. The work shows an AUC of 0.84 for distinguishing patients with and without Alzheimer's Disease using phosphorylated tau proteins when using a highly trained ML model (Arjun et al. 2025). The AUC drops 0.81 when traditional fitting methods are used (Arjun et al. 2025). ML can be used to make biosensors truly high-performance by reducing the variability and easing data analytics through automation.

3.7 Conclusion

The integration of nanostructured materials has unequivocally catalyzed a paradigm shift in electrochemical biosensing, moving beyond incremental improvements to fundamentally redefine the performance and potential of these analytical platforms. This chapter has delineated the multifaceted roles that nanomaterials play in this revolution. We have explored how their exceptional surface-area-to-volume ratios and unique electronic properties are harnessed for critical signal amplification (e.g., AuNPs, nanoporous gold) and how their tunable surfaces provide robust scaffolds that enhance bioreceptor loading and stability. Furthermore, we have detailed strategies to engineer the bio-interface, using nanomaterials to create anti-fouling surfaces (e.g., PEGylated or zwitterionic coatings) that maintain sensor function in complex biological media. Perhaps most significantly, we highlighted the emergence of nanomaterials as direct sensing elements, where their intrinsic nanozymatic (e.g., CeO_2, Fe_3O_4 NPs) or electrocatalytic (e.g., CuNPs, PtNPs) activities enable the development of robust, enzyme-free sensors for critical biomarkers.

Despite this remarkable progress, the translation from laboratory innovation to widespread clinical or field application faces significant hurdles. Challenges in reproducibility across synthesis and fabrication, ensuring long-term operational stability, and navigating the complexities of device integration and biocompatibility remain paramount. The scalability and safety of certain fabrication processes, such as the use of hazardous etchants for MXene synthesis, also require careful consideration.

Nevertheless, the future of the field is exceptionally bright, driven by synergistic advancements across multiple disciplines. The rational design of hybrid nanomaterials promises to unlock unprecedented performance characteristics. The convergence of these advanced materials with microfabrication is paving the way for next-generation wearable and minimally invasive platforms, such as microneedle-based sensors, for continuous physiological monitoring. Finally, the integration of artificial intelligence and machine learning offers a powerful toolset to decipher complex sensor outputs, enhancing diagnostic accuracy and enabling predictive health analytics. Collectively, these trajectories ensure that nanomaterials will continue to be the cornerstone of innovation in biosensing, driving the development of transformative tools poised to revolutionize diagnostics, personalized medicine, and environmental monitoring.

Acknowledgments SEM images taken using the ZEISS Gemini 2 at the University of Liverpool Scanning Electron Microscope Shared Research Facility (SEM SRF). The images were colored using ImageJ.

References

Abbina S et al (2017) Hyperbranched polyglycerols: recent advances in synthesis, biocompatibility and biomedical applications. J Mater Chem B 5:9249–9277. https://doi.org/10.1039/c7tb02515g

Agraja PS, Sreelekshmi PJ, Devika V, Devu C, Rejithamol R (2025) Molecular imprinted polymer decorated electrochemical sensors for diabetes biomarkers: a critical review. Crit Rev Anal Chem:1–18. https://doi.org/10.1080/10408347.2025.2492385

Amarh FA, Kangmennaa A, Agorku ES, Voegborlo RB (2024) A state-of-the-art review of trends in molecularly imprinted polymers in the clean-up of pesticides in environmental samples. Sustain Environ 10:2298067. https://doi.org/10.1080/27658511.2023.2298067

Arjun A, M, Deshpande S, Tom Dunlop BN, Oliviera D, Vulpe G, Moreira F, Sharma S (2024) Alzheimer's diagnosis beyond cerebrospinal fluid: probe-free detection of tau proteins using MXene based redox systems and molecularly imprinted polymers. Biosens Bioelectron: X 20. https://doi.org/10.1016/j.biosx.2024.100513

Arjun AM et al (2025) Low-cost polyphenol–polypyrrole molecularly imprinted sensor for point-of-care Alzheimer's detection. ACS Sens. https://doi.org/10.1021/acssensors.5c01816

Ashwini R, Mohanta Z, Kumar MKP, Santosh MS, Srivastava C (2021) Enhanced heterogeneous electron transfer kinetics in graphene oxide produced from mechanically milled graphite. Carbon Trends 5:100095. https://doi.org/10.1016/j.cartre.2021.100095

Atta NF, Galal A, El-Gohary ARM (2021) Novel designed electrochemical sensor for simultaneous determination of linezolid and meropenem pneumonia drugs. J Electroanal Chem 902:115814. https://doi.org/10.1016/j.jelechem.2021.115814

Attia AK, Al-Ghobashy MA, El-Sayed GM, Kamal SM (2018) Voltammetric monitoring of linezolid, meropenem and theophylline in plasma. Anal Biochem 545:54–64. https://doi.org/10.1016/j.ab.2018.01.009

Baruch-Shpigler Y, Avnir D (2021) Entrapment of glucose oxidase within gold converts it to a general monosaccharide-oxidase. Sci Rep 11:10737. https://doi.org/10.1038/s41598-021-90242-2

Ben Hassine A, Raouafi N, Moreira FTC (2023) Novel biomimetic Prussian blue nanocubes-based biosensor for Tau-441 protein detection. J Pharm Biomed Anal 226:115251. https://doi.org/10.1016/j.jpba.2023.115251

Bezuneh TT, Fereja TH, Kitte SA, Li H, Jin Y (2022) Gold nanoparticle-based signal amplified electrochemiluminescence for biosensing applications. Talanta 248:123611. https://doi.org/10.1016/j.talanta.2022.123611

Bollella P (2020) Porous gold: a new frontier for enzyme-based electrodes. Nanomaterials (Basel) 10. https://doi.org/10.3390/nano10040722

Bollella P, Sharma S, Cass AEG, Tasca F, Antiochia R (2019) Minimally invasive glucose monitoring using a highly porous gold microneedles-based biosensor: characterization and application in artificial interstitial fluid. Catalysts 9:580

Boobphahom S, Ruecha N, Rodthongkum N, Chailapakul O, Remcho VT (2019) A copper oxide-ionic liquid/reduced graphene oxide composite sensor enabled by digital dispensing: non-enzymatic paper-based microfluidic determination of creatinine in human blood serum. Anal Chim Acta 1083:110–118. https://doi.org/10.1016/j.aca.2019.07.029

Canfarotta F, Poma A, Guerreiro A, Piletsky S (2016) Solid-phase synthesis of molecularly imprinted nanoparticles. Nat Protoc 11:443–455. https://doi.org/10.1038/nprot.2016.030

Che PP et al (2022) Biodegradable ultrasmall-in-nano architectures loaded with cisplatin prodrug in combination with ionizing radiation induces DNA damage and apoptosis in pancreatic ductal adenocarcinoma. Cancer 14:3034

Chen Q et al (2019) Impact of antifouling PEG layer on the performance of functional peptides in regulating cell behaviors. J Am Chem Soc 141:16772–16780. https://doi.org/10.1021/jacs.9b07105

Chen A-H et al (2023) Fabrication of modified electrode by reduced graphene oxide (rGO) and polyaniline (PANI) for enhancing azo dye decolorization in bio-electrochemical systems (BESs). Environ Res 231:116042. https://doi.org/10.1016/j.envres.2023.116042

Dahlgren J et al (2025) Investigation of amphiphilic PDMS-hyperbranched polyglycerol copolymers to tune the fouling-release properties in a moisture curable coating system. Langmuir 41:3377–3391. https://doi.org/10.1021/acs.langmuir.4c04338

Deshpande S et al (2025) Redox-Active Polyphenol Red Molecularly Imprinted Polymers on Porous Gold Electrodes for Ultrasensitive, AI-Assisted Detection of Alzheimer's Biomarkers in Undiluted Biofluids. Adv. Healthcare Mater. https://doi.org/10.1002/adhm.202503155

Eduarda Schneider M, Guillade L, Correa-Duarte MA, Moreira FTC (2022) Development of a biosensor for phosphorylated tau 181 protein detection in early-stage Alzheimer's disease. Bioelectrochemistry 145:108057. https://doi.org/10.1016/j.bioelechem.2022.108057

Flemming HC (2002) Biofouling in water systems—cases, causes and countermeasures. Appl Microbiol Biotechnol 59:629–640. https://doi.org/10.1007/s00253-002-1066-9

Ghasemi A et al (2018) Optical assays based on colloidal inorganic nanoparticles. Analyst 143:3249–3283. https://doi.org/10.1039/c8an00731d

Han M, Jung S, Lee Y, Jung D, Kong SH (2021) PEI-functionalized carbon nanotube thin film sensor for CO(2) gas detection at room temperature. Micromachines (Basel) 12. https://doi.org/10.3390/mi12091053

Himawan A et al (2022) Where microneedle meets biomarkers: futuristic application for diagnosing and monitoring localized external organ diseases. Adv Healthc Mater 12. https://doi.org/10.1002/adhm.202202066

Huang Y, Xu J, Liu J, Wang X, Chen B (2017) Disease-related detection with electrochemical biosensors: a review. Sensors 17:2375

Huang W, Yang Y, Xu Y, Xiao F, Wang L (2025) Sweat wearable sensor based on confined Pt nanoparticles in 2D conductive metal–organic frameworks for continuous glucose monitoring. Adv Sci:e07212. https://doi.org/10.1002/advs.202507212

Jannath KA, Saputra HA (2025) A review on recent developments in transition metal and heteroatom-doped carbon catalysts for oxygen reduction reaction. Electrochem Sci Adv 5:e202400033. https://doi.org/10.1002/elsa.202400033

Jia X, Chen X, Han J, Ma J, Ma Z (2014) Triple signal amplification using gold nanoparticles, bienzyme and platinum nanoparticles functionalized graphene as enhancers for simultaneous multiple electrochemical immunoassay. Biosens Bioelectron 53:65–70. https://doi.org/10.1016/j.bios.2013.09.021

Karuppaiah G et al (2025) Nanoengineered hybrid hydrogel-based 3D nanocomposite as an antifouling coating interface for enhanced electrochemical aptasensing of estradiol. Talanta 293:128105. https://doi.org/10.1016/j.talanta.2025.128105

Kim S-K et al (2019) Hyaluronate–gold nanoparticle/glucose oxidase complex for highly sensitive wireless noninvasive glucose sensors. ACS Appl Mater Interfaces 11:37347–37356. https://doi.org/10.1021/acsami.9b13874

Kimling J et al (2006) Turkevich method for gold nanoparticle synthesis revisited. J Phys Chem B 110:15700–15707. https://doi.org/10.1021/jp061667w

Lee J-C et al (2024) Micrometer-thick and porous nanocomposite coating for electrochemical sensors with exceptional antifouling and electroconducting properties. Nat Commun 15:711. https://doi.org/10.1038/s41467-024-44822-1

Li X, Cai T, Chung TS (2014) Anti-fouling behavior of hyperbranched polyglycerol-grafted poly(ether sulfone) hollow fiber membranes for osmotic power generation. Environ Sci Technol 48:9898–9907. https://doi.org/10.1021/es5017262

Li M, Zeng Y, Huang Z, Zhang L, Liu Y (2023) Vertical graphene-based printed electrochemical biosensor for simultaneous detection of four Alzheimer's disease blood biomarkers. Biosensors 13:758

Liu Z et al (2021) A review on molecularly imprinted polymers preparation by computational simulation-aided methods. Polymers (Basel) 13. https://doi.org/10.3390/polym13162657

Liu T et al (2023) Functionalized carbon nanotubes enabled flexible and scalable CO2 sensors. Carbon Trends 12:100291. https://doi.org/10.1016/j.cartre.2023.100291

Liu KW et al (2025) Enhanced SERS performance through defect-guided growth of 2D/3D AuAg nanoplates for chemical sensing and cellular imaging applications. Anal Chim Acta 1353:343940. https://doi.org/10.1016/j.aca.2025.343940

Luc V-S et al (2023) Antifouling properties of amine-oxide-containing zwitterionic polymers. Biomacromolecules 24:5467–5477. https://doi.org/10.1021/acs.biomac.3c00948

Lucisano JY, Routh TL, Lin JT, Gough DA (2017) Glucose monitoring in individuals with diabetes using a long-term implanted sensor/telemetry system and model. IEEE Trans Biomed Eng 64:1982–1993. https://doi.org/10.1109/TBME.2016.2619333

Magar HS, Hassan RYA, Abbas MN (2023) Non-enzymatic disposable electrochemical sensors based on CuO/Co3O4@MWCNTs nanocomposite modified screen-printed electrode for the direct determination of urea. Sci Rep 13:2034. https://doi.org/10.1038/s41598-023-28930-4

Manuel BA, Sterling SA, Sanford AA, Heemstra JM (2022) Systematically modulating aptamer affinity and specificity by guanosine-to-inosine substitution. Anal Chem 94:6436–6440. https://doi.org/10.1021/acs.analchem.2c00422

McCormick W, McCrudden D (2020) Development of a highly nanoporous platinum screen-printed electrode and its application in glucose sensing. J Electroanal Chem 860:113912. https://doi.org/10.1016/j.jelechem.2020.113912

Mehrotra P (2016) Biosensors and their applications - a review. J Oral Biol Craniofac Res 6:153–159. https://doi.org/10.1016/j.jobcr.2015.12.002

Nath S (2024) Advancements in food quality monitoring: integrating biosensors for precision detection. Sustain Food Technol 2:976–992. https://doi.org/10.1039/D4FB00094C

Navarro-Nateras L et al (2023) Development of a redox-polymer-based electrochemical glucose biosensor suitable for integration in microfluidic 3D cell culture systems. Biosensors (Basel) 13. https://doi.org/10.3390/bios13060582

Noguchi T, Nishitani S, Sakata T (2024) Anti-biofouling effect of nanoporous gold electrode on nonspecific signal reduction for electrochemical biosensors. J Electrochem Soc. https://doi.org/10.1149/1945-7111/ad5d9c

Saxena S, Sen P, Soleymani L, Hoare T (2024) Anti-fouling polymer or peptide-modified electrochemical biosensors for improved biosensing in complex media. Adv Sensor Res 3:2300170. https://doi.org/10.1002/adsr.202300170

Tang W, Li L, Wu L, Gong J, Zeng X (2014) Glucose biosensor based on a glassy carbon electrode modified with polythionine and multiwalled carbon nanotubes. PLoS One 9:e95030. https://doi.org/10.1371/journal.pone.0095030

Tang S et al (2024) A signal-amplification electrochemical aptasensor based on porous Pt nanotubes and tetrahedral DNA nanostructures for ultrasensitive detection of citrinin. Sens Actuators B 408:135519. https://doi.org/10.1016/j.snb.2024.135519

Tieu M-V, Choi SH, Le HTN, Cho S (2023) Electrochemical impedance-based biosensor for label-free determination of plasma P-tau181 levels for clinically accurate diagnosis of mild cognitive impairment and Alzheimer's disease. Anal Chim Acta 1273:341535. https://doi.org/10.1016/j.aca.2023.341535

Velický M et al (2014) Electron transfer kinetics on mono- and multilayer graphene. ACS Nano 8:10089–10100. https://doi.org/10.1021/nn504298r

Vora LK et al (2024) Microneedle-based biosensing. Nat Rev Bioeng 2:64–81. https://doi.org/10.1038/s44222-023-00108-7

Wang S et al (2024) High-performance plasma biomarker panel for Alzheimer's disease screening using a femtomolar-level label-free biosensing system. ACS Nano 18:2117–2130. https://doi.org/10.1021/acsnano.3c09311

Yang F et al (2025) Target-triggered enzymatic cascade LF-NMR biosensor for the detection of circulating tumor cells. Anal Chem 97:6175–6181. https://doi.org/10.1021/acs.analchem.4c06901

Yola BB et al (2022) Electrochemical tau protein immunosensor based on MnS/GO/PANI and magnetite-incorporated gold nanoparticles. Electroanalysis 34:1519–1528. https://doi.org/10.1002/elan.202200159

Yu Y, Guo M, Yuan M, Liu W, Hu J (2016) Nickel nanoparticle-modified electrode for ultrasensitive electrochemical detection of insulin. Biosens Bioelectron 77:215–219. https://doi.org/10.1016/j.bios.2015.09.036

Zhang Y et al (2020) A flexible non-enzymatic glucose sensor based on copper nanoparticles anchored on laser-induced graphene. Carbon 156:506–513. https://doi.org/10.1016/j.carbon.2019.10.006

Zhang W et al (2021) PtS(2) nanosheets as a peroxidase-mimicking nanozyme for colorimetric determination of hydrogen peroxide and glucose. Mikrochim Acta 188:174. https://doi.org/10.1007/s00604-021-04826-w

Zhu Y, Qi Y, Xu M, Luo J (2023) Flexible biosensor based on signal amplification of gold nanoparticles-composite flower clusters for glucose detection in sweat. Colloids Surf A Physicochem Eng Asp 661:130908. https://doi.org/10.1016/j.colsurfa.2022.130908

Advances in Nanocomposites and Their Applications in Medical Diagnostics

4

Mark Woollam, Eray Schulz, Yeshwant Kasa, Akanksha Tipparti, Shivaum Heranjal, Akshay Mane, and Mangilal Agarwal

Abstract

Nanomaterial composites can be employed not only as contrast agents for diagnostic biomedical imaging but also as integral components of biosensing devices that detect biomarkers in minimally invasive fluids such as blood. This chapter explores the different methods for nanocomposite fabrication and characterization, along with advancements made in the context of biomedicine. Materials incorporated into nanocomposites, along with their key properties enabling medical diagnostics, are discussed. Recent advancements include but are not limited to the development of superparamagnetic iron oxide nanoparticles for biomedical imaging, as well as gold nanoparticle composites for liquid biopsy and theranostics. Despite these advancements, there are still challenges for clinical translation. Future studies should prioritize thorough nanomaterial characterization, standardization of methods for analysis, development of multifunctional platforms, and clinical trials to validate performance. Overall, this chapter aims to promote ongoing discussion within the nanomedicine domain and encourage continued exploration as well as innovative solutions.

M. Woollam · E. Schulz
Integrated Nanosystems Development Institute, Indiana University Indianapolis, Indianapolis, IN, USA

Department of Chemistry & Chemical Biology, Indiana University Indianapolis, Indianapolis, IN, USA

Y. Kasa
Integrated Nanosystems Development Institute, Indiana University Indianapolis, Indianapolis, IN, USA

Department of Computer Science, Purdue University Indianapolis, Indianapolis, IN, USA

V. Patel et al. (eds.), *Biosensor Technology in Translating Novel Materials into Practical Devices*, https://doi.org/10.1007/978-981-95-5519-2_4

Keywords

Nanocomposites · Medical diagnostics · Biomedical imaging · Glucose monitoring · Liquid biopsy

4.1 Introduction

The first nanomaterial to be identified is considered to be colloidal gold, which was discovered in 1857 by renowned physicist Michael Faraday (Edwards and Thomas 2007). However, nanomaterials have been used historically even before this point in time. For example, carbon nanotubes (CNTs) and cementite nanowires were incorporated into Damascus steel around 900 AD. Another example of this is that artisans from Mesopotamia utilized metallic-based nanoparticles for pottery as early as the ninth century (Deshmukh 2019). The field of nanotechnology was first introduced by Richard Feynman in the 1950s during his "There's Plenty of Room at the Bottom" lecture at the California Institute of Technology. The term was first used by Norio Taniguchi in the 1970s, a pioneering researcher in the field of nanotechnology (Akgöl et al. 2021). Nanomaterials are characterized by having structural elements that are less than 100 nanometers in size in at least one dimension (Malhotra and Ali 2018). These materials possess distinct physical, chemical, and biological properties compared to larger-scale materials, primarily due to their increased surface area relative to volume and the influence of quantum effects. One of the most important inventions that propelled the field of nanoscience in the early 1980s was the advent of scanning tunneling microscopy (STM). This technology allows the investigation and characterization of materials at the atomic level through high-resolution imaging (Granek and Hon 2008).

A. Tipparti
Integrated Nanosystems Development Institute, Indiana University Indianapolis, Indianapolis, IN, USA

Department of Biomedical Engineering & Informatics, Indiana University Indianapolis, Indianapolis, IN, USA

S. Heranjal · A. Mane
Integrated Nanosystems Development Institute, Indiana University Indianapolis, Indianapolis, IN, USA

Department of Electrical & Computer Engineering, Purdue University Indianapolis, Indianapolis, IN, USA

M. Agarwal (✉)
Integrated Nanosystems Development Institute, Indiana University Indianapolis, Indianapolis, IN, USA

Department of Chemistry & Chemical Biology, Indiana University Indianapolis, Indianapolis, IN, USA

Department of Biomedical Engineering & Informatics, Indiana University Indianapolis, Indianapolis, IN, USA
e-mail: agarwal@iu.edu

Since then, the field has exploded with significant advancements such as the discovery of CNTs and fullerene-based structures. Nanotechnology-based research has become a vital component in many different areas because these materials are not only low-cost but also safe, clean, and demonstrate unique physicochemical properties. This field of technology and science is geared toward various applications in textiles, defense, the chemical industry, electronics, the energy sector, and biomedical fields (Khan et al. 2019). Of particular relevance, biomedical engineering/applications are a significant and rapidly expanding area of research within nanotechnology (El Naschie 2006). Beyond individual nanomaterials, nanocomposites incorporate nanoparticles within a matrix of more standardized materials. The standard definition of a composite is any new material that is created using two or more types of materials with unique chemical functionality/structure (Breuer and Sundararaj 2004). Nanocomposites represent a novel category of composite materials. They are utilized across various material groups, including ceramics, metals, and plastics. These materials are characterized by their molecular-level structural arrangement and consist of two or more distinct phases, with at least one phase having dimensions in the nanometer range (Reduwan 2019). The two main classifications or categories of nanocomposites are polymer-based and non-polymer-based (Fig. 4.1 (Gupta et al. 2024)). They can be further broken down into ceramic-based, metal-based, and polymer-ceramic-based nanocomposites (Sen 2020).

More specifically, nano-based composites have been used in many areas of biomedicine, especially with regard to the development of medical diagnostic technologies. Nanobiomedicine is an emerging field in engineering that has led to the development of potentially impactful technologies in healthcare. Nanomaterials and nanocomposites represent very powerful tools in biomedicine, owing to their highly tunable structures that can be functionalized. Certain nanomaterials and composites can be utilized in specialized applications due to their unique properties tailored to specific use cases (Gutierrez et al. 2022; Kannan and Maduraiveeran 2024). In applications for medical diagnostics, nanocomposite-based technology is well positioned to develop biosensors or imaging agents that can be administered in vivo. One example of this is that quantum dots can be implemented in biomedical

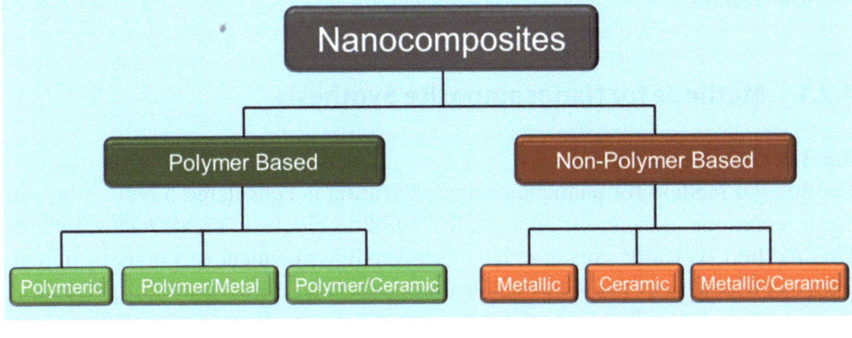

Fig. 4.1 Schematic representation of the nanocomposite categories (Gupta et al. 2024)

imaging since they have unique optical properties, relatively high yields, and long-term stability (Gil et al. 2021). Gold nanoparticles (AuNPs) as well as certain metal oxide (MOx) nanomaterials have ideal absorption properties and therefore can also be used in different biological imaging applications. Nano-based biosensors, on the other hand, enable biomarker detection rapidly with high sensitivity/specificity and involve an array of nanomaterials and composites (Andoh et al. 2024).

The purpose of this chapter is to dive into advances in nanocomposites specifically for medical diagnostic applications. Various aspects of nanotechnology-based approaches are explored, including but not limited to the different types of materials utilized, methods for synthesis and fabrication, specific physicochemical properties enabling enhanced medical diagnostics, and a variety of emerging applications. Not only will the fundamental principles be discussed, but cutting-edge applications in biomedicine will be presented, which include but are not limited to imaging, glucose sensing, and cancer biomarker detection. The novelty of this chapter lies in its comprehensive overview of developments in nanocomposite-based materials, specifically highlighting their roles in biomedical imaging and sensor technologies for diagnostic and theranostic applications. By thoroughly examining these topics, we hope to add valuable perspectives to current discussions in the field, shed light on the various uses of nanocomposites in medical diagnostics, and encourage continued research and innovation.

4.2 Nanocomposite Fabrication and Characterization

Nanomaterials and composites for medical diagnostics can be synthesized using an array of different methods and typically involve integrating nanoparticles into more traditional materials, including polymers. The three main methods for nanocomposite synthesis are the sol–gel method, in situ polymerization, and Layer-by-layer (LbL) assembly (Chauhan et al. 2022; Carrera Espinoza et al. 2023). After synthesis, characterization of nanomaterials and composites is crucial in ensuring that certain nanomaterial properties (physical and chemical) are achieved for proper functionality. Therefore, this section will be dedicated to describing and discussing different methods for nanocomposite synthesis and physicochemical characterization.

4.2.1 Methods for Nanocomposite Synthesis

4.2.1.1 Sol–Gel Method

The sol–gel method for nanocomposite fabrication is considered a bottom-up synthesis technique, meaning it uses smaller building blocks to create nanostructures. This method typically uses a series of irreversible chemical reactions to initially form a colloidal suspension through hydrolysis (called the sol), which can be transformed into a three-dimensional gel through a condensation reaction (Verma et al. 2017; Singh and Birajdar 2017). Typically, inorganic alkoxide monomers are utilized. Metal alkoxides are favored since they easily undergo reactions with water. The most used are alkoxysilanes like tetramethoxysilane (TMOS) and tetraethoxysilane (TEOS). Additionally, other alkoxides such as aluminates, titanates, zirconates, and borates are frequently utilized in the sol–gel process, either on their own or mixed with other alkoxides like TEOS (Young 2002). Once the wet gel is formed through hydrolysis/condensation, it must be dried to remove residual water. Briefly, different methods for drying will directly influence the type of gel formation that is achieved. For example, to produce a relatively porous aerogel, supercritical drying of the wet gel is performed through conditions that prevent or limit capillary stress (Basak and Singhal 2023).

Thermal drying through solvent evaporation will produce xerogels, which are relatively less porous and denser compared to aerogels. This is because thermal drying results in a larger degree of gel shrinkage (Kiciński et al. 2011). Finally, cryogels can be developed using methods such as freeze-drying and are more typically used in applications including regenerative medicine, owing to their robustness and elasticity (Rana et al. 2023). Taken as a whole, drying conditions are important because they can be harnessed to develop gels with nanoporosity. Nanoporous gels have unique properties, primarily their relatively high surface area, but also have other benefits, including but not limited to high yield/purity, uniformity, and homogeneity in pore size (Ju et al. 2014; Yue et al. 2009). Importantly, this technique can produce uniform, high-quality nanocomposites on an industrial scale. It should also be recognized that the sol–gel process is a powerful and flexible method for creating nanooxides with tailored properties, enabling advancements in numerous scientific and industrial fields (Shinde et al. 2012; Shinde et al. 2013). Research has also focused on utilizing this method to develop thin films with thicknesses in the nanometer range, and these can be deposited onto an array of different substrates using different methods such as dip coating, spin coating, flow coating, capillary coating, and more (Habte et al. 2019; Setiawan et al. 2018; Ferraz et al. 2019).

4.2.1.2 In Situ Polymerization

In situ polymerization is a common method for the synthesis of polymer-based nanocomposites. This method is also considered a bottom-up approach for synthesis. Using this method, a homogeneous solution of nanomaterials is synthesized and dispersed in a solution with monomers as well as cross-linkers. A variety of nanomaterials and composites can be used here, including but not limited to metallics and ceramics. A radical initiator is also added to the solution, and the polymerization reaction is induced using light or heat. The polymer chains develop around the nanoparticles, creating a composite material in which the polymer matrix is closely integrated with the nanoparticles. Thus, a thermoset polymer nanocomposite can be synthesized. Different curing procedures for the nanocomposite can be undertaken (using a hardener or catalyst), which have the potential to impact not only the physical but also the chemical properties of the resulting material (Masoumi et al. 2022). In-situ polymerization offers significant benefits, including excellent thermodynamic compatibility at the interface between the matrix and reinforcement, as well as the ability to produce reinforcement surfaces that are free from contamination.

This method is particularly effective for creating insoluble polymer composites, as it ensures a high degree of miscibility for various types of polymers. Additionally, in situ polymerization allows for the uniform distribution of nanoparticles within the polymer matrix, enhancing the mechanical and thermal properties of the resulting composites (Julius et al. 2025).

4.2.1.3 Layer-by-Layer (LbL) Assembly Techniques

LbL assembly techniques, too, are bottom-up approaches, and this method involves sequentially immersing a substrate in solutions of oppositely charged polyelectrolytes or other materials. The charged layers stick to the substrate as well as subsequent layers because of the electrostatic attraction between surfaces with opposite charges. It should be noted that different forces can be used to create LbL assembly structures beyond electrostatic, including but not limited to covalent bonding (Decher et al. 1992; Cassagneau et al. 1998; Cui et al. 2016; Ai et al. 2002; Lee et al. 2019). Through repeated cycles, a multilayer film with precisely managed thickness and composition can be constructed incrementally. The number of assembled components or layers in this process is impacted by the concentration of materials, the strength of molecular interactions, as well as the deposition time and layer number. When assembling composite structures through electrostatic interactions, additional considerations must be paid to ionic strength as well as pH (Dubas et al. 2001; Cho and Char 2004). Of particular importance, metallic and/or MOx nanomaterials can be paired with oppositely charged polymers to develop nanocomposites. Nonetheless, it should be noted that nanoparticles will display electrostatic repulsion and potentially cause aggregation. In turn, this could cause challenges regarding the increase in nanoparticle loading. Additionally, high-density packing of nanomaterials is difficult to achieve (Grabar et al. 1996; Schmitt et al. 1997). Finally, LbL assemblies can be prepared through covalent bonding in organic media (Tettey et al. 2010). This tends to synthesize polymer composites with hydrophobic metals or metal oxides.

4.2.2 Nanocomposite Characterization

4.2.2.1 Dynamic Light Scattering (DLS)

DLS is a very useful and established technique for the characterization of nanomaterial composites, specifically for quantifying the size distribution of particles in a solution. Particles can be immersed in a variety of solvents, and DLS measurements only require viscosity and refractive index inputs to account for instrumental readouts (Rodriguez-Loya et al. 2023). The advantages of this technique over others for size determination (such as electron microscopy techniques, which will be discussed below) are that it is rapid and non-destructive (Ross et al. 1999). Suspended small particles experience random thermal movement called Brownian motion, which is described by the Stokes-Einstein equation (Michaelides 2015). All DLS instruments use a laser as a light source, which illuminates the suspended nanomaterial in a cell. As particles undergo diffusion through Brownian motion, the electric field and associated optical signal will fluctuate. These variations in the signal are caused by the movement of particles and can be utilized to determine their size. Unlike laser diffraction, DLS measurements are generally conducted at a single angle. However, collecting data at multiple angles can provide additional insights and improve the accuracy of the particle size analysis (Naiim et al. 2015). Instruments equipped for DLS frequently have the capability to measure zeta potential at the same time. This dual functionality enables the simultaneous determination of both particle size and surface charge within a single experimental setup. By integrating these measurements, researchers can gain comprehensive insights into the physical and electrochemical properties of nanoparticles and composites.

4.2.2.2 Scanning Electron Microscopy (SEM)

SEM is one of the most widely utilized instrumental characterization techniques across nanotechnology for imaging purposes. SEM is considered to be an optimal imaging technique because it has extremely high resolution equal to approximately 10 nanometers, with more advanced instrumentation even achieving lower values down to about 2.5 nanometers (Webb and Holgate 2003). Another benefit of this technology is that it is often coupled with energy-dispersive X-ray microanalysis (EDAX). Together, this piece of instrumentation can achieve elemental analysis at the nanoscale, thus differentiating differences in nano-composition from those observed in the bulk material (Sleeman and Carter 2005). To generate electrons for SEM, tungsten filaments or a field emission gun are used as a source. The electron beam is produced, and a high voltage is applied to accelerate the electrons. Different lenses are utilized to narrow and focus the beam on the surface of the sample. Through the use of coils, the beam is used to scan the surface of the specimen, thus generating backscattered and secondary electrons that travel to the detector. Examining a sample at high magnification significantly enhances the analysis of surface topography, providing superior spatial resolution. This high magnification allows for detailed observation of fine surface features, enabling precise characterization of the sample's morphology. By utilizing advanced imaging techniques at these magnification levels, researchers can achieve a more accurate and comprehensive understanding of the sample's structural properties, which is crucial for applications in materials science, nanotechnology, and other fields requiring meticulous surface analysis (Anekwe et al. 2024).

4.2.2.3 Transmission Electron Microscopy (TEM)

TEM is an imaging technique that is very similar to that of SEM, but is better suited to image the internal nanostructures of materials rather than the surface. Instead of detecting secondary or backscattered electrons off the sample's surface, this technique relies on detecting transmitted electrons (Wang and Lee 2008). Because electrons are detected after they pass through the sample itself, samples need to be less than 100 nanometers thick (Houck 2023). Another large difference between these two techniques is that TEM can achieve atomic resolution (less than 1 nanometer with up to 50 million times magnification). SEM techniques generally can only reach down to anywhere between 0.5 and 5 nanometers with 2 million times magnification. In addition to higher resolution and the ability to observe internal nanostructures within materials themselves, TEM also has the advantage of performing electron diffraction, which can aid scientists in determining the crystallographic structure of novel nanomaterials (Souza Junior et al. 2021). However, SEM is more available for more diverse sample types, is easier to use, and provides high-resolution images in three-dimensional space.

4.2.2.4 Fourier Transform Infrared Spectroscopy (FTIR)

Aside from physical characterization, including imaging methods, chemical characterization of nanomaterials and composites is also very important to ensure ultimate functionality. FTIR is a technique that is widely used in nanomaterials characterization to understand the functional groups present in the material. Using this technique, infrared (IR) radiation is directed toward the nanocomposite. Depending on the vibrational frequencies arising from the unique molecular structure, specific IR wavelengths are absorbed by the sample. Thus, as transmission/absorbance values are plotted across the wavenumbers scanned, a unique spectral fingerprint is generated, where specific peaks can be attributed to different functional groups of the composite (Eid 2022). One of the main limitations of FTIR is that if there is non-homogeneity or slight differences in chemical structure among nanomaterials, this method may not have the required specificity to detect these differences (Faghihzadeh et al. 2016). Other potential challenges for this method of characterization include the fact that careful attention needs to be paid during sample preparation, as any slight amount of contamination may interfere with analysis.

4.2.2.5 Atomic Force Microscopy-Infrared Spectroscopy (AFM-IR)

Although not discussed in previous sections, atomic force microscopy (AFM) is also a widely utilized technique for the morphological characterization of nanomaterials, although they are not as popular as electron microscopies because it is much more complex and difficult to run. Briefly, AFM is a very powerful nanocomposite characterization method that allows the three-dimensional visualization of an array of surfaces on sample types such as polymers, ceramics, and even biological samples. By principle, AFM is designed with an ultra-thin and sharp tip that is 10–20 nm in diameter and immobilized to a cantilever, allowing both continuous and tapping modes. Tapping mode is the most typical, where the cantilever vibrates right above the surface of the sample, intermittently making contact. The AFM is used not only to image but also to alter atoms and structures on diverse surface types. The atom on the apex of the tip undergoes chemical interactions with the surface, in turn altering the vibrational frequency which can be detected and localized. AFM provides a true three-dimensional view of nanocomposite topological features and has the additional benefit of operating in an ambient environment (not under vacuum) (Sinha Ray 2013).

AFM-IR merges the precise spatial resolution of AFM with the robust chemical analysis capabilities of IR spectroscopy. This integration facilitates detailed chemical imaging and spectroscopy at the nanoscale, enabling researchers to visualize and analyze the molecular composition and interactions within materials with exceptional clarity. This technology is an emerging field and is gaining attention from multiple interdisciplinary experts; and therefore the true potential and scope of applications is still to be determined. AFM-IR operation and function are relatively simple, as it utilizes an IR tunable pulsed laser to induce a photothermal effect within the sample (Mathurin et al. 2022). This effect causes the sample to expand mechanically. AFM is used to detect this expansion through its cantilever tip, which remains in contact with the sample. This process allows for precise measurement and analysis of the sample's chemical and physical properties at the nanoscale. The main benefit of this technology is the fact that chemical compositional mapping can be achieved with a resolution of sub-10 nanometers. This enables the method to identify chemical differences on the nanoscale that may not be revealed using other techniques (dos Santos et al. 2023).

4.2.2.6 X-Ray Diffraction (XRD)

XRD is another very important method for chemical characterization of nanomaterials, since it is used to identify crystalline structure by measuring the intensity of X-rays scattered through the sample at different angles of diffraction. XRD is viable for the characterization of both amorphous and semi-crystalline polymers, and it is very useful for studying the microstructure. Critical parameters that can be measured include lattice constants, the presence of defects or imperfections in the nanomaterial composite, crystallographic orientations, as well as the proportion of a composite that is crystalline. Using this technique, the sample containing the nanocomposite is exposed to X-ray radiation, which is usually produced through electron bombardment of a metallic-based target. As an X-ray beam passes through a specimen, its intensity decreases exponentially. Consequently, the penetration depth of the X-ray is influenced by both the material properties and the energy of the X-ray source. A portion of the incident beam is absorbed, another part is scattered, and the remaining is transmitted through the sample. X-ray scattering occurs when the incident beam interacts with the electrons in the nanocomposite, and the scattered/diffracted X-rays undergo interactions with each other to produce a diffraction pattern that can be used to deduce an array of parameters, including the ones listed above (Adams 2005). Nonetheless, this technique faces challenges in nanocomposite characterization as it is relatively less effective in identifying small crystalline structures. Also, developing a representative sample type can be difficult due to the non-homogeneity of materials and composites (Mourdikoudis et al. 2018; Holder and Schaak 2019).

4.2.2.7 Other Characterization Techniques

Although some primary techniques have been discussed in previous subsections, there are other characterization modes that can be used for the efficient physicochemical characterization of nanomaterial composites. One alternative to AFM, which is used for imaging, is STM, using a conductive tip instead of a mechanical probe. Therefore, STM is ideal for providing high-resolution images on conductive surfaces at the atomic level and can also be used to reveal specific electronic properties of a nanocomposite (Rudd et al. 2005). AFM provides more information on

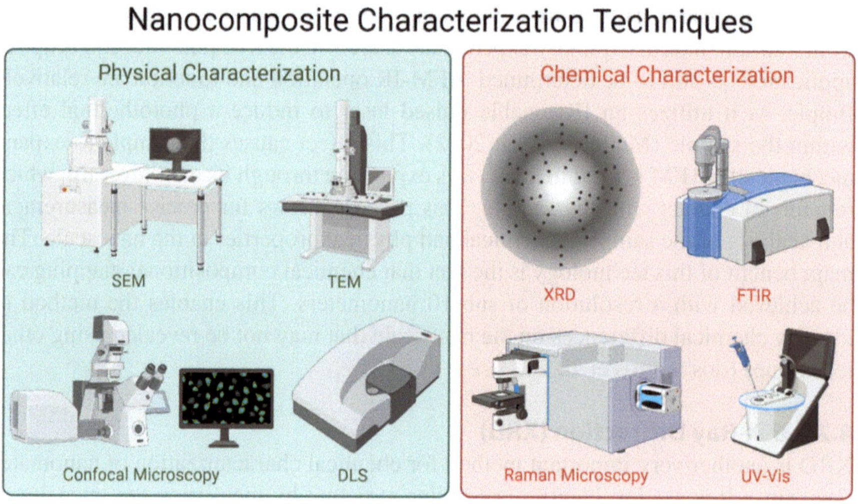

Fig. 4.2 Overview of different physicochemical characterization techniques that can be used to ensure nanocomposite properties and ultimate function (Woollam 2025a)

surface morphology and topography. In addition to SEM, TEM, AFM, and SPM, confocal-laser scanning microscopy can also be used as an imaging technique, and it has significant benefits, such as imaging relatively thick sample types as well as providing detailed information on nanomaterial size, morphology, and distribution throughout a matrix (Elliott 2020). Other spectroscopic-based methods not discussed in previous sections include Raman microscopy for characterizing the distribution of nanomaterials within a composite (along with the chemical interactions), UV–Vis for the characterization of optical properties like absorption, and nuclear magnetic resonance (NMR) to provide more comprehensive information on chemical structures. It should also be noted that goniometry (contact angle measurements) is useful for characterization when the goal is to develop hydrophobic nanocomposites. An overview of the physical and chemical characterization techniques is provided in Fig. 4.2 (Woollam 2025a).

4.3 Key Properties Enabling Medical Diagnostic Applications

4.3.1 Biocompatibility

Nanocomposites in certain applications need to be developed to be biocompatible, as some studies have shown they can be used as imaging agents, and therefore, they need to be determined as safe to not cause inadvertent damage to healthy tissues. Many different parameters of the nanomaterial composite can impact its biocompatibility, including but not limited to size, surface functional groups, shape/

morphology, and the distribution of nanoparticles within the composite (Kyriakides et al. 2021; Chiticaru et al. 2023). Recent findings indicate that biodegradable and biocompatible polymer nanocomposites are becoming increasingly popular in the biomedical field. These materials are frequently utilized in diagnostic tools and drug delivery systems due to their compatibility with biological environments, which helps minimize the likelihood of adverse reactions (Saikia and Karak 2023). Another example of biocompatibility is with MOx nanocomposites, including but not limited to zinc oxide (ZnO) and titanium dioxide (TiO_2), which have demonstrated excellent properties and can be used for detecting an array of different targets in biosensing applications. Carbon-based nanocomposites have also been significantly useful in this regard. Degradable nanocomposites are especially attractive for diagnostic applications because they can be broken down by the body after they have served their purpose. This degradation process reduces the risk of long-term accumulation in the body, which can otherwise lead to potential complications (Liu et al. 2019a). Additionally, their ability to be safely metabolized makes them ideal for use in various medical diagnostics, ensuring that they do not interfere with the body's natural processes over time (Zhang et al. 2020). This property enhances their overall safety and effectiveness in biomedical applications. Nanocomposite research with a focus on biocompatibility is still ongoing, and there are many innovations still to be made to develop materials with superior biocompatibility. As research continues and the understanding of how specific nanocomposite properties impact biocompatibility expands, safer and more effective material composites will be developed in future research endeavors.

4.3.2 Elevated Surface Area

Well-dispersed nanoparticles, including those incorporated into composites, have a significantly high surface area-to-volume ratio, which makes them ideal for applications in biosensing or the delivery of diagnostic-based imaging agents. The high surface area also contributes to significant enhancements in physicochemical properties, including but not limited to mechanical properties (strength/stiffness), thermal conductivity, permeability, and catalytic activity (Ashraf et al. 2018; Harmer et al. 1996). One example of this is that in an array of different polymer composites, carbon-based nanomaterials such as CNTs can be enhanced through the addition of clay nanoparticles to bolster mechanical strength. In these materials, the large surface area enhances load transfer within the matrix, resulting in superior mechanical properties (Sabet 2024). CNTs can also be incorporated into an array of composites and are known for their outstanding thermal conductivity. For example, when they are integrated into a polymer-based nanocomposite, the high surface area of this nanomaterial leads to efficient transfer of heat between them (Yang et al. 2010). Moreover, TiO_2 nanocomposites, known for their widespread use as photocatalysts, can be integrated into nanocomposites to boost their photocatalytic performance. Both TiO_2 and zeolite-polymer nanocomposites, which are porous crystalline aluminosilicates, possess extensive surface areas. This characteristic offers more active sites for photocatalysis, leading to enhanced separation and catalytic properties (Abla et al. 2023; Cheng et al. 2023). Specifically for biosensor applications, an increased surface area of materials can facilitate the functionalization of a higher density of sensing layers, thereby enhancing sensor performance and sensitivity.

4.3.3 Agents for Improved Imaging

Nanocomposites also have unique and enhanced permeability properties and retention effect, making them indispensable tools for emerging applications in diagnostic-based imaging. Small-sized nanoparticles can take advantage of the permeable blood vessels in tumors, enabling them to penetrate and gather within the tumor tissue (Xie et al. 2023). Nanocomposites designed for targeted imaging can integrate a range of imaging agents, including fluorescent dyes, radioisotopes, and magnetic nanoparticles. These agents enable the visualization of tumors through various imaging modalities, such as fluorescence imaging, positron emission tomography (PET), and magnetic resonance imaging (MRI). By incorporating these diverse imaging agents, nanocomposites can provide detailed and precise images of tumor locations and structures. Furthermore, a key property of nanoparticles in imaging applications is that they can be uniquely functionalized with antibodies that specifically target and image cancer cells (Qamar 2021). Compared to traditional materials and agents, nanomaterial-based composites result in imaging with deeper penetration and higher resolution capabilities (Liu et al. 2023). The unique optical, magnetic, and chemical properties of nanoscale materials facilitate the creation of imaging probes with superior contrast, increased sensitivity, controlled biodistribution, enhanced spatial and temporal resolution, multifunctional capabilities, and the potential for multimodal imaging (Alrushaid et al. 2023).

4.3.4 Magnetic Separation

Magnetic-based nanomaterials and composites can be uniquely manipulated through the implementation of magnetic fields. When magnetic nanomaterials are exposed to a magnetic field, they align within the field, which allows their isolation from other non-magnetic components. This is very important in the context of medical diagnostics, since they can be functionalized with antibodies or other biomolecules that specifically bind to cancer cells or specific biomarkers. When subjected to a magnetic field, these magnetic nanoparticles will concentrate at the tumor site, aiding in their separation and detailed analysis. Magnetic nanomaterials are commonly used in tumor imaging applications. Their magnetic properties enhance the quality of MRI scans, enabling the production of high-resolution images (Yigit et al. 2012). Hybrid magnetic nanostructures are utilized in various applications, including magnetic separation, diagnostics, and targeted cancer drug delivery. These versatile nanocomposites allow for the efficient isolation of cancer cells from complex biological samples through magnetic separation, thereby aiding in subsequent analysis and diagnostic procedures (Govindan et al. 2023). Magnetic nanocomposites can also be utilized to capture and purify circulating tumor cells (CTCs) from samples of blood. One example of this is that ferroplatinum iron oxide magnetic nanocomposites have been successfully employed for the capture and isolation of CTCs (Liu et al. 2019b). Multimodal imaging can be achieved using these composites since they can be loaded with various imaging agents, thereby facilitating diagnosis as well as a deeper understanding of the tumor and its microenvironment (Andoh et al. 2024; Yin et al. 2024). They can also be tuned and functionalized to detect an array of different biomarkers, including but not limited to proteins, nucleic acids, and metabolites (Alromi et al. 2021).

4.3.5 Enhancement of Electrochemical Biosensing Capabilities

Nanomaterial-based composites have also been utilized in the development of electrochemical biosensors that target cancer cells or other biomarkers for an array of different medical conditions. This is mostly due to their high surface area as well as their excellent properties regarding electrical conductivity to facilitate electron transfer (Agrahari et al. 2022; Khazaei et al. 2023). Graphene is one popular example of this, as it is a very versatile nanomaterial that is employed for the diagnosis of cancer and other human diseases, including diabetes. These sensors show promise for quick, sensitive, and affordable detection of biomarkers (Andoh et al. 2024). Nanocomposites have been utilized for the precise electrochemical detection of various cancer biomarkers. These include circulating tumor cells, proteins, DNA mutations, non-coding RNAs such as microRNA, glycoproteins, and metabolites. Recently, there has been a lot of research focusing on polymer-based nanocomposites embedded with metallic and carbon nanomaterials to significantly enhance the performance and sensitivity of existing biosensor systems (Mohammadpour-Haratbar et al. 2022a). Moreover, electrochemical sensing enables the detection of cancer-related molecules without the need for labeling. Label-free detection enhances the versatility and efficiency of these platforms, allowing for the rapid and straightforward identification of biomarkers. By eliminating the need for additional labeling steps, these sensors streamline the detection process, reduce costs, and minimize potential interferences, making them highly effective tools in medical diagnostic applications (Sanko and Kuralay 2023).

4.4 Nanocomposites in Medical Imaging Applications

Detection and diagnosis of disease at the earliest stage is important in the clinical standard of care, and this especially holds true for cancer. Often, more times than not, diagnostic imaging modalities are not only crucial for identifying if a patient has cancer, but also to determine tumor response to therapy. Currently employed imaging techniques encompass MRI, X-ray radiography, computed tomography (CT), ultrasound (US), PET, single photon emission computed tomography

(SPECT), and fluorescence imaging methods (Ryvolova et al. 2012). In order to improve accuracy and provide more information on the tumor, clinical imaging contrast agents are used to distinguish tumor tissues specifically. Additionally, clinicians tend to use more than one imaging modality to more accurately interpret cancer diagnoses (Fan et al. 2014). In conventional clinical imaging techniques, the effectiveness of contrast agents in detecting tumors is constrained by the spatial resolution capabilities of the imaging equipment (Cuccurullo et al. 2018). This limitation means that smaller tumors or fine details may not be adequately visualized, potentially impacting the accuracy of diagnosis and treatment planning. Additionally, although the current agents used for contrast are small molecules that demonstrate rapid metabolism, their distribution in the context of cancer cells is relatively nonspecific. These agents can also exhibit inadvertent toxicities to the patient (Chronos et al. 1993; Han et al. 2019).

Recent advancements have shown the potential for nanomaterials and composites to be incorporated into these detection modalities, since they have unique/enhanced permeability and retention effects in tumors (Oh et al. 2013). The relatively small size of nanomaterials has a profound impact on their properties regarding biodistribution, blood circulation half-life, cellular uptake, tumor penetration, as well as targeting (Hoshyar et al. 2016). Nanoparticles smaller than 10 nm are swiftly eliminated by the renal excretion system due to the average size of renal filtration pores being 10 nm. Conversely, nanoparticles larger than 100 nm are readily recognized by macrophages and tend to accumulate in organs associated with the mononuclear phagocyte system (MPS), such as the lymph nodes, liver, spleen, and lungs (Longmire et al. 2008; Zhou and Dai 2018). There have been several other reports that show that nanoparticles with sizes between 10 and 60 nanometers demonstrate enhanced cellular uptake properties (Hoshyar et al. 2016; Huang et al. 2012). Nanocomposite surfaces can be labeled and functionalized with a diverse set of ligands or sensing elements to specifically target receptors and thereby increase contrast agent localization (Chen et al. 2012; Ke et al. 2010). One example of this is that gold nanoparticles can be functionalized with an aptamer that targets the prostate-specific antigen. This agent has been shown to provide a higher CT density for prostate cancer diagnosis through imaging (Kim et al. 2010). Furthermore, nano-sized superparamagnetic iron oxide agents, when coated with a high-affinity antibody, have demonstrated the ability to specifically target lung tumors during MRI scans (Wang et al. 2017a).

Antibodies and antibody fragments are the most common and efficient ligands for active targeting, since they have a relatively high affinity for antigens that can increase nanomaterial concentration in a localized fashion (Alibakhshi et al. 2017). Another class of common ligands that is used for targeting are aptamers, which is a single sequence of nucleic acids that have high affinity toward cell surface receptors and undergo conformational change (folding of the secondary structure). Compared to antibodies, aptamers show significant benefit since they are easy to make, small, and reduce immunogenicity (Jo and Ban 2016). However, there are downfalls, including the fact that they are rapidly excreted and degraded by nucleases, meaning they do not have the desired blood circulation time to localize at the tumor site before they are cleared from the body (Alshaer et al. 2018). Peptides can also be a targeting moiety, as they are not only stable, but are also easy to synthesize and demonstrate a significantly reduced immunogenicity (Inaba and Matsuura 2019). The arginine-glycine-aspartic acid (RGD) peptide is a key integrin-binding domain capable of interacting with various integrin types. It is frequently used in nanoparticle applications (Bellis 2011; Li et al. 2019a). Additionally, other proteins and molecules that play active targeting roles include transferrin, folic acid, and biotin (Zhong et al. 2014).

It is also important to note that a diverse set of stimuli can also play a significant role in nanocomposite-based imaging applications. In these approaches, external sources, including electromagnetic fields, can guide the transportation of nanomaterials toward the target site. They can also precisely control release processes, as demonstrated by photothermal and magnetic hyperthermia therapy (Yu et al. 2016). Endogenous stimuli include pH changes, temperature fluctuations, enzyme activity, and redox gradients, while external stimuli encompass light, magnetic fields, and ultrasound (Yang et al. 2018). Nanomaterial-based contrast agents, compared to traditional agents, have a prolonged time in blood circulation, and this plays a significant role in their mechanisms for enhancement. Therefore, it is of the utmost importance and interest to chemically functionalize or modify the nanomaterial composite to increase the time in blood circulation (Han et al. 2019). One of the most common approaches is to encapsulate hydrophobic nanomaterials within a layer of polyethylene glycol (PEG) (Wang et al. 2018), which increases solubility and therefore blood circulation time. The hydrophilic nature of PEG's backbone reduces the binding of nanoparticles to opsonins and their recognition by macrophages, thereby decreasing their clearance by the reticuloendothelial system (Mozar and Chowdhury 2018). Chitosan, hyaluronic acid, and fucoidan can also be utilized and can have a similar effect on enhancing the time the nanocomposite is in circulation (Abdollah et al. 2018). Modification through zwitterionic interactions also results in nanomaterials with enhanced binding properties, macrophage uptake, and aggregation resistance (Liu et al. 2014; Xiao et al. 2012).

Due to these specific properties, nanocomposites have been studied in imaging applications for early disease detection and diagnosis. These materials have been incorporated into medical imaging diagnostics through three different avenues. First and foremost, nanomaterial-based contrast agents have been widely employed with existing imaging methods. Additionally, nanoparticles can serve as targeted delivery systems, carrying various imaging agents to detect cancers. Finally, nanomaterial composites can also be used for biomarker detection and quantification (Andoh et al. 2024). In imaging-based applications, nanotechnology has the potential to develop nano-imaging agents that have a relatively high surface area, which facilitates surface labeling to increase biocompatibility, decrease toxicity, and improve the quality of biomedical images (Liu and Grodzinski 2021). Imaging nanoparticles offer additional advantages, such as enabling the functional visualization and monitoring of biological processes. For instance, they can be used to detect macrophages in atherosclerotic lesions via CT scans and to perform molecular imaging of angiogenesis using MRI (Quillard and Libby 2012). The fact that nanomaterial-based imaging agents have increased circulation time bolsters their biodistribution and ultimately leads to a more intense and more detectable signal that is specific to cancer cells. The shapes and sizes of nanomaterials within composites can also be controlled, and this can be used to optimize imaging agent loading (Dong et al. 2019).

Given the limitations of existing imaging contrast agents and the promising benefits of nanoparticles for early diagnosis and detailed visualization of microstructures, there is a growing interest in utilizing nanotechnology for biomedical imaging. Nanoparticles offer enhanced contrast, improved sensitivity, and the ability to target specific tissues or cells, making them highly effective for detecting and monitoring diseases at an early stage. This increased interest is driven by the potential of nanotechnology to revolutionize imaging techniques, providing more accurate and comprehensive insights into biological processes and disease progression.

4.4.1 Imaging Modalities: Benefits and Disadvantages

MRI is one of the most common imaging modalities used in the clinic for medical diagnostics and is based on the fact that protons spin when in the presence of an external magnetic field and are excited using a radio frequency pulse. MRI, which relies on the nuclear magnetic resonance signals from protons within the human body, offers exceptional spatial and temporal resolution. This imaging technique is renowned for its superior intrinsic contrast of soft tissues, making it highly effective for detailed visualization of anatomical structures (Florkow et al. 2022). Additionally, MRI can generate three-dimensional tomographic images, providing comprehensive and precise anatomical information. It is also beneficial since this method does not rely on the use of radiotracers. Although MRI and its contrasting agents aid clinicians in diagnosing lesions, there are limitations, which include the fact that it is costly and requires long wait times to generate results. Additionally, this technique can also be sensitive to noise arising from artifacts relating to motions and bodily implants (Murali et al. 2024).

CT, on the other hand, uses variations in tissue X-ray absorption and thickness to produce cross-sectional and 3D images. Because this technology has a relatively rapid testing speed, decreased cost, and improved accuracy/efficiency through higher spatial resolution, it has emerged as a very useful technique even though it involves higher exposure to ionizing radiation compared to other modalities. Contrast agents used for CT play a significant role in isolating tissues with similar attenuation coefficients, and the most common agent used in clinical practice is iodine. It should be noted that employing iodine as a contrast agent has its challenges, given that it is rapidly cleared from the body and can potentially have inadvertent toxic effects on kidney function (Han et al. 2019). Therefore, in CT imaging applications, nanomaterial-based contrast agents may be able to overcome some of these limitations, owing to their unique physicochemical properties discussed above.

US imaging stands out as one of the most prevalent techniques in medical diagnostics. Its popularity stems from several key advantages: it is portable, noninvasive, and offers high spatial resolution. Additionally, US imaging is cost-effective and provides real-time visualization, making it highly practical for various medical applications (Klibanov and Hossack 2015). To further improve the quality of ultrasound images, specialized contrast agents have been developed. These agents work by amplifying the differences in acoustic signals between healthy tissues and areas of concern, such as lesions, thereby enhancing the clarity and diagnostic accuracy of the images. The US contrast agents that are currently employed in the clinic include microbubbles that have diameters in the range of 1 to 8 microns. These larger particles are limited to providing contrast signals within the blood pool and do not get absorbed by cells. Because of their size, they have a short circulation lifespan and are not very stable (Yusefi 2022). Nanomaterials and composites have been of focus to overcome these challenges, but it should be noted that these materials need to be relatively larger (in the range of hundreds to thousands of nanometers in diameter) for them to generate sufficient acoustic reflection/signal (Sakamoto et al. 2005; Seo et al. 2010).

Finally, PET is another imaging modality that is a very powerful tool often used in nuclear medicine technology. This method not only achieves a high tissue penetration depth but also is highly sensitive and facilitates quantitative imaging analyses in real-time. Besides providing highly detailed anatomic information, this technology is also well posed to generate biomolecular information through tracking nuclides. SPECT, on the other hand, is also another technique that is widely utilized in nuclear medicine and offers similar benefits as PET. The main difference in these two techniques is that PET uses positron-emitting tracers, while SPECT uses gamma-emitting tracers. PET provides as a high-resolution imaging platform, while SPECT is a relatively more cost-effective and widely available technology. However, it should be discussed that both PET and SPECT techniques have downfalls, including cost and exposure to potentially harmful radiation (Han ct al. 2019).

4.4.2 Nanomaterials in Biomedical Imaging

4.4.2.1 Quantum Dots

Quantum dots are a class of nanomaterials that are fluorescent semiconductors with enhanced optical and electrical properties (Smith et al. 2008; Gao et al. 2004). Quantum dots, compared to traditional materials like organic dyes or fluorescent biomolecules, have higher brightness intensity and can achieve near-unity quantum yields. These nanomaterials and their composites have also demonstrated desirable optical properties such as broad absorption, narrow linewidth emission spectrum, and a long lifetime for fluorescence (Resch-Genger et al. 2008). Therefore, once quantum dots are conjugated with specific bifunctionality, they can be a very useful type of nanomaterial for in vivo targeting and biomedical imaging applications (Zhang et al. 2008). In these types of studies, researchers can manipulate the size and chemical composition of quantum dots, which in turn will impact and vary the observed optical properties (characteristics of absorption and emission). This can allow the specific tailoring of these materials for cell labeling, biosensing, and nucleic acid detection.

For biomedical imaging applications, it must be considered that quantum dot synthesis requires hydrophobic conditions, and this is problematic given that biological molecules have limited solubility in nonpolar or organic solvents (Gerion et al. 2001). Therefore, prior to implementation, quantum dots must be functionalized or modified with surface stabilizers through ligand exchange or surface conjugation (Smith et al. 2008; Daniel and Astruc 2004). In the ligand exchange process, heterobifunctional ligands like mercaptoacetic acid or 3-mercaptopropyl trimethoxy silane, which contain thiol groups, are utilized. These thiol groups can form covalent bonds with quantum dots. Additionally, the acid groups present in these ligands enhance the hydrophilicity of the quantum dots (Bruchez et al. 1998). However, a significant challenge in these approaches is that they may induce aggregation as well as decrease the intensity/efficiency of fluorescence. To enhance stability and solubility in water, another very effective method is to stabilize the surface using amphiphilic polymers (Xu et al. 2007; Jańczewski et al. 2011). Quantum dots that have been modified for better water stability can then be linked with specific ligands, such as peptides, antibodies, or small molecules, to achieve targeted specificity (Liang et al. 2021). One very common example of this is that quantum dots can be conjugated with PEG to not only reduce nonspecific adsorption/binding of interfering biomolecules, but also to increase blood circulation time (Warnement et al. 2008).

Specifically in biomedical applications, quantum dots are receiving a lot of attention as fluorophores for in vivo imaging using fluorescence-based methods. It should be noted that since this is an optical method, its ability to penetrate deep into tissues may be limited (Nune et al. 2009). Nonetheless, a diverse set of studies has been published demonstrating the potential benefit of utilizing quantum dots. In type I quantum dots, the shell is composed of a material with a high band gap, where the conduction band is at a higher energy level than the core, and the valence band is at a lower energy level than the core. Conversely, type II quantum dots consist of core-shell materials with staggered band gaps (Singh et al. 2020). One of the first publications to emphasize the use of quantum dots in biomedical imaging was conducted by Gao et al. in the early 2000s. This study developed multifunctional quantum dots for in vivo imaging of prostate cancer using murine models. Nanomaterials in this study were fabricated through encapsulating quantum dots functionalized with PEG using an ABC triblock copolymer and linking it to the multiple functionalities, including a tumor-targeting antibody that is specific for the prostate-specific antigen. Through employing subcutaneous injections of quantum dot-tagged cancer cells alongside systemic injections of multifunctional probes, sensitive and multicolor fluorescence images of cancer cells in live animal models were achieved (Gao et al. 2004).

There has also been work that has shown multiple alternative components, including but not limited to gadolinium and manganese, can be integrated into quantum dot-based nanocomposites to facilitate multimodal imaging agents and modalities. One previous example of this is that Jin et al. fabricated hybrid quantum dots that incorporated Gd^{3+} in order to develop a dual-mode imaging modality (fluorescence and magnetic resonance). The hydrophobic quantum dots composed of CdSeTe/CdS were initially modified with glutathione to enhance their biocompatibility. Following this, they underwent further functionalization with Gd^{3+}-1,4,7,10-tetraazacyclododecane-1,4,7,10-tetraacetic acid, which is a gadolinium-based contrast agent. This dual functionalization process not only improves the compatibility of the quantum dots with biological systems but also equips them with properties suitable for advanced imaging applications (Jin et al. 2008). Another more recent study had the goal of doping metals (iron oxide, silver, thulium, neodymium, cerium oxide, cerium chloride, and molybdenum disulfide) into nitrogen-containing graphene quantum dots (NGQDs) that show high-contrast features in US brightness mode and possess visible and/or near-infrared fluorescence imaging abilities. Results from this study showed that not only do the materials demonstrate practical cell viability in toxicity assays, but also facilitate successful bioaccumulation and signal enhancement. The integration of non-invasive ultrasound imaging with precise fluorescence tracking capabilities renders these metal-doped NGQDs highly effective for a range of biomedical applications (Valimukhametova et al. 2022).

4.4.2.2 Gold Nanoparticles

AuNPs are inorganic materials that are significantly valuable tools in the field of biomedical imaging, thanks to their unique physicochemical properties (Mahato et al. 2019) (Fig. 4.3 (Bagheri et al. 2018; Woollam 2025b)). They have good biocompatibility, relatively safe toxicological profiles, as well as high absorption of incident X-rays (Mieszawska et al. 2013). Therefore, most of the applications involving AuNPs undertake CT imaging modalities for detection. Because gold nanoparticles are not stable in solution after synthesis/fabrication, they require stabilizing agents to be added. Here, there are two different methods that can be employed for functionalization. In the first method, ligand exchange is accomplished through replacing synthesis stabilizers with thiols using the mercaptan strategy (Daniel and Astruc 2004). In the second approach, biomolecules can be attached to the stabilizer molecules already present on gold nanoparticles. This often involves modifying the amino acid end groups of the stabilizer through covalent bonding with ligands, using methods such as EDC (1-ethyl-3-(3-dimethylaminopropyl carbodiimide-HCl) chemistry (Heuer-Jungemann et al. 2019). Gold nanoparticles can also be functionalized with tumor-specific biomolecules. The characteristics of the targeting ligand or stabilizer on nanoparticles play a crucial role in determining the particle size, size distribution, and polydispersity of metallic-based nanoparticles/composites (Kesharwani et al. 2023). As a result, there has been significant interest in creating stable, functionalized AuNPs designed to specifically target cancerous tissues. This focus aims to enhance the precision and effectiveness of cancer treatments by ensuring that therapeutic agents are delivered directly to the tumor site, minimizing damage to healthy tissues and improving overall treatment outcomes.

Because AuNPs and composites demonstrate high X-ray attenuation and K-edge energy, they can deliver superior imaging contrast at elevated X-ray tube voltages compared to iodinated CT contrast agents at the same concentration (Mahan and Doiron 2018). Moreover, the shape and size of gold nanoparticles are highly

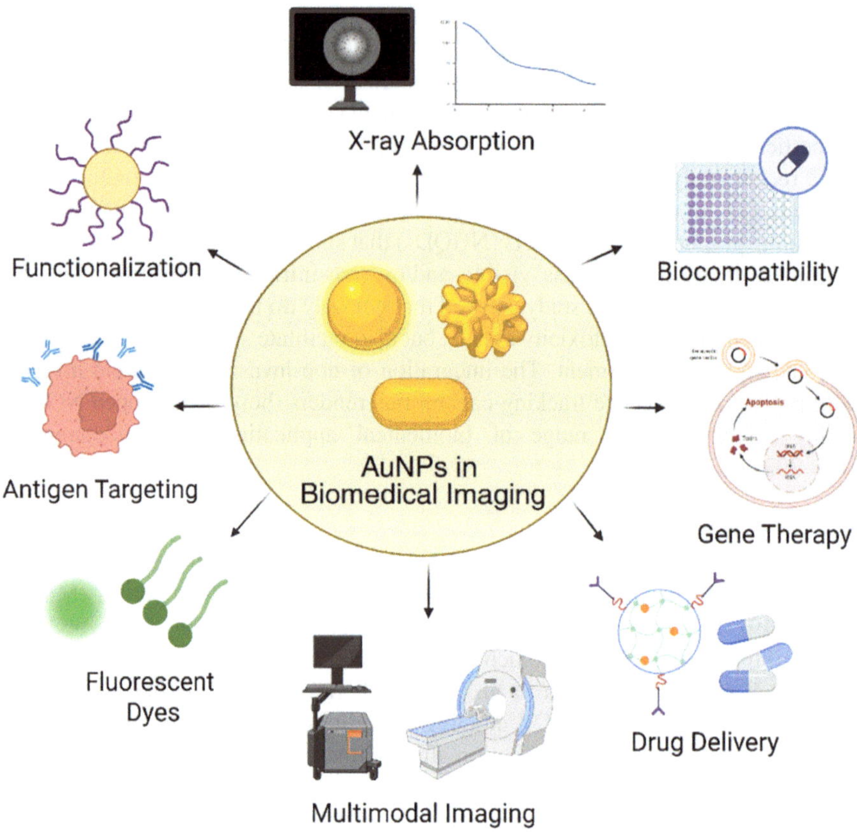

Fig. 4.3 Gold nanoparticle properties and applications regarding biomedical imaging-based diagnostics and theranostics (Bagheri et al. 2018; Woollam 2025b)

tunable, as a myriad of different morphologies have been synthesized and applied over the course of time: nanospheres, nanorods, nanostars, nanoplates, nanocages, nanoshells, nanoprisms, and even nanodisks (Wall et al. 2017). Previous studies have shown that although nanoparticle size does not impact X-ray attenuation properties, an enhanced in vivo CT signal can be facilitated through developing nanomaterials that specifically aggregate in the regions of interest, thus increasing concentrations inside the tumor. One example of this is that a previous study synthesized gold nanospheres functionalized with PEG at different sizes ranging from 4 to 152 nanometers in diameter. The results analyzed CT contrast properties in the context of nanomaterial size, and this showed that relatively smaller gold nanoparticles had stronger CT contrast signals. Smaller nanomaterials were enriched in the blood pool, where relatively larger gold nanoparticles were deposited in the liver and spleen. Therefore, gold nanoparticles with a higher diameter can offer high CT contrast imaging of liver and spleen regions (Dong et al. 2019).

Compared to spherical gold nanoparticles, it is well understood that gold nanorods facilitate enhanced CT imaging and performance, since they not only achieve a higher time in circulation but also demonstrate better intratumor enrichment. One example of this is that Qu et al. synthesized gold nanorods functionalized with RGD peptides to target integrin $\alpha_v\beta_3$, which is dysregulated by certain cancer types. The nanoprobe was evaluated using both in vivo and in vitro approaches, with results showing that conjugated RGD nanorods were not cytotoxic and exhibited enhanced biocompatibility as well as stability (Qu et al. 2016). In addition to nanorods, gold nanostars have also been employed in biomedical imaging. Nanostars contain multiple sharp tips, which can be uniquely functionalized with polydopamine-targeting peptides to improve contrasts in CT imaging through high surface area and extended half-life in the blood (Liu et al. 2015; Wei et al. 2016). Additionally, another study previously engineered triangular gold nanoplates modified with P75, a novel peptide that targets the epidermal growth factor receptor (EGFR). These modified nanoplates are designed to specifically bind to the overexpressed EGFR found in non-small cell lung cancer (Zhao et al. 2018). This targeted approach enables precise CT imaging of cancerous tissues in live animal models, enhancing the accuracy and effectiveness of diagnostic imaging.

Beyond these specific applications, AuNPs and composites have played a crucial role in advancing theranostic technologies, which combine diagnostic and therapeutic functions. These nanoparticles can serve as imaging agents that specifically target cancer sites. Additionally, they can be engineered to release various therapies once they reach their target, enhancing both the precision and effectiveness of cancer treatment. For these theranostic applications, gold nanocages and gold nanoshells are often employed due to their hollow structures and porous walls (Shi et al. 2012; Wang et al. 2014). The surfaces of these gold nanomaterials can be readily modified with a variety of molecules and ligands through the mercaptan strategy. This versatility in surface modification makes them highly promising candidates for drug delivery systems and CT contrast agents (Topete et al. 2025). One example of this in current scientific literature is the use of gold nanocages that incorporate doxorubicin and microRNA for achieving a dual functionality material that can not only be used as CT contrast agents but also facilitates chemotherapy and gene therapy (Huang et al. 2018). Nonetheless, it should be noted that even with the addition of nanomaterials, including composites, CT-based imaging technologies still can struggle with the differentiation of tissue densities (Jiang et al. 2023).

Therefore, AuNPs have been used for multimodal imaging as contrast agents, as these approaches address the limitations of single CT imaging modalities, provide complementary benefits, and expand the scope of molecular imaging techniques (Fu et al. 2019). AuNP composites have been integrated into multimodal approaches that integrate CT with photoacoustic imaging technologies. However, it is well recognized in the research community that the introduction of MRI can overcome limitations in discriminating tissue density more directly (Luo et al. 2021). Therefore, gold nanoparticles have been modified to be compatible for dual-mode imaging through both CT and MRI technologies to facilitate the development of enhanced methods. Multifunctional gold nanoprisms have been previously synthesized and decorated with gadopentetic acid for this specific application, given the high X-ray attenuation of gold nanomaterials and desirable magnetic properties of gadolinium. The nanocomposite demonstrated efficient longitudinal relaxivity as well as a high X-ray absorption coefficient; thus it is a very promising material for dual imaging through CT and MRI (Liu et al. 2017a). It can also be noted that there have also been strides to leverage the unique characteristics of the tumor microenvironment (including but not limited to hypoxia, pH, or responsiveness to H_2O_2) in the design and assembly of gold nanoparticle composites. In short, this in turn can improve the performance of CT contrast agents due to increased accumulation within the tumor microenvironment (Yu et al. 2021).

4.4.2.3 Carbon Nanotubes (CNTs)

Simply put, CNTs are monolayers of graphite that are rolled into tubes, and they demonstrate unique electrical, mechanical, and optical properties. Both single-walled and multi-walled structures can be fabricated, allowing for a variety of biomedical applications. Single-walled structures are composed of a single sheet of rolled-up graphene composed of hexagonal benzene rings, where multi-walled structures contain a stack of graphene sheets that are rolled into concentric circles (Alshammari et al. 2023). Both types of CNTs have significantly high mechanical strength, as well as thermal and electrical conductivity. Single-walled CNTs exhibit distinctive electronic properties, being either metallic or semiconducting based on their chirality. Additionally, they emit near-infrared (NIR) fluorescence, which is influenced by environmental factors such as pH, temperature, and the presence of oxidizing agents. Historically, this is the reason single-walled CNTs have been used in biomedical imaging applications (Nune et al. 2009), where NIR absorption properties or surface functionalization have been of primary focus. The range of the IR spectrum between 900 and 1300 nanometers has relevance in the context of biomedical applications, due to low photo-absorption and auto-fluorescent background. Therefore, in this band, a greater depth of optical penetration can be achieved. It can also be noted that these materials and composites also have desirable photostability properties.

CNTs can be used in the development of probes for exploring stem-cell differentiation and proliferation, given that they are highly hydrophobic and can be highly retained by cells for multiple repeated iterations of cell division (Lee and Parpura 2009). CNTs hold promise as imaging contrast agents across various techniques, including optical detection, MRI, Raman scattering, photoacoustic imaging, fluorescent video imaging, and nuclear imaging. Therefore, applications for CNT composites have emerged and are ever-expanding (Gong et al. 2013). One of the main considerations when employing these nanomaterials is that they are insoluble in many different solvents, including water. Additionally, there is concern that CNTs with certain dimensions or concentrations may induce undesirable toxic effects on biological organisms. Therefore, it is imperative to functionalize the surface of nanomaterials to increase their solubility and ability to evade immune response. Surface functionalization can also be undertaken to form supramolecular complexes with biological macromolecules and substrates through electrostatic interactions

(Al-Jamal et al. 2008). No cytotoxic effects tend to be observed when nanomaterials with these unique functionalities are employed to transport various cargoes across cellular membranes (Bianco et al. 2005). CNT composites have been developed for cancer diagnosis, imaging, and therapy, mostly using single-walled CNTs and confocal microscopy. One of the first studies in this area characterized the uptake of single-walled CNTs functionalized with streptavidin conjugates in human promyelocytic leukemia cells (Shi Kam et al. 2004).

Fluorescence imaging techniques are the most common for CNTs, given their physicochemical properties. Another previous study showed that single-walled CNTs can be used as contrast agents for NIR-II (1100–1400 nanometers) imaging. Through real-time fluorescence imaging using murine models, the study found that CNTs begin circulation in the lungs and kidneys within just several seconds after administration (spleen and liver circulation were observed at later points in time). After employing unsupervised multivariate chemometric approaches to analyze the fluorescent signal, it was realized that there was a high resolution to distinguish organs through imaging, including the pancreas (Welsher et al. 2011). Another report showed that single-walled CNTs can be functionalized with PEG as well as Rituximab (monoclonal antibody for CD20 cell surface proteins) and Transtuzumab (monoclonal antibody for HER2 receptors located on breast cancer cells). The novel nanocomposite not only exhibited selective binding to breast cancer cell lines but also demonstrated photoluminescence of single-walled CNTs, thus offering a highly sensitive imaging approach. A notable benefit of using CNTs was their ability to circumvent cellular autofluorescence, enabling the detection of cells with minimal expression of surface receptors (Welsher et al. 2008).

Although they are not as commonly used as often in biomedical imaging, multiwalled CNTs have been employed in previous studies. For example, multiwalled CNTs were decorated with polyethylenimine (PEI), which was further conjugated with fluorescein isothiocyanate and a prostate stem cell antigen (PSCA) monoclonal antibody. Not only did toxicity assessment deem the materials to be biocompatible, but flow cytometry and confocal luminescence imaging showed that the nanocomposites could bind to the cancer target with high sensitivity/specificity. The probes can be detected using US imaging techniques, with results suggesting that the novel nanocomposite has great potential as a contrast agent. Beyond this, the nanomaterial may also function as a carrier for targeted drug delivery (Wu et al. 2014). There have also been studies that incorporate CNTs into a multimodal imaging approach to increase diagnostic accuracy. One example of this is the use of single-walled structures for in vivo imaging of lung cancer. To ensure the proper magnetic properties required for MRI, gadolinium and copper were integrated using sonication. It was noted that rapid clearance and significant accumulation of this nanocomposite was observed in the pulmonary system, and therefore, these contrast agents may be potentially useful in tracking lung diseases, including cancer. Through the use of a hybrid PET/MRI approach, this contrast agent provides a very promising avenue for developing sophisticated imaging probes with versatile multimodal imaging functionalities (Cisneros et al. 2014).

More recently, there have been advancements in CNT design and development in biomedical applications. One example of this is that they can be coated with different polymers to enhance performance. CNTs coated with poly(2-methacryloyloxyethyl phosphorylcholine-co-n-butyl methacrylate) (PMB) can generate high-quality biomedical images of brown fat through PET with relatively higher brightness and intensity. Brown adipose tissue, known for its heat-generating properties, is gaining considerable interest as a novel therapeutic target for treating metabolic disorders linked to obesity. Due to the incorporation of the amphiphilic and biocompatible polymer, the nanomaterial composite specifically accumulates on capillary endothelial cells desirably and not larger vessels in adipose tissue. Therefore, the brightness of the adipose tissue image is a direct reflection of capillary density (as well as thermogenicity and brownness) (Yudasaka et al. 2017). It has also been shown that CNTs can be integrated with persistent luminescent nanoparticles (PLNPs) to enhance the performance of a multifunctional nanoplatform. The integration of PLNPs with CNTs markedly decreased the recombination efficiency of photogenerated carriers within PLNPs, expanded the specific surface area, and amplified light absorption intensity in the NIR spectrum. The platform was optimized through varying the ratio of PLNPs and CNTs in the composite, which led to the development of a platform that can perform photocatalytic degradation, photocatalytic therapy, photothermal therapy, and drug delivery (Li et al. 2025).

4.4.2.4 Metal Oxides

MOx nanomaterials and composites have also received a lot of attention regarding biomedical imaging applications, given their unique magnetic, optical, and electronic properties. Similar to metallic nanoparticles, metal oxides have adequate biocompatibility when dosed at low concentrations. Metal oxides also present surfaces that can easily functionalized with an array of different molecules, including but not limited to antibodies, nucleosides, proteins and enzymes (Mujahid et al. 2022). Conjugation with these types of biomolecules allows precise cancer targeting in biomedical imaging applications. Some nanomaterial-based metal oxides, such as iron oxide, demonstrate superparamagnetic properties as well as high field irreversibility (Musielak et al. 2019). Superparamagnetic iron oxide nanoparticles (SPIONs) are frequently utilized as the core material, while biocompatible polymers like dextran are often employed as coating materials. It is critical to coat or functionalize metal oxide nanomaterials prior to application, as this will play a key role in determining how the nanocomposite performs in vivo. Coating MOx nanomaterial composites with the right functionality can have positive effects including decreased uptake, increased time while in circulation, and enhanced accumulation of the agent at the targeted site of interest (Wahajuddin and Arora 2012). Other monomer-based molecules can also be coated on MOx materials, and these include bisphosphonates and alkoxysilanes (Wahajuddin and Arora 2012). Similar to other nanomaterials, metal oxides can also be coated with PEG which can drastically increase the stability of colloidal nanomaterials (Schubert and Chanana 2018).

SPIONs have emerged as an interesting nanomaterial that can be employed in MR imaging applications, due to their relatively large magnetic moment. When SPIONs are administered inside the human body, they distort local magnetic fields which ultimately lead to voids in signals and allows for the detection of pathologically relevant areas or specific biological targets (Shen et al. 2024). There have been many different studies that have used SPIONs for T_2-weighted MRI, but they can also be modified physically and chemically for T_1-weighted MRI application (Rahman 2023). T_1-weighted MRI is often favored for its ability to produce positive contrast in images. Conversely, T_2-weighted MRI can encounter issues related to magnetic susceptibilities, bleeding, and calcification (Kawahara and Nagata 2021). Without any chemical modification, SPIONs can be fabricated with extremely low diameter for T_1 and T_2-weighted MRI. A previous study has synthesized extremely small-sized SPIONs with diameters equal to 1.5–3.7 nanometers through oleate reduction. The compact structure of these nanomaterials facilitated the establishment of T_1 contrast, attributed to its high relative surface area with unpaired electrons and a weak magnetic moment (Kim et al. 2011). To further improve the imaging capabilities of SPIONs, previous work has also optimized procedures to reduce magnetic coupling. The introduction of SiO_2 into the nanocomposite was performed through flame aerosol synthesis, and this ultimately reduced the magnetic coupling by providing additional space between the SPIONs (Teleki et al. 2009).

There has also been work done to study how various factors, such as size, crystallinity, surface chemistry, and morphology, impact the performance of SPIONs. Decreases in nanocluster sizes not only result in the specific paramagnetic properties but also correlate to higher saturation magnetization as well as T_2 relaxivities (Li et al. 2017a; Nguyen et al. 2021). Chemical composition of nanomaterials and composites is also very important, as it contributes to water solubility and hydrophobicity, which are critical parameters when the goal is to achieve relaxivity for MRI applications. Different polymers, including polyacrylic acid (PAA), PEI, and polyvinylpyrrolidone (PVP), can be coated onto SPIONs, but previous studies have shown that PAA results in the highest relaxivity (Anderson et al. 2019). The ability and performance of SPION contrast agents can be enhanced through conjugating them with biomolecules, including but not limited to folic acid, hyaluronic acid, or specific antibodies (Zhi et al. 2020). For example, SPION nanoclusters can be conjugated with PEG cross-linked to a pH-low insertion peptide (pHLIP). The SPION nanoclusters were generated, and because the tumor microenvironment is relatively acidic, the pHLIP undergoes a conformational change for membrane insertion. In addition to its primary role as a model for studying membrane protein folding, pHLIP serves as a valuable agent for targeting diseased tissues and transporting molecules across cell membranes into the cytoplasm in environments with high extracellular acidity, such as those found in cancer and inflammation (Wei et al. 2017).

Strategically designing and modifying nanomaterials can imbue them with multifunctional properties, enabling multimodal imaging and concurrent therapeutic applications. This advancement is highly advantageous as it reduces the necessity for multiple contrast agents and streamlines the theranostic process (Xue et al. 2021). Previous work has demonstrated that carbon-encapsulated SPIONs can be developed that are capable of imaging purposes through optical fluorescence and MRI. This nanocomposite was produced using a solvothermal reaction involving ferrocene, and the generated nanomaterials had a relatively smaller size when compared to previous SPION-carbon composites. Moreover, the material is removed from major organs rapidly and shows enhanced relaxivity compared to traditional agents currently used in clinical practice. The nanocomposite also had the capability of optical-based in vivo imaging of tumors (640-nanometer excitation wavelength). Additionally, the NIR of composited SPIONs achieved a photothermal conversion efficiency of 20.03%, effectively inhibiting tumors through photothermal therapy (Anderson et al. 2019). In another approach, gold nanostars were grown on Fe_3O_4@Ag seeds for multimodal imaging through CT and MRI. In addition, PEI was immobilized on the surface of the nanostars, which allowed modification with hyaluronic acid and specific targeting of CD44-overexpressing tumors. High T_2 relaxivity was achieved using this material, and the gold nanostar surface allowed a high degree of X-ray attenuation for CT imaging. Finally, the multifunctional SPIONs also demonstrate photothermal effects, as tumor ablation was observed in murines as the temperature increased from 32.8 to 58.9 °C within the tumor region (Li et al. 2015).

4.5 Nanocomposite-Based Biosensors for Medical Diagnostic Applications

4.5.1 Continuous Glucose Monitoring

Diabetes mellitus, impacting millions worldwide, is a metabolic disorder characterized by chronic high blood sugar levels. This condition presents significant public health challenges due to its prevalence and associated complications. Effective diabetes management requires a multifaceted approach, including medication, lifestyle modifications, and regular monitoring of blood glucose levels to prevent both immediate and long-term health issues (Seewoodhary 2020). Continuous glucose monitoring (CGM) systems have dramatically transformed diabetes management by offering real-time insights into glucose levels. This advanced technology enables patients to make more accurate insulin dosing decisions and better manage their condition. By continuously tracking glucose levels, CGM systems provide valuable data that helps both type 1 and type 2 diabetes patients achieve better glycemic control. Additionally, these systems have been instrumental in reducing the incidence of hypoglycemia, thereby enhancing the overall quality of life for those living with diabetes (Cappon et al. 2019). The ability to monitor glucose levels in real-time allows for timely interventions and more personalized treatment plans, ultimately leading to improved health outcomes. CGMs can also be suited for longitudinal tracking and blood glucose prediction through advanced machine learning algorithms (Sen 2025).

CGMs function as they are placed right under the skin to measure glucose levels in interstitial fluid, which is correlated to blood glucose concentrations. There are also alternative sample types that have been explored for noninvasive glucose monitoring, including sweat, saliva, and tears. However, CGMs are most accurate when sampling interstitial fluid as they are more closely correlated with blood glucose levels (Shang et al. 2022). Additionally, interstitial fluids are generally more available for glucose detection over the alternative sample types. CGMs utilize an enzymatic-based sensing mechanism, in which glucose oxidase (GOx) is immobilized as a sensing element on an electrode. Upon exposure to glucose, GOx catalyzes the oxidation of glucose into gluconic acid as well as hydrogen peroxide (H_2O_2). Hydrogen peroxide is then oxidized at the surface of the electrode and generates a measurable electric current that is proportional to the concentration of glucose in the interstitial fluids (Yoo and Lee 2010). First-generation glucose sensors use molecular oxygen as a cofactor and therefore are subject to variation from interferences of other electroactive chemical species (Lee et al. 2018). Second-generation biosensors overcame these limitations in oxygen dependence and therefore integrate a ferrocene-based redox mediator. Other redox mediators have also been explored, including but not limited to hydroquinone, tetrathiafulvalene, methylene blue, ferricyanide, thionine, transition metal complexes, or osmium-containing redox hydrogels (Chaubey and Malhotra 2002).

While second-generation biosensors are ideal for finger-prick test strips (in vitro), they are not compatible with CGMs (in vivo) due to the leaching of the toxic redox mediator. There have been efforts to alleviate this issue through developing the third generation of biosensors that are designed to directly transfer electrons from the active site of the enzyme to the electrode (Saha et al. 2023). However, the protein has a relatively large insulating layer acting as a potential barrier for electrons, and therefore electrons directly tunnel from the redox active center of the enzyme to the electrode (Guo and Li 2010). Compared to the first and second generations, third-generation biosensors have limited sensitivity as well as a relatively smaller dynamic linear range for quantification. Third-generation sensors are continuously being designed and tested for improvements in analytical performance (Saha et al. 2023). Beyond enzymatic electrochemical-based sensors, there are reasons to explore alternative sensor types for CGM applications. For example, GOx is unstable at pH levels less than 2 and greater than 8. Moreover, increases in relative humidity above 40% can drastically reduce enzymatic activity and associated sensor sensitivity. Traditional glucose biosensors also have relatively high costs for fabrication (Zaidi and Shin 2016; Adeel et al. 2021). Non-enzymatic biosensors can be designed to operate by directly oxidizing glucose on an electrode that has electrocatalytic properties and includes a transition metal center (Duan et al. 2019; Mohammadpour-Haratbar et al. 2022b).

The development of non-enzymatic electrochemical biosensors for glucose detection represents the fourth generation of devices. These sensors are not only easier to fabricate since they negate challenges in enzyme immobilization, but they are also far more stable (Gamessa et al. 2018). Of utmost importance, fourth-generation biosensors have incorporated functionalized nanomaterials, including polymer nanocomposites, that show outstanding potential in increasing the performance of glucose biosensors. These materials not only can act as catalysts for electron transfer but can also serve as immobilization platforms for additional sensing elements (Gorle et al. 2021; Osuna et al. 2022). The most important step in designing a non-enzymatic biosensor is the choice of a catalyst for glucose detection, and there has been extensive research studying the performance and properties of different materials (Waqas et al. 2020). Non-enzymatic electrocatalysts come in various forms, including metallic nanoparticles, MOx nanoparticles, bimetallic or alloy nanostructures, carbon-based nanomaterials, and nanocomposites that combine metallic and carbon-based nanomaterials (Mohammadpour-Haratbar et al. 2022b). It should be noted that although nanomaterial composites are required for non-enzymatic biosensors, they can also be used in the development of enzymatic-based sensors as well, since they can be utilized for immobilizing GOx or other biological sensing elements (Wang et al. 2022).

4.5.1.1 Overview of Nanomaterial Function in Glucose Biosensors

Different nanostructured materials have been implemented in enzymatic and non-enzymatic glucose biosensors, including but not limited to carbon-based materials such as CNTs, metallic nanoparticles, metal oxides, as well as nano-hybrids. First and foremost, nanomaterials can be used as a platform for the immobilization of enzyme-based sensing elements, including GOx. Enzyme immobilization is a key step in the development of biosensors, and many different nanomaterials of different chemical composition, shape, and size have been implemented as electrode materials for this purpose (Zhu et al. 2015). The sophisticated design of nanomaterials opens numerous opportunities for tailoring their properties, thereby enhancing their effectiveness and functionality in enzyme immobilization. By manipulating the structural and chemical characteristics of these nanomaterials, scientists can optimize their interaction with enzymes, leading to improved stability, activity, and reusability (Batool et al. 2019). Because nanomaterials have unique biocompatible properties, enzyme immobilization does not lead to denaturation or associated loss of bioactivity. Many nanomaterial composites possess some surface charge, thus enzyme-based sensing elements may, in some cases, be able to be non-covalently immobilized through electrostatic adsorption. Other nanomaterials, including but not limited to AuNPs and CNTs, allow enzymes to be covalently immobilized to the surface directly (Gole et al. 2001, 2002).

Beyond immobilization of sensing elements, nanomaterials and composites can also act as mediators, thus facilitating the electron transfer between the biomolecules and the electrode surface (Hayat et al. 2014). The traditionally used mediators discussed above can be replaced with metallic nanoparticles that ultimately increase sensor sensitivity as well as response time. Although metallic nanomaterials are widely integrated, non-metallic materials can also be used to enrich the flow rate of electron transfer. The enhancement of electron transfer is highly dependent not only on the conductivity of the nanomaterial, but also on the arrangement they are developed (Xiao et al. 2003). Because nanomaterials and composites demonstrate a high order of organization in their arrangement, analytes such as glucose are transported rapidly on the surface of the transducer. In turn, this enhances the catalytic activity, response times, as well as sensitivity of the biosensor device. The high degree of organization also results in more homogenous immobilization of the sensing elements, which reduces the variability of the measured signal (Hayat et al. 2014). Finally, nanomaterials can also act as signal amplifiers to facilitate ultra-sensitive detection using biosensors (Lei and Ju 2012). These approaches generally utilize novel labels with signal amplification processes to increase overall performance. The most widely utilized method is the integration of nano-signal amplification, using materials including but not limited to carbon nanomaterials like CNTs, metallic nanoparticles, and metal oxides (Ding et al. 2013). Nanomaterials implemented here can enhance the signal of the recognition event, as well as ensure that electrons are produced through the electrochemical reaction (Xiao and Li 2008).

4.5.1.2 Carbon Nanomaterials and Composites

Over the years, carbon-based materials have garnered much attention in the noninvasive and continuous analysis of glucose (Fang and Wang 2013; Huang et al. 2010). These materials exhibit a wide range of morphologies, including one-dimensional structures like CNTs, two-dimensional forms such as graphene and graphitic carbons, and zero-dimensional entities like fullerenes and carbon quantum dots. This diversity in structure results in a variety of electrochemical properties (Batool et al. 2019; Liu et al. 2007). Because CNTs have a very high surface-to-volume ratio and can facilitate rapid electron transfer, they have been widely utilized for electrochemical glucose sensors. In enzyme-based sensors specifically, graphene can overcome challenges in protein hindrances that obstruct the biologically active site through facilitating the direct flow of electrons (Kang et al. 2009). For example, single layers of reduced graphene oxide can be utilized to functionalize the sensing element GOx, which in turn facilitates direct electron transfer into the sensor electrode (Wang et al. 2009). To further bolster the electrochemical properties of the biosensor, carbon-based materials can also be tailored through the modification of both chemical and physical properties. One example of this is that doping heteroatoms within the carbon nanomaterial structure can enhance overall catalytic properties. A microwave-treated N-functionalized doped graphene sensing layer was implemented as an enzyme-free biosensor for glucose detection, and it showed low limit of detection, high sensitivity, and a relatively wide linear dynamic range (Rahsepar et al. 2019).

The performance of carbon-based biosensors for glucose detection can be further enhanced through incorporation polymers, ionic liquids, biomolecules, or other types of materials. In this, a popular route is to functionalize CNTs or graphene with chitosan, a biocompatible polymer that is widely utilized in glucose biosensing applications. Not only is it biocompatible, making it ideal for biomedical applications, but it also has a high concentration of primary amines, which can interact with glucose analytes (Batool et al. 2019). A chitosan core-shelled CNT sensing layer was previously fabricated onto an indium tin oxide electrode to develop an enzyme-based glucose biosensor. In this case, GOx was employed as the sensing layer, and the nanomaterial composite acted as the mediator. Upon characterization and testing, the optimal composition of the layer was identified, and the developed glucose biosensor had a high capability for electron transfer (rate constant (k_s) equal to 8.2 s^{-1}) (Choi et al. 2019). Similar approaches using chitosan-based nano-hybrids have also been employed in non-enzymatic biosensors. A previous study prepared a novel composite of copper nanoparticles deposited onto CNTs and chemically modified with ferrocene-branched chitosan. The specific incorporation of ferrocene-based derivatives improves sensor conductivity, given that ferrocenes in general have appropriate electrochemical properties, including reversibility, stability, and suitable regeneration of electrochemically active species (Wang et al. 2020).

Ionic liquids have also been integrated with carbon-based nanomaterials to increase sensor performance. A glucose biosensor incorporating an ionic liquid functionalized with reduced graphene oxide and bi-metallic Ni-Pd nanoparticles was synthesized and immobilized to a glassy carbon electrode in a basic medium. The Ni-based nanoparticles demonstrate high electro-catalytic activity for glucose detection, and this is further improved through the incorporation of Pd nanoparticles. The specific incorporation of the ionic liquid not only facilitated a more controlled synthesis of the metallic nanoparticles but also prohibited graphene oxide aggregation. Further, the results demonstrated that the biosensor had a wide dynamic linear range between 0.0002 and 10.0 mM, with a limit of detection equal to 0.03 μM (Naeim et al. 2018). To enhance film formation on the surface of the biosensor without dampening the ability for electron transfer, conductive polymer composites have been used with carbon nanomaterials in glucose biosensors. One example of this is the fabrication of a polyaniline (PANI) grafted multiwalled CNT onto a Nafion–silica nanocomposite with immobilized GOx. The novel biosensor had increased catalytic activity, owing to the electrochemical properties of Nafion, silica, CNTs, and the conducting polymer (Gopalan et al. 2009).

4.5.1.3 Metallic Nanoparticles and Metal Oxides

In addition to carbon-based nanostructures, metallic nanoparticles and MOx nanomaterials have also been used significantly in glucose biosensor fabrication for immobilization of sensing elements. Not only do they exhibit high surface area, but they also demonstrate high biocompatibility, chemical stability, and conductivity (Rhouati et al. 2018). Through providing an increased surface area for GOx immobilization and increasing the ability for electron transfer between the sensing element and the electrode, these materials are well suited to increase performance (Li et al. 2009). Metallic nanoparticles used to date for this application include, but are not limited to, copper, zinc, silver, iron, palladium, gold, and platinum, along with their alloys. By integrating two different metallic nanoparticles into a nano-hybrid, several properties can be enhanced that could not be obtained by only using one of the metallic nanoparticles. One example of this is that the limited catalytic efficiency of gold can be improved by incorporating platinum alloys, which work together to boost the overall catalytic performance (Mott et al. 2007). Polymers and other thin films can also be integrated into a metallic-based nanocomposite to prevent leaching of the sensing elements, increase surface stability, and maintain the chemical and conformational integrity of the biosensor components (Saei et al. 2013).

AuNPs are the most common metallic nanomaterials incorporated into electrochemical-based sensors for glucose detection, given they have a relatively high affinity for GOx. Gold nanoparticles are often integrated into the biosensor matrix with ZnO nanomaterials, given that they are biocompatible and have a high surface-to-bulk ratio, electrochemical activity, and stability. Moreover, the high isoelectric point (IEP) of ZnO creates a positively charged environment, making it suitable for immobilizing enzymes with low IEP, such as glucose oxidase (Tian et al. 2002; Rodriguez et al. 2000). Nanocomposites of gold and ZnO can be used to encapsulate the GOx sensing element and facilitate rapid electron transfer. Mandal et al. reported the creation of gold nanoelectrode ensembles to boost the sensitivity of electrochemical glucose biosensors. They incorporated ZnO nanorods to transform the active reaction area from a flat, two-dimensional surface to a more complex, three-dimensional structure, thereby enhancing electron transfer. The study demonstrated that the gold ensemble-based working electrode produced a higher current response and faster response time compared to previously reported enzymatic electrochemical sensors (Mandal et al. 2017). It should also be noted that gold can also be complexed with silver nanoparticles (AgNPs), given that Ag demonstrates desirable catalytic properties that Au lacks. Research in electrochemistry has highlighted the importance of Au-Ag nanoparticles in improving glucose biosensing. These nanoparticles enhance electron transfer, boost stability, and increase the sensitivity of the sensors, making them more effective for glucose detection (Ren et al. 2005).

AuNPs are also often integrated with chitosan into nanocomposites, given that chitosan is a very biocompatible material, and metallic nanoparticles enhance stability, catalytic activity, as well as electron transfer for the detection of electrochemically active species (Luo et al. 2004). Various techniques have been explored for glucose detection, including the straightforward electrochemical deposition of biofilms, single-step electrodeposition, and LbL assembly protocols. These methods have demonstrated remarkable analytical performance, exhibiting high stability and rapid electrochemical response times. Among these approaches, the single-step electrodeposition method has proven to be the most sensitive, offering superior detection capabilities (Du et al. 2007; Wu et al. 2007a). AuNP-chitosan composites can also be deposited onto platinum electrodes that have been chemically modified using Prussian blue to increase sensor performance (Xue et al. 2006). In a similar fashion, iron oxide nanoparticles can also be integrated with chitosan to deposit thin films onto an indium tin oxide electrode. The composite was used to adsorb GOx as a sensing element, and the specific incorporation of chitosan prohibits the agglomeration of MOx nanomaterials without infringing on the desirable catalytic properties (Kaushik et al. 2008). Chemically modified tin oxide nanotube arrays can also be utilized to immobilize the GOx/chitosan sensing matrix. The nanotubes serve as a great route for sensing layer immobilization, given that they have a relatively large surface area and a high degree of uniformity (Benvenuto et al. 2009).

Metallic nanoparticles have also been integrated with conducting polymers, including but not limited to PANI and polypyrrole (PPy). GOx enzymes can be easily immobilized onto the backbone of the conducting polymer, and therefore, these materials are widely used in biosensing applications for glucose (Gerard et al. 2002). One example of this is that AuNPs can be composited with PANI to synthesize nanofibers that immobilize GOx for electrochemical-based sensing of glucose. The methods for encapsulation, which are implemented, allow for the promotion of lateral growth rather than polymeric branching, and in turn, this increases the concentration of GOx immobilized on the sensing layer (Mazeiko et al. 2013). A more recent study examined the fabrication of enzyme-based AuNP sensors, where PANI or PPy was used to immobilize GOx on a graphite rod electrode. The study synthesized dendritic gold nanostructures and determined that utilizing PPy for enzyme immobilization was optimal, since it was 1.35 times more sensitive. The developed biosensor had a relatively low limit of detection (0.070 mmol/L), a wide linear range, adequate reproducibility (8.01%), and long storage time (33 days) (German et al. 2022). Researchers have also developed copper-platinum nanoparticles, which can be successfully modified on a glassy carbon electrode to fabricate non-enzymatic glucose biosensors. Platinum is a widely utilized nanomaterial in biosensor development, since they have unique catalytic properties as well as high electron conductivity. Incorporating additional metals to form bimetallic alloys can prevent catalyst poisoning and enhance electrocatalytic activity through synergistic interactions. Specifically, copper can reduce the cost of platinum electrocatalysts and enhance biosensor performance by modifying the D-band center of platinum (Wang et al. 2023).

4.5.2 Liquid Biopsy for Cancer Diagnosis

Cancer is an overarching challenge in global health, given that in 2025, it is projected that there will be 21 million newly diagnosed cancer cases. Moreover, the global cancer mortality rate is approximately 100 deaths per 100,000 cases, with a total of around 10 million deaths annually (Siegel et al. 2025). The relatively high mortality rate is because many patients do not have access to adequate healthcare resources, and cancer cases tend to be diagnosed at an advanced stage. Moreover, tumor heterogeneity contributes to variations in cancer growth, invasiveness, and susceptibility to treatment (Li et al. 2019b). The gold standard for cancer diagnosis is tissue biopsy, but this technique has challenges in determining cancer subtype/stage and therefore is only equipped to provide a general overview of malignancy (Vaidyanathan et al. 2019). Multiple biopsies could provide more precise and accurate information, but this is not practical, given that it is difficult to abstract samples and the procedure itself is invasive. Tissue biopsies face several other challenges, including but not limited to patient inconvenience, clinical risks, sample preparation issues, sensitivity and precision concerns, potential surgical complications, and financial considerations. It should also be noted that the pathological results from a single biopsy may not reflect the whole genome of the entire tumor (Heitzer et al. 2019).

Due to the limitations of tissue biopsies as described above, researchers have been seeking to develop new approaches to monitor tumor dynamics as well as genetics. As a result of technological advancements in cancer research and biomedical innovation, new screening methods have been developed that utilize body fluid samples instead of tissue samples. This approach is commonly known as a liquid biopsy (Bratulic et al. 2021). Viable sample types for liquid biopsy include urine, saliva, and cerebrospinal fluid, but blood is by far the most common sample matrix. These emerging techniques develop platform technologies that facilitate sensitive and selective detection of target biomarkers in bodily fluids. Circulating targets could include, but are not limited to, nucleic acids, proteins, extracellular vesicles (EVs), and microRNAs. Beyond simply diagnosing cancer, liquid biopsies are also well suited for prognosis as well as treatment monitoring scenarios. Liquid biopsy, in general, has the potential to offer a noninvasive method for early cancer diagnosis, monitoring tumor progression in real-time, and predicting/monitoring the efficacy of treatments (McCartney et al. 2019; Wang et al. 2017b). The overarching vision is for liquid biopsies to spatially and temporally resolve tumor heterogeneity, in turn bolstering patient care and clinical outcomes (Wan et al. 2017).

Even though liquid biopsies can revolutionize the way cancer is diagnosed and treated, this technology has not been adopted into clinical practice for several reasons. A primary challenge in detecting cancer biomarkers in these sample types is that they have relatively low molecular weight and significantly low concentration levels while in circulation. Another issue is that liquid biopsy sample types often constitute a very complex sample matrix containing a multitude of biomolecules, which could cause noise and interference. Therefore, liquid biopsy platforms require biomarker signal amplification (Kalogianni 2021; Singh et al. 2023). Even though there are existing benchtop instruments that have the capability of achieving high sensitivity/selectivity, these devices tend to be expensive, occupy a relatively large footprint, and require trained personnel to run high-quality assays. In addition, biomarker analyses require sample pretreatment procedures, including the isolation of CTCs (Park et al. 2018). Recent advancements in architecture, design, and technology have significantly enabled noninvasive point of-care solutions. The integration of liquid biopsies with innovative miniaturized platforms, utilizing engineered nanomaterials and biosensing techniques, has resulted in the development of point-of-care systems that are easy to use and economical. Research in nanomaterials and composites has significantly elevated the profile of liquid biopsy platforms, as they can act as signal enhancers without using enzymatic reactions or multiple preparation steps for enhancement. This is because of their unique and excellent electrical, electrochemical, and optical properties (Ma et al. 2024). An overview of liquid biopsy approaches using nanocomposite biosensor technology is shown in Fig. 4.4 (Woollam 2025c).

4.5.2.1 Cancer Biomarker Types

As previously discussed, liquid biopsies most often analyze blood samples for the detection of different biomarkers, including but not limited to CTCs, microRNA, proteins, circulating tumor DNA (ctDNA), and exosomes (Adhit et al. 2023). When developing a cancer biosensor for liquid biopsy, there are benefits and disadvantages to different types of biomarkers. For example, although CTCs show benefits

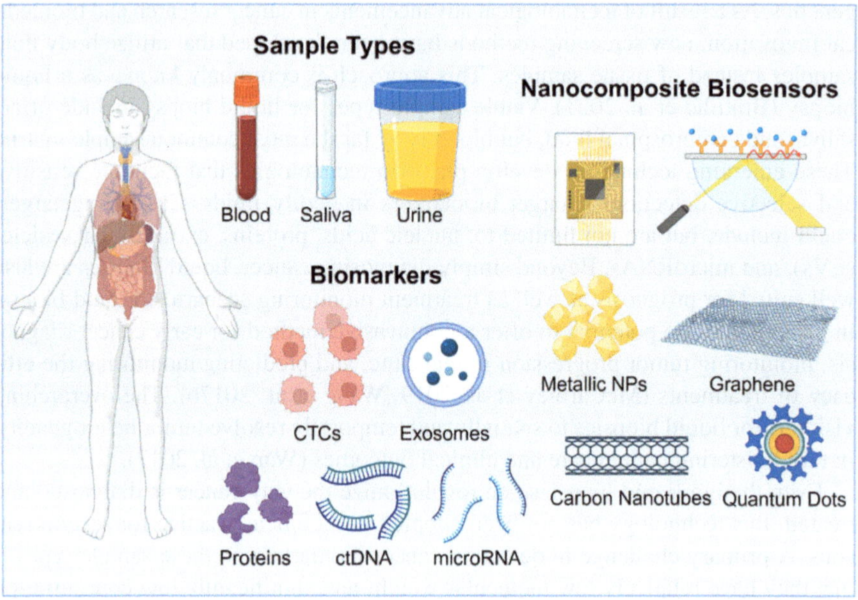

Fig. 4.4 Illustration summarizing different nanocomposite-based approaches for liquid biopsy (Woollam 2025c)

such as the fact that they can be detected noninvasively, these cells are often presented at very low concentration/abundance, which makes isolation and detection challenging. Other challenges with CTCs include that they can display heterogeneity, which could complicate the analysis and conclusions drawn from the results. Nonetheless, CTCs hold important biochemical information that could be used for both diagnostic and prognostic applications in cancer research and liquid biopsy (Ju et al. 2022). ctDNA technology, on the other hand, is more mature compared to CTCs, given they are relatively more stable and easier to isolate from blood. ctDNA biomarkers in general are more sensitive for cancer detection and provide an unprecedented amount of biomolecular information on the tumor. Nonetheless, ctDNA assays also have challenges, including the fact that they provide limited information beyond genomics. Furthermore, in cases where cancer induces a low level of genetic mutations, these assays could have difficulty with accuracy. It should also be noted that these assays also have difficulty in differentiating ctDNA from DNA fragments originating from necrotic/apoptotic cells, and this can significantly confound the analysis (Singh et al. 2023; Hofman et al. 2019).

EVs, including exosomes have also been targeted for cancer biomarkers in different applications, since they provide a rich source of biomolecular information on DNA, RNA, proteins, lipids, and even metabolites. Exosomes also demonstrate outstanding biological stability, which in turn helps preserve the molecular components. Nonetheless, the biggest challenge in EV and exosome analysis is the fact that they have a relatively small size, and therefore they are difficult to isolate

(Kumar et al. 2024). MicroRNA has been widely utilized in liquid biopsies for cancer diagnosis, as they can be used as early-stage biomarkers before the appearance of any symptoms. These biomolecules are clinically relevant, since they are intricately involved in cellular metabolic processes in both normal and diseased conditions. However, microRNA profiling in liquid biopsies also has inherent limitations. The biggest challenge in harnessing the potential of microRNA biomarkers is stability. Not only can microRNA rapidly degrade in various biological sample types, but this is further complicated by the fact that storage conditions can also introduce heterogeneity in analyte degradation (Das et al. 2024; Suárez et al. 2022). Finally, different proteins have also been targeted for detection by liquid biopsy platforms. Benefits here include the fact that proteins are easy to isolate, along with the fact that methods for sample preparation and analysis are or can be easily standardized. However, a challenge that remains is protein stability. Over the course of time, proteins in samples may aggregate and therefore lose biological functionality. Native proteins may undergo significant conformational changes as well, which can also lead to agglomeration (Hu et al. 2022).

4.5.2.2 Sample Pretreatment and Biomarker Purification

Prior to detection, in traditional analyses, it is first required to undertake sample preparation procedures to isolate the analytes of interest (cancer biomarkers). Many different technologies and methods have been developed for isolation/purification (Soda et al. 2019), and these will be discussed briefly. Immunomagnetic purification techniques have been developed over the years to isolate CTCs, and the only commercialized test for this application is the CellSearch CTCs System, which uses immunomagnetic nanoparticles that target Epithelial Cell Adhesion Molecule (EpCAM) to isolate/preconcentrate tumor cells (Eslami et al. 2020). However, a downfall of this technique is that EpCAM and Cytokeratin target antigens in general can demonstrate significant heterogeneity on the surface of tumor cells, and this will directly impact isolation efficiency and purity. More highly specific techniques can be harnessed through developing strategies that target proteins or receptors that present themselves within the exosome membrane (Eslami et al. 2020). Size-based enrichment techniques can also be employed to separate cells and isolate CTCs by taking advantage of the physical differences between CTCs and healthy blood cells. Size exclusion chromatography, on the other hand, can be used to separate exosomes from other macromolecules present in the sample matrix (Dilsiz 2024).

However, ultracentrifugation is the most widely used isolation technique for exosomes, and therefore is regarded as the gold standard. This technique has distinct benefits over other methods, including the fact that they do not require extensive sample preparation or treatment procedures prior to analysis. Filtration can also be coupled with ultracentrifugation, as it can directly remove undesirable cellular debris. Polymer precipitation methods can also be employed for the isolation of exosomes from complex sample matrices, which can be resuspended in buffers for quantitative analysis. Research indicates that commercially available kits provide the highest yield of isolated exosomes from clinical samples and are more straightforward and efficient than other methods (Coughlan et al. 2020; Li et al. 2017b).

Finally, microfluidic devices have been fabricated for sample pretreatment, since they allow efficient control over the transport of fluids, including liquid-based biological sample types (blood, urine, saliva, etc.). For example, to isolate CTCs using a microfluidic device, anti-EpCAM antibodies can be functionalized onto microposts within the system. Beyond CTCs, there have also been efforts to develop microfluidic platforms for the enhanced purification of exosomes, but current technologies are at a relatively early stage (Descamps et al. 2022).

4.5.2.3 Traditional Methods for Cancer Biomarker Detection

Sequencing and amplification technologies, such as the polymerase chain reaction (PCR), are the gold standard and most widely utilized method for the characterization/detection of CTCs. PCR-based technology was initially developed over two decades ago, and since then, they have been widely utilized for CTC detection. Specifically, reverse transcription-PCR (RT-PCR) and quantitative RT-PCR (qRT-PCR) are ideal for the detection of transcription factors related to cancer cells, including microRNA biomarkers (Labib and Kelley 2021). Several methods have been devised to enhance sensitivity for nucleic acid detection, such as Allele-Specific Amplification (AS) PCR, Peptide Nucleic Acid-Locked Nucleic Acid (PNA-LNA) PCR, and Co-Amplification at Lower Denaturation Temperatures (COLD) PCR. Digital PCR (dPCR), on the other hand, is an advanced technique for quantification and amplification of nucleic acids, and this method is widely utilized for detecting ctDNA point mutations. This method presents several benefits, but the most important is the fact that this technique partitions the sample into droplets which enables a more sensitive and robust analysis. It should also be noted that next-generation sequencing (NGS) technology is also emerging as a technique to detect and quantify DNA and RNA, which expands coverage across the genome and allows untargeted approaches to be undertaken for biomarker discovery purposes (Soda et al. 2019).

Microfluidic devices can also be used as an alternative for the development of cancer biomarker detection modalities and have shown great potential for benefit across liquid biopsy platforms. Microfluidics is a popular solution since it facilitates rapid sample processing and accurate control over the flow of biofluids. To date, in scientific literature, there have been a wide array of strategies integrating microfluidic approaches for the detection of multiple biomarker types (CTCs, ctDNA, microRNA, etc.). There are multiple strategies to isolate and detect cancer biomarkers, one of which includes the previously described CTC chip, which uses EpCAM antibodies to bind cancer cells that can be detected and quantified using digital cameras (Habli et al. 2020). Magnetic particles can also be integrated within microfluidic platforms, which can be utilized to isolate biomarkers and analyze them through confocal fluorescence microscopy. There have also been recent advancements in developing microfluidic devices that specifically isolate/detect exosomes, and these strategies have been shown to be rapid, efficient, and produce high purification yields (Liu et al. 2024).

Some of the most widely utilized methods for cancer biomarker detection include the use of immunoassays (Kumar et al. 2019). The enzyme-linked immunosorbent assay (ELISA) is a very popular technique that is used for detection, where exosomes in circulation are immobilized on a well plate. After the plate is treated with blocking agents, a recognition antibody is introduced to the sample and binds to the target if present. Subsequently, an enzyme-conjugated antibody is added, which binds to the target complex and reacts with a specific substrate to produce a measurable signal (Wu et al. 2007b). Aside from ELISA, there are also other immunoassay techniques that can be used for cancer biomarker detection. The previously described CellSearch system not only isolates CTCs through EpCAM antibodies, but samples can also be treated with a nuclear stain (4′,6-diamidino-2-phenylindole, DAPI) as well as a fluorescent cytokeratin stain for detection via automated imaging techniques. Recently, there have also been advancements in immunohistochemical approaches to analyze CTCs through implementation antibodies that achieve a highly sensitive and selective detection. However, these methods are still considered premature and a major challenge that exists is the fact that most cancer types do not have well-defined tumor biomarkers for isolation/detection (Soda et al. 2019; Habli et al. 2020).

4.5.2.4 Nanocomposite Biosensors for Liquid Biopsy

Nanomaterial science has recently become a popular area of investigation in the field of medical diagnostics, given its unique and outstanding physicochemical properties (Azad and Chandra 2025). These properties include, but are not limited to, high surface-to-volume ratio, adequate biocompatibility, and desirable catalytic properties (Kalogianni 2021). Nanoparticles and materials have been incorporated into several different types of biosensors with various modes of transduction, including optical, chemiresistive, piezoelectric, acoustic, and, most importantly, electrochemical. Although all transducer types are used throughout the literature, electrochemical biosensors represent unique benefits, since they are cost-effective to fabricate, offer high sensitivity, and only require the use of straightforward instrumentation to translate an analog signal (Mikaeeli Kangarshahi et al. 2024). More specifically, nanomaterials can be integrated into liquid biopsy biosensors as surface modifiers of the electrodes, as well as signaling labels. For example, modification of the electrode surface using functionalized nanomaterials facilitates signal enrichment through increased catalytic activity and conductivity. Nanomaterials could also provide more transient interactions between analytes and sensing elements to facilitate electron transfer during the biological recognition event. Beyond electrode surface modification, nanoparticles can also be conjugated with signaling molecules (redox-active species or enzymes) for signal enrichment (Kalogianni 2021). There have been tremendous efforts in research and development focusing on utilizing unique nanostructured materials to enhance the analytical detection of cancer biomarkers in liquid biopsy platforms. These integrated materials play a crucial role in advancing technology platforms for diagnostics, prognostics, continuous health monitoring, and various biomedical applications. Recent publications demonstrate the wide use of nanomaterials to enrich biosensor signaling and transduction methods. Many different types of materials have been explored, and among these, the most popular in literature are magnetic nanoparticles, metallic nanoparticles, carbon-based nanomaterials, and conductive polymer composites (Wang et al. 2024a). These can be utilized in various detection and transduction methods to immobilize sensing elements effectively. For example, metallic nanoparticles, including AuNPs have unique physicochemical properties (large surface area, high catalytic activity, biocompatibility) which allow them to be used in electronic- and optical-based biosensor devices for signal enrichment (Malik et al. 2023).

4.5.2.4.1 Electrochemical Biosensors

Biosensors involving electrochemical transduction methods have been widely implemented in the field of liquid biopsy using an array of different approaches (Azad and Chandra 2023). For example, there has been much attention in the development of electrochemical sensor platforms that employ biological recognition elements that capture exosomes and selectively detect surface antigens related to cancer. Here, antibodies are tagged with electroactive compounds and function as electrochemical biosensors. One example of this is the integrated magnetic-electrochemical exosome (iMEX) platform, which is a miniaturized system that can efficiently isolate and detect exosomes related to cancer cells from human plasma with very high sensitivity (Fig. 4.5 (Woollam 2025d; Jeong et al. 2016)). To do this, analysis using the iMEX platform requires two steps: magnetic isolation and electrochemical-based detection. In the first step, cancer cell-specific exosomes can be captured using immunomagnetic beads. Secondary antibodies that also bind to the target exosome are utilized with a conjugated enzyme, in this case, horseradish peroxidase (HRP). The immunomagnetic beads are homogenized with a chromogenic electron-mediator (3,3′,5,5′-tetramethylbenzidine, TMB). The HRP catalyzes the oxidation of TMB, which in turn generates an electrical current as a measurable signal (Jeong et al. 2016). Beyond iMEX, recent advances have shown that nanomaterials may not only aid in the electrochemical detection, but also isolation of exosomes. For example, MOx nanoparticles such as TiO_2 and ZrO_2 can be used to selectively enrich phosphorylated peptides via reversible binding of phosphate groups (Fang et al. 2022). For exosome detection, a variety of different nanomaterials have been employed for signal enrichment and enhanced analysis. For example, a previous study showed that quantum dots can be functionalized with

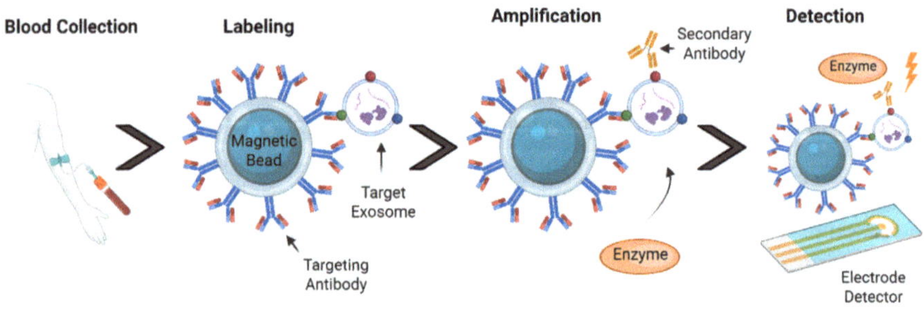

Fig. 4.5 Illustration of the different steps required to isolate and detect exosomes in human plasma using the IMEX platform (Woollam 2025d; Jeong et al. 2016)

cancer-specific antibodies. Using this assay, target exosomes are captured using immunomagnetic beads and they are quantified using CdSe quantum dots functionalized with biotinylated antibodies relating to breast and colon cancer (Boriachek et al. 2017).

Electrochemical sensors are frequently engineered to identify various microRNA biomarkers associated with cancer. This is achieved by immobilizing a receptor probe on the sensor's surface, which binds with the target microRNA on the electrode, generating a detectable signal. Due to the small size of microRNAs, the sensitivity of electrochemical platforms can be improved by labeling the target miRNA and using electrocatalytic amplification. The detection process is powered by electrochemically active reporter species, which alter interfacial properties upon microRNA hybridization. The most common types of electrochemical reporters in these types of biosensors are enzymes/substrates, but can also include a range of small molecules (El Aamri et al. 2020). One example of this is that previous research has developed an electrochemical biosensor that targets microRNA 199a-5p as a biomarker for triple-negative breast cancer. The biosensor initially immobilizes graphene oxide on a glassy carbon electrode. Gold nanorods are deposited at the surface and functionalized with a complementary locked nucleic acid (LNA) probe through the mercaptan strategy. The optimized biosensor platform had very high capability for microRNA 199a-5p detection, demonstrating a dynamic linear range of 15 fM to 148 pM and a limit of detection equal to 4.5 fM. Overall, this study demonstrated that the nanobiosensor is highly sensitive and selective for the detection of miR-199a-5p, making it suitable for measuring low levels of this biomarker in blood (Ebrahimi et al. 2018).

4.5.2.4.2 Optical-Based Approaches

Nanoplasmonic-based sensing platforms, such as surface plasmon resonance (SPR), have emerged as valuable technology for liquid biopsy applications. SPR sensors utilize optical transduction (optical spectral shifts) to produce a measurable change in signal induced by local refractive index changes at the surface of the nanosensor (Fig. 4.6 (Woollam 2025e)). Unlike electrochemical methods, SPR and other

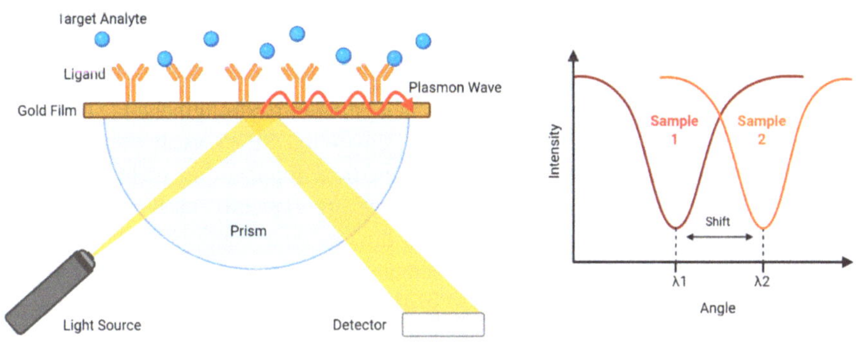

Fig. 4.6 Depiction of SPR technology utilized in optical nanosensing applications, accompanied by exemplary data (Woollam 2025e)

nanoplasmonic biosensors do not require labeling and can also be multiplexed in a facile fashion to detect an array of different cancer biomarkers. SPR has recently become a versatile method for studying molecular interactions by measuring changes in the refractive index on a chip surface (Islam and Masson 2025). This technique involves functionalizing a metal film's surface, which supports a surface plasmon, with specific biorecognition elements such as complementary nucleic acid strands or antibodies. When analyte molecules contact the SPR sensor, they bind to the biorecognition elements, increasing the refractive index at the sensor surface, which is measured optically. The refractive index change caused by the captured biomolecules is highly dependent on the target's concentration and properties. During measurement, the angular shift in the SPR spectrum is tracked over time, indicating the amount of bound target (Soda et al. 2019). Previous research has developed versatile biosensors for the detection of a multitude of microRNA biomarkers. One example of this is that a hairpin loop functionalized with a thiol group can be immobilized on a film of gold. As the target microRNA is exposed, the stem-loop structure of the hairpin unfolds, and AuNPs functionalized with nucleic acids form a DNA super sandwich when additional DNA reporters are added. Because the localized plasmon of the AuNP electronically couples with the plasmon at the sensor surface, the sensitivity for biomarker detection was significantly enhanced (Liu et al. 2017b). There are many other different nanomaterials and composites that have been integrated into SPR biosensors, but functionalized AuNPs are some of the most widely utilized.

There are other nanotechnology-based approaches regarding optical biosensors in detecting cancer biomarkers, such as surface-enhanced Raman scattering (SERS). These biosensor types have been widely studied in recent years, since they provide a robust platform for the recognition and transduction of biomolecular interactions. Overall, SERS is a facile and noninvasive method that can be used to detect and characterize molecular conformational changes induced by several types of phenomena. SERS combines the structural specificity and experimental versatility of traditional Raman spectroscopy, creating an ultrasensitive detection platform for biomolecules with the ability to perform multiplexed analyses. SERS labels can be attached to specific ligands, enabling the selective detection and localization of their target molecules. The key benefit of using nanomaterials and composites in these types of sensors is that there is significant signal enhancement. For example, when target molecules interact with nanomaterial-based sensing elements, the localized electromagnetic field of the nanoparticles is significantly strengthened (Soda et al. 2019). Because of this drastic increase in sensitivity, SERS assays tend to only require minimal amounts of sample. For biomedical applications, including cancer biomarker detection, three nanomaterial types are typically used for biosensor development: colloidal nanoparticles, two-dimensional nanomaterial structures, and SERS tags (Ilyas et al. 2023). Two-dimensional nanomaterials, as well as colloidal nanoparticles, are typically used in the development of biosensors that are tuned to detect native SERS signals correlating to the analyte being detected, where nano-based tags are usually implemented with antibodies or other sensing elements for biomarker detection. One example of this is that Choi et al. developed highly robust SERS nanotags to detect multiple protein-based analytes that are expressed on the surface of breast cancer cells. Hollow nanospheres of Ag encapsulated with Au were fabricated to enhance the electromagnetic field of the reporting molecules. Furthermore, the signal was amplified by the localization of surface electromagnetic fields via the pinholes on the surface of Au hollow nanospheres. The surface of the hybrid nanospheres was also deposited with a PEG layer, to increase the platform's durability and robustness. The results showed that these SERS nanotags enable multiplexed analysis of proteins for breast cancer cell imaging (Choi et al. 2020).

4.5.3 Other Diseases and Applications

4.5.3.1 Neurodegenerative Diseases

Neurodegenerative diseases, such as Alzheimer's and Parkinson's, are a group of progressive disorders that adversely affect the central nervous system (CNS). These conditions often begin with subtle, nonspecific symptoms that can easily go unnoticed, making early diagnosis particularly difficult (Lamptey et al. 2022). Compounding this challenge is the current lack of dedicated diagnostic tools and the absence of a universally accepted gold standard for early detection. Research has demonstrated that early intervention slows disease progression, and therefore, it is necessary to improve technologies that facilitate early detection. Moreover, neurodegenerative diseases in general place a substantial strain on healthcare systems, largely due to aging populations, prolonged disease progression, and the complexity of long-term care needs (Deuschl et al. 2020). A promising area of research that may be able to overcome these challenges is the development of nanocomposite-based biosensors that are noninvasive and cost-effective. Biosensors incorporating nanomaterials and their composites are often configured to target specific biomarkers that are circulating in bodily fluids including but not limited to blood and urine. Biomarkers for different medical conditions can be challenging to detect due to their inherent low concentrations and potentially high variability in samples collected from humans. Nanobiosensors leverage the high surface area and reactivity of nanomaterials to boost biomarker interactions, enabling earlier and more sensitive detection. The use of this technology also allows for a multiplexed detection of multiple biomarkers simultaneously and, therefore is well equipped to provide more comprehensive information for disease monitoring (Yadav et al. 2025; Dhahi et al. 2024).

Over the years, there has been a wide array of research projects that undertake nanobiosensor development for the detection of Alzheimer's and Parkinson's disease, two key neurodegenerative diseases prevalent in older adults. Alzheimer's disease is marked by progressive memory loss and cognitive decline, primarily due to the accumulation of amyloid plaques and tau tangles that damage brain cells. This leads to symptoms such as disorientation, language difficulties, mood swings, and behavioral changes (Subramanian et al. 2020). In contrast, Parkinson's disease is characterized by the gradual loss of dopamine-producing neurons, resulting in motor impairments like tremors, muscle stiffness, and slowed movement (Meder et al. 2019). For Alzheimer's, amyloid-beta and its toxic oligomers can be monitored in cerebrospinal fluid (CSF) or even other bodily fluids like blood. Beyond this specific marker, other studies have also indicated that the tau protein may also be useful clinically. Subcortical cholinergic nuclei share structural traits and are early sites of tau accumulation, forming neurofibrillary tangles. Elevated tau in CSF, coupled with neuroimaging markers, provides valuable tools for early detection and understanding disease progression. Other biomarkers for Alzheimer's can also include neuroinflammatory indicators, including but not limited to cytokines and activated microglia (Hunter et al. 2025). In Parkinson's disease research, on the other hand, nanobiosensors have been engineered to identify various structural forms of alpha-synuclein, such as oligomers, protofibrils, and fibrils. These sensors typically utilize highly specific recognition elements like antibodies or aptamers, allowing for sensitive detection of alpha-synuclein variants in biological fluids (Yadav et al. 2025; Dhahi et al. 2024).

A previous study sought to develop an electrochemical immunosensor tuned to detect beta-amyloid peptides in serum for the early detection of Alzheimer's disease (Ranjan and Khan 2022). Through the fabrication of gold nanoparticle functionalized chitosan-aligned carbon nanotube (CS-aCNT-Au) nanocomposites on glassy carbon electrodes, the antibody for beta-amyloid can be immobilized on the sensor surface. The presence of hydroxyl and amine groups promotes stable antibody attachment and helps secure the nanocomposite on the modified electrode by creating a more adhesive and retention-friendly surface. Even though native CNTs already display a relatively high conductivity and surface area, the incorporation of gold nanoparticles improved these properties even further. Signal transduction for the sensor is performed through differential pulse voltammetry (DPV), which showed that the sensor had outstandingly high sensitivity over a broad range (10 pg/mL–100 μg/mL) with low limits of detection (0.87 pg/mL). Experiments were also undertaken, spiking the target analyte into serum, with results demonstrating dynamic ranges (10 pg/mL–1 ng/mL) and limit of detections (0.95 pg/mL) that are clinically relevant. Finally, the authors also assessed sensor selectivity against potential interferents (dopamine, cortisol, and other biomolecules), which demonstrated high affinity of the immunosensor for analyte detection. Therefore, the authors conclude that this novel nanobiosensor holds promise for point-of-care detection of beta-amyloid in clinical specimens (Ranjan and Khan 2022).

Aside from Alzheimer's, there has also been work on developing a miniaturized nanocomposite-based biosensor for the early detection of Parkinson's disease. For example, a novel electrochemical immunosensor was engineered using graphene modified with gold nanoparticles to facilitate efficient bioconjugation with a biotin-labeled antibody, serving as the biorecognition element. This advanced platform enables highly sensitive and selective detection of alpha-synuclein, a key biomarker associated with Parkinson's disease. Complementing graphene with gold nanoparticles drastically increases the conductivity and surface area of the sensing layer to facilitate a rapid and sensitive detection mode. In this study, for the first time, alpha-synuclein was quantitatively detected in human plasma using the nanobiosensor.

This platform demonstrated a reliable linear detection range from 4 to 128 ng/mL, with a lower limit of quantification of 4 ng/mL. Given its high sensitivity and specificity, this sensing strategy holds strong potential for future clinical deployment, particularly in point-of-care and large-scale screening of Parkinson's disease (Aminabad et al. 2022). In a different study, a disposable electrochemical neurobiosensor was developed on indium tin oxide-coated polyethylene terephthalate (ITO-PET) electrodes. The electrode surface was functionalized with 11-amino-1-undecanethiol and enhanced with a nanocomposite of multiwalled CNTs and AuNPs to improve conductivity, stability, and biomolecule immobilization. This device was specifically developed to monitor the DJ-1 protein biomarker in CSF or saliva. The results showed that the sensor system could detect the target in the concentration range of 4.7–4700 fg/mL with a limit of detection equal to 0.5 fg/mL. Given the relevance of DJ-1 expression in CSF and saliva, the neurobiosensor's ability to detect DJ-1 in these samples was evaluated using the standard addition method. Results suggest that the biosensor offers selective and reliable detection of the DJ-1 protein (Sonuç Karaboğa and Sezgintürk 2021).

4.5.3.2 Infectious Diseases

Infectious diseases are illnesses caused by pathogens (such as viruses, bacteria, fungi, or parasites) that can be transmitted from one host to another (Lim et al. 2020). Detecting human exposure to these pathogens is essential, as infectious diseases not only pose direct health risks but can also trigger secondary complications and long-term disorders. One example of this was seen during the COVID-19 pandemic, where accurate diagnostic testing was the only way to determine if an individual was exposed to the virus. The gold standard for viral diagnostics is RT-PCR, but this method requires assay reagents, is time-consuming, and necessitates trained personnel to run and interpret test results. During the time of the pandemic, this caused a significant bottleneck in delivering diagnostic results to patients to inform social decision-making. The development of accurate, rapid, noninvasive, and cost-effective technologies is crucial, not only for detecting pathogen exposure before symptoms emerge, but also for informing timely decisions on isolation and containment. Moreover, these diagnostic technologies can also enable early intervention through early detection, be used to understand patterns of transmission, and provide data for evidence-based policymaking. Thanks to their outstanding optical, electrical, magnetic, and chemical characteristics, nanomaterial-based composites can be used to overcome these challenges through the development of novel biosensors that target specific biomarkers relating to infection, including but not limited to proteins, antigens, and nucleic acids (Sheikhzadeh et al. 2021).

In studies focusing on biosensor development for COVID-19 specifically, there have been a wide array of sensing elements to detect diverse analytes, including spike proteins, single-stranded RNA, inflammatory cytokines, and other biomarker types. Moreover, there have also been many different transduction techniques that have been undertaken, which include electrochemical, optical, colorimetric, SPR, localized surface plasmon coupled fluorescence (LSPCF), field-effect transistor (FET), as well as many others (Tewari et al. 2025). Of these transduction methods, colorimetric nanobiosensors can be attractive since pathogens can be detected simply via the naked eye (or smartphone) through color transformation. Compared to other nanocomposite biosensor types, they are also relatively easy to use and cost-effective. Incorporation of nanomaterials into colorimetric sensors drastically increases the sensitivity of these assays. AuNPs are often incorporated into biosensors, since they can be synthesized in a facile manner and have desirable biocompatibility, optoelectronic, and other properties, including the ability to be functionalized with a diverse set of chemistries through the mercaptan strategy (Yang et al. 2023). A low-cost, instrument-free colorimetric biosensor was previously developed for SARS-CoV-2 detection using AuNP-functionalized plasmonic sensors conjugated with polyclonal antibodies. Upon binding to the virus in human saliva, the formation of AuNP clusters induced visible color changes due to plasmonic coupling, achieving a detection limit of 0.28 plaque-forming units (PFU)/mL. The biosensor demonstrated high specificity, showing no cross-reactivity with influenza or dengue viruses. A smartphone-based image analysis app, enhanced with machine learning, achieved 100% diagnostic accuracy. Additionally, the sensor detected viral particles in untreated river water, requiring only 20 μL of sample, making it highly suitable for point-of-care and field-based epidemiological applications (Materón et al. 2022).

Beyond viruses, there have also been efforts in the field to develop biosensors that can sense bacteria (Xia et al. 2024). The current technologies and techniques for diagnosing bacterial infections include smear microscopy, isolation culture, and biochemical reactions. Nonetheless, these techniques are inefficient, slow, and often lack the sensitivity/specificity needed for accurate diagnosis, leading to frequent clinical errors. Thanks to the distinctive antimicrobial and physicochemical characteristics of nanomaterials and their composites, these advanced materials frequently serve dual roles in medical applications. Specifically, they enable theranostic approaches, integrating both therapeutic and diagnostic functions, thereby enhancing the precision, efficiency, and responsiveness of treatment strategies. To achieve these goals, many different methods and approaches have been employed for these applications. Among the most prominent are electrochemical techniques, photodynamic therapy, and photothermal approaches. Electrochemical approaches offer key advantages (low cost, minimal power requirements, and facile miniaturization), which make them well suited for rapid/quantitative bacterial detection. Their performance is further enhanced by integration with microfluidic and nanotechnologies, enabling sensitive, point-of-care analysis of bacteria in complex sample types (Xia et al. 2024). One example of this is that immunomagnetic nanoparticles can be coupled with urease-based signal amplification to isolate and detect *Escherichia coli* O157:H7 through microfluidics and electrochemical impedance detectors. Streptavidin-coated magnetic nanoparticles bound to biotinylated antibodies were used to isolate *E. coli* O157:H7, which were then labeled with urease- and aptamer-functionalized AuNPs. The resulting complexes catalyzed urea hydrolysis, thus reducing electrochemical impedance. The sensor's impedance response showed a stable linear relationship with a detection limit as low as 12 colony-forming units (CFU)/mL (Yao et al. 2018).

4.5.3.3 Cardiovascular Health

Cardiovascular diseases (CVDs) are defined as medical conditions that narrow the arteries that transport blood to the heart (Soler-Botija et al. 2019). According to the World Health Organization, CVDs are the leading cause of death around the globe (Organization, W. H 2017) and mainly include coronary artery disease, cardiomyopathies, atherosclerosis, high blood pressure, cerebrovascular accidents, and congestive heart failure. The current standard of care methods for diagnosing CVD in the clinic include a series of tests: electrocardiograms, measuring blood pressure, and biomedical imaging (CT and MRI). Although these tests are accurate and clinically relevant, they do not facilitate modalities for early detection of CVDs (Tang et al. 2022). Therefore, it is important to develop technologies for early-stage diagnosis that are accurate, rapid, and widely deployable. Previous studies have elucidated a range of potential target biomarkers for CVD that are present in bodily fluids. Several biomarkers associated with CVD (such as cardiac troponins, C-reactive protein (CRP), tumor necrosis factor-alpha (TNF-α), and myoglobin) have demonstrated strong potential as early indicators of cardiac dysfunction (Bakirhan et al. 2018). These biological molecules reflect various pathological processes, including myocardial injury, systemic inflammation, and oxidative stress, making them valuable tools for early diagnosis, risk stratification, and timely intervention in cardiovascular conditions.

Nanotechnology and advanced composite materials have been leveraged to develop biosensors that can detect these biomarkers with relevant measures of sensitivity and specificity. Integrating nanomaterials with diverse sensing platforms has led to the development of a wide range of nanosensors that exhibit superior attributes, including high sensitivity, strong photostability, and excellent biocompatibility. These synergistic combinations enhance detection performance across various analytical applications (Tang et al. 2022). Among the different approaches for sensor development and signal transduction, electrochemical and optical remain some of the most widely implemented approaches. An electrochemical nanobiosensor was previously developed through coating gold electrodes with a suspension of TiO_2 that can detect phosphopeptide biomarkers that are associated with cardiac health and function. Prior to detection, samples containing the targets are pretreated with AuNPs, which can bind directly to the polypeptide. TiO_2 nanoparticles selectively interact with phosphate groups on peptides, and the modified AuNPs enhance electron transfer efficiency, enabling effective detection of phosphopeptides (Chen et al. 2021). Other studies have focused on electrochemical nanosensor development for targeting cardiac troponin I (cTnI), a biomarker for CVD, which regulates muscle contractions within the heart (Chen et al. 2024). Flexible electrochemical nanocomposites have also been developed for applications in wearable technology. For example, a previous study showed that fabrication of CNT/PDMS composites functionalized with gold nanomaterials facilitates real-time detection of H_2O_2, which is linked to oxidative stress and CVD. The sensor's sandwich-like nano-Au/CNT network structure imparts strong mechanical integrity and superior electrochemical properties. The resulting nanobiosensor enables sensitive H_2O_2 detection, offering a broad linear range (20 nM–25.8 μM) and a low detection threshold of 8 nM (Li et al. 2021).

Optical biosensors have also been developed for the detection of CVD biomarkers, which often incorporate QDs that emit light in the NIR region of the electromagnetic spectrum. Due to their broad absorption spectrum, sharp emission peaks, and strong resistance to photobleaching, NIR quantum dots are well suited for extended-duration cellular imaging. Red-emitting fluorescent probes can be utilized to minimize background interference and tissue damage, enhancing detection sensitivity and enabling real-time imaging of molecular events in CVDs (Tang et al. 2022). In a previous study, a molecularly imprinted cellulose membrane was functionalized onto cadmium telluride QDs for the sensitive and selective detection of myoglobin in biological media. As the sensing elements bind to myoglobin, fluorescent quenching of the membrane is observed as the concentration of the target increases. In human serum samples, which were diluted by a fold of 1000, the nanocomposite biosensor showed outstanding sensitivity over a dynamic linear range of 7.39–291.3 pg/mL. The optimized membrane exhibited a linear detection profile below the myocardial infarction threshold (23 ng/mL), with an ultra-low detection limit of 3.08 pg/mL. The biosensors also demonstrated outstanding selectivity toward myoglobin compared to non-imprinted sensing elements. In summary, coupling imprinted sensing elements with QDs boosts sensitivity for myoglobin detection in bodily fluids, thus allowing clinically relevant, label-free optical detection in complex protein mixtures such as human serum (Piloto et al. 2021).

4.6 Conclusions and Future Perspectives

4.6.1 Biomedical Imaging Applications

In this chapter, we describe and discuss the importance of nanomaterial composite properties and applications in biomedical imaging using a diverse set of modalities, including fluorescence imaging, MRI, CT, US, and PET. Across these detection modes, nanomaterials and composites have been demonstrated to be enhanced contrast agents for imaging compared to conventional chemicals/materials. Their superior performance can mainly be attributed to improvement in signal intensity, but it should also be noted that these materials can be uniquely functionalized or conjugated to improve not only the targeting ability but also to induce longer circulation times in the body (Han et al. 2019). Nanotechnology has enhanced the capabilities of individual imaging techniques, making them more powerful. Additionally, combining multiple imaging modalities has shown great potential. Across the US Food and Drug Administration (FDA) as well as the European Medicines Agency (EMA), there are over 100 nanomaterial-based drugs (including nanoimaging agents) that are already being marketed. With modest estimations, there are also over 500 new nanomedicines that are currently undergoing clinical trials (Thapa and Kim 2023). It should be noted that historically, it has been observed that there is a significant delay in clinical translation of these technologies, given that there is an array of different factors that impact biological distribution, toxicity, and biosafety.

Properties such as size, shape, surface charge, and surface labeling influence the distribution of nanoparticles in the body. Additionally, the potential toxicity of nanoparticles after they are metabolized is not yet fully understood. Some nanoparticles may damage normal cells due to their native properties (Mitchell et al. 2021). One prominent example of this is that it is well understood that quantum dots are biologically harmful, and even though there are techniques to reduce undesirable toxic effects (encapsulation or surface labeling), there is future research that needs to be undertaken to facilitate a deeper understanding within this area prior to translation (Han et al. 2019). In the future, it is also anticipated that there will be more investigations that seek to develop theranostic nanocomposite platforms that can simultaneously diagnose a medical condition and deliver treatments. As vehicles that can be functionalized for enhanced targeting, nanomaterials and composites can not only be used for imaging but also for the encapsulation of a wide variety of therapies for delivery. In recent studies, various therapeutic approaches have been explored for integration into theranostic approaches. These have been mostly employed in the context of cancer research and include chemotherapy, photothermal therapy, radiotherapy, photodynamic therapy, gene therapy, and more. However, these agents too experience hurdles in clinical translation, which is partially due to variations in fabrication methods (Al-Thani et al. 2024).

To be more efficient and speed up the clinical translation of nanomaterial composites in biomedical imaging applications, comprehensive characterization needs to be undertaken during each phase of development and fabrication. Properties that are recommended to be qualified include, but are not limited to, chemical composition/formulation, shape/morphology, size (including hydrodynamic diameters), stability, solubility, biological distribution in the human body, metabolism, excretion, and biotoxicological characteristics. Only after these characteristics are adequate for biomedical application can studies be undertaken in clinical trials to test the safety and overall performance of the nanodrug. These steps will be very challenging, but they are critical to determine that these agents/materials are not only safe for biological administration but also effective in their application. It is generally recommended that improvements in the development process should focus on increasing the affinity to bind to a specific cancer target and decreasing any inadvertent toxicological effects (Han et al. 2019). Many studies using nano-based imaging agents utilize in vivo models using animals other than humans, and it is important to note that not all results will be translatable between the two. Regardless of the animal models being studied, the nanocomposite's pharmacokinetic profile in humans must be well understood (Mukherjee et al. 2022). Developing nanoparticles for biomedical imaging necessitates collaboration among multiple disciplines, including but not limited to chemists, pharmacists, biologists, physicists, engineers, and physicians. Despite the complexities involved, nanoparticles hold transformative potential as innovative imaging agents for numerous clinical applications.

4.6.2 Nanocomposites for Glucose Monitoring

Nanotechnology has propelled methods for continuous glucose monitoring due to its unique physicochemical properties. In this chapter, we explore how an array of different nanomaterials and composites can be utilized to enhance the performance of sensors that are developed for glucose monitoring. Nonetheless, there is still a lot of future work that needs to be done. One area for advancement in this field is the use of smart plastic nanocomposites (Mahato et al. 2018) that respond to different stimuli, including the introduction of glucose. For instance, glucose-responsive polymer nanocomposites are being developed to release insulin in response to rising blood sugar levels. This technology mimics the body's natural insulin regulation, potentially reducing the need for frequent insulin injections and improving blood sugar control (Sen 2025; Volpatti et al. 2020). Moreover, the integration of an array of different nanocomposites, including polymers, into CGM devices can improve glucose detection and facilitate drug delivery. It is also anticipated that advancements in techniques for nanocomposite fabrication, such as electrospinning nanofibers or 3D printing, will enable the development of intricate and highly tailored nanocomposite structures. They allow for precise control over the material's properties, facilitating the development of devices capable of performing in theranostic applications. One specific example of this is that nanocomposites can be electrospun to develop nanofibers that demonstrate antimicrobial properties and therefore, can be implemented in diabetic wound healing (Jang et al. 2023).

Enhanced clinical information is obtained when implementing nanotechnology for glucose detection, as it can drastically increase the accuracy of assays. Beyond building multi-functional platforms, it is also anticipated that in the future, nanocomposite-based biosensors will be coupled with digital health technology platforms. The biosensor data from nanocomposites will not only be processed but also visualized using smart device applications (or integrated into telemedical practices). Integrating polymer nanocomposites with digital health technologies not only enhances patient outcomes but also lowers healthcare expenses. Remote monitoring reduces the need for frequent hospital visits, easing the burden on healthcare systems and improving patient access to care (Sen 2025). A booming area of research is to utilize pattern recognition through machine learning on biometrics/physiological parameters for blood glucose tracking and predicting hypo- or hyperglycemic events (Marcus et al. 2020). Through integrating biometric and glucose data from nanocomposite biosensors, enhanced performance is projected to be achieved. In turn, this will not only result in a platform that can predict deviations from the normal/healthy blood glucose range but can also be used to make recommendations to improve medical outcomes and overall quality of life.

4.6.3 Liquid Biopsies for Cancer Diagnostics

As described and discussed in previous sections, liquid biopsy using nanomaterial-based composites has emerged as a very popular technique since it is minimally invasive (or noninvasive, depending on the sample type) and can provide clinically relevant information that can be used to accurately diagnose a variety of different types of cancer. A host of different nanoparticles and nanocomposites have been detailed in this chapter, which has demonstrated that compared to more traditional methods, they provide an enhanced mode for analysis when optimized for performance. Specifically, many different materials and approaches have been implemented for signal enhancement and improved efficiency for biomolecule detection. Integrating specific bio-recognition molecules, such as aptamers, peptides, and DNA probes, with innovative nanomaterials has significantly enhanced detection efficiency. These bio-recognition molecules bind selectively to target analytes, while the nanomaterials amplify the signal, resulting in more accurate and sensitive detection (Kalogianni 2021). Nonetheless, there are still significant barriers that exist, which have limited the clinical translation of this approach. First and foremost, it is recognized that nanocomposite-based liquid biopsy platforms cannot distinguish the grade or location of a given tumor. Beyond this, there are also challenges in analyte detection, given that proteomes have a very dynamic nature, CTCs can be rare, and other biomarker types can have indeterminate levels in biological samples. Compared to CTCs, ctDNA offers benefits such as higher concentration and abundance, but it needs to be noted that they can still be present at concentrations below the limits of detection for current liquid biopsy platforms. This especially holds true in patients with early-stage cancer diagnoses (Singh et al. 2023; Wang et al. 2024b).

Another grand challenge is that cancer detection based on liquid biopsy-based quantification of cancer biomarkers requires clinical trials involving diverse sets of patients in different locations with heterogeneous characteristics. Clinical trials are the only way that diagnostic tests, along with their clinical impact, can be assessed. It should also be noted that among all the different sample and analyte types, there is no gold standard method for purification or isolation. Methods for isolation are particularly heterogenous for the purification of exosomes (Dilsiz 2024). Not only will inferior methods negatively impact results, but heterogeneous applications of these techniques can lead to disparate results across published studies. Establishing standardized analytical procedures for isolation and analysis is essential in overcoming these challenges. All of these factors discussed can have negative impacts on diagnostic sensitivity/specificity. It is also noted that clinical translation of liquid biopsy platforms is of challenge, since there is no dedicated pathway or regulatory mechanism for approval and commercialization (Goodsaid 2019).

In the future, developing nanocomposite-based liquid biopsies that can perform multiplexed detection may be able to overcome some of these challenges. For example, a multiplexed approach that probes the measurement of biomarkers encompassing multiple "omics" may not only be able to increase diagnostic accuracy (sensitivity/specificity) but may also be able to distinguish different tumor grades and facilitate an earlier detection of cancer. It will also allow researchers to gain deeper insights into tumor heterogeneity as well as cancer metastasis. Multiplexing in liquid biopsies also has the potential to significantly reduce healthcare costs, given that they can provide biomolecular information that would require several tests in a clinical environment (Choi et al. 2020; Dell'Olio 2021; Goswami et al.

2024). Future research in liquid biopsy technology will also see the integration of machine learning approaches, as they can be used to analyze large and complex data sets collected using these platforms to more accurately diagnose cancer through identifying subtle but consistent changes in cancer biomarkers. Not only can machine learning and artificial intelligence be used to enhance diagnostic accuracy through analyzing a collective response of multiplexed sensors, but they may also be used to identify novel cancer biomarkers and targets. Pattern recognition techniques will also facilitate the implementation of personalized treatment regimens, as they can be implemented on an individual level and used to predict the efficacy of different treatments (Alum 2025).

References

Abdollah MRA, Carter TJ, Jones C, Kalber TL, Rajkumar V, Tolner B, Gruettner C, Zaw-Thin M, Baguña Torres J, Ellis M et al (2018) Fucoidan prolongs the circulation time of Dextran-coated iron oxide nanoparticles. ACS Nano 12(2):1156–1169. https://doi.org/10.1021/acsnano.7b06734

Abla F, Elsayed Y, Abu Farha N, Obaideen K, Mohamed AA, Lee H, Han C, Egilmez M, Kanan S (2023) Fabrication of high surface area TiO2-MoO3 nanocomposite as a photocatalyst for organic pollutants removal from water bodies. Catalysts 13(2):362

Adams F (2005) X-ray absorption and diffraction | overview. In: Worsfold P, Townshend A, Poole C (eds) Encyclopedia of analytical science, 2nd edn. Elsevier, pp 365–377

Adeel M, Asif K, Rahman MM, Daniele S, Canzonieri V, Rizzolio F (2021) Glucose detection devices and methods based on metal–organic frameworks and related materials. Adv Funct Mater 31(52):2106023. https://doi.org/10.1002/adfm.202106023

Adhit KK, Wanjari A, Menon S, K, S. (2023) Liquid biopsy: an evolving paradigm for non-invasive disease diagnosis and monitoring in medicine. Cureus 15(12):e50176. https://doi.org/10.7759/cureus.50176. From NLM

Agrahari S, Kumar Gautam R, Kumar Singh A, Tiwari I (2022) Nanoscale materials-based hybrid frameworks modified electrochemical biosensors for early cancer diagnostics: an overview of current trends and challenges. Microchem J 172:106980. https://doi.org/10.1016/j.microc.2021.106980

Ai H, Fang M, Jones SA, Lvov YM (2002) Electrostatic layer-by-layer nanoassembly on biological microtemplates: platelets. Biomacromolecules 3(3):560–564. https://doi.org/10.1021/bm015659r

Akgöl S, Ulucan-Karnak F, Kuru Cİ, Kuşat K (2021) The usage of composite nanomaterials in biomedical engineering applications. Biotechnol Bioeng 118(8):2906–2922. https://doi.org/10.1002/bit.27843

Alibakhshi A, Abarghooi Kahaki F, Ahangarzadeh S, Yaghoobi H, Yarian F, Arezumand R, Ranjbari J, Mokhtarzadeh A, de la Guardia M (2017) Targeted cancer therapy through antibody fragments-decorated nanomedicines. J Control Release 268:323–334. https://doi.org/10.1016/j.jconrel.2017.10.036

Al-Jamal WT, Al-Jamal KT, Bomans PH, Frederik PM, Kostarelos K (2008) Functionalized-quantum-dot–liposome hybrids as multimodal nanoparticles for cancer. Small 4(9):1406–1415

Alromi DA, Madani SY, Seifalian A (2021) Emerging application of magnetic nanoparticles for diagnosis and treatment of cancer. Polymers 13(23):4146

Alrushaid N, Khan FA, Al-Suhaimi EA, Elaissari A (2023) Nanotechnology in cancer diagnosis and treatment. Pharmaceutics 15(3):1025

Alshaer W, Hillaireau H, Fattal E (2018) Aptamer-guided nanomedicines for anticancer drug delivery. Adv Drug Deliv Rev 134:122–137

Alshammari BH, Lashin MMA, Mahmood MA, Al-Mubaddel FS, Ilyas N, Rahman N, Sohail M, Khan A, Abdullaev SS, Khan R (2023) Organic and inorganic nanomaterials: fabrication, properties and applications. RSC Adv 13(20):13735–13785. https://doi.org/10.1039/D3RA01421E

Al-Thani AN, Jan AG, Abbas M, Geetha M, Sadasivuni KK (2024) Nanoparticles in cancer theragnostic and drug delivery: a comprehensive review. Life Sci 352:122899. https://doi.org/10.1016/j.lfs.2024.122899

Alum EU (2025) AI-driven biomarker discovery: enhancing precision in cancer diagnosis and prognosis. Discov Oncol 16(1):313. https://doi.org/10.1007/s12672-025-02064-7

Aminabad ED, Mobed A, Hasanzadeh M, Hosseinpour Feizi MA, Safaralizadeh R, Seidi F (2022) Sensitive immunosensing of α-synuclein protein in human plasma samples using gold nanoparticles conjugated with graphene: an innovative immuno-platform towards early stage identification of Parkinson's disease using point of care (POC) analysis. RSC Adv 12(7):4346–4357. https://doi.org/10.1039/D1RA06437A

Anderson D, Anderson T, Fahmi F (2019) Advances in applications of metal oxide nanomaterials as imaging contrast agents. Phys Status Solidi A 216(16):1801008. https://doi.org/10.1002/pssa.201801008

Andoh V, Wiredu ODK, Hassan N, Naijian W, Liang C, Keping C, Mao F (2024) The advancing role of nanocomposites in cancer diagnosis and treatment. Int J Nanomedicine 19(null):6099–6126. https://doi.org/10.2147/IJN.S471360

Anekwe IMS, Akpasi SO, Enemuo EM, Ashiegbu D, Mustapha SI, Isa YM (2024) Innovations in catalytic understanding: a journey through advanced characterization. Mater Today Catal 7:100061. https://doi.org/10.1016/j.mtcata.2024.100061

Ashraf MA, Peng W, Zare Y, Rhee KY (2018) Effects of size and aggregation/agglomeration of nanoparticles on the interfacial/interphase properties and tensile strength of polymer nanocomposites. Nanoscale Res Lett 13(1):214. https://doi.org/10.1186/s11671-018-2624-0

Azad UP, Chandra P (2023) Handbook of nanobioelectrochemistry: application in devices and biomolecular sensing. Springer Nature (London, UK)

Azad UP, Chandra P (2025) Handbook of material engineering in nanobiomedicine and diagnostics. Springer Nature

Bagheri S, Yasemi M, Safaie-Qamsari E, Rashidiani J, Abkar M, Hassani M, Mirhosseini SA, Kooshki H (2018) Using gold nanoparticles in diagnosis and treatment of melanoma cancer. Artif Cells Nanomed Biotechnol 46(sup1):462–471. https://doi.org/10.1080/21691401.2018.1430585

Bakirhan NK, Ozcelikay G, Ozkan SA (2018) Recent progress on the sensitive detection of cardiovascular disease markers by electrochemical-based biosensors. J Pharm Biomed Anal 159:406–424. https://doi.org/10.1016/j.jpba.2018.07.021

Basak S, Singhal RS (2023) The potential of supercritical drying as a "green" method for the production of food-grade bioaerogels: a comprehensive critical review. Food Hydrocoll 141:108738. https://doi.org/10.1016/j.foodhyd.2023.108738

Batool R, Rhouati A, Nawaz MH, Hayat A, Marty JL (2019) A review of the construction of nanohybrids for electrochemical biosensing of glucose. Biosensors 9(1):46

Bellis SL (2011) Advantages of RGD peptides for directing cell association with biomaterials. Biomaterials 32(18):4205–4210. https://doi.org/10.1016/j.biomaterials.2011.02.029

Benvenuto P, Kafi AKM, Chen A (2009) High performance glucose biosensor based on the immobilization of glucose oxidase onto modified titania nanotube arrays. J Electroanal Chem 627(1):76–81. https://doi.org/10.1016/j.jelechem.2008.12.022

Bianco A, Kostarelos K, Partidos CD, Prato M (2005) Biomedical applications of functionalised carbon nanotubes. Chem Commun 5:571–577. https://doi.org/10.1039/B410943K

Boriachek K, Islam MN, Gopalan V, Lam AK, Nguyen N-T, Shiddiky MJA (2017) Quantum dot-based sensitive detection of disease specific exosome in serum. Analyst 142(12):2211–2219. https://doi.org/10.1039/C7AN00672A

Bratulic S, Gatto F, Nielsen J (2021) The translational status of cancer liquid biopsies. Regen Eng Transl Med 7(3):312–352. https://doi.org/10.1007/s40883-019-00141-2

Breuer O, Sundararaj U (2004) Big returns from small fibers: a review of polymer/carbon nanotube composites. Polym Compos 25(6):630–645. https://doi.org/10.1002/pc.20058

Bruchez M, Moronne M, Gin P, Weiss S, Alivisatos AP (1998) Semiconductor nanocrystals as fluorescent biological labels. Science 281(5385):2013–2016. https://doi.org/10.1126/science.281.5385.2013

Cappon G, Vettoretti M, Sparacino G, Facchinetti A (2019) Continuous glucose monitoring sensors for diabetes management: a review of technologies and applications. Diabetes Metab J 43(4):383–397. https://doi.org/10.4093/dmj.2019.0121

Carrera Espinoza MJ, Lin K-S, Weng M-T, Kunene SC, Lin Y-S, Wu C-M (2023) Synthesis and characterization of supermagnetic nanocomposites coated with Pluronic F127 as a contrast agent for biomedical applications. Pharmaceutics 15(3):740

Cassagneau T, Mallouk TE, Fendler JH (1998) Layer-by-layer assembly of thin film zener diodes from conducting polymers and CdSe nanoparticles. J Am Chem Soc 120(31):7848–7859

Chaubey A, Malhotra BD (2002) Mediated biosensors. Biosens Bioelectron 17(6):441–456. https://doi.org/10.1016/S0956-5663(01)00313-X

Chauhan S, Al-Dayan N, Kumar R, Chander Chabattula S, Sahni M, Ranjithkumar R, Kumar Gupta P (2022) Synthesis and characterization of novel bimetallic-semi-aromatic polyester nanocomposite for possible biomedical use. Mater Lett 306:130943. https://doi.org/10.1016/j.matlet.2021.130943

Chen LQ, Xiao SJ, Hu PP, Peng L, Ma J, Luo LF, Li YF, Huang CZ (2012) Aptamer-mediated nanoparticle-based protein labeling platform for intracellular imaging and tracking endocytosis dynamics. Anal Chem 84(7):3099–3110

Chen Y, Liu B, Chen Z, Zuo X (2021) Innovative electrochemical sensor using TiO2 nanomaterials to detect Phosphopeptides. Anal Chem 93(30):10635–10643. https://doi.org/10.1021/acs.analchem.1c01973

Chen JN, Hasabnis GK, Akin E, Gao G, Usha SP, Süssmuth R, Altintas Z (2024) Developing innovative point-of-care electrochemical sensors empowered by cardiac troponin I-responsive nanocomposite materials. Sensors Actuators B Chem 417:136052. https://doi.org/10.1016/j.snb.2024.136052

Cheng S, Yang M, Fu J, Wang R, He J, Li Q (2023) Surface-coated polymer nanocomposites containing z-aligned high-k nanowires as high-performance dielectrics at elevated temperatures. IET Nanodielectrics 6(4):237–245. https://doi.org/10.1049/nde2.12060

Chiticaru EA, Damian CM, Pilan L, Ioniţă M (2023) Label-free DNA biosensor based on reduced graphene oxide and gold nanoparticles. Biosensors 13(8):797

Cho J, Char K (2004) Effect of layer integrity of spin self-assembled multilayer films on surface wettability. Langmuir 20(10):4011–4016

Choi Y-B, Kim H-S, Jeon W-Y, Lee B-H, Shin US, Kim H-H (2019) The electrochemical glucose sensing based on the chitosan-carbon nanotube hybrid. Biochem Eng J 144:227–234. https://doi.org/10.1016/j.bej.2018.10.021

Choi N, Dang H, Das A, Sim MS, Chung IY, Choo J (2020) SERS biosensors for ultrasensitive detection of multiple biomarkers expressed in cancer cells. Biosens Bioelectron 164:112326. https://doi.org/10.1016/j.bios.2020.112326

Chronos NA, Goodall AH, Wilson DJ, Sigwart U, Buller NP (1993) Profound platelet degranulation is an important side effect of some types of contrast media used in interventional cardiology. Circulation 88(5):2035–2044. https://doi.org/10.1161/01.CIR.88.5.2035. Acccessed 2025/04/04

Cisneros BT, Law JJ, Matson ML, Azhdarinia A, Sevick-Muraca EM, Wilson LJ (2014) Stable confinement of positron emission tomography and magnetic resonance agents within carbon nanotubes for bimodal imaging. Nanomedicine 9(16):2499–2509. https://doi.org/10.2217/nnm.14.26

Coughlan C, Bruce KD, Burgy O, Boyd TD, Michel CR, Garcia-Perez JE, Adame V, Anton P, Bettcher BM, Chial HJ et al (2020) Exosome isolation by ultracentrifugation and precipitation and techniques for downstream analyses. Curr Protoc Cell Biol 88(1):e110. https://doi.org/10.1002/cpcb.110

Cuccurullo V, Di Stasio GD, Mazzarella G, Cascini GL (2018) Microvascular invasion in HCC: the molecular imaging perspective. Contrast Media Mol Imaging 2018(1):9487938. https://doi.org/10.1155/2018/9487938. Acccessed 2025/04/04

Cui J, Richardson JJ, Björnmalm M, Faria M, Caruso F (2016) Nanoengineered templated polymer particles: navigating the biological Realm. Acc Chem Res 49(6):1139–1148. https://doi.org/10.1021/acs.accounts.6b00088

Daniel M-C, Astruc D (2004) Gold nanoparticles: assembly, supramolecular chemistry, quantum-size-related properties, and applications toward biology, catalysis, and nanotechnology. Chem Rev 104(1):293–346. https://doi.org/10.1021/cr030698+

Das S, Dey MK, Devireddy R, Gartia MR (2024) Biomarkers in cancer detection, diagnosis, and prognosis. Sensors 24(1):37

Decher G, Hong JD, Schmitt J (1992) Buildup of ultrathin multilayer films by a self-assembly process: III. Consecutively alternating adsorption of anionic and cationic polyelectrolytes on charged surfaces. Thin Solid Films 210:831–835

Dell'Olio F (2021) Multiplexed liquid biopsy and tumor imaging using surface-enhanced Raman Scattering. Biosensors 11(11):449

Descamps L, Le Roy D, Deman A-L (2022) Microfluidic-based technologies for CTC isolation: a review of 10 years of intense efforts towards liquid biopsy. Int J Mol Sci 23(4):1981

Deshmukh K (2019) Nanotechnology in ancient era. In: Khoobchandani M, Saxena A (eds) Biotechnology products in everyday life. Springer International Publishing, pp 3–14

Deuschl G, Beghi E, Fazekas F, Varga T, Christoforidi KA, Sipido E, Bassetti CL, Vos T, Feigin VL (2020) The burden of neurological diseases in Europe: an analysis for the Global Burden of Disease Study 2017. Lancet Public Health 5(10):e551–e567. https://doi.org/10.1016/S2468-2667(20)30190-0

Dhahi TS, Yousif Dafhalla AK, Al-Mufti AW, Elobaid ME, Adam T, Gopinath SCB (2024) Application of Nanobiosensor engineering in the diagnosis of neurodegenerative disorders. Results Eng 24:102790. https://doi.org/10.1016/j.rineng.2024.102790

Dilsiz N (2024) A comprehensive review on recent advances in exosome isolation and characterization: toward clinical applications. Transl Oncol 50:102121. https://doi.org/10.1016/j.tranon.2024.102121

Ding L, Bond AM, Zhai J, Zhang J (2013) Utilization of nanoparticle labels for signal amplification in ultrasensitive electrochemical affinity biosensors: a review. Anal Chim Acta 797:1–12. https://doi.org/10.1016/j.aca.2013.07.035

Dong YC, Hajfathalian M, Maidment PSN, Hsu JC, Naha PC, Si-Mohamed S, Breuilly M, Kim J, Chhour P, Douek P et al (2019) Effect of gold nanoparticle size on their properties as contrast agents for computed tomography. Sci Rep 9(1):14912. https://doi.org/10.1038/s41598-019-50332-8

dos Santos VDAC, Hondl N, Ramos-Garcia V, Kuligowski J, Lendl B, Ramer G (2023) AFM-IR for nanoscale chemical characterization in life sciences: recent developments and future directions. ACS Measure Sci Au 3(5):301–314. https://doi.org/10.1021/acsmeasuresciau.3c00010

Du Y, Luo X-L, Xu J-J, Chen H-Y (2007) A simple method to fabricate a chitosan-gold nanoparticles film and its application in glucose biosensor. Bioelectrochemistry 70(2):342–347. https://doi.org/10.1016/j.bioelechem.2006.05.002

Duan X, Liu K, Xu Y, Yuan M, Gao T, Wang J (2019) Nonenzymatic electrochemical glucose biosensor constructed by NiCo2O4@Ppy nanowires on nickel foam substrate. Sensors Actuators B Chem 292:121–128. https://doi.org/10.1016/j.snb.2019.04.107

Dubas ST, Farhat TR, Schlenoff JB (2001) Multiple membranes from "True" polyelectrolyte multilayers. J Am Chem Soc 123(22):5368–5369. https://doi.org/10.1021/ja015774+

Ebrahimi A, Nikokar I, Zokaei M, Bozorgzadeh E (2018) Design, development and evaluation of microRNA-199a-5p detecting electrochemical nanobiosensor with diagnostic application in triple negative breast cancer. Talanta 189:592–598. https://doi.org/10.1016/j.talanta.2018.07.016

Edwards PP, Thomas JM (2007) Gold in a metallic divided state—from Faraday to present-day nanoscience. Angew Chem Int Ed 46(29):5480–5486. https://doi.org/10.1002/anie.200700428

Eid MM (2022) Characterization of nanoparticles by FTIR and FTIR-microscopy. In: Handbook of consumer nanoproducts. Springer Nature Singapore, pp 645–673

El Aamri M, Yammouri G, Mohammadi H, Amine A, Korri-Youssoufi H (2020) Electrochemical biosensors for detection of MicroRNA as a cancer biomarker: pros and cons. Biosensors 10(11):186

El Naschie MS (2006) Nanotechnology for the developing world. Chaos, Solitons Fractals 30(4):769–773. https://doi.org/10.1016/j.chaos.2006.04.037

Elliott AD (2020) Confocal microscopy: principles and modern practices. Curr Protoc Cytom 92(1):e68. https://doi.org/10.1002/cpcy.68. From NLM

Eslami-S Z, Cortés-Hernández LE, Alix-Panabières C (2020) Epithelial cell adhesion molecule: an anchor to isolate clinically relevant circulating tumor cells. Cells 9(8):1836

Faghihzadeh F, Anaya NM, Schifman LA, Oyanedel-Craver V (2016) Fourier transform infrared spectroscopy to assess molecular-level changes in microorganisms exposed to nanoparticles. Nanotechnol Environ Eng 1(1):1. https://doi.org/10.1007/s41204-016-0001-8

Fan Q, Cheng K, Hu X, Ma X, Zhang R, Yang M, Lu X, Xing L, Huang W, Gambhir SS et al (2014) Transferring biomarker into molecular probe: melanin nanoparticle as a naturally active platform for multimodality imaging. J Am Chem Soc 136(43):15185–15194. https://doi.org/10.1021/ja505412p

Fang Y, Wang E (2013) Electrochemical biosensors on platforms of graphene. Chem Commun 49(83):9526–9539. https://doi.org/10.1039/C3CC44735A

Fang X, Wang Y, Wang S, Liu B (2022) Nanomaterials assisted exosomes isolation and analysis towards liquid biopsy. Mater Today Bio 16:100371. https://doi.org/10.1016/j.mtbio.2022.100371

Ferraz E, Gamelas JA, Coroado J, Monteiro C, Rocha F (2019) Recycling waste seashells to produce calcitic lime: characterization and wet slaking reactivity. Waste Biomass Valoriz 10:2397–2414

Florkow MC, Willemsen K, Mascarenhas VV, Oei EHG, van Stralen M, Seevinck PR (2022) Magnetic resonance imaging versus computed tomography for three-dimensional bone imaging of musculoskeletal pathologies: a review. J Magn Reson Imaging 56(1):11–34. https://doi.org/10.1002/jmri.28067. From NLM

Fu Q, Zhu R, Song J, Yang H, Chen X (2019) Photoacoustic imaging: contrast agents and their biomedical applications. Adv Mater 31(6):1805875. https://doi.org/10.1002/adma.201805875

Gamessa TW, Suman D, Tadesse ZK (2018) Blood glucose monitoring techniques: recent advances, challenges and future perspectives. Int J Adv Technol Eng Explor 5(46):335–344

Gao X, Cui Y, Levenson RM, Chung LWK, Nie S (2004) In vivo cancer targeting and imaging with semiconductor quantum dots. Nat Biotechnol 22(8):969–976. https://doi.org/10.1038/nbt994

Gerard M, Chaubey A, Malhotra BD (2002) Application of conducting polymers to biosensors. Biosens Bioelectron 17(5):345–359. https://doi.org/10.1016/S0956-5663(01)00312-8

Gerion D, Pinaud F, Williams SC, Parak WJ, Zanchet D, Weiss S, Alivisatos AP (2001) Synthesis and properties of biocompatible water-soluble silica-coated CdSe/ZnS semiconductor quantum dots. J Phys Chem B 105(37):8861–8871. https://doi.org/10.1021/jp0105488

German N, Popov A, Ramanavicius A, Ramanaviciene A (2022) Development and practical application of glucose biosensor based on dendritic gold nanostructures modified by conducting polymers. Biosensors 12(8):641

Gil HM, Price TW, Chelani K, Bouillard J-SG, Calaminus SDJ, Stasiuk GJ (2021) NIR-quantum dots in biomedical imaging and their future. iScience 24(3):102189. https://doi.org/10.1016/j.isci.2021.102189

Gole A, Dash C, Ramakrishnan V, Sainkar SR, Mandale AB, Rao M, Sastry M (2001) Pepsin–gold colloid conjugates: preparation, characterization, and enzymatic activity. Langmuir 17(5):1674–1679. https://doi.org/10.1021/la001164w

Gole A, Vyas S, Phadtare S, Lachke A, Sastry M (2002) Studies on the formation of bioconjugates of endoglucanase with colloidal gold. Colloids Surf B: Biointerfaces 25(2):129–138. https://doi.org/10.1016/S0927-7765(01)00301-0

Gong H, Peng R, Liu Z (2013) Carbon nanotubes for biomedical imaging: the recent advances. Adv Drug Deliv Rev 65(15):1951–1963. https://doi.org/10.1016/j.addr.2013.10.002. From NLM

Goodsaid FM (2019) The labyrinth of product development and regulatory approvals in liquid biopsy diagnostics. Clin Transl Sci 12(5):431–439. https://doi.org/10.1111/cts.12657

Gopalan AI, Lee KP, Ragupathy D, Lee SH, Lee JW (2009) An electrochemical glucose biosensor exploiting a polyaniline grafted multiwalled carbon nanotube/perfluorosulfonate ionomer–silica nanocomposite. Biomaterials 30(30):5999–6005. https://doi.org/10.1016/j.biomaterials.2009.07.047

Gorle DB, Ponnada S, Kiai MS, Nair KK, Nowduri A, Swart HC, Ang EH, Nanda KK (2021) Review on recent progress in metal–organic framework-based materials for fabricating electrochemical glucose sensors. J Mater Chem B 9(38):7927–7954. https://doi.org/10.1039/D1TB01403J

Goswami S, Samanta P, Adhikari MD (2024) Nanobiotechnology: a smart platform of the future transform liquid biopsy era. J Liquid Biopsy 3:100137. https://doi.org/10.1016/j.jlb.2024.100137

Govindan B, Sabri MA, Hai A, Banat F, Haija MA (2023) A review of advanced multifunctional magnetic nanostructures for cancer diagnosis and therapy integrated into an artificial intelligence approach. Pharmaceutics 15(3):868

Grabar KC, Allison KJ, Baker BE, Bright RM, Brown KR, Freeman RG, Fox AP, Keating CD, Musick MD, Natan MJ (1996) Two-dimensional arrays of colloidal gold particles: a flexible approach to macroscopic metal surfaces. Langmuir 12(10):2353–2361. https://doi.org/10.1021/la950561h

Granek G, Hon G (2008) Searching for asses, finding a kingdom: the story of the invention of the scanning tunnelling microscope (STM). Ann Sci 65(1):101–125. https://doi.org/10.1080/00033790701458769

Guo CX, Li CM (2010) Direct electron transfer of glucose oxidase and biosensing of glucose on hollow sphere-nanostructured conducting polymer/metal oxide composite. Phys Chem Chem Phys 12(38):12153–12159. https://doi.org/10.1039/C0CP00378F

Gupta M, Bala R, Madaan R, Chauhan S, Chawla R, Kaur J, Sharifi-Rad J, Calina D (2024) Unfolding the potential of nanocomposites as drug carriers and their future scenarios. Polym Bull 81(7):5657–5677. https://doi.org/10.1007/s00289-023-04987-z

Gutierrez AM, Frazar EM, Klaus X, Paul P, Hilt JZ (2022) Hydrogels and hydrogel nanocomposites: enhancing healthcare through human and environmental treatment. Adv Healthc Mater 11(7):2101820. https://doi.org/10.1002/adhm.202101820

Habli Z, AlChamaa W, Saab R, Kadara H, Khraiche ML (2020) Circulating tumor cell detection technologies and clinical utility: challenges and opportunities. Cancer 12(7):1930

Habte L, Shiferaw N, Mulatu D, Thenepalli T, Chilakala R, Ahn JW (2019) Synthesis of nano-calcium oxide from waste eggshell by sol-gel method. Sustainability 11(11):3196

Han X, Xu K, Taratula O, Farsad K (2019) Applications of nanoparticles in biomedical imaging. Nanoscale 11(3):799–819. https://doi.org/10.1039/c8nr07769j. From NLM

Harmer MA, Farneth WE, Sun Q (1996) High surface area Nafion Resin/Silica nanocomposites: a new class of solid acid catalyst. J Am Chem Soc 118(33):7708–7715. https://doi.org/10.1021/ja9541950

Hayat A, Catanante G, Marty JL (2014) Current trends in nanomaterial-based Amperometric biosensors. Sensors 14(12):23439–23461

Heitzer E, Haque IS, Roberts CES, Speicher MR (2019) Current and future perspectives of liquid biopsies in genomics-driven oncology. Nat Rev Genet 20(2):71–88. https://doi.org/10.1038/s41576-018-0071-5

Heuer-Jungemann A, Feliu N, Bakaimi I, Hamaly M, Alkilany A, Chakraborty I, Masood A, Casula MF, Kostopoulou A, Oh E et al (2019) The role of ligands in the chemical synthesis and applications of inorganic nanoparticles. Chem Rev 119(8):4819–4880. https://doi.org/10.1021/acs.chemrev.8b00733

Hofman P, Heeke S, Alix-Panabières C, Pantel K (2019) Liquid biopsy in the era of immuno-oncology: is it ready for prime-time use for cancer patients? Ann Oncol 30(9):1448–1459. https://doi.org/10.1093/annonc/mdz196. Acccessed 2025/04/05
Holder CF, Schaak RE (2019) Tutorial on powder X-ray diffraction for characterizing nanoscale materials. ACS Nano 13(7):7359–7365. https://doi.org/10.1021/acsnano.9b05157
Hoshyar N, Gray S, Han H, Bao G (2016) The effect of nanoparticle size on in vivo pharmacokinetics and cellular interaction. Nanomedicine 11(6):673–692
Houck MM (2023) Microscopy: Electron. In: Houck MM (ed) Encyclopedia of forensic sciences, 3rd edn. Elsevier, pp 584–589
Hu C, Jiang W, Lv M, Fan S, Lu Y, Wu Q, Pi J (2022) Potentiality of Exosomal proteins as novel cancer biomarkers for liquid biopsy. Front Immunol 13:Review. https://doi.org/10.3389/fimmu.2022.792046
Huang J, Liu Y, You T (2010) Carbon nanofiber based electrochemical biosensors: a review. Anal Methods 2(3):202–211. https://doi.org/10.1039/B9AY00312F
Huang Y, He S, Cao W, Cai K, Liang X-J (2012) Biomedical nanomaterials for imaging-guided cancer therapy. Nanoscale 4(20):6135–6149
Huang S, Liu Y, Xu X, Ji M, Li Y, Song C, Duan S, Hu Y (2018) Triple therapy of hepatocellular carcinoma with microRNA-122 and doxorubicin co-loaded functionalized gold nanocages. J Mater Chem B 6(15):2217–2229. https://doi.org/10.1039/C8TB00224J
Hunter TR, Santos LE, Tovar-Moll F, De Felice FG (2025) Alzheimer's disease biomarkers and their current use in clinical research and practice. Mol Psychiatry 30(1):272–284. https://doi.org/10.1038/s41380-024-02709-z
Ilyas A, Dyussupova A, Sultangaziyev A, Shevchenko Y, Filchakova O, Bukasov R (2023) SERS immuno- and apta-assays in biosensing/bio-detection: performance comparison, clinical applications, challenges. Talanta 265:124818. https://doi.org/10.1016/j.talanta.2023.124818
Inaba H, Matsuura K (2019) Peptide nanomaterials designed from natural supramolecular systems. Chem Rec 19(5):843–858
Islam MA, Masson J-F (2025) Plasmonic biosensors for health monitoring: inflammation biomarker detection. ACS Sens 10(2):577–601. https://doi.org/10.1021/acssensors.4c03562
Jańczewski D, Tomczak N, Han M-Y, Vancso GJ (2011) Synthesis of functionalized amphiphilic polymers for coating quantum dots. Nat Protoc 6(10):1546–1553. https://doi.org/10.1038/nprot.2011.381
Jang EJ, Patel R, Patel M (2023) Electrospinning nanofibers as a dressing to treat diabetic wounds. Pharmaceutics 15(4):1144
Jeong S, Park J, Pathania D, Castro CM, Weissleder R, Lee H (2016) Integrated magneto–electrochemical sensor for exosome analysis. ACS Nano 10(2):1802–1809. https://doi.org/10.1021/acsnano.5b07584
Jiang Z, Zhang M, Li P, Wang Y, Fu Q (2023) Nanomaterial-based CT contrast agents and their applications in image-guided therapy. Theranostics 13(2):483–509. https://doi.org/10.7150/thno.79625. From NLM
Jin T, Yoshioka Y, Fujii F, Komai Y, Seki J, Seiyama A (2008) Gd3+-functionalized near-infrared quantum dots for in vivo dual modal (fluorescence/magnetic resonance) imaging. Chem Commun (Camb) 44:5764–5766. https://doi.org/10.1039/b812302k. From NLM
Jo H, Ban C (2016) Aptamer–nanoparticle complexes as powerful diagnostic and therapeutic tools. Exp Mol Med 48(5):e230–e230. https://doi.org/10.1038/emm.2016.44
Ju D, Xu H, Zhang J, Guo J, Cao B (2014) Direct hydrothermal growth of ZnO nanosheets on electrode for ethanol sensing. Sensors Actuators B Chem 201:444–451. https://doi.org/10.1016/j.snb.2014.04.072
Ju S, Chen C, Zhang J, Xu L, Zhang X, Li Z, Chen Y, Zhou J, Ji F, Wang L (2022) Detection of circulating tumor cells: opportunities and challenges. Biomark Res 10(1):58. https://doi.org/10.1186/s40364-022-00403-2
Julius A, Malakondaiah S, Pothireddy RB (2025) Polymer and nanocomposite fillers as advanced materials in biomedical applications. Nano Trends 9:100087. https://doi.org/10.1016/j.nwnano.2025.100087

Kalogianni DP (2021) Nanotechnology in emerging liquid biopsy applications. Nano Convergence 8(1):13. https://doi.org/10.1186/s40580-021-00263-w

Kang X, Wang J, Wu H, Aksay IA, Liu J, Lin Y (2009) Glucose oxidase–graphene–chitosan modified electrode for direct electrochemistry and glucose sensing. Biosens Bioelectron 25(4):901–905. https://doi.org/10.1016/j.bios.2009.09.004

Kannan P, Maduraiveeran G (2024) Carbon nanocomposites-based electrochemical sensors and biosensors for biomedical diagnostics. Curr Med Chem 31(25):3870–3881

Kaushik A, Khan R, Solanki PR, Pandey P, Alam J, Ahmad S, Malhotra BD (2008) Iron oxide nanoparticles–chitosan composite based glucose biosensor. Biosens Bioelectron 24(4):676–683. https://doi.org/10.1016/j.bios.2008.06.032

Kawahara D, Nagata Y (2021) T1-weighted and T2-weighted MRI image synthesis with convolutional generative adversarial networks. Rep Pract Oncol Radiother 26(1):35–42. https://doi.org/10.5603/RPOR.a2021.0005. From NLM

Ke R, Yang W, Xia X, Xu Y, Li Q (2010) Tandem conjugation of enzyme and antibody on silica nanoparticle for enzyme immunoassay. Anal Biochem 406(1):8–13. https://doi.org/10.1016/j.ab.2010.06.039

Kesharwani P, Ma R, Sang L, Fatima M, Sheikh A, Abourehab MAS, Gupta N, Chen Z-S, Zhou Y (2023) Gold nanoparticles and gold nanorods in the landscape of cancer therapy. Mol Cancer 22(1):98. https://doi.org/10.1186/s12943-023-01798-8

Khan I, Saeed K, Khan I (2019) Nanoparticles: properties, applications and toxicities. Arab J Chem 12(7):908–931. https://doi.org/10.1016/j.arabjc.2017.05.011

Khazaei M, Hosseini MS, Haghighi AM, Misaghi M (2023) Nanosensors and their applications in early diagnosis of cancer. Sen Bio-Sens Res 41:100569. https://doi.org/10.1016/j.sbsr.2023.100569

Kiciński W, Szala M, Nita M (2011) Structurally tailored carbon xerogels produced through a sol–gel process in a water–methanol–inorganic salt solution. J Sol-Gel Sci Technol 58(1):102–113. https://doi.org/10.1007/s10971-010-2362-y

Kim D, Jeong YY, Jon S (2010) A drug-loaded aptamer– gold nanoparticle bioconjugate for combined CT imaging and therapy of prostate cancer. ACS Nano 4(7):3689–3696

Kim BH, Lee N, Kim H, An K, Park YI, Choi Y, Shin K, Lee Y, Kwon SG, Na HB et al (2011) Large-scale synthesis of uniform and extremely small-sized iron oxide nanoparticles for high-resolution T1 magnetic resonance imaging contrast agents. J Am Chem Soc 133(32):12624–12631. https://doi.org/10.1021/ja203340u. From NLM

Klibanov AL, Hossack JA (2015) Ultrasound in radiology: from anatomic, functional, molecular imaging to drug delivery and image-guided therapy. Investig Radiol 50(9):657–670. https://doi.org/10.1097/rli.0000000000000188. From NLM

Kumar A, Purohit B, Mahato K, Chandra P (2019) Advance engineered nanomaterials in point-of-care immunosensing for biomedical diagnostics. In: Ahmed MU, Zourob M, Tamiya E (eds) Immunosensors. The Royal Society of Chemistry

Kumar MA, Baba SK, Sadida HQ, Marzooqi SA, Jerobin J, Altemani FH, Algehainy N, Alanazi MA, Abou-Samra A-B, Kumar R et al (2024) Extracellular vesicles as tools and targets in therapy for diseases. Signal Transduct Target Ther 9(1):27. https://doi.org/10.1038/s41392-024-01735-1

Kyriakides TR, Raj A, Tseng TH, Xiao H, Nguyen R, Mohammed FS, Halder S, Xu M, Wu MJ, Bao S (2021) Biocompatibility of nanomaterials and their immunological properties. Biomed Mater 16(4):042005

Labib M, Kelley SO (2021) Circulating tumor cell profiling for precision oncology. Mol Oncol 15(6):1622–1646. https://doi.org/10.1002/1878-0261.12901

Lamptey RNL, Chaulagain B, Trivedi R, Gothwal A, Layek B, Singh J (2022) A review of the common neurodegenerative disorders: current therapeutic approaches and the potential role of nanotherapeutics. Int J Mol Sci 23(3):1851

Lee W, Parpura V (2009) Chapter 6 - Carbon nanotubes as substrates/scaffolds for neural cell growth. Prog Brain Res 180:110–125. https://doi.org/10.1016/s0079-6123(08)80006-4. From NLM

Lee H, Hong YJ, Baik S, Hyeon T, Kim D-H (2018) Enzyme-based glucose sensor: from invasive to wearable device. Adv Healthc Mater 7(8):1701150. https://doi.org/10.1002/adhm.201701150

Lee S, Yeom B, Kim Y, Cho J (2019) Layer-by-layer assembly for ultrathin energy-harvesting films: piezoelectric and triboelectric nanocomposite films. Nano Energy 56:1–15. https://doi.org/10.1016/j.nanoen.2018.11.024

Lei J, Ju H (2012) Signal amplification using functional nanomaterials for biosensing. Chem Soc Rev 41(6):2122–2134. https://doi.org/10.1039/C1CS15274B

Li J, Wei X, Yuan Y (2009) Synthesis of magnetic nanoparticles composed by Prussian blue and glucose oxidase for preparing highly sensitive and selective glucose biosensor. Sensors Actuators B Chem 139(2):400–406. https://doi.org/10.1016/j.snb.2009.03.004

Li J, Hu Y, Yang J, Wei P, Sun W, Shen M, Zhang G, Shi X (2015) Hyaluronic acid-modified Fe3O4@Au core/shell nanostars for multimodal imaging and photothermal therapy of tumors. Biomaterials 38:10–21. https://doi.org/10.1016/j.biomaterials.2014.10.065

Li Q, Kartikowati CW, Horie S, Ogi T, Iwaki T, Okuyama K (2017a) Correlation between particle size/domain structure and magnetic properties of highly crystalline Fe3O4 nanoparticles. Sci Rep 7(1):9894. https://doi.org/10.1038/s41598-017-09897-5

Li P, Kaslan M, Lee SH, Yao J, Gao Z (2017b) Progress in exosome isolation techniques. Theranostics 7(3):789–804., Review. https://doi.org/10.7150/thno.18133

Li Y, Xiao Y, Lin H-P, Reichel D, Bae Y, Lee EY, Jiang Y, Huang X, Yang C, Wang Z (2019a) In vivo β-catenin attenuation by the integrin α5-targeting nano-delivery strategy suppresses triple negative breast cancer stemness and metastasis. Biomaterials 188:160–172. https://doi.org/10.1016/j.biomaterials.2018.10.019

Li X, Ye M, Zhang W, Tan D, Jaffrezic-Renault N, Yang X, Guo Z (2019b) Liquid biopsy of circulating tumor DNA and biosensor applications. Biosens Bioelectron 126:596–607. https://doi.org/10.1016/j.bios.2018.11.037

Li J, Jiang M, Su M, Tian L, Shi W, Yu C (2021) Stretchable and transparent electrochemical sensor based on nanostructured au on carbon nanotube networks for real-time analysis of H2O2 release from cells. Anal Chem 93(17):6723–6730. https://doi.org/10.1021/acs.analchem.1c00336

Li H, Tursun M, Aihemaiti A, Yan P, Liu X, Abdukayum A (2025) A multifunctional nanoplatform based on carbon nanotubes loaded with persistent luminescent nanoparticles for photocatalysis, photothermal therapy, and drug delivery applications. ACS Appl Mater Interfaces 17(9):13592–13604. https://doi.org/10.1021/acsami.4c21734

Liang Z, Khawar MB, Liang J, Sun H (2021) Bio-conjugated quantum dots for cancer research: detection and imaging. Front Oncol 11:749970. https://doi.org/10.3389/fonc.2021.749970. From NLM

Lim HJ, Saha T, Tey BT, Tan WS, Ooi CW (2020) Quartz crystal microbalance-based biosensors as rapid diagnostic devices for infectious diseases. Biosens Bioelectron 168:112513. https://doi.org/10.1016/j.bios.2020.112513

Liu CH, Grodzinski P (2021) Nanotechnology for cancer imaging: advances, challenges, and clinical opportunities. Radiol Imaging Cancer 3(3):e200052. https://doi.org/10.1148/rycan.2021200052. From NLM

Liu Q, Lu X, Li J, Yao X, Li J (2007) Direct electrochemistry of glucose oxidase and electrochemical biosensing of glucose on quantum dots/carbon nanotubes electrodes. Biosens Bioelectron 22(12):3203–3209. https://doi.org/10.1016/j.bios.2007.02.013

Liu X, Li H, Chen Y, Jin Q, Ren K, Ji J (2014) Mixed-charge nanoparticles for long circulation, low reticuloendothelial system clearance, and high tumor accumulation. Adv Healthc Mater 3(9):1439–1447. https://doi.org/10.1002/adhm.201300617

Liu Y, Yuan H, Fales AM, Register JK, Vo-Dinh T (2015) Multifunctional gold nanostars for molecular imaging and cancer therapy. Front Chem 3:Perspective. https://doi.org/10.3389/fchem.2015.00051

Liu W, Liu K, Zhao Y, Zhao S, Luo S, Tian Y, Teng Z, Wang S, Lu G (2017a) T 1-Weighted MR/CT dual-modality imaging-guided photothermal therapy using gadolinium-functionalized triangular gold nanoprism. RSC Adv 7(26):15702–15708

Liu R, Wang Q, Li Q, Yang X, Wang K, Nie W (2017b) Surface plasmon resonance biosensor for sensitive detection of microRNA and cancer cell using multiple signal amplification strategy. Biosens Bioelectron 87:433–438. https://doi.org/10.1016/j.bios.2016.08.090

Liu H, Jian R, Chen H, Tian X, Sun C, Zhu J, Yang Z, Sun J, Wang C (2019a) Application of biodegradable and biocompatible nanocomposites in electronics: current status and future directions. Nano 9(7):950

Liu C, Yang B, Chen X, Hu Z, Dai Z, Yang D, Zheng X, She X, Liu Q (2019b) Capture and separation of circulating tumor cells using functionalized magnetic nanocomposites with simultaneous in situ chemotherapy. Nanotechnology 30(28):285706

Liu R, Xu Y, Zhang N, Qu S, Zeng W, Li R, Dai Z (2023) Nanotechnology for enhancing medical imaging. In: Gu N (ed) Nanomedicine. Springer Nature Singapore, pp 99–156

Liu Z, Zhou Y, Lu J, Gong T, Ibáñez E, Cifuentes A, Lu W (2024) Microfluidic biosensors for biomarker detection in body fluids: a key approach for early cancer diagnosis. Biomark Res 12(1):153. https://doi.org/10.1186/s40364-024-00697-4

Longmire M, Choyke PL, Kobayashi H (2008) Clearance properties of nano-sized particles and molecules as imaging agents: considerations and caveats. Nanomedicine 3(5):703–717

Luo X-L, Xu J-J, Du Y, Chen H-Y (2004) A glucose biosensor based on chitosan–glucose oxidase–gold nanoparticles biocomposite formed by one-step electrodeposition. Anal Biochem 334(2):284–289. https://doi.org/10.1016/j.ab.2004.07.005

Luo D, Wang X, Burda C, Basilion JP (2021) Recent development of gold nanoparticles as contrast agents for cancer diagnosis. Cancers (Basel) 13(8). https://doi.org/10.3390/cancers13081825. From NLM

Ma L, Guo H, Zhao Y, Liu Z, Wang C, Bu J, Sun T, Wei J (2024) Liquid biopsy in cancer: current status, challenges and future prospects. Signal Transduct Target Ther 9(1):336. https://doi.org/10.1038/s41392-024-02021-w

Mahan MM, Doiron AL (2018) Gold nanoparticles as X-Ray, CT, and multimodal imaging contrast agents: formulation, targeting, and methodology. J Nanomater 2018(1):5837276. https://doi.org/10.1155/2018/5837276

Mahato K, Baranwal A, Srivastava A, Maurya PK, Chandra P (2018) Smart materials for biosensing applications. Springer International Publishing, Cham, pp 421–431

Mahato K, Nagpal S, Shah MA, Srivastava A, Maurya PK, Roy S, Jaiswal A, Singh R, Chandra P (2019) Gold nanoparticle surface engineering strategies and their applications in biomedicine and diagnostics. 3 Biotech 9(2):57. https://doi.org/10.1007/s13205-019-1577-z

Malhotra BD, Ali MA (2018) Chapter 5 - Nanocomposite materials: biomolecular devices. In: Malhotra BD, Ali MA (eds) Nanomaterials for biosensors. William Andrew Publishing, pp 145–159

Malik S, Singh J, Goyat R, Saharan Y, Chaudhry V, Umar A, Ibrahim AA, Akbar S, Ameen S, Baskoutas S (2023) Nanomaterials-based biosensor and their applications: a review. Heliyon 9(9):e19929. https://doi.org/10.1016/j.heliyon.2023.e19929

Mandal S, Marie M, Kuchuk A, Manasreh MO, Benamara M (2017) Sensitivity enhancement in an in-vitro glucose sensor using gold nanoelectrode ensembles. J Mater Sci Mater Electron 28(7):5452–5459. https://doi.org/10.1007/s10854-016-6207-5

Marcus Y, Eldor R, Yaron M, Shaklai S, Ish-Shalom M, Shefer G, Stern N, Golan N, Dvir AZ, Pele O et al (2020) Improving blood glucose level predictability using machine learning. Diabetes Metab Res Rev 36(8):e3348. https://doi.org/10.1002/dmrr.3348

Masoumi S, O'Shaughnessy S, Pakdel A (2022) Organic-based flexible thermoelectric generators: from materials to devices. Nano Energy 92:106774. https://doi.org/10.1016/j.nanoen.2021.106774

Materón EM, Gómez FR, Almeida MB, Shimizu FM, Wong A, Teodoro KBR, Silva FSR, Lima MJA, Angelim MKSC, Melendez ME et al (2022) Colorimetric detection of SARS-CoV-2 using plasmonic biosensors and smartphones. ACS Appl Mater Interfaces 14(49):54527–54538. https://doi.org/10.1021/acsami.2c15407

Mathurin J, Deniset-Besseau A, Bazin D, Dartois E, Wagner M, Dazzi A (2022) Photothermal AFM-IR spectroscopy and imaging: status, challenges, and trends. J Appl Phys 131(1). https://doi.org/10.1063/5.0063902. Acccessed 4/4/2025

Mazeiko V, Kausaite-Minkstimiene A, Ramanaviciene A, Balevicius Z, Ramanavicius A (2013) Gold nanoparticle and conducting polymer-polyaniline-based nanocomposites for glucose biosensor design. Sensors Actuators B Chem 189:187–193. https://doi.org/10.1016/j.snb.2013.03.140

McCartney DL, Zhang F, Hillary RF, Zhang Q, Stevenson AJ, Walker RM, Bermingham ML, Boutin T, Morris SW, Campbell A et al (2019) An epigenome-wide association study of sex-specific chronological ageing. Genome Med 12(1):1. https://doi.org/10.1186/s13073-019-0693-z. From NLM

Meder D, Herz DM, Rowe JB, Lehéricy S, Siebner HR (2019) The role of dopamine in the brain - lessons learned from Parkinson's disease. NeuroImage 190:79–93. https://doi.org/10.1016/j.neuroimage.2018.11.021

Michaelides EE (2015) Brownian movement and thermophoresis of nanoparticles in liquids. Int J Heat Mass Transf 81:179–187. https://doi.org/10.1016/j.ijheatmasstransfer.2014.10.019

Mieszawska AJ, Mulder WJM, Fayad ZA, Cormode DP (2013) Multifunctional gold nanoparticles for diagnosis and therapy of disease. Mol Pharm 10(3):831–847. https://doi.org/10.1021/mp3005885

Mikaeeli Kangarshahi B, Morteza NS, Rabiee N (2024) DNA/RNA-based electrochemical nanobiosensors for early detection of cancers. Crit Rev Clin Lab Sci 61(6):473–495. https://doi.org/10.1080/10408363.2024.2321202

Mitchell MJ, Billingsley MM, Haley RM, Wechsler ME, Peppas NA, Langer R (2021) Engineering precision nanoparticles for drug delivery. Nat Rev Drug Discov 20(2):101–124. https://doi.org/10.1038/s41573-020-0090-8

Mohammadpour-Haratbar A, Zare Y, Rhee KY (2022a) Electrochemical biosensors based on polymer nanocomposites for detecting breast cancer: recent progress and future prospects. Adv Colloid Interf Sci 309:102795. https://doi.org/10.1016/j.cis.2022.102795

Mohammadpour-Haratbar A, Mohammadpour-Haratbar S, Zare Y, Rhee KY, Park S-J (2022b) A review on non-enzymatic electrochemical biosensors of glucose using carbon nanofiber nanocomposites. Biosensors 12(11):1004

Mott D, Luo J, Njoki PN, Lin Y, Wang L, Zhong C-J (2007) Synergistic activity of gold-platinum alloy nanoparticle catalysts. Catal Today 122(3):378–385. https://doi.org/10.1016/j.cattod.2007.01.007

Mourdikoudis S, Pallares RM, Thanh NTK (2018) Characterization techniques for nanoparticles: comparison and complementarity upon studying nanoparticle properties. Nanoscale 10(27):12871–12934. https://doi.org/10.1039/C8NR02278J

Mozar FS, Chowdhury EH (2018) PEGylation of carbonate apatite nanoparticles prevents Opsonin binding and enhances tumor accumulation of Gemcitabine. J Pharm Sci 107(9):2497–2508. https://doi.org/10.1016/j.xphs.2018.05.020

Mujahid MH, Upadhyay TK, Khan F, Pandey P, Park MN, Sharangi AB, Saeed M, Upadhye VJ, Kim B (2022) Metallic and metal oxide-derived nanohybrid as a tool for biomedical applications. Biomed Pharmacother 155:113791. https://doi.org/10.1016/j.biopha.2022.113791

Mukherjee P, Roy S, Ghosh D, Nandi SK (2022) Role of animal models in biomedical research: a review. Lab Anim Res 38(1):18. https://doi.org/10.1186/s42826-022-00128-1

Murali S, Ding H, Adedeji F, Qin C, Obungoloch J, Asllani I, Anazodo U, Ntusi NAB, Mammen R, Niendorf T et al (2024) Bringing MRI to low- and middle-income countries: directions, challenges and potential solutions. NMR Biomed 37(7):e4992. https://doi.org/10.1002/nbm.4992

Musielak M, Piotrowski I, Suchorska WM (2019) Superparamagnetic iron oxide nanoparticles (SPIONs) as a multifunctional tool in various cancer therapies. Rep Pract Oncol Radiother 24(4):307–314. https://doi.org/10.1016/j.rpor.2019.04.002. From NLM

Naeim H, Kheiri F, Sirousazar M, Afghan A (2018) Ionic liquid/reduced graphene oxide/nickel-palladium nanoparticle hybrid synthesized for non-enzymatic electrochemical glucose sensing. Electrochim Acta 282:137–146. https://doi.org/10.1016/j.electacta.2018.05.204

Naiim M, Boualem A, Ferre C, Jabloun M, Jalocha A, Ravier P (2015) Multiangle dynamic light scattering for the improvement of multimodal particle size distribution measurements. Soft Matter 11(1):28–32. https://doi.org/10.1039/C4SM01995D

Nguyen MD, Tran HV, Xu S, Lee TR (2021) Fe(3)O(4) nanoparticles: structures, synthesis, magnetic properties, surface functionalization, and emerging applications. Appl Sci (Basel) 11(23). https://doi.org/10.3390/app112311301. From NLM.

Nune SK, Gunda P, Thallapally PK, Lin YY, Forrest ML, Berkland CJ (2009) Nanoparticles for biomedical imaging. Expert Opin Drug Deliv 6(11):1175–1194. https://doi.org/10.1517/17425240903229031. From NLM

Oh I-H, Min HS, Li L, Tran TH, Lee Y-K, Kwon IC, Choi K, Kim K, Huh KM (2013) Cancer cell-specific photoactivity of pheophorbide a–glycol chitosan nanoparticles for photodynamic therapy in tumor-bearing mice. Biomaterials 34(27):6454–6463. https://doi.org/10.1016/j.biomaterials.2013.05.017

Organization, W.H (2017) Cardiovascular disease. https://www.who.int/cardiovascular_diseases/en/

Osuna V, Vega-Rios A, Zaragoza-Contreras EA, Estrada-Moreno IA, Dominguez RB (2022) Progress of polyaniline glucose sensors for diabetes mellitus management utilizing enzymatic and non-enzymatic detection. Biosensors 12(3):137

Park ES, Yan JP, Ang RA, Lee JH, Deng X, Duffy SP, Beja K, Annala M, Black PC, Chi KN et al (2018) Isolation and genome sequencing of individual circulating tumor cells using hydrogel encapsulation and laser capture microdissection. Lab Chip 18(12):1736–1749. https://doi.org/10.1039/C8LC00184G

Piloto AML, Ribeiro DSM, Rodrigues SSM, Santos JLM, Sampaio P, Sales G (2021) Imprinted fluorescent cellulose membranes for the on-site detection of myoglobin in biological media. ACS Appl Bio Mater 4(5):4224–4235. https://doi.org/10.1021/acsabm.1c00039

Qamar SUR (2021) Nanocomposites: potential therapeutic agents for the diagnosis and treatment of infectious diseases and cancer. Colloid Interface Sci Commun 43:100463

Qu X, Li X, Liang J, Wang Y, Liu M, Liang J (2016) Micro-CT imaging of RGD-conjugated gold nanorods targeting tumor in vivo. J Nanomater 2016(1):8368154. https://doi.org/10.1155/2016/8368154

Quillard T, Libby P (2012) Molecular imaging of atherosclerosis for improving diagnostic and therapeutic development. Circ Res 111(2):231–244. https://doi.org/10.1161/CIRCRESAHA.112.268144. Acccessed 2025/04/04

Rahman M (2023) Magnetic resonance imaging and iron-oxide nanoparticles in the era of personalized medicine. Nano 7(4):424–449. https://doi.org/10.7150/ntno.86467. From NLM

Rahsepar M, Foroughi F, Kim H (2019) A new enzyme-free biosensor based on nitrogen-doped graphene with high sensing performance for electrochemical detection of glucose at biological pH value. Sensors Actuators B Chem 282:322–330. https://doi.org/10.1016/j.snb.2018.11.078

Rana D, Colombani T, Saleh B, Mohammed HS, Annabi N, Bencherif SA (2023) Engineering injectable, biocompatible, and highly elastic bioadhesive cryogels. Mater Today Bio 19:100572. https://doi.org/10.1016/j.mtbio.2023.100572

Ranjan P, Khan R (2022) Electrochemical immunosensor for early detection of β-Amyloid Alzheimer's disease biomarker based on aligned carbon nanotubes gold nanocomposites. Biosensors 12(11):1059

Reduwan Billah SM (2019) Composites and nanocomposites. In: Jafar Mazumder MA, Sheardown H, Al-Ahmed A (eds) Functional polymers. Springer International Publishing, pp 1–67

Ren X, Meng X, Tang F (2005) Preparation of Ag–Au nanoparticle and its application to glucose biosensor. Sensors Actuators B Chem 110(2):358–363. https://doi.org/10.1016/j.snb.2005.02.016

Resch-Genger U, Grabolle M, Cavaliere-Jaricot S, Nitschke R, Nann T (2008) Quantum dots versus organic dyes as fluorescent labels. Nat Methods 5(9):763–775. https://doi.org/10.1038/nmeth.1248

Rhouati A, Marty J-L, Vasilescu A (2018) Chapter 7 - Metal nanomaterial-assisted Aptasensors for emerging pollutants detection. In: Nikolelis DP, Nikoleli G-P (eds) Nanotechnology and biosensors. Elsevier, pp 193–231

Rodriguez JA, Jirsak T, Dvorak J, Sambasivan S, Fischer D (2000) Reaction of NO2 with Zn and ZnO: photoemission, XANES, and density functional studies on the formation of NO3. J Phys Chem B 104(2):319–328. https://doi.org/10.1021/jp993224g

Rodriguez-Loya J, Lerma M, Gardea-Torresdey JL (2023) Dynamic light scattering and its application to control nanoparticle aggregation in colloidal systems: a review. Micromachines (Basel) 15(1). https://doi.org/10.3390/mi15010024. From NLM

Ross H, Scattering F, Sizing P (1999) Applications. In: Lindon JC (ed) Encyclopedia of spectroscopy and spectrometry. Elsevier, pp 2067–2074

Rudd T, Skidmore MA, Yates EA (2005) Chapter 12 - Surface-based studies of Heparin/Heparan sulfate-protein interactions: considerations for surface immobilisation of HS/Heparin Saccharides and monitoring their interactions with binding proteins. In: Garg HG, Linhardt RJ, Hales CA (eds) Chemistry and biology of Heparin and Heparan Sulfate. Elsevier Science, pp 345–366

Ryvolova M, Chomoucka J, Drbohlavova J, Kopel P, Babula P, Hynek D, Adam V, Eckschlager T, Hubalek J, Stiborova M (2012) Modern micro and nanoparticle-based imaging techniques. Sensors 12(11):14792–14820

Sabet M (2024) Advanced developments in carbon nanotube polymer composites for structural applications. Iran Polym J. https://doi.org/10.1007/s13726-024-01419-1

Saei AA, Dolatabadi JEN, Najafi-Marandi P, Abhari A, de la Guardia M (2013) Electrochemical biosensors for glucose based on metal nanoparticles. TrAC Trends Anal Chem 42:216–227. https://doi.org/10.1016/j.trac.2012.09.011

Saha T, Del Caño R, Mahato K, De la Paz E, Chen C, Ding S, Yin L, Wang J (2023) Wearable electrochemical glucose sensors in diabetes management: a comprehensive review. Chem Rev 123(12):7854–7889. https://doi.org/10.1021/acs.chemrev.3c00078

Saikia A, Karak N (2023) Chapter 1 - Introduction to biodegradable and biocompatible polymer nanocomposites: synthesis, structure, fundamental properties, biocompatibility, and biodegradability. In: Deshmukh K, Pandey M (eds) Biodegradable and biocompatible polymer nanocomposites. Elsevier, pp 1–34

Sakamoto JH, Smith BR, Xie B, Rokhlin SI, Lee SC, Ferrari M (2005) The molecular analysis of breast cancer utilizing targeted nanoparticle based ultrasound contrast agents. Technol Cancer Res Treat 4(6):627–636. https://doi.org/10.1177/153303460500400606

Sanko V, Kuralay F (2023) Label-free electrochemical biosensor platforms for cancer diagnosis: recent achievements and challenges. Biosensors 13(3):333

Schmitt J, Decher G, Dressick WJ, Brandow SL, Geer RE, Shashidhar R, Calvert JM (1997) Metal nanoparticle/polymer superlattice films: fabrication and control of layer structure. Adv Mater 9(1):61–65. https://doi.org/10.1002/adma.19970090114

Schubert J, Chanana M (2018) Coating matters: review on colloidal stability of nanoparticles with biocompatible coatings in biological media, living cells and organisms. Curr Med Chem 25(35):4553–4586. https://doi.org/10.2174/0929867325666180601101859. From NLM

Seewoodhary M (2020) An overview of diabetic retinopathy and other ocular complications of diabetes mellitus. Eye 36:71

Sen M (2020) Nanocomposite materials. In: Sen M (ed) Nanotechnology and the environment. IntechOpen

Sen A (2025) Polymer nanocomposites in diabetes management: advances in biosensors and drug delivery systems. Discov Mater 5(1):26. https://doi.org/10.1007/s43939-025-00210-0

Seo M, Gorelikov I, Williams R, Matsuura N (2010) Microfluidic assembly of monodisperse, nanoparticle-incorporated perfluorocarbon microbubbles for medical imaging and therapy. Langmuir 26(17):13855–13860. https://doi.org/10.1021/la102272d

Setiawan BD, Rizqi O, Brilianti NF, Wasito H (2018) Nanoporous of waste avian eggshell to reduce heavy metal and acidity in water. Sustain Chem Pharm 10:163–167. https://doi.org/10.1016/j.scp.2018.10.002

Shang T, Zhang JY, Thomas A, Arnold MA, Vetter BN, Heinemann L, Klonoff DC (2022) Products for monitoring glucose levels in the human body with noninvasive optical, noninvasive fluid sampling, or minimally invasive technologies. J Diabetes Sci Technol 16(1):168–214. https://doi.org/10.1177/19322968211007212. From NLM

Sheikhzadeh E, Beni V, Zourob M (2021) Nanomaterial application in bio/sensors for the detection of infectious diseases. Talanta 230:122026. https://doi.org/10.1016/j.talanta.2020.122026

Shen S, Koonjoo N, Boele T, Lu J, Waddington DEJ, Zhang M, Rosen MS (2024) Enhancing organ and vascular contrast in preclinical ultra-low field MRI using superparamagnetic iron oxide nanoparticles. Commun Biol 7(1):1197. https://doi.org/10.1038/s42003-024-06884-1

Shi Kam NW, Jessop TC, Wender PA, Dai H (2004) Nanotube molecular transporters: internalization of carbon nanotube–protein conjugates into mammalian cells. J Am Chem Soc 126(22):6850–6851. https://doi.org/10.1021/ja0486059

Shi P, Qu K, Wang J, Li M, Ren J, Qu X (2012) pH-responsive NIR enhanced drug release from gold nanocages possesses high potency against cancer cells. Chem Commun 48(61):7640–7642. https://doi.org/10.1039/C2CC33543C

Shinde SS, Bhosale CH, Rajpure KY (2012) Photocatalytic degradation of toluene using sprayed N-doped ZnO thin films in aqueous suspension. J Photochem Photobiol B Biol 113:70–77. https://doi.org/10.1016/j.jphotobiol.2012.05.008

Shinde SS, Bhosale CH, Rajpure KY (2013) Photoelectrochemical properties of highly mobilized Li-doped ZnO thin films. J Photochem Photobiol B Biol 120:1–9. https://doi.org/10.1016/j.jphotobiol.2013.01.003

Siegel RL, Kratzer TB, Giaquinto AN, Sung H, Jemal A (2025) Cancer statistics, 2025. CA Cancer J Clin 75(1):10–45. https://doi.org/10.3322/caac.21871

Singh I, Birajdar B (2017) Synthesis, characterization and photocatalytic activity of mesoporous Na-doped TiO2 nano-powder prepared via a solvent-controlled non-aqueous sol–gel route. RSC Adv 7(85):54053–54062. https://doi.org/10.1039/C7RA10108B

Singh S, Dhawan A, Karhana S, Bhat M, Dinda AK (2020) Quantum dots: an emerging tool for point-of-care testing. Micromachines (Basel) 11(12). https://doi.org/10.3390/mi11121058. From NLM

Singh S, Podder PS, Russo M, Henry C, Cinti S (2023) Tailored point-of-care biosensors for liquid biopsy in the field of oncology. Lab Chip 23(1):44–61. https://doi.org/10.1039/D2LC00666A

Sinha Ray S (2013) 3 - Structure and morphology characterization techniques. In: Sinha Ray S (ed) Clay-containing polymer nanocomposites. Elsevier, pp 39–66

Sleeman R, Carter J (2005) F. Forensic sciences | Explosives. In: Worsfold P, Townshend A, Poole C (eds) Encyclopedia of analytical science, 2nd edn. Elsevier, pp 400–406

Smith AM, Duan H, Mohs AM, Nie S (2008) Bioconjugated quantum dots for in vivo molecular and cellular imaging. Adv Drug Deliv Rev 60(11):1226–1240. https://doi.org/10.1016/j.addr.2008.03.015

Soda N, Rehm BHA, Sonar P, Nguyen N-T, Shiddiky MJA (2019) Advanced liquid biopsy technologies for circulating biomarker detection. J Mater Chem B 7(43):6670–6704. https://doi.org/10.1039/C9TB01490J

Soler-Botija C, Gálvez-Montón C, Bayés Genís A (2019) Epigenetic biomarkers in cardiovascular diseases. Front Genet 10:Review. https://doi.org/10.3389/fgene.2019.00950

Sonuç Karaboğa MN, Sezgintürk MK (2021) A nano-composite based regenerative neuro biosensor sensitive to Parkinsonism-associated protein DJ-1/Park7 in cerebrospinal fluid and saliva. Bioelectrochemistry 138:107734. https://doi.org/10.1016/j.bioelechem.2020.107734

Souza Junior JB, Schleder GR, Bettini J, Nogueira IC, Fazzio A, Leite ER (2021) Pair distribution function obtained from electron diffraction: an advanced real-space structural characterization tool. Matter 4(2):441–460. https://doi.org/10.1016/j.matt.2020.10.025

Suárez B, Solé C, Márquez M, Nanetti F, Lawrie CH (2022) Circulating MicroRNAs as cancer biomarkers in liquid biopsies. In: Schmitz U, Wolkenhauer O, Vera-González J (eds) Systems biology of MicroRNAs in cancer. Springer International Publishing, pp 23–73

Subramanian J, Savage JC, Tremblay M-È (2020) Synaptic loss in Alzheimer's disease: mechanistic insights provided by two-photon in vivo imaging of Transgenic Mouse Models. Front Cell Neurosci 14:Review. https://doi.org/10.3389/fncel.2020.592607

Tang X, Zhu Y, Guan W, Zhou W, Wei P (2022) Advances in nanosensors for cardiovascular disease detection. Life Sci 305:120733. https://doi.org/10.1016/j.lfs.2022.120733

Teleki A, Suter M, Kidambi P, Ergeneman O, Krumeich F, Nelson B, Pratsinis S (2009) Hermetically coated superparamagnetic Fe2O3 particles with SiO2 nanofilms. Chem Mater:21. https://doi.org/10.1021/cm803153m

Tettey KE, Yee MQ, Lee D (2010) Layer-by-layer assembly of charged particles in nonpolar media. Langmuir 26(12):9974–9980. https://doi.org/10.1021/la1000655

Tewari M, Rana P, Pande V (2025) Nanomaterial-based biosensors for the detection of COVID-19. Indian J Microbiol 65(1):120–136. https://doi.org/10.1007/s12088-024-01336-0

Thapa RK, Kim JO (2023) Nanomedicine-based commercial formulations: current developments and future prospects. J Pharm Investig 53(1):19–33. https://doi.org/10.1007/s40005-022-00607-6

Tian ZR, Voigt JA, Liu J, McKenzie B, McDermott MJ (2002) Biomimetic arrays of oriented helical ZnO nanorods and columns. J Am Chem Soc 124(44):12954–12955. https://doi.org/10.1021/ja0279545

Topete A, Varela A, Navarro-Real M, Rial R, Pardo A, Taboada P (2025) Revisiting gold nanoshells as multifunctional biomedical nanotools. Coord Chem Rev 523:216250. https://doi.org/10.1016/j.ccr.2024.216250

Vaidyanathan R, Soon RH, Zhang P, Jiang K, Lim CT (2019) Cancer diagnosis: from tumor to liquid biopsy and beyond. Lab Chip 19(1):11–34. https://doi.org/10.1039/C8LC00684A

Valimukhametova AR, Zub OS, Lee BH, Fannon O, Nguyen S, Gonzalez-Rodriguez R, Akkaraju GR, Naumov AV (2022) Dual-mode fluorescence/ultrasound imaging with biocompatible metal-doped graphene quantum dots. ACS Biomater Sci Eng 8(11):4965–4975. https://doi.org/10.1021/acsbiomaterials.2c00794

Verma R, Gangwar J, Srivastava AK (2017) Multiphase TiO2 nanostructures: a review of efficient synthesis, growth mechanism, probing capabilities, and applications in bio-safety and health. RSC Adv 7(70):44199–44224. https://doi.org/10.1039/C7RA06925A

Volpatti LR, Matranga MA, Cortinas AB, Delcassian D, Daniel KB, Langer R, Anderson DG (2020) Glucose-responsive nanoparticles for rapid and extended self-regulated insulin delivery. ACS Nano 14(1):488–497. https://doi.org/10.1021/acsnano.9b06395

Wahajuddin, Arora S (2012) Superparamagnetic iron oxide nanoparticles: magnetic nanoplatforms as drug carriers. Int J Nanomedicine 7:3445–3471. https://doi.org/10.2147/ijn.S30320. From NLM

Wall MA, Harmsen S, Pal S, Zhang L, Arianna G, Lombardi JR, Drain CM, Kircher MF (2017) Surfactant-free shape control of gold nanoparticles enabled by unified theoretical framework of nanocrystal synthesis. Adv Mater 29(21). https://doi.org/10.1002/adma.201605622. From NLM

Wan JCM, Massie C, Garcia-Corbacho J, Mouliere F, Brenton JD, Caldas C, Pacey S, Baird R, Rosenfeld N (2017) Liquid biopsies come of age: towards implementation of circulating tumour DNA. Nat Rev Cancer 17(4):223–238. https://doi.org/10.1038/nrc.2017.7

Wang ZL, Lee JL (2008) Chapter 9 - Electron microscopy techniques for imaging and analysis of nanoparticles. In: Kohli R, Mittal KL (eds) Developments in surface contamination and cleaning, 2nd edn. William Andrew Publishing, pp 395–443

Wang Z, Zhou X, Zhang J, Boey F, Zhang H (2009) Direct electrochemical reduction of single-layer graphene oxide and subsequent functionalization with glucose oxidase. J Phys Chem C 113(32):14071–14075. https://doi.org/10.1021/jp906348x

Wang Z, Chen Z, Liu Z, Shi P, Dong K, Ju E, Ren J, Qu X (2014) A multi-stimuli responsive gold nanocage–hyaluronic platform for targeted photothermal and chemotherapy. Biomaterials 35(36):9678–9688. https://doi.org/10.1016/j.biomaterials.2014.08.013

Wang Z, Qiao R, Tang N, Lu Z, Wang H, Zhang Z, Xue X, Huang Z, Zhang S, Zhang G et al (2017a) Active targeting theranostic iron oxide nanoparticles for MRI and magnetic resonance-guided focused ultrasound ablation of lung cancer. Biomaterials 127:25–35. https://doi.org/10.1016/j.biomaterials.2017.02.037

Wang J, Chang S, Li G, Sun Y (2017b) Application of liquid biopsy in precision medicine: opportunities and challenges. Front Med 11(4):522–527. https://doi.org/10.1007/s11684-017-0526-7
Wang J-L, Du X-J, Yang J-X, Shen S, Li H-J, Luo Y-L, Iqbal S, Xu C-F, Ye X-D, Cao J et al (2018) The effect of surface poly(ethylene glycol) length on in vivo drug delivery behaviors of polymeric nanoparticles. Biomaterials 182:104–113. https://doi.org/10.1016/j.biomaterials.2018.08.022
Wang F, Hu S, Shi F, Huang K, Li J (2020) A non-enzymatic sensor based on Fc-CHIT/CNT@Cu nanohybrids for electrochemical detection of glucose. Polymers 12(10):2419
Wang T-T, Huang X-F, Huang H, Luo P, Qing L-S (2022) Nanomaterial-based optical- and electrochemical-biosensors for urine glucose detection: a comprehensive review. Adv Sensor Energy Mater 1(3):100016. https://doi.org/10.1016/j.asems.2022.100016
Wang C, Yang X, Zhu G, Wang T, Yu D, Lu Y, Yu H (2023) One-step synthesis of copper-platinum nanoparticles modified electrode for non-enzymatic salivary glucose detection. Colloids Surf A Physicochem Eng Asp 658:130672. https://doi.org/10.1016/j.colsurfa.2022.130672
Wang B, Hu S, Teng Y, Chen J, Wang H, Xu Y, Wang K, Xu J, Cheng Y, Gao X (2024a) Current advance of nanotechnology in diagnosis and treatment for malignant tumors. Signal Transduct Target Ther 9(1):200. https://doi.org/10.1038/s41392-024-01889-y
Wang X, Wang L, Lin H, Zhu Y, Huang D, Lai M, Xi X, Huang J, Zhang W, Zhong T (2024b) Research progress of CTC, ctDNA, and EVs in cancer liquid biopsy. Front Oncol 14:Review. https://doi.org/10.3389/fonc.2024.1303335
Waqas M, Lan J, Zhang X, Fan Y, Zhang P, Liu C, Jiang Z, Wang X, Zeng J, Chen W (2020) Fabrication of non-enzymatic electrochemical glucose sensor based on Pd–Mn alloy nanoparticles supported on reduced graphene oxide. Electroanalysis 32(6):1226–1236. https://doi.org/10.1002/elan.201900705
Warnement MR, Tomlinson ID, Chang JC, Schreuder MA, Luckabaugh CM, Rosenthal SJ (2008) Controlling the reactivity of Ampiphilic quantum dots in biological assays through hydrophobic assembly of custom PEG derivatives. Bioconjug Chem 19(7):1404–1413. https://doi.org/10.1021/bc800104n
Webb J, Holgate J (2003) H. MICROSCOPY | scanning electron microscopy. In: Caballero B (ed) Encyclopedia of food sciences and nutrition, 2nd edn. Academic Press, pp 3922–3928
Wei P, Chen J, Hu Y, Li X, Wang H, Shen M, Shi X (2016) Dendrimer-stabilized gold nanostars as a multifunctional theranostic nanoplatform for CT imaging, photothermal therapy, and gene silencing of tumors. Adv Healthc Mater 5(24):3203–3213. https://doi.org/10.1002/adhm.201600923
Wei Y, Liao R, Mahmood AA, Xu H, Zhou Q (2017) pH-responsive pHLIP (pH low insertion peptide) nanoclusters of superparamagnetic iron oxide nanoparticles as a tumor-selective MRI contrast agent. Acta Biomater 55:194–203. https://doi.org/10.1016/j.actbio.2017.03.046
Welsher K, Liu Z, Daranciang D, Dai H (2008) Selective probing and imaging of cells with single walled carbon nanotubes as near-infrared fluorescent molecules. Nano Lett 8(2):586–590. https://doi.org/10.1021/nl072949q
Welsher K, Sherlock SP, Dai H (2011) Deep-tissue anatomical imaging of mice using carbon nanotube fluorophores in the second near-infrared window. Proc Natl Acad Sci USA 108(22):8943–8948. https://doi.org/10.1073/pnas.1014501108. From NLM
Woollam M (2025a). https://BioRender.com/qqax65b. Created in Biorender
Woollam M (2025b). https://BioRender.com/a09faqd. Created in Biorender
Woollam M (2025c). https://BioRender.com/zkl40sq. Created in Biorender
Woollam M (2025d). https://BioRender.com/w4w9kkn. Created in Biorender
Woollam M (2025e). https://BioRender.com/fndo3of. Created in Biorender
Wu B-Y, Hou S-H, Yin F, Li J, Zhao Z-X, Huang J-D, Chen Q (2007a) Amperometric glucose biosensor based on layer-by-layer assembly of multilayer films composed of chitosan, gold nanoparticles and glucose oxidase modified Pt electrode. Biosens Bioelectron 22(6):838–844. https://doi.org/10.1016/j.bios.2006.03.009

Wu J, Fu Z, Yan F, Ju H (2007b) Biomedical and clinical applications of immunoassays and immunosensors for tumor markers. TrAC Trends Anal Chem 26(7):679–688. https://doi.org/10.1016/j.trac.2007.05.007

Wu H, Shi H, Zhang H, Wang X, Yang Y, Yu C, Hao C, Du J, Hu H, Yang S (2014) Prostate stem cell antigen antibody-conjugated multiwalled carbon nanotubes for targeted ultrasound imaging and drug delivery. Biomaterials 35(20):5369–5380. https://doi.org/10.1016/j.biomaterials.2014.03.038

Xia Q, Jiang H, Liu X, Yin L, Wang X (2024) Advances in engineered nano-biosensors for bacteria diagnosis and multidrug resistance inhibition. Biosensors 14(2):59

Xiao Y, Li CM (2008) Nanocomposites: from fabrications to electrochemical bioapplications. Electroanalysis 20(6):648–662. https://doi.org/10.1002/elan.200704125

Xiao Y, Patolsky F, Katz E, Hainfeld JF, Willner I (2003) "Plugging into Enzymes": Nanowiring of redox enzymes by a gold nanoparticle. Science 299(5614):1877–1881. https://doi.org/10.1126/science.1080664

Xiao W, Lin J, Li M, Ma Y, Chen Y, Zhang C, Li D, Gu H (2012) Prolonged in vivo circulation time by zwitterionic modification of magnetite nanoparticles for blood pool contrast agents. Contrast Media Mol Imaging 7(3):320–327. https://doi.org/10.1002/cmmi.501

Xie W, Liu Y, Lin J (2023) Advances in organic–inorganic nanocomposites for cancer imaging and therapy. Nanotechnol Rev 12(1):20230133

Xu J, Wang J, Mitchell M, Mukherjee P, Jeffries-El M, Petrich JW, Lin Z (2007) Organic−inorganic nanocomposites via directly grafting conjugated polymers onto quantum dots. J Am Chem Soc 129(42):12828–12833. https://doi.org/10.1021/ja074133x

Xue M-H, Xu Q, Zhou M, Zhu J-J (2006) In situ immobilization of glucose oxidase in chitosan–gold nanoparticle hybrid film on Prussian Blue modified electrode for high-sensitivity glucose detection. Electrochem Commun 8(9):1468–1474. https://doi.org/10.1016/j.elecom.2006.07.019

Xue Y, Gao Y, Meng F, Luo L (2021) Recent progress of nanotechnology-based theranostic systems in cancer treatments. Cancer Biol Med 18(2):336–351. https://doi.org/10.20892/j.issn.2095-3941.2020.0510. From NLM

Yadav S, Bukke SPN, Prajapati S, Singh AP, Chettupalli AK, Nicholas B (2025) Nanobiosensors in neurodegenerative disease diagnosis: a promising pathway for early detection. Digit Health 11:20552076251342457. https://doi.org/10.1177/20552076251342457

Yang W, Ratinac KR, Ringer SP, Thordarson P, Gooding JJ, Braet F (2010) Carbon nanomaterials in biosensors: should you use nanotubes or graphene? Angew Chem Int Ed 49(12):2114–2138. https://doi.org/10.1002/anie.200903463

Yang L, Sun H, Liu Y, Hou W, Yang Y, Cai R, Cui C, Zhang P, Pan X, Li X (2018) Self-assembled aptamer-grafted hyperbranched polymer nanocarrier for targeted and photoresponsive drug delivery. Angew Chem 130(52):17294–17298

Yang J, Wang X, Sun Y, Chen B, Hu F, Guo C, Yang T (2023) Recent advances in colorimetric sensors based on gold nanoparticles for pathogen detection. Biosensors 13(1):29

Yao L, Wang L, Huang F, Cai G, Xi X, Lin J (2018) A microfluidic impedance biosensor based on immunomagnetic separation and urease catalysis for continuous-flow detection of E. coli O157:H7. Sensors Actuators B Chem 259:1013–1021. https://doi.org/10.1016/j.snb.2017.12.110

Yigit MV, Moore A, Medarova Z (2012) Magnetic nanoparticles for cancer diagnosis and therapy. Pharm Res 29(5):1180–1188. https://doi.org/10.1007/s11095-012-0679-7

Yin C, Hu P, Qin L, Wang Z, Zhao H (2024) The current status and future directions on nanoparticles for tumor molecular imaging. Int J Nanomedicine 19:9549–9574. https://doi.org/10.2147/ijn.S484206. From NLM

Yoo E-H, Lee S-Y (2010) Glucose biosensors: An overview of use in clinical practice. Sensors 10(5):4558–4576

Young SK (2002) Overview of sol-gel science and technology

Yu X, Trase I, Ren M, Duval K, Guo X, Chen Z (2016) Design of nanoparticle-based carriers for targeted drug delivery. J Nanomater 2016(1):1087250. https://doi.org/10.1155/2016/1087250

Yu C, Bao H, Chen Z, Li X, Liu X, Wang W, Huang J, Zhang Z (2021) Enhanced and long-term CT imaging tracking of transplanted stem cells labeled with temperature-responsive gold nanoparticles. J Mater Chem B 9(12):2854–2865. https://doi.org/10.1039/D0TB02997A

Yudasaka M, Yomogida Y, Zhang M, Tanaka T, Nakahara M, Kobayashi N, Okamatsu-Ogura Y, Machida K, Ishihara K, Saeki K et al (2017) Near-infrared photoluminescent carbon nanotubes for imaging of Brown fat. Sci Rep 7(1):44760. https://doi.org/10.1038/srep44760

Yue S, Lu J, Zhang J (2009) Synthesis of three-dimensional ZnO superstructures by a one-pot solution process. Mater Chem Phys 117(1):4–8. https://doi.org/10.1016/j.matchemphys.2009.05.010

Yusefi H, Helfield B (2022) Ultrasound contrast imaging: fundamentals and emerging technology. Front Phys 10:Review. https://doi.org/10.3389/fphy.2022.791145

Zaidi SA, Shin JH (2016) Recent developments in nanostructure based electrochemical glucose sensors. Talanta 149:30–42

Zhang H, Douglas Y, Wang C (2008) Quantum dots for cancer diagnosis and therapy: biological and clinical perspectives. Nanomedicine 3(1):83–91. https://doi.org/10.2217/17435889.3.1.83

Zhang A, Meng K, Liu Y, Pan Y, Qu W, Chen D, Xie S (2020) Absorption, distribution, metabolism, and excretion of nanocarriers in vivo and their influences. Adv Colloid Interf Sci 284:102261. https://doi.org/10.1016/j.cis.2020.102261

Zhao Y, Liu W, Tian Y, Yang Z, Wang X, Zhang Y, Tang Y, Zhao S, Wang C, Liu Y et al (2018) Anti-EGFR peptide-conjugated triangular gold nanoplates for computed tomography/photoacoustic imaging-guided photothermal therapy of non-small cell lung cancer. ACS Appl Mater Interfaces 10(20):16992–17003. https://doi.org/10.1021/acsami.7b19013

Zhi D, Yang T, Yang J, Fu S, Zhang S (2020) Targeting strategies for superparamagnetic iron oxide nanoparticles in cancer therapy. Acta Biomater 102:13–34. https://doi.org/10.1016/j.actbio.2019.11.027

Zhong Y, Meng F, Deng C, Zhong Z (2014) Ligand-directed active tumor-targeting polymeric nanoparticles for cancer chemotherapy. Biomacromolecules 15(6):1955–1969

Zhou Y, Dai Z (2018) New strategies in the design of nanomedicines to oppose uptake by the mononuclear phagocyte system and enhance cancer therapeutic efficacy. Chem Asian J 13(22):3333–3340

Zhu C, Yang G, Li H, Du D, Lin Y (2015) Electrochemical sensors and biosensors based on nanomaterials and nanostructures. Anal Chem 87(1):230–249. https://doi.org/10.1021/ac5039863

Nanocomposites in Diagnostics and Therapeutics: Recent Advances and Emerging Applications

5

Rajan Patyal, Kaifi Ali, and Vinay Sharma

Abstract

Nanocomposites play an important role in the advancement of modern biomedical diagnostics. These multifunctional materials exhibit enhanced physicochemical properties, such as a high surface area-to-volume ratio, tunable optical and electrical characteristics, and excellent biocompatibility, which make them highly suitable for various biological applications. They have demonstrated remarkable sensitivity and specificity in detecting cancer biomarkers, infectious disease antigens, and metabolic enzymes. Beyond diagnostics, nanocomposites are increasingly used in theranostics, where they integrate diagnostic imaging with targeted therapy. This is particularly impactful in oncology, where metal and carbon-based nanocomposites enable dual functionality for tumor imaging and localized drug delivery. This chapter explores the major categories of nanocomposites employed in medical diagnostics and highlights their emerging applications in nanotheranostics, advancing the development of next-generation tools for precision medicine.

Keywords

Nanocomposites · Medical diagnostics · Carbon dots · Nanotheranostics, · Biosensors · Imaging

R. Patyal · K. Ali · V. Sharma (✉)
Department of Biosciences and Bioengineering, Indian Institute of Technology Jammu, Jagti, Jammu, Jammu and Kashmir, India
e-mail: vinay.sharma@iitjammu.ac.in

V. Patel et al. (eds.), *Biosensor Technology in Translating Novel Materials into Practical Devices*, https://doi.org/10.1007/978-981-95-5519-2_5

5.1 Introduction

In recent years, nanotechnology has brought significant changes in the healthcare sector, especially in the fields of diagnostics, therapeutics, and personalized medicine. Consequently, nanotechnology, which involves synthesizing and using materials of dimensions in the nanometer range (usually less than 100 nm), gives us the opportunity to create materials and/or devices capable of interacting with biological systems at the molecular level (Chen et al. 2019; Khan et al. 2019). In particular, nanocomposites, as one of the nanostructured materials, have been an efficient and versatile class based on their multifunctionality and better physicochemical properties (Baig et al. 2021).

Nanocomposites are typically categorized according to the nature of the nanofillers employed, as shown in Fig. 5.1. The metal-based nanocomposites consist of gold (Au), silver (Ag), iron oxide (Fe_3O_4), and zinc oxide (ZnO) particles, which have plasmonic, magnetic, and antibacterial properties (Yaqoob et al. 2020; Dar et al. 2011). Polymer-derived nanocomposites involve the use of synthetic or natural

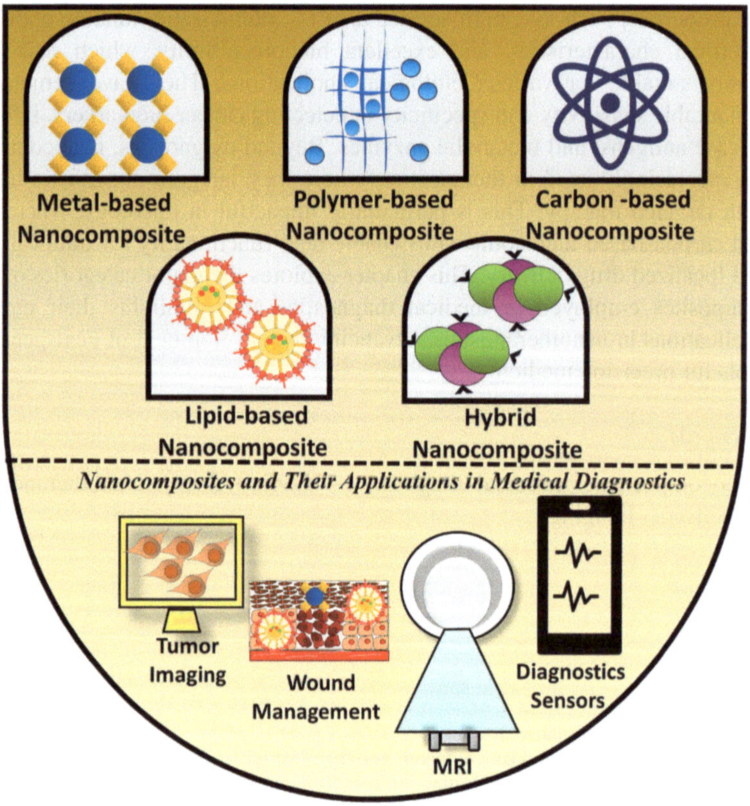

Fig. 5.1 Schematic of different types of nanocomposites and their application in medical diagnostics

polymers with flexibility or easy processability, which are frequently used for biosensors and drug delivery systems (Solangi et al. 2024; Julius et al. 2025). The carbon-based nanocomposites, including carbon dot (CD)–polymer nanocomposite, graphene–metal oxide nanocomposite, and CDs–metal nanoparticle nanocomposite, have high surface area, conductivity, and biocompatibility (Saleh et al. 2025; Mahor et al. 2021). Lipid-based nanocomposites such as liposomes and solid lipid nanoparticles are particularly well-suited for drug- and bio-molecule encapsulation (Puri et al. 2009). Hybrid nanocomposites also combine more than one class of nanomaterial to achieve a synergistic effect in biomedical applications (Mehta et al. 2022; Phadtare et al. 2025). Among carbon-based nanocomposites, CDs are a kind of carbon nanomaterial with a small size (usually <10 nm) and have remarkable fluorescence, water solubility, and low toxicity (Patyal et al. 2025; Warjurkar et al. 2023; Sharma et al. 2018, 2021). CDs, together with other materials, like metal NPs or biopolymers, chemical conjugation of metal NPs or biopolymers templates by forming multifunctional nanocomposites, can be employed in various diagnostics (Vodyashkin et al. 2022; Yaraki et al. 2022; Fazal et al. 2023). Due to their favorable quantum yield and excellent stability, CDs have strong potential for applications in bioimaging, fluorescence resonance energy transfer (FRET)-based techniques, and real-time detection of biomolecules, offering high sensitivity, low toxicity, and reliable performance in complex biological environments (Ge et al. 2025; Kim and Kim 2012; Kaur et al. 2019). Furthermore, their surfaces are easy to modify by the addition of antibodies, aptamers, or peptides for the targeted recognition of certain disease-related biomarkers.

Traditional diagnostic techniques like ELISA, western blot, and PCR are accurate but have several drawbacks. They are often expensive, time-consuming, and require skilled operators and centralized laboratory setups (Hosseini et al. 2018; Ghosh et al. 2014; Khodaparast et al. 2024). These methods may also show low sensitivity or delayed response, and can suffer from non-specific interactions. As a result, they are not always suitable for rapid or affordable diagnosis. On the other hand, nanocomposite-based diagnostic techniques are believed to provide the prospects of fast, highly sensitive, and point-of-care (POC) detection, and are indispensable in the early detection of infectious diseases, cancer, and metabolic diseases (Thwala et al. 2023; He et al. 2022; Wang et al. 2021). Their capability of signal amplification contributes to their successful recognition of biomarkers at an ultralow level. In addition, they can be combined with wearable devices, microfluidic systems, and intelligent biosensors (Thiruvengadam et al. 2025; Chicea and Nicolae-Maranciuc 2025).

Another fast-growing field of application of nanocomposites in medicine is to be found in wound healing and tissue regeneration. Chronic wounds, burns, and diabetic ulcers demand sophisticated treatments, which extend beyond traditional dressings (Renuka et al. 2022; Ezhilarasu et al. 2020). Nanocomposite-enhanced materials, in particular, those readily having antimicrobial additives such as Ag or copper (Cu) NPs, offer increased resistance to infection (Wang et al. 2017; Zhang et al. 2022a). In addition, pH or enzyme-sensitive nanocomposites that release bioactive agents under varying pH or enzyme activity conditions can maintain the controlled and sustainable therapeutic conditions (Espenti et al. 2025; Chu et al. 2022).

This book chapter provides a concise overview of nanocomposites and their growing role in medical diagnostics. It begins by exploring various classes of nanocomposites, their synthesis methods, key properties, and advantages for biomedical applications. The chapter also discusses new applications of nanocomposites, such as in nanotheranostics and showing their wide use in modern healthcare. By bringing together knowledge from materials science, nanotechnology, and biomedical engineering, it highlights that nanocomposites play a key role in both accurate disease detection and tissue repair, with great potential for the future.

5.2 Classification of Nanocomposites

Nanocomposites can be classified based on the materials as shown in Fig. 5.2 and Table 5.1. These can be metal-based, polymer-based, carbon-based, lipid-based, and hybrid nanocomposites.

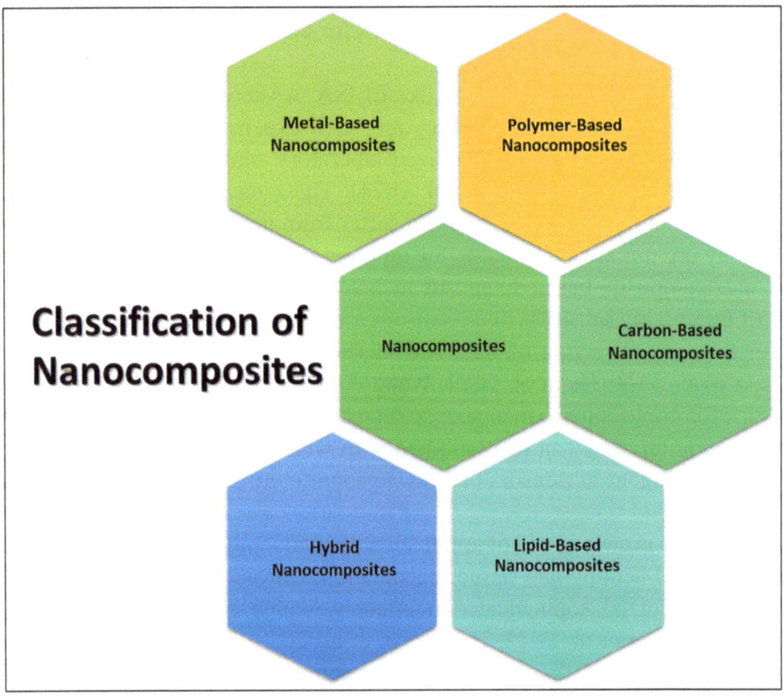

Fig. 5.2 Schematic of classification of nanocomposites

Table 5.1 Comparison of nanocomposite types used in medical diagnostics

Type of nanocomposites	Examples	Properties	Diagnostic applications	References
Metal-based	Au, Ag, Fe_3O_4, ZnO	Plasmonic activity, MRI contrast, antibacterial	Imaging (MRI, CT), biosensing	Chicea and Nicolae-Maranciuc (2025), Kumar et al. (2023a), Li and Chen (2015), Mahardika et al. (2023), Mohammed et al. (2017), and Sha et al. (2022)
Polymer-based	PEG, PLGA, Chitosan	Biocompatible, tunable degradation	Drug delivery, biosensors	Yao et al. (2023), Suk et al. (2016), Jiang and Wu (2019), Majeed et al. (2022), and Singh et al. (2024a)
Carbon-based	CDs, Graphene, CNTs	Fluorescent, conductive, biocompatible	Bioimaging, POC devices	Kumar Krishnan et al. (2019), Lu et al. (2025a), Kumar et al. (2023b), and Lohani et al. (2025)
Lipid-based	Liposomes, SLNs, NLCs	Encapsulation, targeting, and high stability	Drug delivery, diagnostic, imaging	Mall et al. (2024), Viegas et al. (2023), Kostevšek et al. (2020), and Xia et al. (2019)
Hybrid	Metal-polymer, lipid-carbon	Synergistic multifunctionality	Theranostics, wound healing	Shukla et al. (2025), Ewii et al. (2025), Feng and Wang (2022), and Andoh et al. (2024)

5.2.1 Metal-Based Nanocomposites

Metal nanocomposites are usually in the form of a metal or metal oxide nanoparticle phase in a matrix of or combined with a support, such as polymers, silica, and carbon. In such nanocomposites, one of the most used metals is Au; apart from this, Ag, (Cu), Fe_3O_4, and ZnO can also be used. These nanocomposites provide distinctive diagnostic benefits to make them promising sensing, imaging, and therapeutic monitoring nanomaterials (Chicea and Nicolae-Maranciuc 2025; Kumar et al. 2023a; Kaur et al. 2022).

Au-based nanocomposites exhibit surface plasmon resonance (SPR), where conduction electrons in the metal surface oscillate in the presence of light (Li et al. 2025a; Huang and El-Sayed 2010). This makes Au-based nanocomposites with a narrow and redshifted optical absorption peak and renders them well-suited for use as colorimetric biosensors and optical imaging agents (Si et al. 2021; Park et al. 2024). Au-nanocomposites can be applied for highly sensitive detection of cancer biomarkers, pathogens, and environmental toxins following the conjugation with targeting ligands like antibodies or aptamers (Li et al. 2023). Furthermore, Au nanorods and nanoshells have been employed in photoacoustic imaging (PAI) to improve contrast and enable noninvasive diagnostic studies (Sun et al. 2022; Li and Chen 2015).

Antibacterial effects, along with their plasmonic characteristics, have made Ag-based nanocomposites widely recognized. For detection, Ag nanoparticles will increase the signal intensity of surface-enhanced Raman scattering (SERS) assays to achieve ultrasensitive molecular detection (Eskandari et al. 2023; Gao et al. 2024; Abu Bakar and Shapter 2023). Among other applications, Ag-polymer composites have been employed in POC devices for high-performance detection of bacterial DNA or protein markers (Lee et al. 2014; Mahardika et al. 2023; Hou et al. 2023). They have antimicrobial activity, but the cytotoxicity at high concentrations gives rise to concerns, so the size and dose of particles require strict control.

Cu-based nanocomposites have also shown high plasmonic and catalytic properties. Cu is less studied than Au and Ag nanocomposites, but it provides economic alternatives for electrochemical and optical biosensors (Anh et al. 2022; Gawande et al. 2016). Their presence as redox-active species contributes to signal transduction in many sensing technologies, and their low cost enables large-scale production in resource-poor settings.

ZnO composites are semiconducting with a large bandgap, and they show strong luminescence and photocatalytic activity (Zhu and Wang 2025; Sharma et al. 2016). For instance, ZnO composites have been used in UV-based biosensors and optical imaging (Mohammed et al. 2017; Sha et al. 2022). Their piezoelectric characteristics also allow them to be incorporated into nanogenerators and wearable diagnostic platforms (Bhadwal et al. 2023). Comprehensively, metal-based nanocomposites encompass a wide spectrum of functional applications, including signal amplification, molecular recognition, antimicrobial properties, and contrast imaging, which makes them attractive for building sophisticated diagnostic systems.

5.2.2 Polymer-Based Nanocomposites

The polymer-based nanocomposites are composed of a polymer matrix with nanoscale fillers of metal nanoparticles, quantum dots, or carbon nanomaterials, for introducing desirable functions. Polymers such as PEG (polyethylene glycol), PLGA (poly(lactic-co-glycolic acid)), chitosan, and PANI (polyaniline) have been extensively utilized in developing diagnostic platforms, each offering distinct advantageous characteristics.

PEG, a nontoxic hydrophilic polymer is often used to enhance the solubility and stability of nanomaterials in biological applications (Yao et al. 2023; Suk et al. 2016). With the application in nanocomposites, protein absorption and immunogenic clearance could be avoided by PEGylation, and the diagnostic effect of the nanoparticle-based system could be enhanced (Partikel et al. 2019). PEG is an attractive nanocomposite surface modification for optical and magnetic imaging, while it can be made functional with targeting agents for site-specific diagnostics, in particular in the case of oncology (Singh and Lillard 2009; Carregal-Romero et al. 2018; Zhang et al. 2022b).

Chitosan, a naturally occurring polymer obtained from chitin, possesses good mucoadhesive characteristics, and it is characterized by antimicrobial and immunomodulatory activities (Aranaz et al. 2021). The chitosan-based nanocomposites have been used for biosensing with a focus on glucose detection and pathogen sensing (Jiang and Wu 2019). In addition, graphene oxide (GO) enhances chitosan-based delivery systems and can act as a platform for targeted delivery and imaging, including magnetic resonance imaging (MRI) inside cells (Dash et al. 2024; Wang et al. 2013).

PANI and other conductive polymers have been applied in the fabrication of electrochemical biosensors in virtue of their excellent electrical conductivity and stability in the environment (Kale et al. 2024). The conducting PANI-based nanocomposites doped/aggregated with metallic or carbon nanomaterials promote charge transfer and signal amplification, which can give a response to the detection and ultra-sensitive detection of disease biomarkers (Majeed et al. 2022). These systems are especially well-suited for POC diagnostics where rapid signal readout is required.

Surface chemistry of polymer nanocomposites can be precisely adjusted to enhance their targeting ability and interaction with biological targets. Surface functionalization facilitates binding of the composite to target cells or molecules with antibodies, aptamers, or peptides (Wieszczycka et al. 2021; Singh et al. 2024a). This modularity affords the representatives of polymer-based nanocomposites an opportunity to act as smart diagnostic tools that are capable of sensing, reacting, and signaling "real-time" disease monitoring with high accuracy. As the field progresses, numerous new types of biodegradable and stimuli-responsive polymers are incorporated into nanocomposite systems to generate smart diagnostic materials that sense environmental conditions like pH or enzymes and provide dynamic information about physiological phenomena.

5.2.3 Carbon-Based Nanocomposites

Carbon-based nanocomposites have paved the way for a revolutionary class of materials in medical diagnostics, given the excellent electrical, thermal, and optical properties of carbon nanomaterials, as shown in Fig. 5.3. The use of CDs, graphene, and carbon nanotubes (CNT) composites has facilitated the generation of sensitive, rapid, and inexpensive diagnostic platforms (Jayaprakash et al. 2024; Ahmad et al. 2024). Such composites are highly suitable for biosensing, molecular imaging, and disease tracking.

Graphene and its derivatives (such as GO and reduced (rGO)) have been broadly utilized in biosensors because they have good electrical conductivity and a large surface area (Maiti et al. 2019; Kumar Krishnan et al. 2019; Ren 2025). Furthermore, these substances can promote electron transport of biomolecules with electrodes,

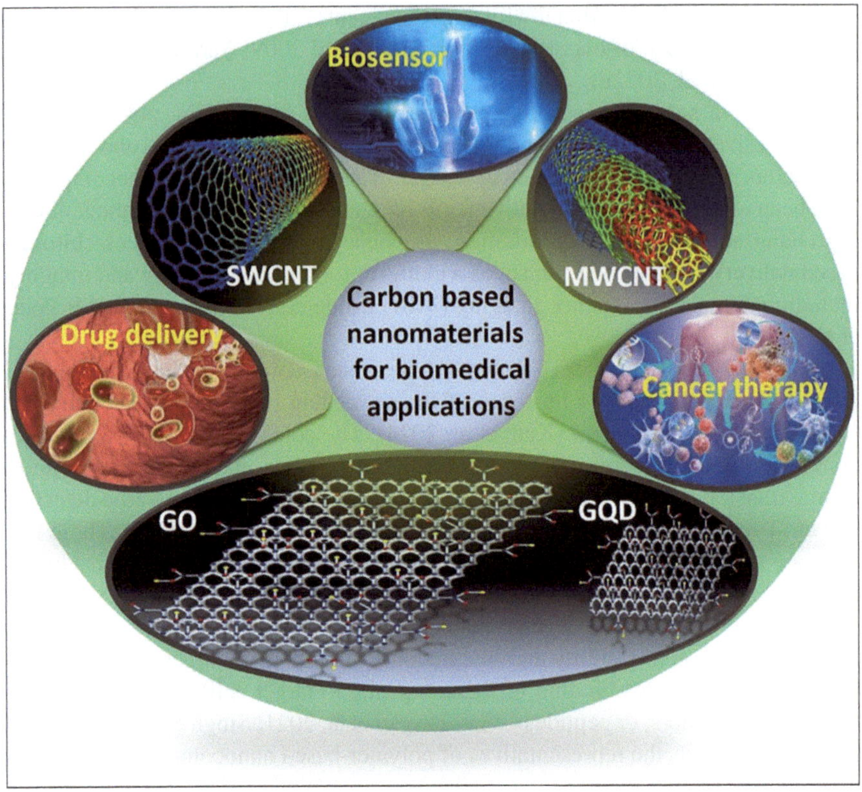

Fig. 5.3 The application of carbon-based nanomaterials in various medical fields, such as drug delivery, cancer therapy, and biosensors. (Reproduced from Maiti et al. (2019) with permission from Frontiers in Pharmacology)

thus providing good performance toward electrochemical biosensing (Kumar Krishnan et al. 2019). Graphene nanocomposites are used for glucose sensors, nucleic acid detection, and real-time pathogen analysis (Song et al. 2025). In addition, their 2D feature provides the immobilization of various bioreceptor types and promotes assay specificity (Mukherjee et al. 2024).

Carbon nanotubes, single-walled (SWCNTs) and multi-walled (MWCNTs), have high aspect ratios, strength, and electrical conductivities. Combined with diagnostic nanocomposites, they increase the signal transduction performance of optical and electrochemical sensors (Lu et al. 2025a; Kumar et al. 2023b). CNTs are further functionalized with DNA, proteins, or antibodies, in a manner that also allows them to selectively sense disease biomarkers (Lohani et al. 2025). Furthermore, CNT–polymer hybrids are used in wearable biosensors for the real-time analysis of physiological levels like pH, glucose, and sweat.

Carbon-based nanocomposites offer many advantages, including low background signals, high stability, and suitability for various detection methods. They are highly versatile and can be used in lab-on-a-chip systems, microfluidic devices, and portable diagnostic tools. In the future, these materials are expected to be developed further using green synthesis approaches and combined with metals or polymers to greatly enhance diagnostic performance.

5.2.4 Lipid-Based Nanocomposites

Lipid-based nanocomposites represent an important group of materials for biomedical diagnostics because of their natural biocompatibility and structural adjustability, as well as their ability to encapsulate drugs and biomolecules (Mehta et al. 2023; Waheed et al. 2024). These hybrid nanocomposites generally consist of nanocarriers made up of a lipid, and these are solid lipid nanoparticles (SLNs), liposomes, and nanostructured lipid carriers (NLCs), with functional nanomaterials to improve the diagnostic performance (Lu et al. 2021; Mall et al. 2024; Viegas et al. 2023). Spherical liposomes are formed of phospholipid bilayers and can encapsulate hydrophilic compounds inside the aqueous content or hydrophobic compounds between the lipid layers. In diagnostics, liposome-based nanocomposites are often surface-functionalized with contrast agents, targeting ligands, or fluorescent probes. These systems are widely used in imaging techniques such as MRI, positron emission tomography (PET), and optical imaging (Kostevšek et al. 2020; Xia et al. 2019).

NLCs are further developed SLN generation using a combination of solid and liquid lipids. Such structural modification would result in higher drug loading capacity and release behavior of the diagnostic agent. NLCs have also been used for the delivery of fluorescent dyes, quantum dots, and radiolabeled compounds for imaging and detection applications (Nguyen et al. 2022; Giordano et al. 2024). Nanomedicines formulated with lipids have several advantages, such as biodegradability, modifiable size, scale-up, and the promise of clinical translation (Kurul et al. 2025). They can conjugate to multiple diagnostic and therapeutic agents, which is convenient for their application to theranostics. Advanced diagnostic units based on lipids (LIPs) may include features of imaging agents, responsive materials, and digital biosensors within a single construct for monitoring patients and delivering personal information (Lu et al. 2017).

5.2.5 Hybrid Nanocomposites

The hybrid nanocomposite is a diverse and fast-developing category of materials that consists of two or more classes of nanomaterials together to leverage their functional performance in synergy. The most widely used hybrid nanocomposites are the metal–polymer system. In the composites, the metal nanoparticles, such as Au/Ag, are embedded in a polymer matrix such as PEG, PLGA, or chitosan, or are coated on the polymer (Singh et al. 2024b). These combinations stabilize metal nanoparticles in biological systems and improve their biocompatibility, and inhibit their agglomeration. For instance, Au-PEG nanocomposites have been used in colorimetric biosensors, where the plasmonic nature of Au induces signal generation while the PEG shell provides prolonged circulation time and minimizes immunogenicity (Shukla et al. 2025). Moreover, these hybrid particles tend to have functional groups on the polymer surface for bioconjugation with antibodies, aptamers, or peptides, providing targeted specificity for specific biomarkers.

Hybrid lipid–metal nanocomposites have also demonstrated the distinctive benefits, especially for imaging and drug-delivering systems (Vargas and Shon 2019). Quantum dots and Au nanoparticle-loaded liposomes for imaging and therapy with POC diagnostics. Such systems can be programmed to break and release their contents by the changes in pH or by the presence of enzymes, or can be set to do so through light or a magnetic field (Ewii et al. 2025; Wang and Chao 2018). This increased responsiveness increases the diagnostic precision of interventions and minimizes off-target effects. Metals provide imaging contrast, and lipids enable encapsulation and biocompatibility; thus, these hybrids are promising for theranostics.

Polymer–carbon hybrids, which include chitosan-GO composites, are being increasingly utilized in biosensor construction (Feng and Wang 2022; Sabzevari et al. 2018).. For instance, nucleic acids or proteins can be immobilized on chitosan as a substrate, and the amplified signals can be realized in GO. These composites are particularly useful in electrochemical sensors detecting trace levels of disease-related DNA or proteins (Tiwari et al. 2015). The hybrid nanocomposites can be designed as multifunctional platforms that could be used as diagnostic probes, imaging agents, and carriers for therapy. For instance, an Au nanoparticle–CDs-biodegradable polymer nanocomposite was prepared for early cancer diagnosis (Andoh et al. 2024). The Au provided the imaging of computed tomography (CT), the CDs for fluorescent tracing, and the polymer wrapped a chemotherapeutic drug. It serves here as a representative example of how the incorporation of different nanomaterial components can result in a versatile, multifunctional diagnostic and therapeutic system. Hybrid nanocomposites help solve some problems seen with single-material systems. For example, metal nanoparticles can work better and become less toxic when mixed into a biocompatible material. Similarly, carbon-based materials often don't mix well in biological systems, but this can be fixed by coating them with polymers or wrapping them in lipids.

5.3 Methods of Synthesis

Preparation and characterization of nanocomposites are crucial for establishing their efficacy, stability, and utility in biomedical diagnosis. Various synthetic protocols are reported to synthesize nanocomposites with controlled size, shape, and composition as shown in Fig. 5.4. They provide different levels of control of physicochemical properties, and consequently, they can control the interaction of the material with biological systems. In addition, precise characterization of these nanocomposites is required for evaluation of their diagnostic capability, biocompatibility, and performance reproducibility.

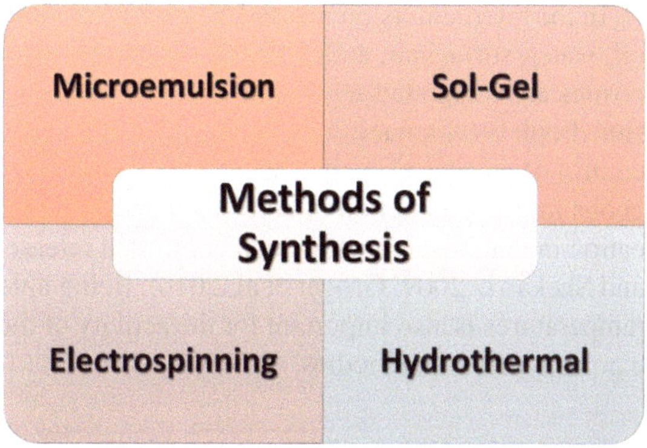

Fig. 5.4 Schematic of different methods of synthesis of nanocomposites

5.3.1 Sol–Gel, Hydrothermal, Electrospinning, and Microemulsion Methods

The sol–gel process is an established wet-chemical process for producing metal oxide nanocomposites, including silica- and titanium-based systems, among others. It is the transformation of a liquid "sol" into a solid "gel" system. Precursors such as metal alkoxides or metal chlorides, for example, undergo hydrolysis and condensation in solution to give a colloid. The gel is further dried and calcinated, and nanocomposite particles are formed (Bokov et al. 2021; Hench and West 1990). This method allows for precise control over particle size, composition, and porosity and hence is particularly well suited to the preparation of nanomaterials with homogeneous properties. Sol–gel derived nanocomposites have been used in the field of biomedicine, especially for biosensing and drug delivery, because of their high surface area and tailorable pore structure (Singh et al. 2014; Owens et al. 2016).

The basic characteristics of the hydrothermal process (crystallization at high temperatures from hot water solutions at high pressures, usually inside sealed autoclaves). This method can be used to make nanocomposites with well-defined morphologies like rods, spheres, or sheets (Tazim et al. 2025). Hydrothermal synthesis is the most common technique for the fabrication of materials such as ZnO, TiO_2, and different-doped nanoparticles. Closed systems enable the production of nanostructures with high purity and crystallinity, which is essential for diagnostic applications requiring stability and reproducibility (Tazim et al. 2025; Anaya-Zavaleta et al. 2025; Tudor et al. 2014).

Electrospinning is a versatile method most commonly employed to produce nanocomposite fibers by means of generating an intense electric field on a polymer solution or melt (Rogina 2014). To facilitate these functions, nanomaterials, including metal nanoparticles, CNTs, or quantum dots, can be integrated with the polymer matrix to produce diagnostic platforms (Gómez et al. 2021). Because of their large surface area-to-volume ratio and porous structure, electrospun nanofibers have superior biomolecule immobilization and signal transduction in biosensing applications (Feng et al. 2021; Lan et al. 2023; Kilic et al. 2024). Such an approach has also been employed in the development of wearable diagnostic tools and wound healing patches with sensing functions.

In the microemulsion method, thermodynamically stable colloidal dispersions of oil, water, surfactant, and co-surfactant are prepared. In this process, the nanocomposites are integrated within the nanoreactors, which are the confined microemulsion droplets (Nikolaev et al. 2023; Suhail et al. 2021). The technique offers accurate control of particle size and shape. Microemulsion synthesis is particularly advantageous for the production of core–shell and hollow nanostructures, which find application in diagnostic imaging and controlled release (Galogahi et al. 2020; Eslamian and Shekarriz 2009; Gröger et al. 2010). Being able to produce nanoparticles at low temperatures is also important for the activity of the biological agents encapsulated, e.g., enzymes or antibodies.

5.3.2 Significance of Surface Functionalization of Nanocomposite

The key factor affecting the interaction with biological systems is the functionalization of the surface of nanocomposites. Functionalization of the nanoparticle surface with functional groups, ligands, or biomolecules that provide the specificity, stability, and biocompatibility. This approach not only provides improved targeted recognition but also better physiological media dispersion and lower nonspecific adsorption, thereby improving the performance of nanocomposites in diagnostic applications.

One of the most popular methods for nanocomposite surface modification is the PEGylation of the surface of the nanocomposite. This functionalization endows the particles with hydrophilic properties, conferring low adsorption of protein and immune recognition. PEGylated nanocomposites have longer circulation times and enhanced accumulation in target tissues that are important for in vivo imaging and diagnosis applications (Suk et al. 2016; Chen et al. 2024). Silane chemistry has also been used for the treatment of silica and metal oxide nanocomposites. For example, silane coupling agents like (3-aminopropyl) triethoxysilane (APTES) also allow functional density to be engineered onto the particle surface and serve as a site for subsequent conjugation (Mallakpour and Madani 2015; Niranjana et al. 2025). Functionalization is also important for enhancing the colloidal stability of the nanocomposites in biofluids, preventing aggregation and guaranteeing a constant performance. Surface charges, often characterized as zeta potential, can be adjusted by pH to ensure stable suspensions in physiological solutions (Gambinossi et al. 2015).

In addition to biological ligands, which are stimuli-responsive moieties that are attached to achieve a smart diagnostic response. Among these, pH-sensitive, redox-sensitive, and enzyme-cleavable linkers have been designed to activate the signal only in specific biological environments like the tumor microenvironment or the site of infection (Wang et al. 2024a; Liu et al. 2024). In general, surface functionalization is critical for extending the physicochemical properties of a nanocomposite to its use in a biomedical application. It ensures the specificity, safety, and compatibility, giving support for the construction of an intelligent diagnostic system that can selectively interact with the biological target but has fewer side effects.

5.4 Nanocomposites in Medical Diagnostics

Various types of nanomaterials can be used to make nanocomposites in the biomedical field, as discussed earlier. These nanomaterials have several advantages and limitations, such as biocompatibility, instability, and other optical properties. In contrast, nanomaterials such as CDs have emerged as promising tools in biodiagnostics because of their special optical and physico-chemical features (Patyal et al. 2025; Kumarasamy and Sharma 2025; Tiwari et al. 2020). One of the most attractive CD properties is their high and stable photoluminescence, which makes them ideal candidates as fluorescent probes (Sharma et al. 2017; Warjurkar et al. 2025; Sharma 2021). Photostability is a characteristic property of CDs, which exhibit resistance against photobleaching even under long irradiation times with visible light. This feature is especially advantageous for the visualization of cellular and tissue structures in real-time and long-term (Wang and Lu 2022; Ozyurt et al. 2023). Furthermore, in comparison to conventional fluorophores, CDs show both excitation-dependent and adjustable fluorescence emission that can be easily modulated by changing the synthetic system, that is, the substrate (precursor), reaction time, and temperature (Alafeef et al. 2024; Lu et al. 2025b). This multifunctionality allows CDs to be used in multiplexed diagnostic assays, where several biomarkers can be simultaneously detected through their unique emission wavelengths. Another major benefit of CDs is their inherent biocompatibility. It has been well reported that CDs, and particularly those obtained from natural sources, have a low cytotoxicity in a range of in vitro and in vivo models (Xu et al. 2024a; González and Romero 2025). Their small size allows for cellular internalization and biodistribution with negligible immunogenicity, which is ideal for systemic delivery for diagnostic imaging (Kaurav et al. 2023; Liu et al. 2020).

CD-derived nanocomposites exhibited significant potential in diverse diagnostic applications, especially in fluorescence-based biosensing and imaging-guided diagnosis. Conjugated with metals, polymers, or other nanostructures, CDs can function as efficient luminescent probes, with high sensitivity and selectivity for the diagnosis of disease biomarkers, pathogens, and cellular disorders (Qi et al. 2024; Kaurav et al. 2023). The integration of CDs with polymers further enhances their functionality and selectivity towards various analytes. Polymer/CDs nanocomposites have shown excellent performance in detecting chemical and biological targets (Kar et al. 2024). Magnetic/light-sensitive CDs are used in the dual-modal or multi-modal imaging technology. For example, CD-magnetic Fe_3O_4 nanocomposites facilitate double imaging based on FLI and MRI for a full understanding of pathological tissues (Thirumalai et al. 2025). The frequent functional groups available on the surface of CDs create reactive sites for the conjugation of specific targeting groups, thus leading to selective interactions with biological targets, such as proteins, nucleic acids, or cellular receptors (Belza et al. 2021; Sharma and Lee 2024; Truskewycz et al. 2022). Aptamer–CD complexes offer high affinity and stability, enabling applications like thrombin detection or tumor targeting (Motaghi et al. 2017). Peptide-conjugated CDs, such as RGD-CDs, provide efficient receptor

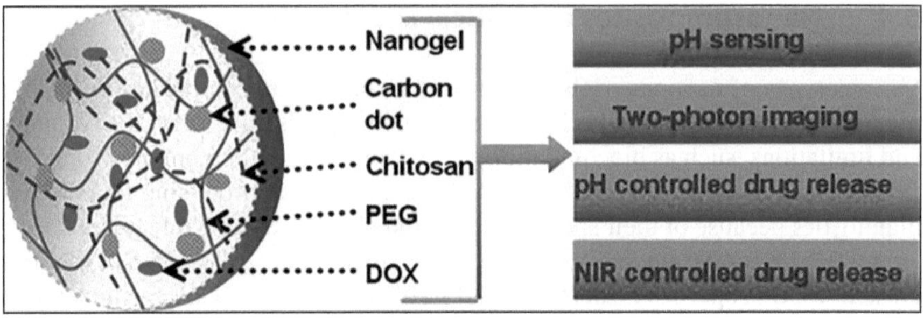

Fig. 5.5 Schematic PEG-chitosan@CDs hybrid nanogel designed for multifunctional applications in the biomedical field. (Reproduced from Wang et al. (2015b) with permission from Wiley-VCH)

targeting due to their small size and deep tissue penetration (Hazra et al. 2023). Surface-modified CDs can further be incorporated into multi-functional nanocomposites, which combine targeting, detection, and therapy. Such convergence anatomy introduces the potential for a real-time monitoring platform and feedback-regulated therapeutic modalities, which significantly advances the realm of personalized medicine.

Wu et al. synthesized a smart electrochemiluminescence (ECL) immunosensor using a material called nanoporous Ag (NPS), which was combined with CDs to form an NPS@CDs composite. The CDs, made by electrooxidizing graphite, helped produce the ECL signal. This sensor, with its 3D porous structure, was able to detect cancer-related proteins like prostate-specific antigen (PSA), showing promise for use in medical diagnosis (Wu et al. 2013). Wang et al. synthesized a composite material by incorporating CDs into flower-shaped NiAl layered double hydroxides (NiAl-LDHs). The resulting structure showed excellent selectivity, making it suitable for use as a non-enzymatic electrochemical sensor to detect neurotransmitters like acetylcholine (Wang et al. 2016).

Glutathione is a vital antioxidant that protects cells from oxidative stress and maintains redox balance in the body. Abnormal GSH levels are linked to diseases like cancer, liver damage, and neurodegenerative disorders. Wang et al. synthesized a FRET-based biosensor by integrating CDs with MnO_2 nanosheets. This sensor possessed high selectivity and sensitivity for glutathione detection in human blood samples (Wang et al. 2015a). Wang et al., synthesized biocompatible PEG–chitosan@CDs hybrid nanogels as shown in Fig. 5.5. The embedded CDs enabled two-photon FLI, pH sensing, and enhanced drug loading. Chitosan provided pH-responsive drug release, while the PEG network responded to NIR light for controlled release. The nanocomposites showed high in vitro therapeutic efficacy via combined chemo–photothermal therapy (Wang et al. 2015b).

5.5 Application of Nanocomposites

5.5.1 Biosensing Applications

Nanocomposites have been used in transforming biosensing by offering superior platforms enabling the detection of biomolecules with high sensitivity, selectivity, and rapid response time (Fu et al. 2024; Sharma et al. 2025). A biosensor is generally composed of a biological recognition element (e.g., enzymes, antibodies, DNA sequences) and a transducer to convert the biological response into a signal (Naresh and Lee 2021).

In order to promote electron transfer, enhance surface area for binding of analyte, and ensure bio-stability, electrochemical biosensors are often based on the use of nanocomposites. Nanoparticles made up of metals, such as Au or platinum, modified graphene or CNTs-based nanocomposites have been used for preparing electrodes with improved conductivity and signal amplification (Fritea et al. 2021; Bas 2015). For example, in glucose biosensing, nanocomposites of Au NPs, glucose oxidase immobilized on a G/ G/chitosan matrix, have been found to quickly and accurately measure glucose in blood and interstitial fluid (Luo et al. 2004).

Optical biosensors provide a method for the optical nature of nanocomposites for label-free or fluorescent detection (Costanzo et al. 2023; Peltomaa et al. 2018). The CD nanocomposite showed high quantum yield and photostability, and was demonstrated to be useful for the detection of cancer biomarkers and viral proteins (Tavan et al. 2025; Pechnikova et al. 2025). In the same way, Au–Ag alloy nanocomposites have also been utilized in SPR-based biosensors for the real-time monitoring of antigen–antibody reactions with an ultra-low detection limit (Yi et al. 2020).

A classic example is the early detection of cancer biomarkers—prostate-specific antigen (PSA) and carcinoembryonic antigen (CEA) (Zhou et al. 2024). As an example, the authors pointed out that nanocomposites decorated with targeted antibodies have enabled electrochemical sensing of these signatures at picomolar levels, which was not possible before for use in clinical diagnosis (Khazaei et al. 2023). Nanocomposite biosensors are being incorporated in infectious disease diagnostics, such as HIV and hepatitis B viral protein detection, in resource-scarce settings, since they could have the capability of portability and low cost (Mokhtarzadeh et al. 2017).

In addition, the construction of multianalyte detecting nanocomposites is forthcoming. Complex diseases also benefit from the utility of these systems, as in the diagnosis of certain complex diseases, multiple biomarkers have to be measured for accurate diagnosis. The coupling of these bio-nanocomposites with microfluidics and smartphone-based readers has been further driving their applications in personalized healthcare for the real-time monitoring of diseases and early interventions.

5.5.2 Molecular Imaging

Molecular imaging is a method that makes it possible to see, characterize, and quantify biological processes at the cellular and molecular level directly in living organisms. Nanocomposites are of great interest for contrast/multi-modal enhancement and selective targeting of diseased tissues for molecular imaging applications. They have been used for a variety of imaging methodologies such as MRI, PET, CT, and fluorescence imaging (FLI).

Nanocomposites for MRI where magnetic materials (e.g., superparamagnetic iron oxide (SPION) nanoparticle) are used as contrast agents. Embedded within a polymer or silica matrix, SPIONs increase the relaxivity of proximate water protons, leading to improved contrast in T2-weighted images, and the modification of targeting ligands (i.e., antibodies or peptides) will enable these nanocomposites to accumulate specifically in the tumor or inflammation sites for accurate imaging and early diagnosis (Neuwelt et al. 2015; Mao et al. 2016; Nelson et al. 2020; Li et al. 2013). The liposomal nanocomposite designed for improved MRI-based tumor imaging, particularly in lung cancer models, was synthesized by Erdogan et al. Liposomes loaded with Gd-PAP showed stronger MRI signals than standard Gd-DTPA-PE liposomes. In lung cancer models, these liposomes reduced tumor T1 values within 4 h, indicating effective targeting. When modified with the 2C5 antibody, they accumulated even more in tumors. 3D angiography further confirmed clear tumor visualization from 4 to 48 h after injection (Erdogan et al. 2008). Luciani et al. synthesized niosomes modified with glucose and PEG to target tumor cells. In vitro studies using PC3 prostate cancer cells showed enhanced uptake, while in-vivo MRI in tumor-bearing mice revealed improved targeting. Niosomes modified with both PEG and glucose achieved the highest tumor-to-muscle contrast, highlighting their potential for precise tumor imaging in lung and other cancers (Luciani et al. 2004).

CDs combined with magnetic materials have been used to create dual-mode MRI and FLI, allowing both structural and functional imaging at the same time during one diagnostic test (Redondo-Fernandez et al. 2023; Lv et al. 2025). In PET and CT imaging, nanocomposites are used to enhance the biodistribution and retention of radiolabeled or x-ray absorbing agents (Jiang et al. 2023; Mutreja et al. 2023). Au-NPs decorated forms are found to be efficient CT contrast agents because of their high atomic number and biocompatibility. These compounds are labeled on cancer-targeting moieties to increase the visualization of primary tumors and metastatic deposits (Jiang et al. 2023; Reuveni et al. 2011; Malekzadeh et al. 2023). PET visualization of metabolism and receptor expression can also be performed with high sensitivity, using nanocomposites labeled with positron-emitting isotopes (Goel et al. 2017). The photostable and size-tunable emission features of nanocomposites (including quantum dots and CDs) make them an ideal candidate for FLI (Qureshi et al. 2024). They are especially used for the cellular uptake, drug delivery monitoring, and real-time protein–protein interaction imaging. Drug-loaded/aggregation-induced emission activated nanocomposite probes for deep-tissue penetration and reduced background signal FLI at near-infrared II (Yan et al. 2023; Li et al. 2021; Hussain et al. 2023).

Multimodal imaging, where two or more imaging modalities are integrated in one platform, is an emerging field with the potential of nanocomposites. When combining magnetic, radioactive, and fluorescent elements in a single nanocomposite, scientists have the potential to get complementary diagnostic information in a manner that can improve accuracy and decrease false positives. Such integration is particularly useful in oncology, in which anatomical, functional, and molecular aspects need to be evaluated simultaneously for the purpose of treating and monitoring therapeutic efficiency.

5.5.3 POC Diagnostics

POC testing represents a significant advancement in healthcare, enabling fast and convenient disease detection directly. Nanocomposites are pivotal for improving the sensitivity, specificity, and utility of POC diagnostic tools. Their integration into paper-based assays, lateral flow devices, microfluidic chips, and so forth has turned traditional assays into smart, sensitive systems for high-throughput screening, which can provide rapid, valid test results in minutes (Tavakoli et al. 2022; Roy et al. 2022).

Paper-based diagnostic devices, such as LFAs, have gained popularity due to their low cost, portability, and simplicity of operation (Sher et al. 2017). Nanocomposites (especially Au or carbon-based) incorporated with LFAs greatly enhance the visibility and sensitivity of the test line (Ardekani and Thulstrup 2022; Porras et al. 2021). For example, Au nanoparticle-polyaniline composites were developed for visual detection of C-reactive protein (CRP) and cardiac troponins, critical biomarkers of inflammatory and cardiac diseases (António et al. 2018; Fukuzumi et al. 2025; Luo et al. 2024; Iwasaki et al. 2014). The detection limits based on these nanocomposite-labeled LFAs were found to be significantly lower than those of the standard colloidal Au-based composite (Wang et al. 2024b). In tuberculosis (TB) and malaria detection, which are still one of the largest global health threats, they can be applied electrochemical paper-based devices with a nanocomposite as a recognition element can be applied, enabling the detection of specific antigens and DNA of the disease with excellent specificity (Mobed et al. 2024; Li et al. 2025b). Furthermore, nanocomposites can be used as a route to multiplexed POC devices (able to screen for several analytes in the same test) (Moulahoum et al. 2023). Such information is indispensable for differential diagnosis, particularly when overlapping symptoms can be observed in different diseases. By pairing nanocomposite biosensors with smartphone applications and cloud-based software for data storage and analysis, this system provides on-spot health monitoring, automatic interpretation of the results, and connection with healthcare practitioners, greatly improving disease surveillance and management (Qian et al. 2022; Xing et al. 2025). With increasing moves towards POC, nanocomposite-based POC diagnostics will play a vital role in addressing disparities in access, timeliness, and quality of diagnostics for different populations.

5.5.4 Wearable and Digital Health Convergence

Integrating nanocomposites into wearable devices and digital health platforms marks the beginning of a new era in diagnostics, enabling continuous, non-invasive monitoring outside of traditional laboratory settings (Hemdan et al. 2024; Mishra and Saha 2024). Their electrical and mechanical characteristics make them flexible, stretchable, and comfortable to wear on the human body with no degradation of signal quality. Nanocomposite-based wearables are also being used to detect volatile organic compounds (VOCs) from breath or skin, helping to identify early signs of diseases such as diabetes, lung infections, and cancer (Chaudhary et al. 2024).. Nanocomposites also have potential for integration with wireless communication modules, which allow real-time transmission of digital health data to smartphones, tablets, or cloud-based systems (Verma et al. 2022; Xu et al. 2024b). Such digital interfaces provide patients and clinicians with instant access to health indicators for timely interventions and regimen customization. With the rapid expansion of telemedicine, nanocomposite-mediated sensors can contribute to remote diagnostics and limit the pressure on the healthcare system, ensuring medical services to people in rural and underdeveloped areas.

5.6 Challenges and Future Perspectives

Nanocomposites have been developed in medical diagnostics and have shown new opportunities for early disease diagnosis, targeted imaging, and integrated therapy. Despite the advances, some key challenges remain, especially in reproducibility, scalability, and compatibility with regulatory standards, which currently preclude meaningful clinical translation of these novel materials (Kurul et al. 2025). A major limitation in the synthesis of nanocomposites is the scalability and reproducibility. The performance of nanocomposites significantly depends upon the synthesis conditions, such as temperature, solvent systems, precursor concentrations, and reaction time. Small differences in these parameters result in large differences in size, shape, surface charge, and bioactivity, which in turn influence accuracy and safety in diagnostic applications. Sometimes, when nanocomposites functionalized with targeting ligands, antibodies, or fluorophores, batch-to-batch variation can lead to instability and non-specific diagnostic responses (Saha et al. 2025). In the future, the development of precision diagnostics and artificial intelligence (AI) may also help to reduce these limitations. Nanocomposites, especially for the tunable properties, can be developed to sense the patient-based biomarkers for patient-specific disease profiling and treatment. Combined with AI-based image analysis or interpretation of biosensor data, nanocomposites can provide an accurate, real-time diagnostic. ML models could predict disease progression, treatment response, or infection severity using nanocomposite interactions and can improve clinical intervention. The next generation of these biosensors for future pandemics is anticipated to draw upon pre-developed libraries of nanocomposite-based biosensors that will be quickly adaptable for newly emerging pathogens. Such systems could be connected to a global digital health architecture for real-time epidemiological surveillance and outbreak management (Akbari Nakhjavani et al. 2024; Sumitha and Suryabai 2024).

In chronic disease maintenance, nanocomposites provide the opportunity to monitor diabetes, CVD (cardiovascular disease), cancer, and so forth continuously. Photo Dressings that contain nanocomposite biosensors can keep track of glucose, identify inflammatory agents, or even recognize early signs of infection in diabetic sores. Likewise, wearables with flexible nanocomposites could constantly monitor the performance of the heart and detect cancer biomarkers without the need for invasive procedures, allowing early intervention and a personalized treatment scheme.

Apart from the biomedical application and diagnosis, the nanocomposite can have scope in food packaging, automobile components, electromagnetic interference (EMI) shielding, anti-microbial coating, and various types of protective garments used during medical diagnostics (Jayakumar et al. 2023; Qamar 2021). In the future, the nanocomposite-based food packaging could be beneficial for reducing contamination and can be used in increasing the shelf life of the food. Protective garments coated with nanocomposites may help in resistance to infection, and if the sensors are incorporated, it will offer both safety and real-time health monitoring.

5.7 Conclusion

Over the past years, there has been an advancement in the synthesis and application of nanocomposites for medical diagnosis, representing a fusion of material science, nanotechnology, biomedicine, and engineering. These hybrids (based on metal, polymers, carbon, lipids, and hybrid systems) have shown potential for enhancing the sensitivity, specificity, and versatility of the next-generation diagnostic systems. In biosensors, imaging modalities, or POC devices, nanocomposites are an important tool in the earlier diagnosis of diseases, improved monitoring, and more targeted therapy (Ali et al. 2023). A remarkable progress is the development of CD-based nanocomposites, which possess an interesting combination of photoluminescence, biocompatibility, as well as low toxicity. In addition, the use of nanocomposites has evolved from the traditional use in diagnostics to multi-functional applications, particularly in nanotheranostics and wound management. In skin wound healing, intelligent nanocomposite dressings have shown promise in the treatment of chronic wounds, burns, and diabetic ulcers via antimicrobial effects, bioimaging, and tissue repair, as well as those containing Ag and CDs.

The use and integration of AI and digital health care bring new horizons to data analysis, prediction, diagnosis, and personalized treatment paths. Finally, despite the potential of nanocomposites to transform diagnostics, their full potential requires ongoing investment in translational research, clinical trials, and regulatory capacity building. It is only through such integrative and iterative engagements that these advanced materials can truly realize their future role in advancing precision medicine and global healthcare innovation.

Acknowledgements The authors wish to acknowledge research support from IIT Jammu. V.S. acknowledges the IIT Jammu Seed Grant for financial assistance. R.P. would like to acknowledge the University Grant Commission (UGC) for the Senior Research Fellowship (221610142183). K.A. acknowledges IIT Jammu for the fellowship.

Competing Interests The authors declare no competing financial interest.

References

Abu Bakar N, Shapter JG (2023) Silver nanostar films for surface-enhanced Raman spectroscopy (SERS) of the pesticide Imidacloprid. Heliyon 9(3):e14686. https://doi.org/10.1016/j.heliyon.2023.e14686

Ahmad F, Mahmood A, Muhmood T (2024) Carbon allotropes: basics, properties and applications. In: Heteroatom-doped carbon allotropes: progress in synthesis, characterization, and applications, ACS symposium series, vol 1491. American Chemical Society, pp 1–18. https://doi.org/10.1021/bk-2024-1491.ch001

Akbari Nakhjavani S, Mirzajani H, Carrara S, Onbaşlı MC (2024) Advances in biosensor technologies for infectious diseases detection. TrAC Trends Anal Chem 180:117979. https://doi.org/10.1016/j.trac.2024.117979

Alafeef M, Srivastava I, Aditya T, Pan D (2024) Carbon dots: from synthesis to unraveling the fluorescence mechanism. Small 20(4):2303937. https://doi.org/10.1002/smll.202303937

Ali F, Neha K, Parveen S (2023) Current regulatory landscape of nanomaterials and nanomedicines: a global perspective. J Drug Delivery Sci Technol 80:104118. https://doi.org/10.1016/j.jddst.2022.104118

Anaya-Zavaleta JC, Ledezma-Pérez AS, Gallardo-Vega C, Rodríguez-Hernández J, Alvarado-Canché CN, García-Casillas PE, de León A, Herrera-May AL (2025) ZnO nanoparticles by hydrothermal method: synthesis and characterization. Technologies 13(1):18. https://doi.org/10.3390/technologies13010018

Andoh V, Ocansey DKW, Naveed H, Wang N, Chen L, Chen K, Mao F (2024) The advancing role of nanocomposites in cancer diagnosis and treatment. Int J Nanomed 19:6099–6126. https://doi.org/10.2147/IJN.S471360

Anh NT, Dinh NX, Van Tuan H, Doan MQ, Anh NH, Khi NT, Trang VT, Tri DQ, Le A-T (2022) Eco-friendly copper nanomaterials-based dual-mode optical nanosensors for ultrasensitive trace determination of amoxicillin antibiotics residue in tap water samples. Mater Res Bull 147:111649. https://doi.org/10.1016/j.materresbull.2021.111649

António M, Nogueira J, Vitorino R, Daniel-da-Silva AL (2018) Functionalized gold nanoparticles for the detection of C-reactive protein. Nanomaterials (Basel) 8(4):200. https://doi.org/10.3390/nano8040200

Aranaz I, Alcántara AR, Civera MC, Arias C, Elorza B, Heras Caballero A, Acosta N (2021) Chitosan: an overview of its properties and applications. Polymers 13(19):3256. https://doi.org/10.3390/polym13193256

Ardekani LS, Thulstrup PW (2022) Gold nanoparticle-mediated lateral flow assays for detection of host antibodies and COVID-19 proteins. Nanomaterials (Basel) 12(9):1456. https://doi.org/10.3390/nano12091456

Baig N, Kammakakam I, Falath W (2021) Nanomaterials: a review of synthesis methods, properties, recent progress, and challenges. Mater Adv 2(6):1821–1871. https://doi.org/10.1039/D0MA00807A

Bas SZ (2015) Gold nanoparticle functionalized graphene oxide modified platinum electrode for hydrogen peroxide and glucose sensing. Mater Lett 150:20–23. https://doi.org/10.1016/j.matlet.2015.02.130

Belza J, Opletalová A, Poláková K (2021) Carbon dots for virus detection and therapy. Microchim Acta 188(12):430. https://doi.org/10.1007/s00604-021-05076-6

Bhadwal N, Ben Mrad R, Behdinan K (2023) Review of zinc oxide piezoelectric nanogenerators: piezoelectric properties, composite structures and power output. Sensors 23(8):3859. https://doi.org/10.3390/s23083859

Bokov D, Turki Jalil A, Chupradit S, Suksatan W, Javed Ansari M, Shewael IH, Valiev GH, Kianfar E (2021) Nanomaterial by sol-gel method: synthesis and application. Adv Mater Sci Eng 2021(1):5102014. https://doi.org/10.1155/2021/5102014

Carregal-Romero S, Plaza-García S, Piñol R, Murillo JL, Ruiz-Cabello J, Padro D, Millán A, Ramos-Cabrer P (2018) MRI study of the influence of surface coating aging on the in vivo biodistribution of iron oxide nanoparticles. Biosensors 8(4):127. https://doi.org/10.3390/bios8040127

Chaudhary V, Taha BA, Lucky, Rustagi S, Khosla A, Papakonstantinou P, Bhalla N (2024) Nose-on-chip nanobiosensors for early detection of lung cancer breath biomarkers. ACS Sens 9(9):4469–4494. https://doi.org/10.1021/acssensors.4c01524

Chen L, Wu Y, Wu H, Li J, Xie J, Zang F, Ma M, Gu N, Zhang Y (2019) Magnetic targeting combined with active targeting of dual-ligand iron oxide nanoprobes to promote the penetration depth in tumors for effective magnetic resonance imaging and hyperthermia. Acta Biomater 96:491–504. https://doi.org/10.1016/j.actbio.2019.07.017

Chen X, Argandona SM, Melle F, Rampal N, Fairen-Jimenez D (2024) Advances in surface functionalization of next-generation metal-organic frameworks for biomedical applications: design, strategies, and prospects. Chem 10(2):504–543. https://doi.org/10.1016/j.chempr.2023.09.016

Chicea D, Nicolae-Maranciuc A (2025) Metal nanocomposites as biosensors for biological fluids analysis. Materials 18(8):1809. https://doi.org/10.3390/ma18081809

Chu S, Shi X, Tian Y, Gao F (2022) pH-responsive polymer nanomaterials for tumor therapy. Front Oncol 12:855019. https://doi.org/10.3389/fonc.2022.855019

Costanzo H, Gooch J, Frascione N (2023) Nanomaterials for optical biosensors in forensic analysis. Talanta 253:123945. https://doi.org/10.1016/j.talanta.2022.123945

Dar AA, Umar K, Mir NA, Haque MM, Muneer M, Boxall C (2011) Photocatalysed degradation of a herbicide derivative, Dinoterb, in aqueous suspension. Res Chem Intermed 37(6):567–578. https://doi.org/10.1007/s11164-011-0299-6

Dash BS, Lu Y-J, Huang Y-S, Chen J-P (2024) Chitosan-coated magnetic graphene oxide for targeted delivery of doxorubicin as a nanomedicine approach to treat glioblastoma. Int J Biol Macromol 260:129401. https://doi.org/10.1016/j.ijbiomac.2024.129401

Erdogan S, Medarova ZO, Roby A, Moore A, Torchilin VP (2008) Enhanced tumor MR imaging with gadolinium-loaded polychelating polymer-containing tumor-targeted liposomes. J Magn Reson Imaging 27(3):574–580. https://doi.org/10.1002/jmri.21202

Eskandari V, Sahbafar H, Karooby E, Heris MH, Mehmandoust S, Razmjoue D, Hadi A (2023) Surface-enhanced Raman scattering (SERS) filter paper substrates decorated with silver nanoparticles for the detection of molecular vibrations of acyclovir drug. Spectrochim Acta A Mol Biomol Spectrosc 298:122762. https://doi.org/10.1016/j.saa.2023.122762

Eslamian M, Shekarriz M (2009) Recent advances in nanoparticle preparation by spray and microemulsion methods. Recent Pat Nanotechnol 3(2):99–115

Espenti CS, Mettu MR, Surendra TV, Srinivas B, Rao KM, Rao KSVK, Laxminarayana E, Mallikarjun A (2025) pH-responsive polymer hydrogel nanocomposites for sensor applications: a review. Sens Actuators A Phys 393:116853. https://doi.org/10.1016/j.sna.2025.116853

Ewii UE, Attama AA, Olorunsola EO, Onugwu AL, Nwakpa FU, Anyiam C, Chijioke C, Ogbulie T (2025) Nanoparticles for drug delivery: insight into *in vitro* and *in vivo* drug release from nanomedicines. Nano TransMed 4:100083. https://doi.org/10.1016/j.ntm.2025.100083

Ezhilarasu H, Vishalli D, Dheen ST, Bay B-H, Srinivasan DK (2020) Nanoparticle-based therapeutic approach for diabetic wound healing. Nanomaterials 10(6):1234. https://doi.org/10.3390/nano10061234

Fazal T, Nazia Murtaza B, Shah M, Iqbal S, Rehman M, Jaber F, A.A. Dera, Awwad NS, Ibrahium HA (2023) Recent developments in natural biopolymer based drug delivery systems. RSC Adv 13(33):23087–23121. https://doi.org/10.1039/D3RA03369D

Feng W, Wang Z (2022) Biomedical applications of chitosan-graphene oxide nanocomposites. iScience 25(1):103629. https://doi.org/10.1016/j.isci.2021.103629

Feng Z, Adolfsson KH, Xu Y, Fang H, Hakkarainen M, Wu M (2021) Carbon dot/polymer nanocomposites: from green synthesis to energy, environmental and biomedical applications. Sustain Mater Technol 29:e00304. https://doi.org/10.1016/j.susmat.2021.e00304

Fritea L, Banica F, Costea TO, Moldovan L, Dobjanschi L, Muresan M, Cavalu S (2021) Metal nanoparticles and carbon-based nanomaterials for improved performances of electrochemical (bio)sensors with biomedical applications. Materials (Basel) 14(21):6319. https://doi.org/10.3390/ma14216319

Fu Y, Liu T, Wang H, Wang Z, Hou L, Jiang J, Xu T (2024) Applications of nanomaterial technology in biosensing. J Sci Adv Mater Devices 9(2):100694. https://doi.org/10.1016/j.jsamd.2024.100694

Fukuzumi N, Nakagawa T, Hirao G, Ogawa A, Maeda M, Asahi T, Zako T (2025) Detection of C-reactive protein using single cluster analysis of gold nanoparticle aggregates using a dark-field microscope equipped with a smartphone. Sens Diagn 4(2):159–165. https://doi.org/10.1039/D4SD00329B

Galogahi FM, Zhu Y, An H, Nguyen N-T (2020) Core-shell microparticles: generation approaches and applications. J Sci Adv Mater Dev 5(4):417–435. https://doi.org/10.1016/j.jsamd.2020.09.001

Gambinossi F, Mylon SE, Ferri JK (2015) Aggregation kinetics and colloidal stability of functionalized nanoparticles. Adv Colloid Interf Sci 222:332–349. https://doi.org/10.1016/j.cis.2014.07.015

Gao T, Yachi T, Shi X, Sato R, Sato C, Yonamine Y, Kanie K, Misawa H, Ijiro K, Mitomo H (2024) Ultrasensitive surface-enhanced Raman scattering platform for protein detection via active delivery to nanogaps as a hotspot. ACS Nano 18(32):21593–21606. https://doi.org/10.1021/acsnano.4c09578

Gawande MB, Goswami A, Felpin F-X, Asefa T, Huang X, Silva R, Zou X, Zboril R, Varma RS (2016) Cu and Cu-based nanoparticles: synthesis and applications in catalysis. Chem Rev 116(6):3722–3811. https://doi.org/10.1021/acs.chemrev.5b00482

Ge C, Pei F, Zhang P, Wang X, Li Z, Sai Z, Ni T, Chang K, Yang Z (2025) Naked-eye and fluorescence resonance energy transfer based ratiometric fluorescent probe for rapid, sensitive and selective detection of hydrazine and its applications in imaging of environmental samples and living systems. J Hazard Mater 484:136781. https://doi.org/10.1016/j.jhazmat.2024.136781

Ghosh R, Gilda JE, Gomes AV (2014) The necessity of and strategies for improving confidence in the accuracy of western blots. Expert Rev Proteomics 11(5):549–560. https://doi.org/10.1586/14789450.2014.939635

Giordano A, Provenza AC, Reverchon G, Baldino L, Reverchon E (2024) Lipid-based nanocarriers: bridging diagnosis and cancer therapy. Pharmaceutics 16(9):1158. https://doi.org/10.3390/pharmaceutics16091158

Goel S, England CG, Chen F, Cai W (2017) Positron emission tomography and nanotechnology: a dynamic duo for cancer theranostics. Adv Drug Deliv Rev 113:157–176. https://doi.org/10.1016/j.addr.2016.08.001

Gómez IJ, Vázquez Sulleiro M, Mantione D, Alegret N (2021) Carbon nanomaterials embedded in conductive polymers: a state of the art. Polymers 13(5):745. https://doi.org/10.3390/polym13050745

González M, Romero MP (2025) Surface-modified carbon dots for cancer therapy: integrating diagnostic and therapeutic applications. Int J Nanomedicine 20:7715–7741. https://doi.org/10.2147/IJN.S508181

Gröger H, Kind C, Leidinger P, Roming M, Feldmann C (2010) Nanoscale hollow spheres: microemulsion-based synthesis, structural characterization and container-type functionality. Materials 3(8):4355–4386. https://doi.org/10.3390/ma3084355

Hazra N, Hazra S, Paul S, Banerjee A (2023) Surface modification of carbon dots via peptide covalent conjugation. Chem Commun 59(33):4931–4934. https://doi.org/10.1039/D2CC06478B

He Y, Hu C, Li Z, Wu C, Zeng Y, Peng C (2022) Multifunctional carbon nanomaterials for diagnostic applications in infectious diseases and tumors. Mater Today Bio 14:100231. https://doi.org/10.1016/j.mtbio.2022.100231

Hemdan M, Ali MA, Doghish AS, Mageed SSA, Elazab IM, Khalil MM, Mabrouk M, Das DB, Amin AS (2024) Innovations in biosensor technologies for healthcare diagnostics and therapeutic drug monitoring: applications, recent progress, and future research challenges. Sensors 24(16):5143. https://doi.org/10.3390/s24165143

Hench LL, West JK (1990) The sol-gel process. Chem Rev 90(1):33–72. https://doi.org/10.1021/cr00099a003

Hosseini S, Vázquez-Villegas P, Rito-Palomares M, Martinez-Chapa SO (2018) Advantages, disadvantages and modifications of conventional ELISA. In: Hosseini S, Vázquez-Villegas P, Rito-Palomares M, Martinez-Chapa SO (eds) Enzyme-linked immunosorbent assay (ELISA): from A to Z. Springer, Singapore, pp 67–115. https://doi.org/10.1007/978-981-10-6766-2_5

Hou F, Sun S, Waheed Abdullah S, Tang Y, Li X, Guo H (2023) The application of nanoparticles in point-of-care testing (POCT) immunoassays. Anal Methods 15(18):2154–2180. https://doi.org/10.1039/D3AY00182B

Huang X, El-Sayed MA (2010) Gold nanoparticles: optical properties and implementations in cancer diagnosis and photothermal therapy. J Adv Res 1(1):13–28. https://doi.org/10.1016/j.jare.2010.02.002

Hussain MM, Khan WU, Ahmed F, Wei Y, Xiong H (2023) Recent developments of red/NIR carbon dots in biosensing, bioimaging, and tumor theranostics. Chem Eng J 465:143010. https://doi.org/10.1016/j.cej.2023.143010

Iwasaki Y, Kimura T, Orisaka M, Kawasaki H, Goda T, Yusa S (2014) Label-free detection of C-reactive protein using highly dispersible gold nanoparticles synthesized by reducible biomimetic block copolymers. Chem Commun 50(42):5656–5658. https://doi.org/10.1039/C4CC01855A

Jayakumar S, Saravanan T, Philip J (2023) A review on polymer nanocomposites as lead-free materials for diagnostic X-ray shielding: recent advances, challenges and future perspectives. Hybrid Adv 4:100100. https://doi.org/10.1016/j.hybadv.2023.100100

Jayaprakash N, Elumalai K, Manickam S, Bakthavatchalam G, Tamilselvan P (2024) Carbon nanomaterials: revolutionizing biomedical applications with promising potential. Nano Mater Sci. https://doi.org/10.1016/j.nanoms.2024.11.004

Jiang Y, Wu J (2019) Recent development in chitosan nanocomposites for surface-based biosensor applications. Electrophoresis 40(16–17):2084–2097. https://doi.org/10.1002/elps.201900066

Jiang Z, Zhang M, Li P, Wang Y, Fu Q (2023) Nanomaterial-based CT contrast agents and their applications in image-guided therapy. Theranostics 13(2):483–509. https://doi.org/10.7150/thno.79625

Julius A, Malakondaiah S, Pothireddy RB (2025) Polymer and nanocomposite fillers as advanced materials in biomedical applications. Nano Trends 9:100087. https://doi.org/10.1016/j.nwnano.2025.100087

Kale RA, Dhawale SC, Mulik BB, Adhikari A, Sathe BR (2024) Polyaniline based highly selective electrochemical sensor for ascorbic acid determination: performance studies towards real sample analysis. J Ind Eng Chem 136:167–176. https://doi.org/10.1016/j.jiec.2024.02.004

Kar DK, V P, Si S, Panigrahi H, Mishra S (2024) Carbon dots and their polymeric nanocomposites: insight into their synthesis, photoluminescence mechanisms, and recent trends in sensing applications. ACS Omega 9(10):11050–11080. https://doi.org/10.1021/acsomega.3c07612

Kaur N, Sharma V, Tiwari P, Saini AK, Mobin SM (2019) "Vigna Radiata" based green C-dots: photo-triggered theranostics, fluorescent sensor for extracellular and intracellular iron (III) and multicolor live cell imaging probe. Sens Actuators B Chem 291:275–286. https://doi.org/10.1016/j.snb.2019.04.039

Kaur N, Sharma R, Sharma V (2022) Chapter 15 - Advances in the synthesis and antimicrobial applications of metal oxide nanostructures. In: Singh S, Kumar P, Mondal DP (eds) Advanced ceramics for versatile interdisciplinary applications, Elsevier series in advanced ceramic materials. Elsevier, pp 339–369. https://doi.org/10.1016/B978-0-323-89952-9.00015-4

Kaurav H, Verma D, Bansal A, Kapoor DN, Sheth S (2023) Progress in drug delivery and diagnostic applications of carbon dots: a systematic review. Front Chem 11:1227843. https://doi.org/10.3389/fchem.2023.1227843

Khan I, Saeed K, Khan I (2019) Nanoparticles: properties, applications and toxicities. Arab J Chem 12(7):908–931. https://doi.org/10.1016/j.arabjc.2017.05.011

Khazaei M, Hosseini MS, Haghighi AM, Misaghi M (2023) Nanosensors and their applications in early diagnosis of cancer. Sens Bio Sens Res 41:100569. https://doi.org/10.1016/j.sbsr.2023.100569

Khodaparast M, Sharley D, Marshall S, Beddoe T (2024) Advances in point-of-care and molecular techniques to detect waterborne pathogens. NPJ Clean Water 7(1):74. https://doi.org/10.1038/s41545-024-00368-9

Kilic NM, Gelen SS, Er Zeybekler S, Odaci D (2024) Carbon-based nanomaterials decorated electrospun nanofibers in biosensors: a review. ACS Omega 9(1):3–15. https://doi.org/10.1021/acsomega.3c00798

Kim GB, Kim Y-P (2012) Analysis of protease activity using quantum dots and resonance energy transfer. Theranostics 2(2):127–138. https://doi.org/10.7150/thno.3476

Kostevšek N, Cheung CCL, Serša I, Kreft ME, Monaco I, Comes Franchini M, Vidmar J, Al-Jamal WT (2020) Magneto-liposomes as MRI contrast agents: a systematic study of different liposomal formulations. Nanomaterials 10(5):889. https://doi.org/10.3390/nano10050889

Kumar Krishnan S, Singh E, Singh P, Meyyappan M, Singh Nalwa H (2019) A review on graphene-based nanocomposites for electrochemical and fluorescent biosensors. RSC Adv 9(16):8778–8881. https://doi.org/10.1039/C8RA09577A

Kumar S, Shukla MK, Sharma AK, Jayaprakash GK, Tonk RK, Chellappan DK, Singh SK, Dua K, Ahmed F, Bhattacharyya S, Kumar D (2023a) Metal-based nanomaterials and nanocomposites as promising frontier in cancer chemotherapy. MedComm 4(2):e253. https://doi.org/10.1002/mco2.253

Kumar S, K. Sidhu H, K. Paul A, Bhardwaj N, S. Thakur N, Deep A (2023b) Bioengineered multi-walled carbon nanotube (MWCNT) based biosensors and applications thereof. Sensors Diagn 2(6):1390–1413. https://doi.org/10.1039/D3SD00176H

Kumarasamy S, Sharma V (2025) Unveiling cellular secrets: illuminating carbon dot lighthouses for improved mitochondrial exploration. Chem Mater 37(1):1–16. https://doi.org/10.1021/acs.chemmater.4c01481

Kurul F, Turkmen H, Cetin AE, Topkaya SN (2025) Nanomedicine: how nanomaterials are transforming drug delivery, bio-imaging, and diagnosis. Next Nanotechnol 7:100129. https://doi.org/10.1016/j.nxnano.2024.100129

Lan H, Jamil M, Ke G, Dong N (2023) The role of nanoparticles and nanomaterials in cancer diagnosis and treatment: a comprehensive review. Am J Cancer Res 13(12):5751–5784

Lee IH, Lee JM, Jung Y (2014) Controlled protein embedment onto Au/Ag core–shell nanoparticles for immuno-labeling of nanosilver surface. ACS Appl Mater Interfaces 6(10):7659–7664. https://doi.org/10.1021/am500960b

Li W, Chen X (2015) Gold nanoparticles for photoacoustic imaging. Nanomedicine (Lond) 10(2):299–320. https://doi.org/10.2217/nnm.14.169

Li L, Jiang W, Luo K, Song H, Lan F, Wu Y, Gu Z (2013) Superparamagnetic iron oxide nanoparticles as MRI contrast agents for non-invasive stem cell labeling and tracking. Theranostics 3(8):595–615. https://doi.org/10.7150/thno.5366

Li Y, Zhuang J, Lu Y, Li N, Gu M, Xia J, Zhao N, Tang BZ (2021) High-performance near-infrared aggregation-induced emission luminogen with mitophagy regulating capability for multimodal cancer theranostics. ACS Nano 15(12):20453–20465. https://doi.org/10.1021/acsnano.1c08928
Li C-H, Chan M-H, Chang Y-C, Hsiao M (2023) Gold nanoparticles as a biosensor for cancer biomarker determination. Molecules 28(1):364. https://doi.org/10.3390/molecules28010364
Li M, Huang Y, Shen C, Wang Y, Lin Y, Wang Z, Chen N, Luo Y (2025a) Application of quantum dots in cancer diagnosis and treatment: advances and perspectives. Nano Res 18(1). https://doi.org/10.26599/NR.2025.94907163
Li M, Shen C, Lv M, Luo Y (2025b) Nanobiosensors enable high-efficiency detection of tuberculosis nucleic acid. JACS Au 5(2):536–549. https://doi.org/10.1021/jacsau.4c01206
Liu J, Li R, Yang B (2020) Carbon dots: a new type of carbon-based nanomaterial with wide applications. ACS Cent Sci 6(12):2179–2195. https://doi.org/10.1021/acscentsci.0c01306
Liu X, He F, Liu M (2024) New opportunities of stimulus-responsive smart nanocarriers in cancer therapy. Nano Mater Sci. https://doi.org/10.1016/j.nanoms.2024.10.013
Lohani AP, Elosta M, Maksoud M, Murshid N (2025) Functionalized carbon nanotubes: emerging nanomaterials for enhanced cancer diagnosis and imaging. Molecules 30(11):2364. https://doi.org/10.3390/molecules30112364
Lu S, Yu T, Wang Y, Liang L, Chen Y, Xu F, Wang S (2017) Nanomaterial-based biosensors for measurement of lipids and lipoproteins towards point-of-care of cardiovascular disease. Analyst 142(18):3309–3321. https://doi.org/10.1039/C7AN00847C
Lu H, Zhang S, Wang J, Chen Q (2021) A review on polymer and lipid-based nanocarriers and its application to nano-pharmaceutical and food-based systems. Front Nutr 8:783831. https://doi.org/10.3389/fnut.2021.783831
Lu Y, Chen X, Lan H, Nag A, Chen Y, Gao J, Deng S (2025a) A review of multi-walled carbon nanotubes-based electrochemical sensors to detect heavy metals for food packaging applications. J Alloys Compd 1017:179106. https://doi.org/10.1016/j.jallcom.2025.179106
Lu F, Xu X, Wan W, Liang X, Xia J, Cao W, Chen Z, Hu M (2025b) Advances in the syntheses, mechanisms and applications of room-temperature phosphorescent carbon dots. J Mater Chem C 13(5):2091–2120. https://doi.org/10.1039/D4TC04759A
Luciani A, Olivier J-C, Clement O, Siauve N, Brillet P-Y, Bessoud B, Gazeau F, Uchegbu IF, Kahn E, Frija G, Cuenod CA (2004) Glucose-receptor MR imaging of tumors: study in mice with PEGylated paramagnetic niosomes. Radiology 231(1):135–142. https://doi.org/10.1148/radiol.2311021559
Luo X-L, Xu J-J, Du Y, Chen H-Y (2004) A glucose biosensor based on chitosan–glucose oxidase–gold nanoparticles biocomposite formed by one-step electrodeposition. Anal Biochem 334(2):284–289. https://doi.org/10.1016/j.ab.2004.07.005
Luo C, Zhang R, Liu J, He X, Li S, Ran C, Ma S, Shen Y (2024) A one step strategy based on hollow gold nanoparticles to detect C-reactive protein with high sensitivity (Hs-CRP) in serum for monitoring cardiovascular disease. Int J Nanomed 19:845–858. https://doi.org/10.2147/IJN.S436391
Lv X, Chen L, Guo R, Yang Y, Liu X, Yu S (2025) Gadolinium functionalized carbon dot complexes for dual-modal imaging: structure, performance, and applications. ACS Biomater Sci Eng 11(4):2037–2051. https://doi.org/10.1021/acsbiomaterials.4c02278
Mahardika IH, Naorungroj S, Khamcharoen W, Kin S, Rodthongkum N, Chailapakul O, Shin K (2023) Point-of-care testing (POCT) devices for DNA detection: a comprehensive review. Adv NanoBiomed Res 3(11):2300058. https://doi.org/10.1002/anbr.202300058
Mahor A, Singh PP, Bharadwaj P, Sharma N, Yadav S, Rosenholm JM, Bansal KK (2021) Carbon-based nanomaterials for delivery of biologicals and therapeutics: a cutting-edge technology. C 7(1):19. https://doi.org/10.3390/c7010019
Maiti D, Tong X, Mou X, Yang K (2019) Carbon-based nanomaterials for biomedical applications: a recent study. Front Pharmacol 9:1401. https://doi.org/10.3389/fphar.2018.01401
Majeed AH, Mohammed LA, Hammoodi OG, Sehgal S, Alheety MA, Saxena KK, Dadoosh SA, Mohammed IK, Jasim MM, Salmaan NU (2022) A review on polyaniline: synthesis, prop-

erties, nanocomposites, and electrochemical applications. Int J Polym Sci 2022(1):9047554. https://doi.org/10.1155/2022/9047554

Malekzadeh R, Ghorbani M, Faghani P, Abdollahi BB, Mortezazadeh T, Farhood B (2023) Fabrication of targeted gold nanoparticle as potential contrast agent in molecular CT imaging. J Radiat Res Appl Sci 16(1):100490. https://doi.org/10.1016/j.jrras.2022.100490

Mall J, Naseem N, Haider MF, Rahman MA, Khan S, Siddiqui SN (2024) Nanostructured lipid carriers as a drug delivery system: a comprehensive review with therapeutic applications. Intell Pharm. https://doi.org/10.1016/j.ipha.2024.09.005

Mallakpour S, Madani M (2015) A review of current coupling agents for modification of metal oxide nanoparticles. Prog Org Coat 86:194–207. https://doi.org/10.1016/j.porgcoat.2015.05.023

Mao X, Xu J, Cui H (2016) Functional nanoparticles for magnetic resonance imaging. Wiley Interdiscip Rev Nanomed Nanobiotechnol 8(6):814–841. https://doi.org/10.1002/wnan.1400

Mehta S, Suresh A, Nayak Y, Narayan R, Nayak UY (2022) Hybrid nanostructures: versatile systems for biomedical applications. Coord Chem Rev 460:214482. https://doi.org/10.1016/j.ccr.2022.214482

Mehta M, Bui TA, Yang X, Aksoy Y, Goldys EM, Deng W (2023) Lipid-based nanoparticles for drug/gene delivery: an overview of the production techniques and difficulties encountered in their industrial development. ACS Mater Au 3(6):600–619. https://pubs.acs.org/doi/10.1021/acsmaterialsau.3c00032. Accessed 29 June 2025

Mishra S, Saha B (2024) Graphene- polymer nanocomposite-based wearable strain sensors for physiological signal monitoring: recent progress and challenges. Curr Opinion Solid State Mater Sci 31:101174. https://doi.org/10.1016/j.cossms.2024.101174

Mobed A, Darvishi M, Kohansal F, Dehfooli FM, Alipourfard I, Tahavvori A, Ghazi F (2024) Biosensors; nanomaterial-based methods in diagnosing of *mycobacterium tuberculosis*. J Clin Tuberc Other Mycobact Dis 34:100412. https://doi.org/10.1016/j.jctube.2023.100412

Mohammed AM, Ibraheem IJ, Obaid AS, Bououdina M (2017) Nanostructured ZnO-based biosensor: DNA immobilization and hybridization. Sens Biosensing Res 15:46–52. https://doi.org/10.1016/j.sbsr.2017.07.003

Mokhtarzadeh A, Eivazzadeh-Keihan R, Pashazadeh P, Hejazi M, Gharaatifar N, Hasanzadeh M, Baradaran B, de la Guardia M (2017) Nanomaterial-based biosensors for detection of pathogenic virus. Trends Analyt Chem 97:445–457. https://doi.org/10.1016/j.trac.2017.10.005

Motaghi H, Mehrgardi MA, Bouvet P (2017) Carbon dots-AS1411 aptamer nanoconjugate for ultrasensitive spectrofluorometric detection of cancer cells. Sci Rep 7(1):10513. https://doi.org/10.1038/s41598-017-11087-2

Moulahoum H, Ghorbanizamani F, Guler Celik E, Zihnioglu F, Timur S (2023) Chapter 6 - Nanoconjugated materials as sensors in point-of-care diagnostic tools: detection of small molecules and viruses. In: Comprehensive analytical chemistry, Verma SK, Das AK (eds) Bioconjugated materials part 1 Preparation, characterization and applications in therapeutics, environmental monitoring and point-of-care diagnostics, vol 102. Elsevier, pp 203–231. https://doi.org/10.1016/bs.coac.2023.02.002

Mukherjee S, Mukherjee A, Bytesnikova Z, Ashrafi AM, Richtera L, Adam V (2024) 2D graphene-based advanced nanoarchitectonics for electrochemical biosensors: applications in cancer biomarker detection. Biosens Bioelectron 250:116050. https://doi.org/10.1016/j.bios.2024.116050

Mutreja I, Maalej N, Kaushik A, Kumar D, Raja A (2023) High atomic number nanoparticles to enhance spectral CT imaging aspects. Mater Adv 4(18):3967–3988. https://doi.org/10.1039/D3MA00231D

Naresh V, Lee N (2021) A review on biosensors and recent development of nanostructured materials-enabled biosensors. Sensors (Basel) 21(4):1109. https://doi.org/10.3390/s21041109

Nelson NR, Port JD, Pandey MK (2020) Use of superparamagnetic iron oxide nanoparticles (SPIONs) via multiple imaging modalities and modifications to reduce cytotoxicity: an educational review. J Nanotheranostics 1(1):105–135. https://doi.org/10.3390/jnt1010008

Neuwelt A, Sidhu N, Hu C-AA, Mlady G, Eberhardt SC, Sillerud LO (2015) Iron-based superparamagnetic nanoparticle contrast agents for MRI of infection and inflammation. AJR Am J Roentgenol 204(3):W302–W313. https://doi.org/10.2214/AJR.14.12733

Nguyen VH, Thuy VN, Van TV, Dao AH, Lee B-J (2022) Nanostructured lipid carriers and their potential applications for versatile drug delivery via oral administration. OpenNano 8:100064. https://doi.org/10.1016/j.onano.2022.100064

Nikolaev B, Yakovleva L, Fedorov V, Li H, Gao H, Shevtsov M (2023) Nano- and microemulsions in biomedicine: from theory to practice. Pharmaceutics 15(7):1989. https://doi.org/10.3390/pharmaceutics15071989

Niranjana VS, Ponnan S, Mukundan A, Prabu AA, Wang H-C (2025) Emerging trends in silane-modified nanomaterial–polymer nanocomposites for energy harvesting applications. Polymers (Basel) 17(10):1416. https://doi.org/10.3390/polym17101416

Owens GJ, Singh RK, Foroutan F, Alqaysi M, Han C-M, Mahapatra C, Kim H-W, Knowles JC (2016) Sol–gel based materials for biomedical applications. Prog Mater Sci 77:1–79. https://doi.org/10.1016/j.pmatsci.2015.12.001

Ozyurt D, Kobaisi MA, Hocking RK, Fox B (2023) Properties, synthesis, and applications of carbon dots: a review. Carbon Trends 12:100276. https://doi.org/10.1016/j.cartre.2023.100276

Park S, Nguyen VP, Wang X, Paulus YM (2024) Gold nanoparticles for retinal molecular optical imaging. Int J Mol Sci 25(17):9315. https://doi.org/10.3390/ijms25179315

Partikel K, Korte R, Stein NC, Mulac D, Herrmann FC, Humpf H-U, Langer K (2019) Effect of nanoparticle size and PEGylation on the protein corona of PLGA nanoparticles. Eur J Pharm Biopharm 141:70–80. https://doi.org/10.1016/j.ejpb.2019.05.006

Patyal R, Warjurkar K, Sharma V (2025) Advancements in tumor diagnostics through carbon dot-assisted photoacoustic imaging. Adv Opt Mater 13(4):2402343. https://doi.org/10.1002/adom.202402343

Pechnikova NA, Domvri K, Porpodis K, Istomina MS, Iaremenko AV, Yaremenko AV (2025) Carbon quantum dots in biomedical applications: advances, challenges, and future prospects. Aggregate 6(3):e707. https://doi.org/10.1002/agt2.707

Peltomaa R, Glahn-Martínez B, Benito-Peña E, Moreno-Bondi MC (2018) Optical biosensors for label-free detection of small molecules. Sensors (Basel) 18(12):4126. https://doi.org/10.3390/s18124126

Phadtare P, Viswapriya V, Shinde V, Mathure D, Salunke MR (2025) Hybrid bionanocomposites as the advancements in biomedical utility. Hybrid Adv 8:100365. https://doi.org/10.1016/j.hybadv.2024.100365

Porras JC, Bernuz M, Marfa J, Pallares-Rusiñol A, Martí M, Pividori MI (2021) Comparative study of gold and carbon nanoparticles in nucleic acid lateral flow assay. Nanomaterials (Basel) 11(3):741. https://doi.org/10.3390/nano11030741

Puri A, Loomis K, Smith B, Lee J-H, Yavlovich A, Heldman E, Blumenthal R (2009) Lipid-based nanoparticles as pharmaceutical drug carriers: from concepts to clinic. Crit Rev Ther Drug Carrier Syst 26(6):523–580. https://doi.org/10.1615/critrevtherdrugcarriersyst.v26.i6.10

Qamar SUR (2021) Nanocomposites: potential therapeutic agents for the diagnosis and treatment of infectious diseases and cancer. Colloid Interface Sci Commun 43:100463. https://doi.org/10.1016/j.colcom.2021.100463

Qi J, Zhang P, Zhang T, Zhang R, Zhang Q, Wang J, Zong M, Gong Y, Liu X, Wu X, Li B (2024) Metal-doped carbon dots for biomedical applications: from design to implementation. Heliyon 10(11):e32133. https://doi.org/10.1016/j.heliyon.2024.e32133

Qian S, Cui Y, Cai Z, Li L (2022) Applications of smartphone-based colorimetric biosensors. Biosens Bioelectron X 11:100173. https://doi.org/10.1016/j.biosx.2022.100173

Qureshi ZA, Dabash H, Ponnamma D, Abbas MKG (2024) Carbon dots as versatile nanomaterials in sensing and imaging: efficiency and beyond. Heliyon 10(11):e31634. https://doi.org/10.1016/j.heliyon.2024.e31634

Redondo-Fernandez G, Cigales Canga J, Soldado A, Ruiz Encinar J, Costa-Fernandez JM (2023) Functionalized heteroatom-doped carbon dots for biomedical applications: a review. Anal Chim Acta 1284:341874. https://doi.org/10.1016/j.aca.2023.341874

Ren H (2025) Graphene and its derivatives for electrochemical sensing. Sensors 25(7):1993. https://doi.org/10.3390/s25071993

Renuka RR, Julius A, Yoganandham ST, Umapathy D, Ramadoss R, Samrot AV, Vijay DD (2022) Diverse nanocomposites as a potential dressing for diabetic wound healing. Front Endocrinol (Lausanne) 13:1074568. https://doi.org/10.3389/fendo.2022.1074568

Reuveni T, Motiei M, Romman Z, Popovtzer A, Popovtzer R (2011) Targeted gold nanoparticles enable molecular CT imaging of cancer: an in vivo study. Int J Nanomed 6:2859–2864. https://doi.org/10.2147/IJN.S25446

Rogina A (2014) Electrospinning process: versatile preparation method for biodegradable and natural polymers and biocomposite systems applied in tissue engineering and drug delivery. Appl Surf Sci 296:221–230. https://doi.org/10.1016/j.apsusc.2014.01.098

Roy L, Buragohain P, Borse V (2022) Strategies for sensitivity enhancement of point-of-care devices. Biosens Bioelectron X 10:100098. https://doi.org/10.1016/j.biosx.2021.100098

Sabzevari M, Cree DE, Wilson LD (2018) Graphene oxide–chitosan composite material for treatment of a model dye effluent. ACS Omega 3(10):13045–13054. https://doi.org/10.1021/acsomega.8b01871

Saha R, Munshi MH, Akter M, Shikder AAR, Islam T (2025) Synthesis techniques, fundamental properties, and emerging applications of nanocomposites: a comprehensive review. SPE Polym 6(2):e70004. https://doi.org/10.1002/pls2.70004

Saleh M, Gul A, Nasir A, Moses TO, Nural Y, Yabalak E (2025) Comprehensive review of carbon-based nanostructures: properties, synthesis, characterization, and cross-disciplinary applications. J Ind Eng Chem 146:176–212. https://doi.org/10.1016/j.jiec.2024.11.052

Sha R, Basak A, Maity PC, Badhulika S (2022) ZnO nano-structured based devices for chemical and optical sensing applications. Sens Actuator Rep 4:100098. https://doi.org/10.1016/j.snr.2022.100098

Sharma V (2021) The emergence of carbon-dots for optical molecular electronics: from sensors to logic gates, memory devices, and security. J Mater Chem C 9(47):16828–16842. https://doi.org/10.1039/D1TC03859A

Sharma AS, Lee NY (2024) Comprehensive review on fluorescent carbon dots and their applications in nucleic acid detection, nucleolus targeted imaging and gene delivery. Analyst 149(16):4095–4115. https://doi.org/10.1039/D4AN00630E

Sharma V, Mohammad A, Mishra V, Chaudhary A, Kapoor K, Mobin SM (2016) Fabrication of innovative ZnO nanoflowers showing drastic biological activity. New J Chem 40(3):2145–2155. https://doi.org/10.1039/C5NJ02391B

Sharma V, Tiwari P, Mobin SM (2017) Sustainable carbon-dots: recent advances in green carbon dots for sensing and bioimaging. J Mater Chem B 5(45):8904–8924. https://doi.org/10.1039/C7TB02484C

Sharma V, Kaur N, Tiwari P, Mobin SM (2018) Full color emitting fluorescent carbon material as reversible pH sensor with multicolor live cell imaging. J Photochem Photobiol B Biol 182:137–145. https://doi.org/10.1016/j.jphotobiol.2018.04.006

Sharma V, Tiwari P, Kaur N, Mobin SM (2021) Optical nanosensors based on fluorescent carbon dots for the detection of water contaminants: a review. Environ Chem Lett 19(4):3229–3241. https://doi.org/10.1007/s10311-021-01241-8

Sharma M, Mahajan P, Alsubaie AS, Khanna V, Chahal S, Thakur A, Yadav A, Arya A, Singh A, Singh G (2025) Next-generation nanomaterials-based biosensors: real-time biosensing devices for detecting emerging environmental pollutants. Mater Today Sustain 29:101068. https://doi.org/10.1016/j.mtsust.2024.101068

Sher M, Zhuang R, Demirci U, Asghar W (2017) Paper-based analytical devices for clinical diagnosis: recent advances in the fabrication techniques and sensing mechanisms. Expert Rev Mol Diagn 17(4):351–366. https://doi.org/10.1080/14737159.2017.1285228

Shukla N, Das R, Rodriguez CYC, Mukhanova E, Soldatov A, Bathla A, kumari I, Hauserao N, Belbekhouche S (2025) Optimizing near-infrared-activated gold nanostructures for targeted combination cancer therapy. Colloids Surf B Biointerfaces 253:114687. https://doi.org/10.1016/j.colsurfb.2025.114687

Si P, Razmi N, Nur O, Solanki S, Pandey CM, Gupta RK, Malhotra BD, Willander M, de la Zerda A (2021) Gold nanomaterials for optical biosensing and bioimaging. Nanoscale Adv 3(10):2679–2698. https://doi.org/10.1039/d0na00961j

Singh R, Lillard JW (2009) Nanoparticle-based targeted drug delivery. Exp Mol Pathol 86(3):215–223. https://doi.org/10.1016/j.yexmp.2008.12.004

Singh LP, Bhattacharyya SK, Kumar R, Mishra G, Sharma U, Singh G, Ahalawat S (2014) Sol-gel processing of silica nanoparticles and their applications. Adv Colloid Interf Sci 214:17–37. https://doi.org/10.1016/j.cis.2014.10.007

Singh R, Srinivas SP, Kumawat M, Daima HK (2024a) Ligand-based surface engineering of nanomaterials: trends, challenges, and biomedical perspectives. OpenNano 15:100194. https://doi.org/10.1016/j.onano.2023.100194

Singh S, Banerjee R, Pal K (2024b) Emerging trends in biodegradable polymer-metal nanoconjugates for cancer therapeutics. Eur Polym J 207:112835. https://doi.org/10.1016/j.eurpolymj.2024.112835

Solangi NH, Karri RR, Mubarak NM, Mazari SA (2024) Mechanism of polymer composite-based nanomaterial for biomedical applications. Adv Ind Eng Poly Res 7(1):1–19. https://doi.org/10.1016/j.aiepr.2023.09.002

Song J, Luo Y, Hao Z, Qu M, Huang C, Wang Z, Yang J, Liang Q, Jia Y, Song Q, Zhang Q, Luo S (2025) Graphene-based wearable biosensors for point-of-care diagnostics: from surface functionalization to biomarker detection. Mater Today Bio 32:101667. https://doi.org/10.1016/j.mtbio.2025.101667

Suhail N, Alzahrani AK, Basha WJ, Kizilbash N, Zaidi A, Ambreen J, Khachfe HM (2021) Microemulsions: unique properties, pharmacological applications, and targeted drug delivery. Front Nanotechnol 3. https://doi.org/10.3389/fnano.2021.754889

Suk JS, Xu Q, Kim N, Hanes J, Ensign LM (2016) PEGylation as a strategy for improving nanoparticle-based drug and gene delivery. Adv Drug Deliv Rev 99(Pt A):28–51. https://doi.org/10.1016/j.addr.2015.09.012

Sumitha MNSK, Suryabai XT (2024) Sensing the future—frontiers in biosensors: exploring classifications, principles, and recent advances. ACS Omega 9(50):48918–48987. https://doi.org/10.1021/acsomega.4c07991

Sun J-P, Ren Y-T, Wei K, He M-J, Gao B-H, Qi H (2022) Photoacoustic response optimization of gold nanorods in the near-infrared region. Results Phys 34:105209. https://doi.org/10.1016/j.rinp.2022.105209

Tavakoli H, Mohammadi S, Li X, Fu G, Li X (2022) Microfluidic platforms integrated with nano-sensors for point-of-care bioanalysis. Trends Analyt Chem 157:116806. https://doi.org/10.1016/j.trac.2022.116806

Tavan M, Yousefian Z, Bakhtiar Z, Rahmandoust M, Mirjalili MH (2025) Carbon quantum dots: multifunctional fluorescent nanomaterials for sustainable advances in biomedicine and agriculture. Ind Crop Prod 231:121207. https://doi.org/10.1016/j.indcrop.2025.121207

Tazim TQ, Kawsar M, Sahadat Hossain M, Bahadur NM, Ahmed S (2025) Hydrothermal synthesis of nano-metal oxides for structural modification: a review. Next Nanotechnol 7:100167. https://doi.org/10.1016/j.nxnano.2025.100167

Thirumalai A, Sharmiladevi P, Girigoswami K, Prabhu AD, Girigoswami A (2025) Tuneable carbon dots coated iron oxide nanoparticles as superior T1 contrast agent for multimodal imaging. ADMET DMPK 13(3):2790. https://doi.org/10.5599/admet.2790

Thiruvengadam M, Chi H-Y, Choi H-J, Jung B-S, Lee S-B, Park Y, Jeon D, Ciftci F, Shariati MA, Kim S-H (2025) Sustainable and smart nano-biosensors: integrated solutions for healthcare, environmental monitoring, agriculture, and food safety. Ind Crop Prod 233:121337. https://doi.org/10.1016/j.indcrop.2025.121337

Thwala LN, Ndlovu SC, Mpofu KT, Lugongolo MY, Mthunzi-Kufa P (2023) Nanotechnology-based diagnostics for diseases prevalent in developing countries: current advances in point-of-care tests. Nanomaterials (Basel) 13(7):1247. https://doi.org/10.3390/nano13071247

Tiwari I, Singh M, Pandey CM, Sumana G (2015) Electrochemical genosensor based on graphene oxide modified iron oxide–chitosan hybrid nanocomposite for pathogen detection. Sens Actuators B Chem 206:276–283. https://doi.org/10.1016/j.snb.2014.09.056

Tiwari P, Kaur N, Sharma V, Mobin SM (2020) A spectroscopic investigation of carbon dots and its reduced state towards fluorescence performance. J Photochem Photobiol A Chem 403:112847. https://doi.org/10.1016/j.jphotochem.2020.112847

Truskewycz A, Yin H, Halberg N, Lai DTH, Ball AS, Truong VK, Rybicka AM, Cole I (2022) Carbon dot therapeutic platforms: administration, distribution, metabolism, excretion, toxicity, and therapeutic potential. Small 18(16):2106342. https://doi.org/10.1002/smll.202106342

Tudor IA, Petriceanu M, Piticescu RR, Piticescu RM, Predescu C (2014) Hydrothermal synthesis of doped zno and tio2 nanomaterials: oppurtunities for textile applications. UPB Sci Bull Ser B 76:207–215

Vargas KM, Shon Y-S (2019) Hybrid lipid–nanoparticle complexes for biomedical applications. J Mater Chem B 7(5):695–708. https://doi.org/10.1039/C8TB03084G

Verma D, Singh KR, Yadav AK, Nayak V, Singh J, Solanki PR, Singh RP (2022) Internet of things (IoT) in nano-integrated wearable biosensor devices for healthcare applications. Biosens Bioelectron X 11:100153. https://doi.org/10.1016/j.biosx.2022.100153

Viegas C, Patrício AB, Prata JM, Nadhman A, Chintamaneni PK, Fonte P (2023) Solid lipid nanoparticles vs. nanostructured lipid carriers: a comparative review. Pharmaceutics 15(6):1593. https://doi.org/10.3390/pharmaceutics15061593

Vodyashkin AA, Kezimana P, Vetcher AA, Stanishevskiy YM (2022) Biopolymeric nanoparticles–multifunctional materials of the future. Polymers 14(11):2287. https://doi.org/10.3390/polym14112287

Waheed I, Ali A, Tabassum H, Khatoon N, Lai W-F, Zhou X (2024) Lipid-based nanoparticles as drug delivery carriers for cancer therapy. Front Oncol 14:1296091. https://doi.org/10.3389/fonc.2024.1296091

Wang Q, Chao Y (2018) Multifunctional quantum dots and liposome complexes in drug delivery. J Biomed Res 32(2):91–106. https://doi.org/10.7555/JBR.31.20160146

Wang B, Lu S (2022) The light of carbon dots: from mechanism to applications. Matter 5(1):110–149. https://doi.org/10.1016/j.matt.2021.10.016

Wang C, Ravi S, Garapati US, Das M, Howell M, Mallela J, Alwarappan S, Mohapatra SS, Mohapatra S (2013) Multifunctional chitosan magnetic-graphene (CMG) nanoparticles: a theranostic platform for tumor-targeted co-delivery of drugs, genes and MRI contrast agents. J Mater Chem B 1(35):4396–4405. https://doi.org/10.1039/C3TB20452A

Wang Y, Jiang K, Zhu J, Zhang L, Lin H (2015a) A FRET-based carbon dot–MnO2 nanosheet architecture for glutathione sensing in human whole blood samples. Chem Commun 51(64):12748–12751. https://doi.org/10.1039/C5CC04905A

Wang H, Di J, Sun Y, Fu J, Wei Z, Matsui H, del C. Alonso A, Zhou S (2015b) Biocompatible PEG-chitosan@carbon dots hybrid nanogels for two-photon fluorescence imaging, near-infrared light/pH dual-responsive drug carrier, and synergistic therapy. Adv Funct Mater 25(34):5537–5547. https://doi.org/10.1002/adfm.201501524

Wang L, Chen X, Liu C, Yang W (2016) Non-enzymatic acetylcholine electrochemical biosensor based on flower-like NiAl layered double hydroxides decorated with carbon dots. Sens Actuators B Chem 233:199–205. https://doi.org/10.1016/j.snb.2016.04.062

Wang L, Hu C, Shao L (2017) The antimicrobial activity of nanoparticles: present situation and prospects for the future. Int J Nanomedicine 12:1227–1249. https://doi.org/10.2147/IJN.S121956

Wang J, Sui L, Huang J, Miao L, Nie Y, Wang K, Yang Z, Huang Q, Gong X, Nan Y, Ai K (2021) MoS2-based nanocomposites for cancer diagnosis and therapy. Bioact Mater 6(11):4209–4242. https://doi.org/10.1016/j.bioactmat.2021.04.021

Wang J, Liu M, Zhang X, Wang X, Xiong M, Luo D (2024a) Stimuli-responsive linkers and their application in molecular imaging. Exploration (Beijing) 4(4):20230027. https://doi.org/10.1002/EXP.20230027

Wang K, Yu D, Liang X, Lu W, Jiang X, Tashpulatov K, Zeng J, Wen C-Y (2024b) Janus Fe3O4-Au@Pt nanozymes based lateral flow assay for enhanced-sensitive colorimetric detection of influenza A virus. Microchem J 204:111104. https://doi.org/10.1016/j.microc.2024.111104

Warjurkar K, Panda S, Sharma V (2023) Red emissive carbon dots: a promising next-generation material with intracellular applicability. J Mater Chem B 11(37):8848–8865. https://doi.org/10.1039/D3TB01378B

Warjurkar K, Patyal R, Sharma V (2025) Multifunctional Tradescantia Pallida derived copper–nitrogen codoped green carbon dots as nanozyme, dual sensor, and fluorescent ink for anticounterfeiting and smart textiles. ACS Appl Bio Mater 8(6):4779–4790. https://doi.org/10.1021/acsabm.5c00150

Wieszczycka K, Staszak K, Woźniak-Budych MJ, Litowczenko J, Maciejewska BM, Jurga S (2021) Surface functionalization – the way for advanced applications of smart materials. Coord Chem Rev 436:213846. https://doi.org/10.1016/j.ccr.2021.213846

Wu L, Li M, Zhang M, Yan M, Ge S, Yu J (2013) Ultrasensitive electrochemiluminescence immunosensor for tumor marker detection based on nanoporous sliver@carbon dots as labels. Sens Actuators B Chem 186:761–767. https://doi.org/10.1016/j.snb.2013.06.092

Xia Y, Xu C, Zhang X, Ning P, Wang Z, Tian J, Chen X (2019) Liposome-based probes for molecular imaging: from basic research to the bedside. Nanoscale 11(13):5822–5838. https://doi.org/10.1039/C9NR00207C

Xing E, Chen H, Xin X, Cui H, Dou Y, Song S (2025) Recent advances in smart phone-based biosensors for various applications. Chemosensors 13(7):221. https://doi.org/10.3390/chemosensors13070221

Xu J, Huang B-B, Lai C-M, Lu Y-S, Shao J-W (2024a) Advancements in the synthesis of carbon dots and their application in biomedicine. J Photochem Photobiol B Biol 255:112920. https://doi.org/10.1016/j.jphotobiol.2024.112920

Xu Z, Hao Y, Luo A, Jiang Y (2024b) Technologies and applications in wireless biosensors for real-time health monitoring. Med-X 2(1):24. https://doi.org/10.1007/s44258-024-00041-3

Yan D, Qin Y, Yan S, Sun P, Wang Y, Wang D, Tang BZ (2023) Near-infrared emissive AIE nanoparticles for biomedical applications: from the perspective of different nanocarriers. Particuology 74:103–118. https://doi.org/10.1016/j.partic.2022.06.001

Yao X, Qi C, Sun C, Huo F, Jiang X (2023) Poly(ethylene glycol) alternatives in biomedical applications. Nano Today 48:101738. https://doi.org/10.1016/j.nantod.2022.101738

Yaqoob AA, Ahmad H, Parveen T, Ahmad A, Oves M, Ismail IMI, Qari HA, Umar K, Mohamad Ibrahim MN (2020) Recent advances in metal decorated nanomaterials and their various biological applications: a review. Front Chem 8:341. https://doi.org/10.3389/fchem.2020.00341

Yaraki MT, Zahed Nasab S, Zare I, Dahri M, Moein Sadeghi M, Koohi M, Tan YN (2022) Biomimetic metallic nanostructures for biomedical applications, catalysis, and beyond. Ind Eng Chem Res 61(22):7547–7593. https://doi.org/10.1021/acs.iecr.2c00285

Yi R, Zhang Z, Liu C, Qi Z (2020) Gold-silver alloy film based surface plasmon resonance sensor for biomarker detection. Mater Sci Eng C 116:111126. https://doi.org/10.1016/j.msec.2020.111126

Zhang S, Lin L, Huang X, Lu Y-G, Zheng D-L, Feng Y (2022a) Antimicrobial properties of metal nanoparticles and their oxide materials and their applications in oral biology. J Nanomater 2022(1):2063265. https://doi.org/10.1155/2022/2063265

Zhang D, Liu L, Wang J, Zhang H, Zhang Z, Xing G, Wang X, Liu M (2022b) Drug-loaded PEG-PLGA nanoparticles for cancer treatment. Front Pharmacol 13. https://doi.org/10.3389/fphar.2022.990505

Zhou Y, Tao L, Qiu J, Xu J, Yang X, Zhang Y, Tian X, Guan X, Cen X, Zhao Y (2024) Tumor biomarkers for diagnosis, prognosis and targeted therapy. Signal Transduct Target Ther 9(1):132. https://doi.org/10.1038/s41392-024-01823-2

Zhu C, Wang X (2025) Nanomaterial ZnO synthesis and its photocatalytic applications: a review. Nanomaterials 15(9):682. https://doi.org/10.3390/nano15090682

Integrated Microfluidics-Based Sensing Chip for Biomedical Applications

6

Sreekant Damodara and Krishna Jangid

Abstract

Microfluidics has found widespread application in the development of biosensors due to the numerous advantages gained from miniaturization and the numerous techniques available to leverage these advantages to improve biosensing capabilities. This chapter first describes these advantages broadly, including reduction in sample volume, advantages gained from scaling down, multiplexing, cost reduction, enhanced mass transport, accelerated kinetics, and additional preconcentration possibilities. Then, the various methods of fluid manipulation are described with examples of their commercialized applications. These methods include pneumatic microfluidics, centrifugal microfluidics, capillary microfluidics, lateral flow tests, paper/textile/thread microfluidics, digital Electrowetting-on-Dielectric (EWOD)-based microfluidics, and others. Following this, various modalities of biosensors, including electrochemical, optical, magnetic, and emerging technologies, are described, along with their integration into microfluidic devices, accompanied by examples of commercial biosensors. Finally, a short discussion on the challenges with integrating microfluidics with biosensors and prospective applications, and a perspective on microfluidic biosensors is presented.

Keywords

Microfluidics · Paper · Textile · Electrowetting · Biosensors

S. Damodara
Verv Technologies, Sudbury, ON, Canada

K. Jangid (✉)
Volta Labs Inc., Boston, MA, USA

V. Patel et al. (eds.), *Biosensor Technology in Translating Novel Materials into Practical Devices*, https://doi.org/10.1007/978-981-95-5519-2_6

Microfluidics is the manipulation and control of microvolumes of fluids in channels with at least one of the characteristic dimensions being on the order of a few hundred micrometers or smaller. The reduction of volume compared to conventional fluidics and the resultant increase in relative surface area of the fluid result in several advantages for their use in biosensors and other applications. In addition, the reduction in size improves portability of the final device and allows deployment of the resultant biosensors in areas that would be challenging with traditional techniques (Olanrewaju et al. 2018). As a result, microfluidics has often been suggested in the development of biosensors that meet WHO's "ASSURED" (Bhardwaj et al. 2022) (Affordable, Sensitive, Specific, User-friendly, Rapid and robust, Equipment-free, and Delivered) and more recently, "REASSURED" (Land et al. 2019) criteria for the development of diagnostic biosensors for resource-limited locations.

Microfluidics is a multidisciplinary technology that utilizes, links, and leverages advancements in several different fields of research, including biochemistry, engineering, physics, nanotechnology, and electronics, among others (Luka et al. 2015), which lead to rapid advancements in design and a reduction in cost.

6.1 Advantages of miniaturization

The advantages of miniaturization in microfluidics can broadly be summarized as below.

6.1.1 Reduction in Sample Volume

Microfluidic biosensors work with sample and reagent volumes on the order of a few hundred microliters or below in comparison to conventional biosensors that operate on the order of a few milliliters or above. The reduction in sample volume presents advantages not just in the raw reduction of reagents required for analysis but also in the ability to store and dispense reagents in automated aliquots within the device, multiplexed analysis, and increased throughput due to faster reaction times that enable the use of microfluidics for the development of an integrated assay design.

6.1.2 Scaling

The reduction in fluid volume in microfluidic environments results in changes to the physical behaviour of fluids as the forces responsible for fluid behavior respond differently to the reduction in scale. As microfluidic devices shrink, the forces that scale by volume, such as gravity and inertia, decrease faster than forces that scale by surface area (such as electrostatic forces) and length (capillary force). This is applied in microfluidic device fabrication by using non-conventional methods for moving fluids within the system. These trends are called scaling laws and are represented using the characteristic length scale of the device (L). Therefore, forces that scale

Table 6.1 Dimensionless numbers

Dimensionless number	Formula	Description
Reynolds number	$\rho UL/\eta$	Inertial effects/viscous effects
Peclet number	UL/D	Convection/diffusion
Capillary number	$\eta U/\gamma$	Viscous effects/interfacial effects
Knudsen number	β/L	Slip length/characteristic length

w.r.t the volume of the device are represented by *L*3, while those that scale by surface area are represented as *L*2 and so forth. Conventional pressure-based systems scale poorly when miniaturized, as represented by the Euler number that compares pressure to inertial forces.

$$\text{Eu} = \text{Pressure} / \text{Inertia} = \Delta P.L^2 \; / \; \rho.U^2.L^2$$

At constant velocity, Eu scales as L^{-1} and at constant pressure head, Eu scales as L^{-2}. This implies that as the device is scaled down, a larger pressure gradient is necessary to drive flow, making it a less efficient method to drive fluid movement in microfluidic flows. In contrast, other forces that scale well, such as capillary forces and Coulomb forces, are used more often in microfluidic flows. A list of commonly used dimensional numbers is shown below (Table 6.1).

When scaled down for microfluidics, the Reynolds number decreases greatly as viscous forces dominate, meaning flow is highly laminar, and inducing turbulence for mixing in microfluidics is challenging. Reynolds numbers for common microfluidic devices with water as a working fluid and a flow rate of 1 μm/s^{-1} cm s^{-1} in channels with a radius of 1–100 μm result in a Reynolds number on the order of ~10^{-6} and 10.

In the absence of turbulence due to the low Reynolds number, the Peclet number is used to characterize the relative effects of convection and diffusion in microfluidic flows. Most typically represented by a T junction with fluid inlets on either side merging into a central inlet. The Peclet number defines the length of the channel necessary for mixing between the two streams in terms of the width of the channel. Capillary number is used to represent the relative impact of capillary force when competing with viscous forces, such as when a liquid enters a hydrophilic capillary or is on a surface where a drop saddles areas with different hydrophilicities. A low capillary number in these cases indicates that surface tension dominates viscous forces and the liquid moves rapidly into the capillary or onto the hydrophilic side of the surface. Conversely, a high capillary number would indicate slower entry and slow or no movement of the liquid on the surface. Similar observations can be made for the other dimensionless numbers, which can be read about in the paper by Squires and Quake (2005).

6.1.3 Multiplexing

Multiplexing is the measurement of multiple analytes with a single sample. Microfluidics is primed for applications that require multiplexing due to its ability to integrate complete assays in a single platform, the limited use of reagents, and the numerous ways available for sample transport and control; as a result of which numerous "lab-on-a-chip" (LOC) platforms have been developed using microfluidics. Multiplexing in microfluidics is of particular importance in the development of clinical diagnostic assays as it can help with differential diagnosis and screening of disease biomarkers on a single panel instead of requiring multiple individual tests (Araz et al. 2013).

6.1.4 Cost

Microfluidics was first developed through the use of silicon and glass microfabrication (Nge et al. 2013) techniques implemented for fluid control, and was expensive due to the high cost of photolithography. Over time, advances in microfluidics led to the development of soft lithography, where soft polymers such as poly dimethyl siloxane (PDMS) were cast in molds made from conventional methods to reduce the cost of fabrication in prototyping devices. Eventually, conventional mass fabrication techniques were integrated into microfluidic fabrication and methods such as injection molding of PMMA (Yu et al. 2002), cyclic olefin copolymer (COC), cyclic olefin polymer (COP), and other polymeric materials (Agha et al. 2022) were used to fabricate microfluidic devices. This reduced the cost of fabrication of microfluidic devices compared to the first generation of glass and silicon microfluidic devices. In addition to these, paper microfluidic devices first suggested by Martinez et al. (2007a) as a low cost medium for microfluidic devices in the form of a microfluidic paper-based analytical device (μPAD) led to the development of a number of low cost microfluidic devices using paper and textile/fabric as a medium for controlling microfluidic flows with over a thousand publications being released between 2007 and 2014 (Cate et al. 2015). These devices further reduced the cost of microfluidic devices and enhanced their appeal for application that necessitated portability and lowered fabrication cost.

Beyond the generalized benefits of microfluidic systems in fluid handling, the distinctive characteristics inherent to microfluidic environments impart profound advantages that directly enhance the performance, sensitivity, and functional attributes of biosensors. These specific advantages include:

6.1.5 Enhanced Mass Transport and Accelerated Reaction Kinetics

Microfluidic devices work with sample volumes from microliters to nanoliters (Dittrich et al. 2006; Zhang et al. 2019). The inherent scaling of microfluidics results in high surface-to-volume ratios, enabling precise control of mass transfer (Fig. 6.1).

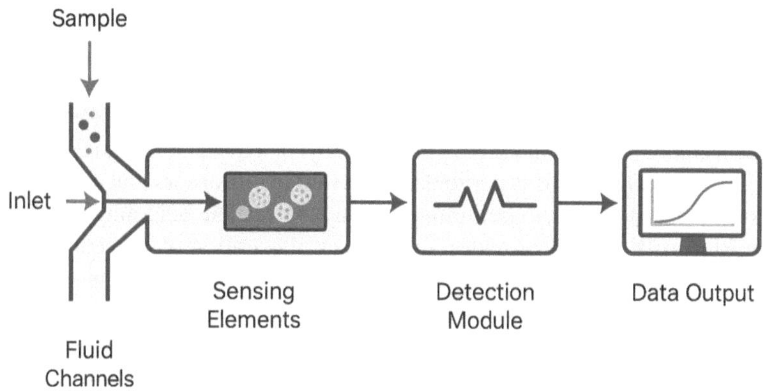

Fig. 6.1 General schematic of a microfluidic biosensing system

Subsequently, it requires less reagent and sample volume, which ensures cost-effectiveness and enhances the sensor's portability (Seymour et al. 2017). Moreover, as discussed in the next section, the small size of microfluidic channels facilitates the efficient transport of microvolumes of target analytes across the active surface area of the biosensor, resulting in accelerated transport and enhanced binding kinetics, which amplify the detectable signal (Erickson and Li 2004; Sackmann et al. 2014). In resource-limited or point-of-care (POC) settings, rapid detection is crucial for both rapid diagnostic applications and real-time biological monitoring. Moreover, being able to perform diagnostics with minimal sample input is vital for accessibility, speed, and deployment outside traditional laboratory environments (Chin et al. 2011).

One prominent example is the Abbott ID NOW™ device, whose platform integrates isothermal nucleic acid amplification chemistry in a self-contained microfluidic cartridge for qualitative molecular results in under 15 min (Iglesias-Ussel Maria et al. 2025). Designed for POC use, it requires only a nasal or throat swab. With automated sample lysis and accelerated nucleic acid amplification from a reduction in reaction volume, leading to faster and more cost-effective target detection in point-of-care (POC) settings. Due to its compact size and minimal cold chain requirements, the device is particularly effective for urgent care clinics, emergency departments, and remote areas. The ID NOW system shows how microfluidics can enable decentralized testing. The commercialization of this platform during the COVID-19 pandemic demonstrated the importance of microfluidic point-of-care (POC) diagnostics in managing public health responses where lab infrastructure is limited (Nguyen et al. 2020).

6.1.6 Mass Transport and Kinetics

The small size of microfluidic channels facilitates the efficient transport of microvolumes of target analytes across the active surface area of the biosensor, resulting from reduced analyte diffusion distances. In conventional systems, the mass transport of the analyte to the sensor surface influences the rate-limiting step, particularly for analytes of low concentration (Jangid et al. 2022a). Conversely, a microfluidics system provides higher control over both diffusion and convective flow, resulting in an enhancement of reaction kinetics and, thereby, in a detectable signal (Stone et al. 2004; Tabeling 2023). This is particularly relevant to biosensors that employ surface reactions, such as affinity-based immunoassays or nucleic acid amplification. The Cytiva Biacore™ system provides a prominent illustration of this enhanced mass transport for affinity-based immunoassays (Abdiche et al. 2009). Through its integrated microfluidic design of the flow cells for its Surface Plasmon Resonance (SPR) technology, analytes are introduced into narrow channels next to the sensor chip with immobilized molecules. The reduced diffusion distance of the analytes and continuous solution replenishment via precise laminar flow facilitate their faster transport to the chip surface, ensuring the prevention of analyte-depleted boundary layers. Consequently, it enables the Cytiva Biacore™ system to provide accurate real-time determination of kinetic parameters for comprehensive immunoassay characterization (Rich and Myszka 2001).

6.1.7 Preconcentration Capabilities

The biosensor sensitivity is influenced by its capability to detect analytes at low concentrations (Jangid et al. 2021, 2022b). Enabling preconcentration of analytes in the biosensor system enhances its analytical sensitivity and thereby detection capability at significantly lower concentrations. Microfluidics provides passive and active preconcentration techniques to enrich analytes, as illustrated in Fig. 6.2. Passive preconcentration in microfluidics utilizes the inherent geometry of the channel to concentrate target analytes near the sensing surface, eliminating the need for external energy fields or complex instrumentation (Chen et al. 2011). These methods are driven by fluid dynamics and diffusion in the microscale. Key structural elements, including narrow constrictions, serpentine paths, and dead-end chambers, are engineered to manipulate the flow (Stroock et al. 2002). Narrow constrictions slow down the flow, increasing the analyte residence time in specific areas. Serpentine channels lengthen the path and promote transverse diffusion by repeatedly changing the flow direction, which mixes and pushes the target molecules toward the sensor interface (Ahmed et al. 2009). Dead-end chambers or recessed pockets are low-flow or stagnant areas where analytes can be temporarily trapped or accumulate due to reduced convective washout (Liu et al. 2002). The local enrichment of analytes near the detection zones boosts the signal-to-noise ratio and overall sensitivity. Importantly, these designs do not require pumps, electric fields, or magnetic forces, making them ideal for portable, low-cost diagnostic devices where power consumption, footprint, and robustness are crucial (Kaigala et al. 2012). Hence, passive preconcentration is an excellent strategy for commercial microfluidic biosensors for point-of-care testing, environmental monitoring, and resource-limited settings (Martinez et al. 2007b).

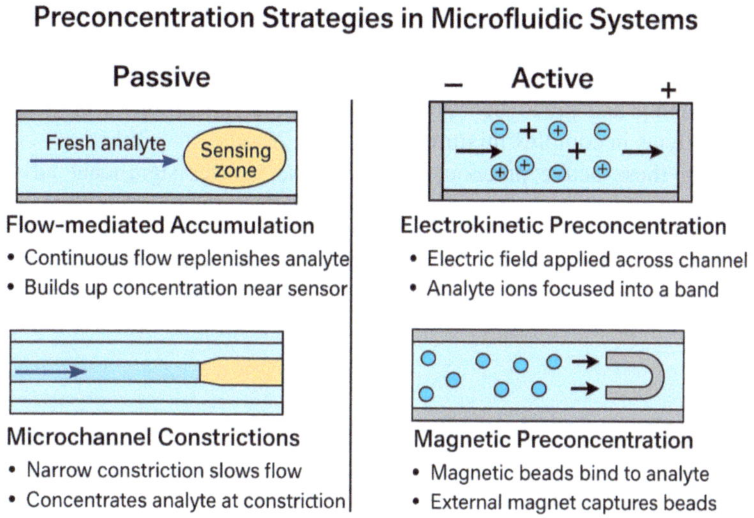

Fig. 6.2 Integrated preconcentration strategies in microfluidic biosensing, including passive and active preconcentration methods. Passive strategies include flow-mediated accumulation and microchannel constrictions, which enrich analytes through geometric or hydrodynamic control. Active approaches leverage electrokinetic gradients or magnetic fields to focus and isolate analytes upstream of the detection zone

Conversely, active preconcentration techniques in microfluidic systems use externally applied fields, including electric, magnetic, or dielectrophoretic forces, to precisely manipulate and enrich analytes in microscale environments (Pethig 2010). These are particularly effective for charged or polarizable biomolecules and are increasingly being integrated into advanced diagnostic platforms due to their enhanced detection sensitivity and analytical throughput. Among these, electrokinetic methods, such as isotachophoresis (ITP), use electric fields to create dynamic interfaces between leading and trailing electrolytes (Gascoyne and Vykoukal 2002). Charged analytes migrate and concentrate sharply at the boundary of these zones and form very narrow bands. This focused migration allows for efficient delivery of preconcentrated analytes to downstream sensing elements. ITP in microfluidic channels has been demonstrated for pathogen detection (Nelson and Patten 2009), so it is relevant for both clinical diagnostics and environmental monitoring. Magnetic preconcentration uses magnetic beads conjugated to specific antibodies that bind to target analytes. Once captured, the analyte-bead complexes can be manipulated and localized near sensor surfaces using externally applied magnetic fields (Basu 2013). This is particularly useful for isolating low-abundance analytes from large volumes or complex biological samples. Commercial implementations include Thermo Fisher's Pathatrix®, which recirculates food samples over antibody-coated magnetic beads to capture pathogens, and Siemens' Atellica VTLi (Magnotech), a point-of-care platform that utilizes magnetically actuated nanoparticles for the rapid detection of cardiac biomarkers, such as troponin (Aubret 2023; Fedio et al. 2011).

Dielectrophoresis (DEP) is another active technique that uses non-uniform electric fields to induce differential motion in particles based on their dielectric properties (Green et al. 2000). DEP allows for label-free, frequency-tunable control over particle positioning and preconcentration, enabling the separation or enrichment of specific analytes in complex mixtures (Kim et al. 2018).

Together, these active preconcentration methods offer significant advantages over passive methods, including increased sensitivity, reduced assay time, and precise spatial control of target species. Therefore, their integration into lab-on-a-chip and point-of-care diagnostic systems enables improved sample enrichment and biosensor performance without compromising the compact and user-friendly system designs.

6.2 Methods for Fluid Manipulation

The impact of scaling laws and the need for reduction in costs and higher throughput led to the development of several methods for controlling fluid movement in microfluidic biosensors that are not possible for conventional biosensors. A few of these are described in Table 6.2 with examples of commercial devices.

Table 6.2 Methods of fluid manipulation

Method	Pros	Cons
Pneumatic microfluidics	Established methods of flow control based on macroscale devices Wide range of viable materials allows the use of injection molding to reduce cost	Scales poorly to smaller volumes Requires pumps to drive fluid flow
Centrifugal microfluidics	Wide range of forces and flow control methods viable	Complex channel geometry Requires a single large rotor in the base station
Capillary microfluidics	Scale well for miniaturization Lower cost with modern fabrication methods Passive, can be run without external actuation	Limited materials due to requirements of hydrophilicity/hydrophobicity
Lateral flow tests	Simple construction Low-cost fabrication Passive, can be run without external actuation	Limited types of tests viable Mostly limited to qualitative and semi-quantitative tests with recent forays into quantitative tests
Paper/textile/thread microfluidics	Low cost of fabrication More viable tests than with lateral flow Passive, can be run without external actuation	More complex than lateral flow Challenging environment for quantitative measurement
Digital microfluidics (EWOD)	Discrete droplet control enables a wide range of tests Fully electronic control reduces the number of moving parts Enables dynamic reconfiguration of the testing protocol without changing the geometry of the device	Complex fabrication of both chips and base station

6.2.1 Pneumatic Microfluidic Device

While pneumatic pressure scales poorly down to microfluidic scales, it is still used in the development of microfluidic devices due to its well-developed fluid control techniques. While using external manual pumps for microfluidic devices would make the overall device unwieldy, miniaturized, program-controlled pumps integrated into a base station have been used to control movement in disposable cartridges. Using this format for pneumatic actuation of fluids, solenoid valves for controlling fluid pathways, and blisters for controlled dispense of stored reagent, a microfluidic device for point of care applications was developed by Binx Biomedical (Ben Arlett and Tom Edwards 2022). A figure from their patent is shown in Fig. 6.3 and shows the various layers used for implementing a cartridge with pneumatic actuation, including the blister subassembly for reagent storage is 112, the pneumatic control layer 114, the fluid transport layer 115, among others.

Due to the pneumatic actuation being less dependent on surface properties of the cartridge, a wide array of materials could potentially be used with conventional mass fabrication techniques like injection molding to manufacture pneumatic microfluidic devices at scale at the cost of complexity in the base station due to the need for pumps and valves for flow control.

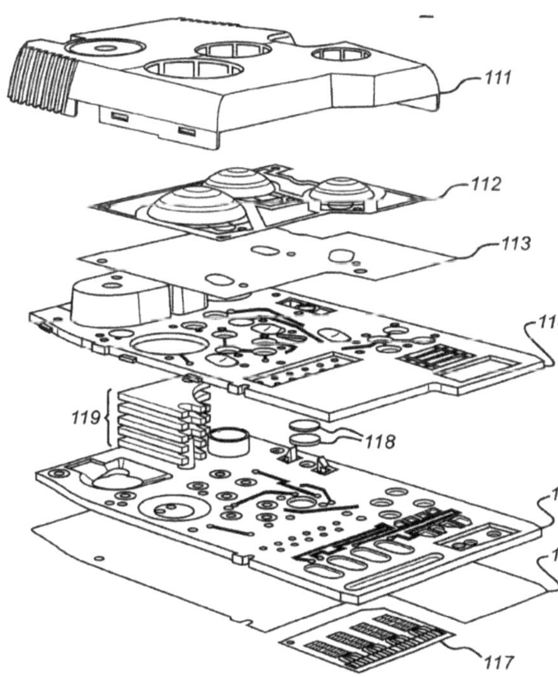

Fig. 6.3 The different layers used in the making of pneumatic microfluidic chip (Ben Arlett, Bristol (GB); Tom Edwards, Salisbury (GB), 2022)

6.2.2 Centrifugal Microfluidics

Centrifugal microfluidics simplifies the need for multiple pumps that are needed in pneumatic microfluidic devices and instead uses centrifugal forces generated on a disc-shaped substrate to move fluids within patterned channels. This reduces the complexity of the base station to one single large motor to drive fluid flow in the cartridge. The device uses a combination of centrifugal, Coriolis, Euler, capillary, and viscous forces to control fluid movement through the pathways to enable sample mixing, preparation, and sensing. They have found widespread use in point of care applications and have been accepted as gold standard tests in these applications, with devices such as Piccolo Xpress (2025) from Abbott offering a full complement of CLIA-waived blood chemistry tests, and are currently used in a variety of settings, both inpatient and outpatient, including urgent care clinics in the United States. There is also continued development in this space by companies such as Vital Biosciences which has raised a capital of $48 million USD (Sarah 2023) from venture capital firms in Silicon Valley, based on their centrifugal microfluidic device that is integrated with computer vision and fluorescence imaging.

Figure 6.4 shows a cross section of a section of the centrifugal microfluidic cassette patented by Vital Biosciences (Barreiros et al. 2024) and shows the reagent

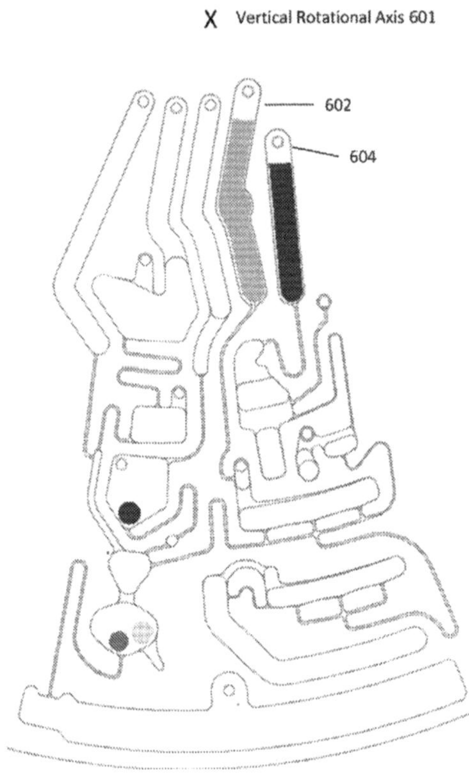

Fig. 6.4 Cross section of the section of a centrifugal microfluidic cassette

storage chambers and complexity of pathways that can be utilized using centrifugal microfluidics. A large number of valving techniques are viable in centrifugal microfluidics due to the number of forces that can be leveraged for fluid control (Peshin et al. 2022). They can be broadly classified as active, hybrid, and passive valves. The active valves use an external stimulus to initiate the valving action, such as pH-controlled hydrogel valves that respond to changes in the pH of the solution, thermally actuated membrane valves that respond to the temperature of the solution, Laser packs that (Shin et al. 2022) release liquid due to a laser shining on it, and so on. These valves respond quickly to changes in the environment, but add complexity to the overall system due to the need for external stimulating systems. Passive valves do not require external systems for actuation and actuate based on spin speed, channel dimensions, channel surface characteristics, and similar innate features of the fluid pathways. Some examples of this are siphon valves, Coriolis force microvalves, and hydrophobic microvalves, among others. They have slower response times compared to their active counterparts (Peshin et al. 2022).

6.2.3 Capillary Microfluidics

Capillary forces in microfluidic channels are controlled by the interplay between the surface energy of the liquid, the surface energy of the interacting material surface, and its geometry. As a result of the scaling laws described earlier, these forces scale extremely well when miniaturized, and due to their "passive" nature, that can result in automated movement with no external input, they are highly sought after for low-cost, autonomous microfluidic biosensors. In particular, this section focuses on open microcondiuts carved in a material like glass, silicon, polymers, or other materials that enable capillary forces as a result of the interaction between the walls of the conduit and the working fluid.

When a hydrophilic capillary is placed horizontally in contact with a liquid, the extent to which it is filled can be described using the Washburn equation (Washburn 1921).

$$L = \sqrt{\gamma r t \cos(\phi) / 2\eta}$$

where γ is the surface tension of the fluid, r is the radius of the capillary, t is the time since the liquid was introduced, ϕ is the contact angle between the fluid and the walls of the capillary, and η is the dynamic viscosity of the fluid. The rate of liquid entering the capillary slows over time in uniformly sized capillaries and increases with a decrease in the diameter of the capillary.

Several techniques have been developed to control movement in capillaries, including capillary pumps to avoid the reduction in flow rate over time. This was done to ensure consistent filling times and was done by narrowing the air vent, which adds a new regime of flow dominated by the gas viscosity and is characterized by a constant flow rate (Guo et al. 2016). In addition, micro-structures to control flow direction, stop valves (Glière and Delattre 2006) and timing valves using hydrophobic surfaces (McNeely et al. 1999), integration with electrostatic and electrochemical forces for finer flow regulation, leveraging Marangoni forces for flow control (Damodara et al. 2021a) among others. Numerous methods for flow control have been designed over time for flow reservoirs, reaction chambers, flow resistors, capillary pumps, filling front guides, stop valves, capillary trigger valves, capillary retention valves, capillary burst valves, and delay valves that are described in more detail by (Olanrewaju et al. 2018).

The materials used for capillary microfluidics are emblematic of the field of microfluidics at large, changing from Silicon and glass photolithography-based devices to mass-fabricated polymer-based and recently devices made from patterned laser-cut plastic sheets/tapes. Each of these materials and fabrication techniques presents their unique advantages, such as high dimensional accuracy (photo-lithography), scalability (injection molding), or rapid prototyping (laser cut plastic, 3d printing) that make them viable in different scenarios. A detailed description of the advancements in capillary microfluidics and the materials used can be obtained from a review by Olanrewaju et al. (2018), a summarization of which is provided in Fig. 6.5.

Capillary microfluidic biosensors have found great success in the commercial space with implementations by a range of companies, including 1drop Diagnostics, Mfluidx, among others, and can be custom-ordered and available from microfluidic chip shops such as Dolomite Microfluidics, Micronit, and others. Due to the wide acceptance, high reliability, and relative lack of reliance on gravity of capillary microfluidics, 1Drop Diagnostics was even able to develop a biosensor for testing on the International Space Station (ISS) (Patrick 2020) and currently has numerous tests available for purchase.

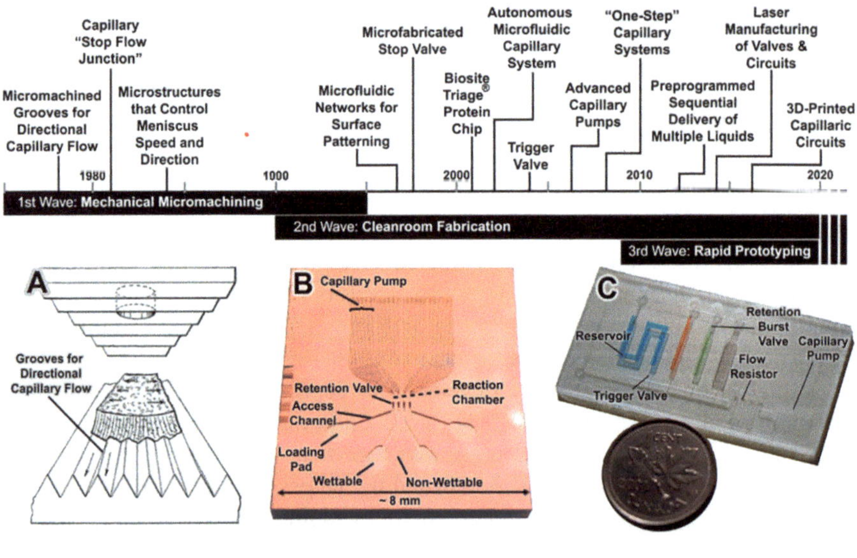

Fig. 6.5 Advances in capillary microfluidics

6.2.4 Lateral Flow Tests

Lateral flow tests are immunochromatographic tests that use capillary forces in a porous membrane to drive fluid unidirectionally through predeposited reagents for a no-wash immunoassay (Di Nardo et al. 2021). Qualitative lateral flow tests are widely used microfluidic devices that successfully meet the "ASSURED" criteria and are popularized for home testing and can be most recognized in their applications as pregnancy tests and for at-home COVID-19 testing. Their popularity stems from their simple fabrication, resultant low cost, and no requirement for equipment or technical expertise, resulting in improved usability in resource-limited areas.

The porous membrane used in lateral flow tests ranges from cellulose, to nitrocellulose, glass fiber membranes, and synthetic proprietary fibers that minimally interact with the sample solution to reduce interference. Different media are chosen based on the role they perform within the device. For example, a sampling pad may be used to draw liquid into the device rapidly, a wicking pad may be used to drive faster movement of fluid through the lateral flow strip. These membranes are then encased in a housing that makes it easy for a consumer to identify the qualitative result. The porous membrane can currently be easily purchased from a range of suppliers, including Cytiva, Radetec Diagnostic, and Porex, among others, which enables companies to quickly prototype and test new biosensors using lateral flow. Lateral flow assays have been developed for clinical, food safety, veterinary, environmental, agricultural, industrial forensic applications, among others (Di Nardo et al. 2021).

Quantitative lateral flow is a developing field that uses external readers to analyze the intensity of the signal generated by the lateral flow strip. This was originally led by the development of colorimetric sensors, often using smartphone cameras, but have since diversified through the addition of different methods of detection, including fluorescence, chemiluminescence. Colorimetric detection, which dominated detection techniques and was present in 93.7% of publications in 2010, dropped to 78.1% of publications in 2019 (Di Nardo et al. 2021). Companies, such as Bloom Diagnostics have released commercially available fluorescent quantitative lateral flow test kits for biomarkers in blood Figure 6.6. Figure 6.6a shows the quantitative lateral flow strip with its various components, including sampling pad (15), conjugate pad (162), and wicking pad (161) with the reagents (13, 14) appropriately placed as patented by Bloom diagnostics. Figure 6.6b shows the lateral flow strip illustrated within a schematic of their measurement device that uses cameras (22, 23) for obtaining a quantitative measurement.

6.2.5 Paper/Textile/Thread Microfluidics

Paper microfluidic devices also use capillary forces in a porous medium to drive fluid flow, but consist of patterned geometries and have more complicated flow paths compared to lateral flow assays. As a result, they enable a much wider range

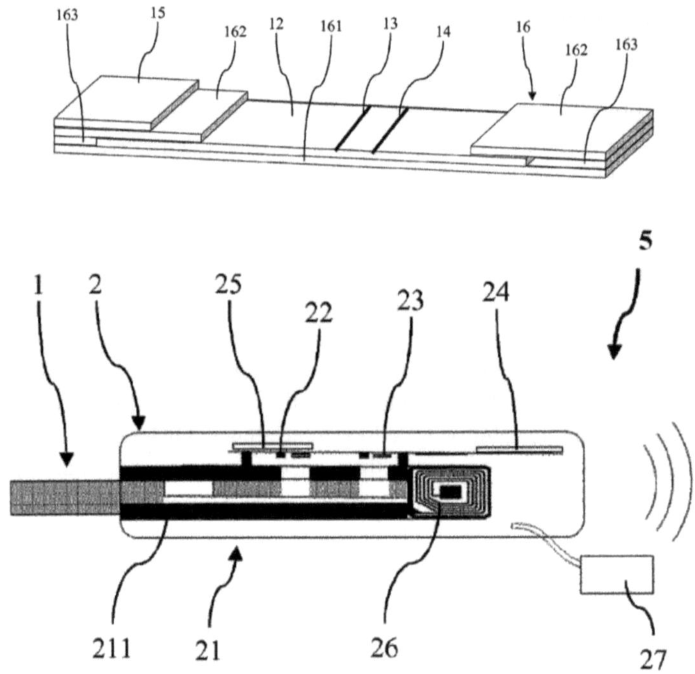

Fig. 6.6 Lateral flow assays schematics as patented by Bloom Diagnostics (Patent US11740181B2)

of tests at the cost of higher complexity. Textile microfluidics uses threads in place of a 2D paper-based porous medium and presents the advantages of having a wider range of materials, including cotton, rayon, hemp, nylon, polyester, wool, acrylic, and natural silk, among others (Nilghaz et al. 2013). As a result of this, they possess better wet strength than paper microfluidic devices but face additional challenges in patterning and modeling fluid physics within the fabric that are still being studied (Ballerini et al. 2011). Thread microfluidics uses individual threads as channels for fluid flow.

Flow within paper microfluidic devices follows a slightly modified version of the Washburn equation in 1 dimension when the capillary diameter is accurately estimated (Masoodi and Pillai 2010). The volumetric flow rate through porous media can also be described using Darcy's law, which states that

$$Q = k.A.\Delta P / \mu L$$

where Q is the volumetric flow rate, k is the permeability of the porous media, A is the cross-sectional area, ΔP is the pressure drop, L is the distance over which the pressure drop is computed, and μ is the dynamic viscosity of the fluid. Darcy's law enables simulation and prediction of 2D and 3D wicking compared to the Washburn equation, which is limited to 1D wicking (Masoodi and Pillai 2010).

6.2.5.1 Fabrication

Patterning of paper microfluidic devices can be done in a number of ways, some of which are shown in Fig. 6.7 (Cate et al. 2015). These methods generate channels by establishing hydrophobic barriers that force liquids to wick in specific directions. Of the methods shown, the most commonly used method for patterning paper microfluidic devices uses a wax printer to print the channel shape on the surface of the paper which is then baked to allow the pattern to penetrate through the thickness of the paper, establishing hydrophilic capillary channels with a height dependent on the thickness of the paper, and width controlled by the resolution of the printer and wicking rate of wax (Martinez et al. 2007b). Three dimensional channels could then be made by folding a patterned 2D paper with double sided tape as an intermediary and holes allowing passage of fluid between vertically separated layers (Martinez et al. 2010). Alternate methods for making 3D paper microfluidic devices include the use of origami to fold a patterned 2D paper (Ding et al. 2016) and 3D printing using a digital light processing-based 3D printer to pattern within a thick paper embedded in the resin and washing off the excess resin (Park et al. 2018). The use of wax printer improved the reproducibility of paper microfluidic devices compared to more manual methods like stamping without requiring expensive photolithographic techniques and led to a spurt in development of micro paper-based

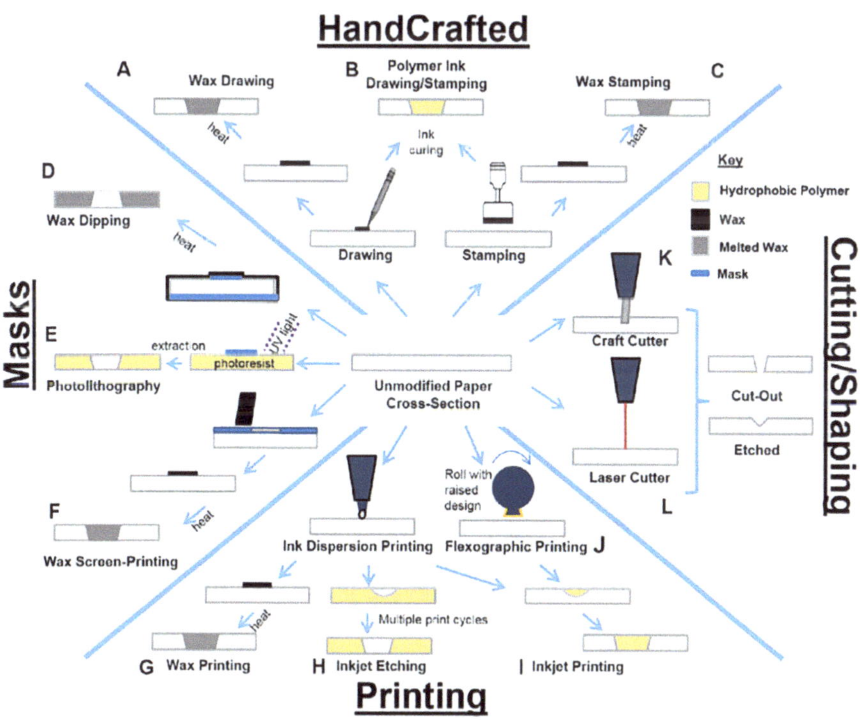

Fig. 6.7 Summary of methods of patterning paper microfluidic devices

analytical devices (μPADs). Reagents were dropped and dried within specific chambers of the 2D and 3D paper microfluidic devices to enable complex assays. Textile microfluidics show similar characteristics to paper microfluidic devices and can use several of the fluid control methods described above with a wider range of materials that allow weaving hydrophilic and hydrophobic threads to be woven together to create channels (Bhandari et al. 2011). Thread/textile devices have also been frequently integrated with a paper microfluidic device to leverage the advantages of both (Dossi et al. 2018; Neris et al. 2019; Zhou et al. 2012). Similarly, threads have been integrated with PDMS (Damodara et al. 2021b) and plastic laminated (Tomimuro et al. 2020) microfluidic devices. A summary of some of the recent advances in thread/textile microfluidic devices can be found in the reviews by Farajikhah et al. (2019) and Mostafalu et al. (2016).

6.2.5.2 Flow Control

Fluid is controlled within paper microfluidic devices using geometric, mechanical, or chemical means. Geometric flow control is based on altering the geometry of the channels to control flow. For example, using longer flow paths for delaying samples in some channels compared to others, varying the width of the channels (Eriksson et al. 2019) laminating the paper microfluidic device with hydrophilic plastic to increase flow rate (Channon et al. 2018) and semi-filled wax channels were used to control flow rate through channels (Strong et al. 2019). Chemical methods use various hydrophilic, hydrophobic, dissolvable, or surfactant molecules to control fluid flow. For example, a surfactant on one side of a hydrophobic barrier was used to create a one-directional fluid valve (Chen et al. 2012) and dissolvable sugar bridges were used to make a delayed stop valve that depends on the dissolution time of the sugar (Houghtaling et al. 2013). Mechanical methods use the physical movement of components on the μPAD to control fluid flow, such as by using the deformation of paper to enable or disable flow paths (Kong et al. 2017). These and several other methods for flow control can be found described in more detail by Lim et al. (2019).

Flow control in thread microfluidics using one dimensional movement across the thread was achieved using threads held in tension and knots being used for mixing and flow control. Binary switches were made by coating a section of thread with a hydrophobic coating and using a sliding knot to engage or disengage from the wetted portion of that thread. This was also used to select between two sample sources. The threads were woven into a plastic backing for rigidity and another form of suggested on/off switch was using a pull tab to allow a wetted thread to contact a previously blocked thread segment on pulling of the tab (Masoodi and Pillai 2010). The twists per inch of the strands within a thread can also be modulated to change the porosity of the thread and was used for separating RBCs from blood (Ulum et al. 2016; Yazdani et al. 2015). Threads were also integrated with metallic fibers for electrophoretic protein separation (Tanya et al. 2015).

Commercial fabric microfluidic devices were developed by companies such as Achira Labs, which used woven silk microfluidic devices for biomarker sensing and are targeted at low-cost personal healthcare in resource-poor locations. Their device, shown in Fig. 6.8, uses silk (42) and cotton (36, 40) to conduct a sample down

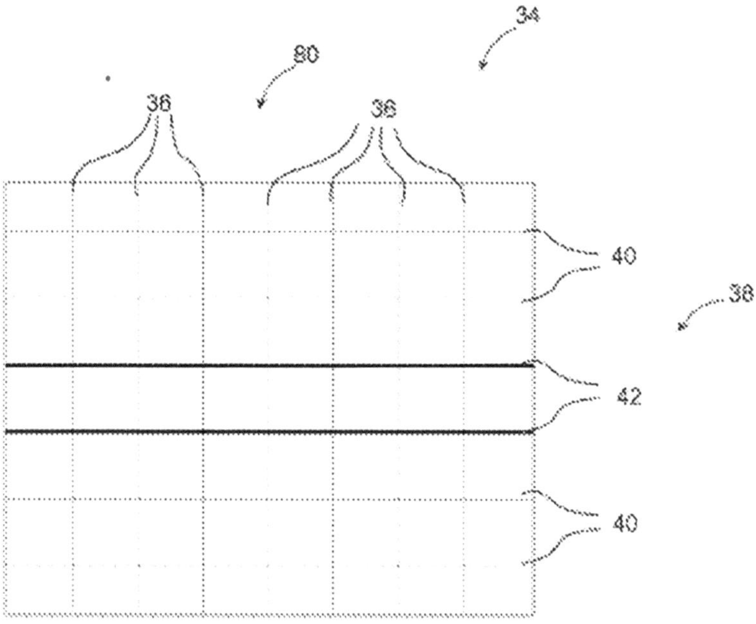

Fig. 6.8 Silk microfluidic device patented by Achira Labs (adapted from Patent WO2012150487A1)

specific paths for detection. The overall sheet shown is made from silk, with threads (42) specifically being made to be hydrophilic. The use of weaving reduced their cost of production and allowed them to produce devices at scale.

6.2.6 Digital Microfluidic Devices

Digital microfluidic devices use the Marangoni forces that result from exposure to an electric field to drive fluid movement. In its most common form, it is applied using electrowetting on dielectric (EWOD), where a fluid droplet is exposed to an electric field generated through a grid of individually addressable electrodes and separated from electrical contact using a dielectric layer. This is then further topped with a hydrophobic layer to prevent the drop from pinning on the surface. A droplet placed on this surface, in the natural state, is hydrophobic due to the coating. When the grid cells under the droplet are turned on, the electric field produces a Debye double layer at the interface with the dielectric, which reduces the apparent contact angle. The change in surface energy as a result of the electric field can be calculated using Lippmann's equation as

$$\gamma = \gamma_0 - CV^2/2$$

where γ is the surface energy with the electric field applied, γ_0 is the surface energy, C is the capacitance per unit area of the electrical double layer, and V is the applied potential (Labeed and Fatoyinbo 2014) and the change in contact angle when combined with Young's equation is

$$\cos\theta = \cos\theta_0 + CV^2 / 2\gamma$$

where θ_0 is the original contact angle on the hydrophobic face, θ is the contact angle when exposed to the electric field, C is the capacitance per unit area of the electrical double layer, V is the applied potential, and γ is the interfacial tension at the fluid-vapor interface (Teng et al. 2020).

EWOD allows for precise and reconfigurable control of individual liquid droplets on a flat surface via electrically controlled surface wettability (Ding et al. 2016). Unlike traditional continuous flow microfluidics, which rely on fixed channel geometries and pressure-driven flow, EWOD systems use arrays of individually addressable electrodes beneath a dielectric layer to control droplet behavior. When an electric potential is applied, the contact angle of a droplet is locally reduced, and the droplet moves toward the activated electrode site (Park et al. 2018). This enables core droplet operations such as dispensing, transport, merging, splitting, and mixing without the need for mechanical pumps, valves, or external plumbing. EWOD microfluidics has advantages in biochemical and biosensing workflows that require dynamic protocol reconfiguration, minimal reagent consumption, and compact system architecture (Eriksson et al. 2019). The digital nature of EWOD enables precise spatiotemporal control over fluidic operations, allowing for multiplexed reactions and parallel processing on a single chip. Additionally, the closed and contamination-free environment of EWOD platforms makes it suitable for sensitive applications such as clinical diagnostics, genomic workflows, and point-of-care testing.

EWOD can be found in either an open configuration or one with parallel plates, one of which acts as a ground. In the open configuration, the ground electrodes are patterned into the electrode grid and have a lower friction due to the reduced contact area. However, this leaves the droplet exposed to air and has a higher evaporation rate compared to parallel plate EWOD. In either configuration, if a droplet of the sample is large enough to straddle two electrodes, one of which is turned on, the contact angle over that electrode is reduced, and the difference in contact angle generates a Marangoni force that pushes the liquid toward the grid cell with the lower contact angle to reduce the surface energy of the drop. A schematic illustrating this in a parallel plate configuration is shown in Fig. 6.9 (Li and Kim 2020).

There are several formats of parallel plate EWOD that have been developed, including water in air, water in oil, oil-encapsulated water in air, oil in air, among others (Nelson and Kim 2012). The oil is used to reduce the voltage necessary for depinning the water drop, reduce biofouling, and allow faster movement across the grid (Yamamoto et al. 2022). The AC voltage applied for EWOD can range from 300 to 400 V in older devices to ~40–75 V in newer devices, with a frequency ranging from <1 kHz to 10 kHz depending on the geometry of the device and the thickness of the dielectric and hydrophobic layers. AC voltage is preferred to DC for EWOD as it reduces dielectric charging over time (Nampoothiri et al. 2018).

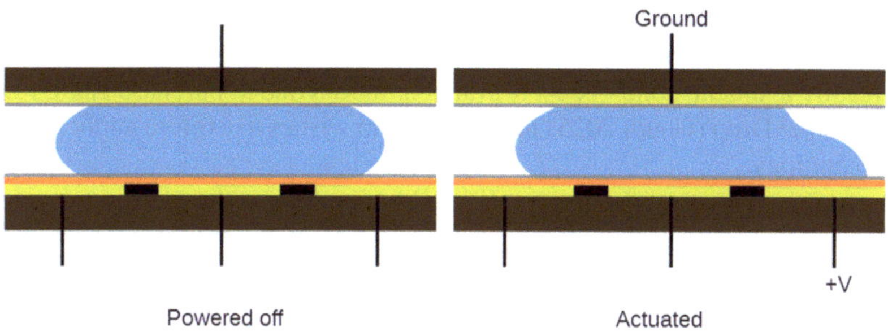

Fig. 6.9 Schematic of the cross-section of EWOD devices

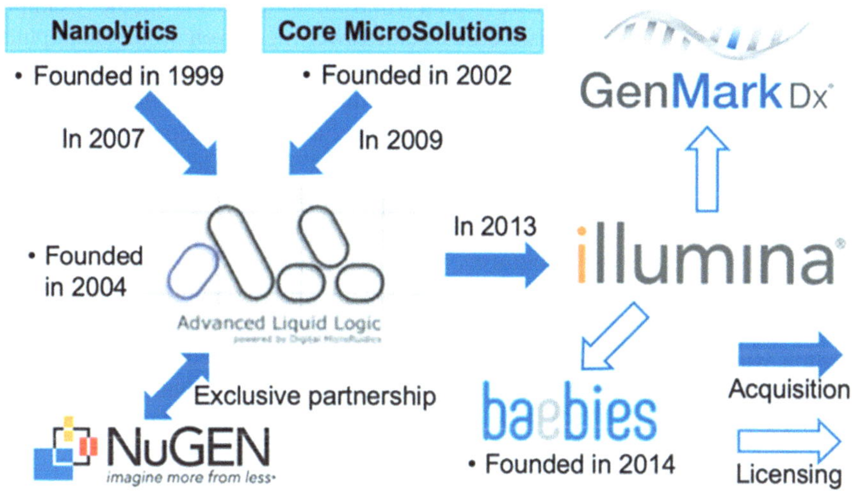

Fig. 6.10 Schematic history of some companies that use EWOD in commercial devices

When placed on a grid of individually addressable electrodes, EWOD allows discrete droplet control using programmable sequences that enable automated control of droplets on the device. Moreover, this control can be adapted rapidly to new protocols that allow the platform to be used for multiple tests and rapidly iterate on tests. Several operations necessary for an assay, such as droplet dispensing from a bulk solution, mixing, splitting, and picking up dried reagents on the hydrophobic surface, have been demonstrated on EWOD (Nikapitiya et al. 2017). As a result of its versatility and reconfigurability for a number of tests, EWOD has been used in commercial applications with a number of companies developing EWOD-based assays (Teng et al. 2020). Figure 6.10 sourced from that paper, shows a schematic history of companies that have used PCB-based EWOD commercially.

Baebies, using its EWOD-based FINDER platform, is currently adopted by hospitals across the United States as a near-patient diagnostic platform for a range of molecular, immunoassay, coagulation, and chemistry tests on human samples, and has received FDA approval for the first point-of-care heparin monitoring assay. In addition, an open source EWOD community project that relies strongly on *low-cost* and readily available components is available for anyone to purchase and try in the form of OpenDrop (Gaudi 2025) for anyone who wishes to explore applications for this technology.

Another commercial example of EWOD technology is the platform developed by Advanced Liquid Logic (Wheeler et al. 2005) using digital microfluidics to automate next-generation sequencing (NGS) library preparation. The system uses droplet-level control to execute multiple enzymatic and purification steps, including fragmentation, end-repair, ligation, and bead-based cleanup, in a disposable cartridge (Srinivasan et al. 2004a). This reduces reagent consumption, processing time, and human error, thereby increasing throughput and reproducibility of NGS workflows. Moreover, the Callisto™ platform from Volta Labs is another example of EWOD microfluidics. Callisto utilizes electrowetting-driven droplet manipulation for mixing, combined with magnetically actuated bead handling, for mixing and cleaning. Designed for automated DNA library preparation, the system performs key molecular biology operations, including fragmentation, ligation, cleanup, and size selection (Umapathi et al. 2018). The modular, programmable architecture allows for rapid protocol customization, reduced sample input, and scalable deployment in synthetic biology and clinical genomics environments. Beyond genomics, EWOD platforms are being explored for broader biosensing applications, including immunoassays, enzymatic kinetics, and real-time protein detection. The platform's ability to miniaturize and control fluid allows for integration with on-chip sensors and electronics, enabling closed-loop automation, real-time feedback, and AI-assisted assay optimization (Barbulovic-Nad et al. 2008; Rhee and Burns 2009). Therefore, incorporating the EWOD technique significantly enhances microfluidic automation, providing a programmable, compact, and scalable solution for droplet-based biochemistry. Platforms like Illumina's digital library prep and Volta Labs' Callisto are examples of how EWOD is redefining the landscape of biosensing, diagnostics, and lab automation (Barbulovic-Nad et al. 2008).

6.2.7 Other Microfluidic Devices

In addition to the commonly used techniques for microfluidic control above, novel methods for implementing assays in the microfluidic regime have been developed using non-traditional methods for controlling the assay. One such method is that developed by Brevitest that uses a gel-based discontinuous fluidic chambers through which magnetic beads are moved using a magnet. Portable immunoassays were developed using this method for coroners and medical examiners to determine the cause of death. A schematic from their patent is shown in Fig. 6.11 and shows the individual chambers that are independently filled with a fluid and are separated by a gel that allows passage of magnetic beads through individual reaction chambers.

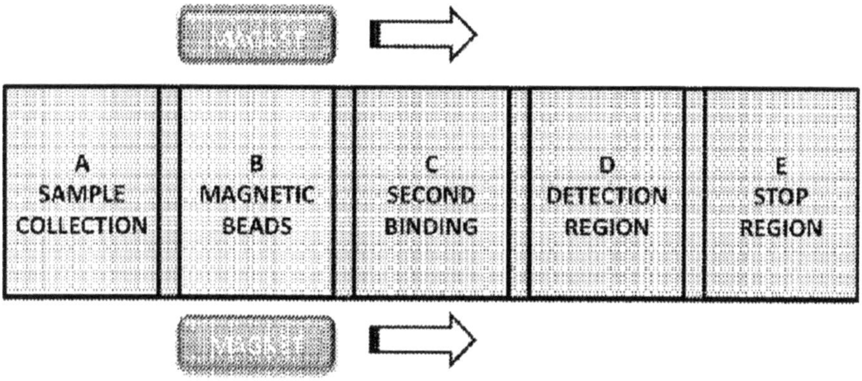

Fig. 6.11 Discontinuous microfluidic device as patented by Brevitest

6.3 Biosensor Modalities Integrated with Microfluidic Systems

Microfluidics is not a biosensing modality itself but rather an enabling technology to enhance the performance, precision, and versatility of a broad range of biosensor platforms. A biosensor modality refers to the physical or chemical transduction principle by which a biosensor converts a biological recognition event into a measurable signal. These modalities include electrochemical, optical, acoustic, magnetic, and mechanical transduction, each with its own signal generation mechanism (e.g., electrical current, optical intensity, acoustic resonance shift) (Turner 2013; Thévenot et al. 2001) as illustrated in Fig. 6.12. Microfluidics combined with these modalities provides a set of functional advantages, including precise fluid handling, rapid and controlled analyte delivery, reduced reagent consumption, and improved reaction kinetics due to enhanced mass transport in confined geometries. The laminar flow and scalability of microfluidic systems also enable multiplexed detection, high-throughput processing, and automation in miniaturized assay formats.

This section illustrates the synergy between microfluidics and biosensor modalities, demonstrating how combining them yields compact, high-performance analytical devices suitable for both central laboratory and point-of-care applications.

6.3.1 Electrochemical Biosensors

Electrochemical biosensors convert biochemical interactions at the sensor surface into electrical signals, typically measured as current (amperometric), potential (potentiometric), impedance (impedimetric), or conductivity (conductometric) changes at functionalized electrodes (Vo-Dinh and Cullum 2000; Homola 2008). Microfluidics integration in the electrochemical biosensors improves their performance by delivering analytes precisely and reproducibly to the electrode surface. In

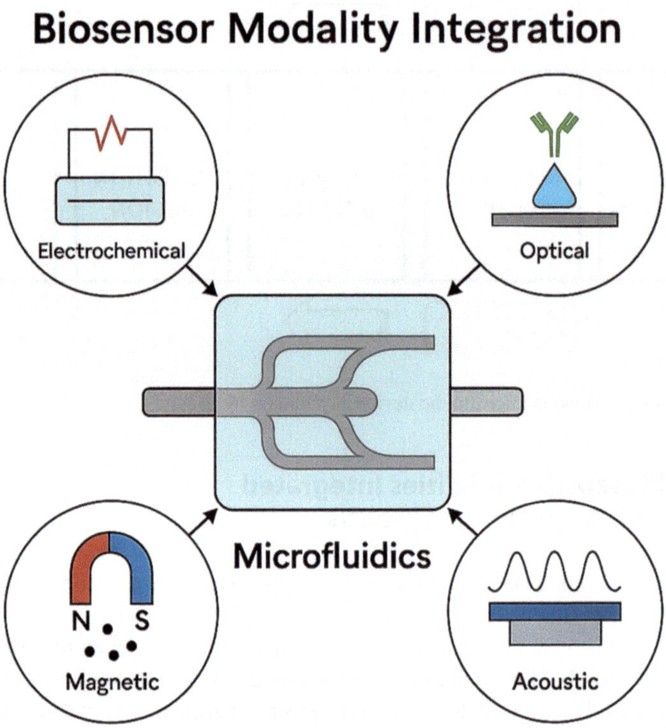

Fig. 6.12 Schematic illustration of integrated biosensing modalities in microfluidic platforms

a microfluidic environment, laminar flow conditions promote uniform mass transport, while the reduced channel dimensions yield high local analyte concentrations, thereby enhancing the signal-to-noise ratio and consequently enabling the sensitive detection of biomarkers at lower concentrations (Sackmann et al. 2014; Ymeti et al. 2007). Furthermore, microfluidic platforms facilitate the incorporation of multiple electrodes within a compact footprint, allowing for multiplexed detection and real-time internal calibration (Chin et al. 2011). The ability to perform automated wash steps and integrate on-chip reference electrodes further improves assay reproducibility and reduces matrix effects.

These advantages are demonstrated in commercial systems such as the *Dexcom G6* and *Abbott FreeStyle Libre*, which utilize miniaturized electrochemical sensors for continuous glucose monitoring in wearable devices (Gaster et al. 2011). For ex vivo diagnostic applications, companies such as *Sensirion* have developed high-precision flow sensors that are increasingly incorporated into electrochemical diagnostic platforms to enhance fluid control and improve measurement reproducibility, enhancing the accuracy and stability of analyte quantification (Osterfeld et al. 2008; Perez et al. 2002). A concrete example of an electrochemical sensor incorporated into a microfluidic platform is described in the patent (Raveendran et al. 2021),

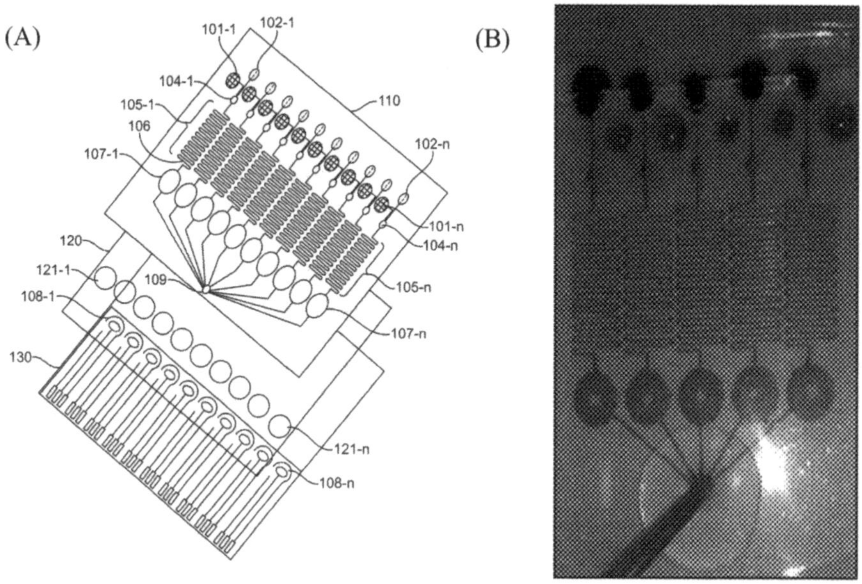

Fig. 6.13 (**a**) A schematic illustration of the microfluidic array device, demonstrating its capability for the simultaneous, multiplexed determination of analyte concentrations across multiple samples. (**b**) A visual representation of the micro-stamp fabricated using soft lithography. The stamp is used to create the intricate microfluidic patterns on the device's surface

titled "Lab on a chip device for multi-analyte detection and a method of fabrication thereof." This patent describes a multi-layered microfluidic chip where an array of non-enzymatic electrochemical sensors is integrated. The device uses a series of wells and channels to control the sequential flow of samples and reagents over the sensor array, enabling the simultaneous detection of multiple analytes such as glucose, cholesterol, and bilirubin, as illustrated in Fig. 6.13. This architecture highlights the ability to perform complex, multiplexed assays on a miniaturized, single use platform.

The fluidic control essential for these multi step assays is often enabled by microfluidic valves. These on-chip valves, typically pneumatic, function as gates that are actuated by external pressure to control the flow of liquids. They allow for the sequential delivery of reagents, automating the entire immunoassay protocol from sample loading and incubation to washing and detection. This automated process ensures the rapid and efficient removal of unbound reagents, significantly reducing background noise and improving the assay's signal-to-noise ratio (Azizian et al. 2023). By isolating different reaction chambers, valves also prevent cross-contamination in multiplexed assays and create a closed, contamination-free diagnostic system (Fu et al. 2019). This integration of valves simplifies the user interface, reduces reagent consumption, and enhances the overall reliability and reproducibility of the immunoassay, making it suitable for compact, portable diagnostic devices.

6.3.2 Optical Biosensors

Optical biosensors function by transducing specific biological recognition events into measurable optical signals, including changes in absorbance, fluorescence intensity, luminescence, refractive index, or surface plasmon resonance (SPR) (Tan and Takeuchi 2007). These modalities are particularly advantageous for their high sensitivity, real-time monitoring capabilities, and potential for label-free detection. The integration of microfluidics into optical biosensing platforms significantly enhances their analytical and operational performance (Wanunu 2012). Microfluidic channels can serve as precisely engineered optical paths or reaction chambers, enabling controlled and reproducible interaction between the analyte and the optical transduction surface. The microscale manipulation of fluid volumes and geometries enables rapid reagent mixing and uniform sample illumination, two key factors that reduce signal variability and photobleaching in fluorescence-based assays (Dekker 2007).

In the case of SPR and localized-SPR biosensors, microfluidic flow cells maintain continuous and laminar flow of analytes across functionalized metal surfaces, enabling real-time kinetic analysis of biomolecular interactions under controlled conditions. This offers higher sensitivity and temporal resolution, allowing for label-free operation by eliminating the need for secondary signal amplification (Zhang and Ning 2012). Additionally, microfluidic integration allows for the miniaturization of complex optical setups by embedding waveguides, lenses, and detectors directly within the chip architecture (Gao et al. 2015). This reduces the need for bulky external optics and aligns with the requirements of portable and point-of-care devices, where compactness, automation, and robustness are crucial. A prominent commercial realization of microfluidic-optical integration is the Biacore SPR systems (developed by GE Healthcare Life Sciences, now Cytiva), which utilize microfluidic delivery to precisely control the exposure of sensor surfaces to biomolecular samples (Malmqvist 1993). These platforms illustrate the capabilities of microfluidics to support label-free, high-throughput, and highly sensitive detection in a real-time format (Campbell and Kim 2007). Such developments are paving the way for compact, integrated optical biosensors capable of delivering rapid and accurate results across a wide range of biomedical and environmental applications.

6.3.3 Magnetic Biosensors

Magnetic biosensors operate by detecting the presence and concentration of target biomolecules through the magnetic properties of functionalized magnetic nanoparticles (MNPs), which serve as labels or transduction elements (Becker and Gärtner 2008). Upon binding to the target analyte, these MNPs generate measurable magnetic signals, which are typically captured using transducers such as giant magnetoresistance (GMR) sensors, tunnel magnetoresistance (TMR) sensors, Hall effect sensors, or, in some advanced applications, Superconducting Quantum Interference Devices (SQUIDs) (Xia and Whitesides 1998; Reyes et al. 2002). Magnetic biosensing offers high sensitivity, minimal interference from biological media (due to the absence of magnetic background in most samples), and compatibility with label-based assay formats. When coupled with microfluidic systems, the performance of magnetic biosensors can be significantly enhanced in terms of analyte manipulation, preconcentration, and signal accuracy (Weigl et al. 2003).

Microfluidic integration allows for the spatial and temporal control needed to manipulate MNPs within confined flow channels (Nguyen et al. 2019). By applying external magnetic fields or embedding micro-scale electromagnetic coils on-chip, MNP-analyte complexes can be efficiently guided, mixed, and concentrated within specific microfluidic regions (Pamme 2006). This targeted preconcentration increases the local analyte density at the sensing surface, substantially lowering the limit of detection for trace biomarkers. Furthermore, microfluidic platforms enable automated and rapid wash steps that effectively remove unbound MNPs, thereby reducing non-specific background signals and enhancing the signal-to-noise ratio, which improves assay reproducibility. Being able to localize and control magnetic bead motion within a closed microfluidic environment also enables the development of compact, automated, and contamination-free diagnostic systems (Zhong et al. 2023). These advantages are exemplified by platforms such as MIAtek, developed by Magnisense, which employs microfluidic magnetic immunoassay technology for rapid and sensitive detection of various analytes (Gas et al. 2016). Another study outlines methods for manipulating magnetic particles within microfluidic environments, showcasing the technical feasibility and versatility of magnetic biosensing in lab-on-chip formats. Collectively, the convergence of magnetic transduction and microfluidic precision offers a powerful solution for developing highly sensitive, rapid, and miniaturized diagnostic systems suitable for both centralized laboratories and point-of-care applications.

6.3.4 Emerging Biosensing Technologies

In addition to established transduction mechanisms, a growing class of emerging biosensing modalities, such as nanopore sensing and field-effect transistor (FET)-based biosensors, has gained prominence for their ability to achieve label-free, highly sensitive, and miniaturized detection of biomolecules (Wei et al. 2024). These advanced modalities rely on nanoscale sensing elements whose function critically depends on the controlled delivery and interaction of analytes within confined environments (Tahvildari et al. 2015). In this context, microfluidics plays a crucial role by providing precise sample handling, isolation, and delivery systems that enable reproducible and high-throughput analysis at the single-molecule or single-cell level (Vanderpoorten et al. 2019).

Nanopore sensors, in particular, detect biomolecules, most notably nucleic acids, by measuring changes in ionic current as individual molecules translocate through nanoscale pores embedded in a membrane (Zhang et al. 2017). Accurate detection in such systems requires stringent control over sample volume, flow rate, and electrical conditions, all of which are facilitated by the integration of microfluidics (Jain et al. 2013). A prominent example is the platform developed by Oxford Nanopore

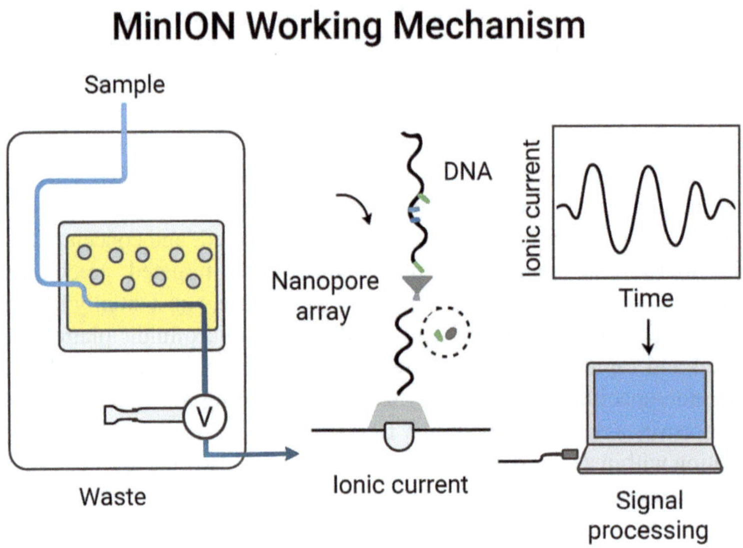

Fig. 6.14 Schematic representation of the Oxford Nanopore MinION flow cell and its working mechanism. The flow cell (left) contains a nanopore array embedded in a membrane, across which a voltage is applied. DNA molecules pass through individual nanopores, producing characteristic ionic current disruptions (center) that are detected and converted into electrical signals. These signals are processed in real time by MinKNOW software (right) to generate nucleotide sequence information

Technologies, whose commercial devices (e.g., *MinION*, *GridION*) utilize microfluidics to guide DNA or RNA molecules through individual protein or solid-state nanopores for real-time sequencing. The microfluidic interface in these systems enables stable, low-noise electrical measurements and continuous analyte delivery, which are essential for sustained high-resolution signal acquisition during translocation events (Fig. 6.14). Similarly, field-effect transistor (FET) biosensors, including those based on graphene or silicon nanowires, detect changes in electrical conductivity or surface potential resulting from biomolecular binding at the gate region of the transistor. These sensors offer high sensitivity, fast response times, and a pathway to ultra-miniaturized, label-free diagnostic devices (Noor and Krull 2014). However, their performance is highly dependent on the consistency of analyte exposure and the minimization of nonspecific interactions, both of which are addressed effectively through microfluidic integration (Oliveira et al. 2023). By enabling regulated fluid flow, localized reagent delivery, and integration with electrical readout components, microfluidics enhances the stability, reproducibility, and scalability of FET-based biosensing systems. Numerous applications reflect the integration of microfluidic channels with nanomaterial-based FETs, reflecting the technological convergence of microfluidics and nanoelectronics in next-generation diagnostics (Sengupta and Hussain 2021). Collectively, the fusion of microfluidics with novel biosensing modalities not only expands the scope of measurable analytes and assay formats but also supports the development of compact, high-resolution, and field-deployable biosensing technologies.

6.4 Challenges in Implementation and Manufacturing Scale-Up

Despite their transformative potential, microfluidic-based biosensors face several persistent challenges that have impeded their broad clinical translation and large-scale commercialization. These barriers span technical, material, operational, and regulatory dimensions, often arising at the critical interfaces between device design, user interaction, and manufacturing scalability (Cong and Zhang 2022).

A primary technical hurdle is achieving precise and reproducible fluidic control at the microscale. Devices such as the Abaxis Piccolo Xpress biochemical analyzer have demonstrated the clinical utility of microfluidics but rely on carefully tuned pressure and rotational forces to ensure consistent flow. Variability in flow performance across cartridges has necessitated strict manufacturing tolerances and extensive calibration (Strohmeier et al. 2015). Additionally, evaporation-induced fluidic drift has posed challenges in open-format devices such as early-generation electrowetting-based systems, where evaporative loss altered droplet volume and concentration over time, requiring improved sealing strategies and humidity control (Srinivasan et al. 2004b).

Surface fouling and non-specific adsorption also continue to degrade signal quality and sensor lifetime. For instance, in the Biacore SPR systems (Cytiva), precise microfluidic delivery is critical for label-free detection; however, repeated use can result in gradual fouling of flow cells, necessitating surface regeneration protocols or disposable cartridges (Chatelier et al. 1995). Similarly, in Siemens' Atellica® VTLi magnetic immunoassay platform, non-specific bead aggregation has been documented as a factor requiring careful tuning of washing and magnetic actuation steps (Chatelier et al. 1995). Material compatibility and chemical resistance remain concerns in platforms utilizing PDMS or soft lithography. Early microfluidic prototypes developed for point-of-care nucleic acid testing suffered from PDMS absorption of small hydrophobic molecules and dye leaching, prompting a shift toward cyclic olefin copolymer (COC) and other solvent-resistant thermoplastics in commercial devices (Toepke and Beebe 2006). System integration challenges are evident in devices like the Cepheid GeneXpert®, which, although highly successful, required significant engineering to integrate temperature control, fluidics, optics, and mechanical actuation within a compact disposable cartridge (Ulrich et al. 2006). The complexity of integrating upstream sample preparation steps, especially in applications such as whole blood or stool diagnostics, is also highlighted in platforms such as the BioFire FilmArray®, where lysis, purification, and amplification are all managed within a single pouch (Babady 2013). While effective, these systems require complex multilayer manufacturing and precise reagent stabilization, which increases cost and production complexity.

User interface complexity has posed challenges for devices targeting resource-limited settings or self-testing markets. For instance, early iterations of the mChip HIV diagnostic device required manual steps that introduced variability. Subsequent designs had to incorporate passive flow controls and automated readouts to improve usability (Chin et al. 2012). Similarly, the Cue Health Monitoring System, while successful in securing FDA Emergency Use Authorization for COVID-19 testing, received user complaints related to ambiguous error codes and sample handling difficulties, highlighting the importance of intuitive, user-centered design (Bruijns et al. 2022). From a production standpoint, manufacturing reproducibility and cost control remain major barriers. Even established systems like *Illumina's Nextera XT library prep kits*, when miniaturized for microfluidic use, require meticulous volume control and bead handling strategies to ensure consistent performance across batches (Sinkala and Riba n.d.).

In summary, while the integration of microfluidics with biosensing technologies continues to enable compact, automated, and sensitive diagnostic solutions, successful translation requires coordinated efforts to address fluidic stability, material robustness, and user-friendliness. Case studies from both successful and troubled platforms provide critical insights into overcoming these multidimensional challenges during product development and scale-up.

6.5 Prospective Applications and Future Perspectives in Microfluidic Biosensing

As microfluidics continues to evolve as a foundational platform in biosensing, its convergence with emerging digital, material, and manufacturing technologies is catalyzing a profound shift in how diagnostics are designed, deployed, and experienced. The demand for decentralized, real-time, and personalized healthcare solutions is driving the field toward more intelligent, accessible, and integrative systems. Looking forward, several key directions, ranging from artificial intelligence (AI) integration to wearable platforms, are expected to define the next generation of microfluidic biosensing technologies (Apoorva et al. 2024).

One of the most transformative trajectories involves the integration of artificial intelligence and machine learning with microfluidic systems. Microfluidic biosensors are capable of generating complex, high-dimensional data, particularly in real-time kinetic assays, droplet-based platforms, or multiplexed systems. AI algorithms, whether embedded in on-chip firmware or connected through cloud infrastructure, can interpret this data in real time to identify subtle diagnostic patterns, correct for sensor drift, and predict abnormal trends (Antonelli et al. 2024). For instance, Bio-Rad Laboratories has explored machine learning-enhanced diagnostic tools that could significantly improve accuracy and reduce reliance on expert interpretation (Malic et al. 2025). A recent study describes AI-driven systems for analyzing microfluidic droplet images, highlighting the growing push toward automated signal interpretation (Guo et al. 2024). In addition to data analysis, AI can also support real-time self-calibration and environmental adaptation, enabling biosensors to compensate for changes in temperature, humidity, or reagent degradation over extended use, thus improving long-term reliability and reducing the need for manual recalibration (Zhang et al. 2023).

Another major frontier is the integration of microfluidic biosensors with smartphone platforms, offering an unprecedented pathway for widespread, low-cost diagnostic access. Modern smartphones provide high-resolution imaging, robust processors, and cloud connectivity, making them ideal as portable readers for microfluidic chips. Devices are increasingly being developed to interface directly with smartphone cameras for colorimetric or fluorescence-based assays, while electrochemical sensors can connect via a compact potentiostat using USB or Bluetooth (Zhang et al. 2022). Cloud connectivity enables remote diagnosis by clinicians, centralized data logging, and integration with telemedicine infrastructures. While commercial diagnostic tools exclusively based on smartphones are still under refinement, numerous prototypes are advancing this concept (Wang et al. 2023). For instance, several studies have demonstrated the use of smartphone-integrated diagnostic platforms employing disposable microfluidic chips for rapid and decentralized analysis (Xing et al. 2025). Moreover, numerous studies have demonstrated proof-of-concept systems for detecting infectious diseases and monitoring environmental water quality using this model (Chandra Kishore et al. 2022; Yang et al. 2016). Although regulatory and reliability hurdles remain, the foundational infrastructure for such platforms is already in place (Mejía-Salazar et al. 2020).

The need for scalable and cost-effective production of microfluidic devices is also driving the adoption of advanced manufacturing approaches. Additive manufacturing techniques, particularly 3D printing, are increasingly being employed to fabricate complex, multilevel fluidic structures with embedded sensors or actuation mechanisms (Thorsen et al. 2002). These methods enable rapid prototyping and customization of devices with non-planar geometries or internal features that would be difficult to produce via traditional photolithography. Meanwhile, roll-to-roll manufacturing, which is well-established in the packaging and electronics industries, is being adapted for large-scale fabrication of paper-based or polymeric microfluidic systems (Hiltunen et al. 2018). Companies targeting mass screening applications, such as pandemic diagnostics or environmental surveillance, are investing in these high-throughput, low-cost processes to facilitate population-scale deployment (Tsaloglou et al. 2025).

In parallel, microfluidic systems are being miniaturized and optimized for continuous physiological monitoring via wearable or implantable formats. The low volume requirements and compact nature of microfluidic sensors make them well-suited for integration into transdermal patches, smart textiles, and even implantable capsules (Gao et al. 2023; Pour et al. 2024). These devices enable real-time, non-invasive tracking of biomarkers in biofluids such as sweat, interstitial fluid, or tears (Hosseinzadeh Fakhr et al. 2024). Epicore Biosystems, for example, has successfully commercialized sweat-sensing wearables that leverage microfluidic channels to quantify hydration and electrolyte loss in athletes and industrial workers (Ghaffari et al. 2023). The advancement of microfluidic biosensors is also tightly coupled to innovations in materials science. The incorporation of functional nanocomposites, such as graphene, quantum dots, MXenes, and responsive hydrogels, has significantly enhanced the sensitivity, selectivity, and versatility of biosensors (Krishnan et al. 2019). These materials offer improved electrical conductivity, enhanced optical properties, and dynamic responsiveness to stimuli such as temperature, pH, or light (Zambry et al. 2022). Moreover, their surface properties can be engineered to resist fouling, self-clean, or dynamically actuate fluid flow. For instance, conductive hydrogels integrated into microfluidic channels enable real-time electrochemical sensing with enhanced biocompatibility, while graphene oxide layers have been shown to facilitate label-free detection of nucleic acids with sub-picomolar range (Thirumalai et al. 2024). A growing body of research highlights the integration of advanced functional materials into lab-on-chip systems, underscoring the critical role of interdisciplinary materials engineering in the evolution of microfluidic device design and performance (Ma et al. 2017).

Altogether, the convergence of microfluidics with artificial intelligence, mobile platforms, advanced fabrication, wearable systems, and innovative materials is setting the stage for a new generation of biosensors that are not only analytically powerful but also accessible, autonomous, and adaptable. These integrations are enabling diagnostics that are continuous rather than episodic, decentralized rather than centralized, and proactive rather than reactive. The expanding landscape of intellectual property and early commercial successes across each of these fronts suggests a robust pipeline from research to real-world application. Continued interdisciplinary collaboration, spanning bioengineering, data science, materials chemistry, and industrial design, will be essential in ensuring these innovations reach their full potential in addressing global health challenges.

References

Abdiche YN, Malashock DS, Pinkerton A, Pons J (2009) Exploring blocking assays using Octet, ProteOn, and Biacore biosensors. Anal Biochem 386(2):172–180. https://doi.org/10.1016/j.ab.2008.11.038

Agha A, Waheed W, Alamoodi N, Mathew B, Alnaimat F, Abu-Nada E, Abderrahmane A, Alazzam A (2022) A review of cyclic olefin copolymer applications in microfluidics and microdevices. Macromol Mater Eng 307(8):2200053. https://doi.org/10.1002/mame.202200053. Accessed 30 June 2025. 18:27:55. From DOI.org (Crossref)

Ahmed D, Mao X, Shi J, Juluri BK, Huang TJ (2009) A millisecond micromixer via single-bubble-based acoustic streaming. Lab Chip 9(18):2738–2741. https://doi.org/10.1039/B903687C

Antonelli G, Filippi J, D'Orazio M, Curci G, Casti P, Mencattini A, Martinelli E (2024) Integrating machine learning and biosensors in microfluidic devices: a review. Biosens Bioelectron 263:116632. https://doi.org/10.1016/j.bios.2024.116632

Apoorva S, Nguyen N-T, Sreejith KR (2024) Recent developments and future perspectives of microfluidics and smart technologies in wearable devices. Lab Chip 24(7):1833–1866. https://doi.org/10.1039/D4LC00089G

Araz MK, Tentori AM, Herr AE (2013) Microfluidic multiplexing in bioanalyses. SLAS Technol 18(5):350–366. https://doi.org/10.1177/2211068213491408. Accessed 11 July 2025. 02:36:57. From DOI.org (Crossref)

Aubret M (2023) Point-of-Care medical device development for high sensitivity multiplexed detection of blood biomarkers for health care management of cardiac patients. Université Grenoble Alpes. https://theses.hal.science/tel-04480275

Azizian P, Casals-Terré J, Ricart J, Cabot JM (2023) Diffusion-free valve for preprogrammed immunoassay with capillary microfluidics. Microsyst Nanoeng 9(1):91. https://doi.org/10.1038/s41378-023-00568-2

Babady NE (2013) The FilmArray® respiratory panel: an automated, broadly multiplexed molecular test for the rapid and accurate detection of respiratory pathogens. Expert Rev Mol Diagn 13(8):779–788. https://doi.org/10.1586/14737159.2013.848794

Ballerini DR, Li X, Shen W (2011) Flow control concepts for thread-based microfluidic devices. Biomicrofluidics 5(1):014105. https://doi.org/10.1063/1.3567094. Accessed 27 June 2025. 00:58:00. From DOI.org (Crossref)

Barbulovic-Nad I, Yang H, Park PS, Wheeler AR (2008) Digital microfluidics for cell-based assays. Lab Chip 8(4):519–526. https://doi.org/10.1039/B717759C

Barreiros M, Santos DPDS, Perez PSE, Masum F, Barbosa LMM, Koussa M (2024) Pneumatic siphon valves and reaction chambers for sample analysis. WO 2024/184867 A1. Accessed 9 March 2024

Basu AS (2013) Droplet morphometry and velocimetry (DMV): a video processing software for time-resolved, label-free tracking of droplet parameters. Lab Chip 13(10):1892–1901. https://doi.org/10.1039/C3LC50074H

Becker H, Gärtner C (2008) Polymer microfabrication technologies for microfluidic systems. Anal Bioanal Chem 390(1):89–111

Ben Arlett B, Tom Edwards S (2022) Instrument for performing a diagnostic test on a fluidic cartridge. U.S. Patent No. US12465919B2

Bhandari P, Narahari T, Dendukuri D (2011) Fab-chips': a versatile, fabric-based platform for low-cost, rapid and multiplexed diagnostics. Lab Chip 11(15):2493–2499. https://doi.org/10.1039/C1LC20373H. Accessed 6 July 2025. 22:11:25. From pubs.rsc.org

Bhardwaj T, Ramana LN, Sharma TK (2022) Current advancements and future road map to develop ASSURED microfluidic biosensors for infectious and non-infectious diseases. Biosensors 12(5):357. https://doi.org/10.3390/bios12050357. Accessed 7 June 2025. 19:02:51. From DOI.org (Crossref)

Bruijns B, Folkertsma L, Tiggelaar R (2022) FDA authorized molecular point-of-care SARS-CoV-2 tests: a critical review on principles, systems and clinical performances. Biosens Bioelectron X 11:100158. https://doi.org/10.1016/j.biosx.2022.100158

Campbell CT, Kim G (2007) SPR microscopy and its applications to high-throughput analyses of biomolecular binding events and their kinetics. Biomaterials 28(15):2380–2392

Cate DM, Adkins JA, Mettakoonpitak J, Henry CS (2015) Recent developments in paper-based microfluidic devices. Anal Chem 87(1):19–41. https://doi.org/10.1021/ac503968p. Accessed 27 June 2025. 00:56:11. From DOI.org (Crossref)

Chandra Kishore S, Samikannu K, Atchudan R, Perumal S, Edison TNJI, Alagan M, Sundramoorthy AK, Lee YR (2022) Smartphone-operated wireless chemical sensors: a review. Chemosensors 10(2):55

Channon RB, Nguyen MP, Scorzelli AG, Henry EM, Volckens J, Dandy DS, Henry CS (2018) Rapid flow in multilayer microfluidic paper-based analytical devices. Lab Chip 18(5):793–802. https://doi.org/10.1039/C7LC01300K. Accessed 6 July 2025. 20:27:29. From DOI.org (Crossref)

Chatelier RC, Gengenbach TR, Griesser HJ, Brighamburke M, Oshannessy DJ (1995) A general method to recondition and reuse Biacore sensor chips fouled with covalently immobilized protein/peptide. Anal Biochem 229(1):112–118. https://doi.org/10.1006/abio.1995.1386

Chen Y-A, King AD, Shih H-C, Peng C-C, Wu C-Y, Liao W-H, Tung Y-C (2011) Generation of oxygen gradients in microfluidic devices for cell culture using spatially confined chemical reactions. Lab Chip 11(21):3626–3633. https://doi.org/10.1039/C1LC20325H

Chen H, Cogswell J, Anagnostopoulos C, Faghri M (2012) A fluidic diode, valves, and a sequential-loading circuit fabricated on layered paper. Lab Chip 12(16):2909–2913. https://doi.org/10.1039/C2LC20970E. Accessed 6 July 2025. 20:31:04. From pubs.rsc.org

Chin CD, Laksanasopin T, Cheung YK, Steinmiller D, Linder V, Parsa H, Wang J, Moore H, Rouse R, Umviligihozo G et al (2011) Microfluidics-based diagnostics of infectious diseases in the developing world. Nat Med 17(8):1015–1019. https://doi.org/10.1038/nm.2408

Chin CD, Linder V, Sia SK (2012) Commercialization of microfluidic point-of-care diagnostic devices. Lab Chip 12(12):2118–2134

Cong H, Zhang N (2022) Perspectives in translating microfluidic devices from laboratory prototyping into scale-up production. Biomicrofluidics 16(2):021301

Damodara S, Dwivedi DJ, Liaw PC, Fox-Robichaud AE, Selvaganapathy PR (2021a) Single step separation and concentration of biomarker proteins using agarose based miniaturized isoelectric gates for point of care diagnostics. Sensors Actuators B Chem 330:129265. https://doi.org/10.1016/j.snb.2020.129265. Accessed 27 June 2025. 00:51:12. From DOI.org (Crossref)

Damodara S, Zhu Y, Selvaganapathy PR (2021b) Patterned threads as solid-state reagent storage and delivery medium for automated periodic colorimetric monitoring of the environment. Microfluid Nanofluid 25(11):93. https://doi.org/10.1007/s10404-021-02496-x. Accessed 6 July 2025. 22:45:01. From Springer Link

Dekker C (2007) Solid-state nanopores. Nat Nanotechnol 2(4):209–215

Di Nardo F, Chiarello M, Cavalera S, Baggiani C, Anfossi L (2021) Ten years of lateral flow immunoassay technique applications: trends, challenges and future perspectives. Sensors 21(15):5185. https://doi.org/10.3390/s21155185. Accessed 2 July 2025. 00:59:11. From www.mdpi.com

Ding J, Li B, Chen L, Qin W (2016) A three-dimensional origami paper-based device for potentiometric biosensing. Angew Chem Int Ed 55(42):13033–13037. https://doi.org/10.1002/anie.201606268. Accessed 6 July 2025. 18:31:17. From Wiley Online Library

Dittrich PS, Tachikawa K, Manz A (2006) Micro total analysis systems. Latest advancements and trends. Anal Chem 78(12):3887–3908. https://doi.org/10.1021/ac0605602

Dossi N, Toniolo R, Terzi F, Sdrigotti N, Tubaro F, Bontempelli G (2018) A cotton thread fluidic device with a wall-jet pencil-drawn paper based dual electrode detector. Anal Chim Acta 1040:74–80. https://doi.org/10.1016/j.aca.2018.06.061. Accessed 27 June 2025. 00:55:30. From DOI.org (Crossref)

Erickson D, Li D (2004) Integrated microfluidic devices. Anal Chim Acta 507(1):11–26. https://doi.org/10.1016/j.aca.2003.09.019

Eriksson E, Lysell J, Larsson H, Cheung KY, Filippini D, Mak WC (2019) Geometric flow control lateral flow immunoassay devices (GFC-LFIDs): a new dimension to enhance analytical performance. Research 2019. https://doi.org/10.34133/2019/8079561. Accessed 6 July 2025. 20:26:53. From spj.science.org (Atypon)

Farajikhah S, Cabot JM, Innis PC, Paull B, Wallace G (2019) Life-saving threads: advances in textile-based analytical devices. ACS Comb Sci 21(4):229–240. https://doi.org/10.1021/acscombsci.8b00126. Accessed 27 June 2025. 00:55:26. From DOI.org (Crossref)

Fedio WM, Jinneman KC, Yoshitomi KJ, Zapata R, Wendakoon CN, Browning P, Weagant SD (2011) Detection of E. coli O157: H7 in raw ground beef by Pathatrix™ immunomagnetic-separation, real-time PCR and cultural methods. Int J Food Microbiol 148(2):87–92

Fu H, Song P, Wu Q, Zhao C, Pan P, Li X, Li-Jessen NYK, Liu X (2019) A paper-based microfluidic platform with shape-memory-polymer-actuated fluid valves for automated multi-step immunoassays. Microsyst Nanoeng 5(1):50. https://doi.org/10.1038/s41378-019-0091-0

Gao N, Zhou W, Jiang X, Hong G, Fu T-M, Lieber CM (2015) General strategy for biodetection in high ionic strength solutions using transistor-based nanoelectronic sensors. Nano Lett 15(3):2143–2148

Gao F, Liu C, Zhang L, Liu T, Wang Z, Song Z, Cai H, Fang Z, Chen J, Wang J et al (2023) Wearable and flexible electrochemical sensors for sweat analysis: a review. Microsyst Nanoeng 9(1):1. https://doi.org/10.1038/s41378-022-00443-6

Gas F, Baus B, Quere J, Chapelle A, Dreanno C (2016) Rapid detection and quantification of the marine toxic algae, Alexandrium minutum, using a super-paramagnetic immunochromatographic strip test. Talanta 147:581–589

Gascoyne PRC, Vykoukal J (2002) Particle separation by dielectrophoresis. Electrophoresis 23(13):1973–1983. https://doi.org/10.1002/1522-2683(200207)23:13<1973::AID-ELPS1973>3.0.CO;2-1

Gaster RS, Xu L, Han S-J, Wilson RJ, Hall DA, Osterfeld SJ, Yu H, Wang SX (2011) Quantification of protein interactions and solution transport using high-density GMR sensor arrays. Nat Nanotechnol 6(5):314–320

Gaudi L (2025) OpenDrop: An Integrated do-it-yourself platform for personal use of biochips. Bioengineering 4:45. https://doi.org/10.3390/bioengineering4020045

Ghaffari R, Aranyosi AJ, Lee SP, Model JB, Baker LB (2023) The Gx sweat patch for personalized hydration management. Nat Rev Bioeng 1(1):5–7. https://doi.org/10.1038/s44222-022-00005-5

Glière A, Delattre C (2006) Modeling and fabrication of capillary stop valves for planar microfluidic systems. Sens Actuators A Phys 130–131:601–608. https://doi.org/10.1016/j.sna.2005.12.011. Accessed 3 July 2025. 03:50:26. From ScienceDirect

Green NG, Ramos A, Morgan H (2000) Ac electrokinetics: a survey of sub-micrometre particle dynamics. J Phys D Appl Phys 33(6):632. https://doi.org/10.1088/0022-3727/33/6/308

Guo W, Hansson J, Van Der Wijngaart W (2016) Capillary pumping independent of liquid sample viscosity. Langmuir 32(48):12650–12655. https://doi.org/10.1021/acs.langmuir.6b03488. Accessed 27 June 2025. 01:00:01. From DOI.org (Crossref)

Guo K, Song Z, Zhou J, Shen B, Yan B, Gu Z, Wang H (2024) An artificial intelligence-assisted digital microfluidic system for multistate droplet control. Microsyst Nanoeng 10(1):138. https://doi.org/10.1038/s41378-024-00775-5

Hiltunen J, Liedert C, Hiltunen M, Huttunen O-H, Hiitola-Keinänen J, Aikio S, Harjanne M, Kurkinen M, Hakalahti L, Lee LP (2018) Roll-to-roll fabrication of integrated PDMS–paper microfluidics for nucleic acid amplification. Lab Chip 18(11):1552–1559. https://doi.org/10.1039/C8LC00269J

Homola J (2008) Surface plasmon resonance sensors for detection of chemical and biological species. Chem Rev 108(2):462–493

Hosseinzadeh Fakhr M, Lopez Carrasco I, Belyaev D, Kang J, Shin Y, Yeo J-S, Koh W-G, Ham J, Michaelis A, Opitz J et al (2024) Recent advances in wearable electrochemical biosensors towards technological and material aspects. Biosens Bioelectron X 19:100503. https://doi.org/10.1016/j.biosx.2024.100503

Houghtaling J, Liang T, Thiessen G, Fu E (2013) Dissolvable bridges for manipulating fluid volumes in paper networks. Anal Chem 85(23):11201–11204. https://doi.org/10.1021/ac4022677. Accessed 6 July 2025. 20:34:44. From DOI.org (Crossref)

Iglesias-Ussel Maria D, Bowie A, Anderson Jack G, Li Y, Park Lawrence P, Cardona Jose F, Dennis P, Ebuh V, Geller Steven A, Jain M et al (2025) Clinical performance of Abbott ID NOW™ COVID-19 2.0 rapid molecular point-of-care test compared to three real-time RT-PCR assays. Microbiol Spectr 13(3):e02033–e02024. https://doi.org/10.1128/spectrum.02033-24. Accessed 15 July 2025

Jain T, Guerrero RJS, Aguilar CA, Karnik R (2013) Integration of solid-state nanopores in microfluidic networks via transfer printing of suspended membranes. Anal Chem 85(8):3871–3878. https://doi.org/10.1021/ac302972c

Jangid K, Sahu RP, Pandey R, Chen R, Zhitomirsky I, Puri IK (2021) Multiwalled carbon nanotubes coated with nitrogen–sulfur Co-doped activated carbon for detecting fenitrothion. ACS Appl Nano Mater 4(5):4781–4789. https://doi.org/10.1021/acsanm.1c00376

Jangid K, Gupta R, Sahu RP, Zhitomirsky I, Puri IK (2022a) Influence of conductive porous electrodes on the apparent electrode kinetics of fenitrothion. J Electroanal Chem 910:116200

Jangid K, Sahu RP, Sakib S, Zhitomirsky I, Puri IK (2022b) Surface-modified metal oxides for ultrasensitive electrochemical detection of organophosphates, heavy metals, and nutrients. ACS Appl Nano Mater 5(11):17183–17193. https://doi.org/10.1021/acsanm.2c04105

Kaigala GV, Lovchik RD, Delamarche E (2012) Microfluidics in the "open space" for performing localized chemistry on biological interfaces. Angew Chem Int Ed 51(45):11224–11240. https://doi.org/10.1002/anie.201201798. Accessed 15 July 2025

Kim D, Sonker M, Ros A (2018) Dielectrophoresis: from molecular to micrometer-scale analytes. Anal Chem 91(1):277–295

Kong T, Flanigan S, Weinstein M, Kalwa U, Legner C, Pandey S (2017) A fast, reconfigurable flow switch for paper microfluidics based on selective wetting of folded paper actuator strips. Lab Chip 17(21):3621–3633. https://doi.org/10.1039/C7LC00620A. Accessed 6 July 2025. 20:45:35. From DOI.org (Crossref)

Krishnan SK, Singh E, Singh P, Meyyappan M, Nalwa HS (2019) A review on graphene-based nanocomposites for electrochemical and fluorescent biosensors. RSC Adv 9(16):8778–8881. https://doi.org/10.1039/C8RA09577A

Labeed FH, Fatoyinbo HO (2014) Microfluidics in detection science: lab-on-a-chip technologies. Royal Society of Chemistry

Land KJ, Boeras DI, Chen X-S, Ramsay AR, Peeling RW (2019) REASSURED diagnostics to inform disease control strategies, strengthen health systems and improve patient outcomes. Nat Microbiol 4(1):46–54. https://doi.org/10.1038/s41564-018-0295-3. Accessed 7 June 2025. 19:56:30. From www.nature.com

Li J, Kim C-JC (2020) Current commercialization status of electrowetting-on-dielectric (EWOD) digital microfluidics. Lab Chip 20(10):1705–1712. https://doi.org/10.1039/D0LC00144A. Accessed 27 June 2025. 00:53:57. From DOI.org (Crossref)

Lim H, Jafry AT, Lee J (2019) Fabrication, flow control, and applications of microfluidic paper-based analytical devices. Molecules 24(16):2869. https://doi.org/10.3390/molecules24162869. Accessed 6 July 2025. 20:45:50. From www.mdpi.com

Liu RH, Yang J, Pindera MZ, Athavale M, Grodzinski P (2002) Bubble-induced acoustic micro-mixing. Lab Chip 2(3):151–157. https://doi.org/10.1039/B201952C

Luka G, Ahmadi A, Najjaran H, Alocilja E, DeRosa M, Wolthers K, Malki A, Aziz H, Althani A, Hoorfar M (2015) Microfluidics integrated biosensors: a leading technology towards lab-on-a-chip and sensing applications. Sensors (Basel) 15(12):30011–30031. https://doi.org/10.3390/s151229783. Accessed 7 July 2025. 19:02:54. From DOI.org (Crossref)

Ma J, Wang Y, Liu J (2017) Biomaterials meet microfluidics: from synthesis technologies to biological applications. Micromachines 8(8):255

Malic L, Zhang PGY, Plant PJ, Clime L, Nassif C, Da Fonte D, Haney EE, Moon B-U, Sit VM-S, Brassard D et al (2025) A machine learning and centrifugal microfluidics platform for bedside prediction of sepsis. Nat Commun 16(1):4442. https://doi.org/10.1038/s41467-025-59227-x

Malmqvist M (1993) Biospecific interaction analysis using biosensor technology. Nature 361(6408):186–187

Martinez AW, Phillips ST, Butte MJ, Whitesides GM (2007a) Patterned paper as a platform for inexpensive, low-volume, portable bioassays. Angew Chem Int Ed 46(8):1318–1320. https://doi.org/10.1002/anie.200603817. Accessed 27 June 2025. 00:56:15. From DOI.org (Crossref)

Martinez AW, Phillips ST, Butte MJ, Whitesides GM (2007b) Patterned paper as a platform for inexpensive, low-volume, portable bioassays. Angew Chem Int Ed 46(8):1318–1320. https://doi.org/10.1002/anie.200603817. Accessed 15 July 2025

Martinez AW, Phillips ST, Whitesides GM, Carrilho E (2010) Diagnostics for the developing world: microfluidic paper-based analytical devices. Anal Chem 82(1):3–10. https://doi.org/10.1021/ac9013989. Accessed 27 June 2025. 00:54:48. From DOI.org (Crossref)

Masoodi R, Pillai KM (2010) Darcy's law-based model for wicking in paper-like swelling porous media. AIChE J 56(9):2257–2267. https://doi.org/10.1002/aic.12163. Accessed 6 July 2025. 16:43:16. From DOI.org (Crossref)

McNeely MR, Sputea MK, Tusneem NA, Oliphant AR (1999) Sample processing with hydrophobic microfluidics. J Assoc Lab Autom 4(4):30–33. https://doi.org/10.1016/S1535-5535-04-00016-4. Accessed 3 July 2025. 03:47:21. From SAGE Journals

Mejía-Salazar JR, Rodrigues Cruz K, Materón Vásques EM, Novais de Oliveira O Jr (2020) Microfluidic point-of-care devices: new trends and future prospects for ehealth diagnostics. Sensors 20(7):1951

Mostafalu P, Akbari M, Alberti KA, Xu Q, Khademhosseini A, Sonkusale SR (2016) A toolkit of thread-based microfluidics, sensors, and electronics for 3D tissue embedding for medical diagnostics. Microsyst Nanoeng 2(1):16039. https://doi.org/10.1038/micronano.2016.39. Accessed 27 June 2025. 00:57:56. From DOI.org (Crossref)

Nampoothiri KN, Seshasayee MS, Srinivasan V, Bobji MS, Sen P (2018) Direct heating of aqueous droplets using high frequency voltage signals on an EWOD platform. Sens Actuators B Chem 273:862–872. https://doi.org/10.1016/j.snb.2018.06.091. Accessed 7 July 2025. 23:17:47. From ScienceDirect

Nelson WC, Kim C-JC (2012) Droplet actuation by electrowetting-on-dielectric (EWOD): a review. J Adhes Sci Technol 26(12–17):1747–1771. https://doi.org/10.1163/156856111X599562. Accessed 7 July 2025. 02:49:54. From DOI.org (Crossref)

Nelson AC, Patten FW (2009) Automated cell sample enrichment preparation method. U.S. Patent No. 7,494,809

Neris NM, Guevara RD, Gonzalez A, Gomez FA (2019) 3D multilayered paper- and thread/paper-based microfluidic devices for bioassays. Electrophoresis 40(2):296–303. https://doi.org/10.1002/elps.201800383. Accessed 27 June 2025. 00:55:31. From DOI.org (Crossref)

Nge PN, Rogers CI, Woolley AT (2013) Advances in microfluidic materials, functions, integration, and applications. Chem Rev 113(4):2550–2583. https://doi.org/10.1021/cr300337x. Accessed 30 June 2025. 18:16:26. From ACS Publications

Nguyen N-T, Wereley ST, Shaegh SAM (2019) Fundamentals and applications of microfluidics. Artech House

Nguyen TT, Ta QT, Nguyen TK, Nguyen TT, Vo VG (2020) Role of body-fluid biomarkers in Alzheimer's disease diagnosis. Diagnostics 10:326

Nikapitiya NYJB, Nahar MM, Moon H (2017) Accurate, consistent, and fast droplet splitting and dispensing in electrowetting on dielectric digital microfluidics. Micro Nano Syst Lett 5(1):24. https://doi.org/10.1186/s40486-017-0058-6. Accessed 7 July 2025. 03:03:34. From DOI.org (Crossref)

Nilghaz A, Ballerini DR, Shen W (2013) Exploration of microfluidic devices based on multi-filament threads and textiles: a review. Biomicrofluidics 7(5):051501. https://doi.org/10.1063/1.4820413. Accessed 27 June 2025. 00:57:59. From DOI.org (Crossref)

Noor MO, Krull UJ (2014) Silicon nanowires as field-effect transducers for biosensor development: a review. Anal Chim Acta 825:1–25. https://doi.org/10.1016/j.aca.2014.03.016

Olanrewaju A, Beaugrand M, Yafia M, Juncker D (2018) Capillary microfluidics in microchannels: from microfluidic networks to capillaric circuits. Lab Chip 18(16):2323–2347. https://doi.org/10.1039/C8LC00458G. Accessed 25 June 2025. 12:15:54. From DOI.org (Crossref)

Oliveira DCDB, Costa FHM, da Silva JAF (2023) The integration of field effect transistors to microfluidic devices. Micromachines 14(4):791

Osterfeld SJ, Yu H, Gaster RS, Caramuta S, Xu L, Han S-J, Hall DA, Wilson RJ, Sun S, White RL (2008) Multiplex protein assays based on real-time magnetic nanotag sensing. Proc Natl Acad Sci 105(52):20637–20640

Pamme N (2006) Magnetism and microfluidics. Lab Chip 6(1):24–38. https://doi.org/10.1039/B513005K

Park C, Han YD, Kim HV, Lee J, Yoon HC, Park S (2018) Double-sided 3D printing on paper towards mass production of three-dimensional paper-based microfluidic analytical devices (3D-μPADs). Lab Chip 18(11):1533–1538. https://doi.org/10.1039/C8LC00367J. Accessed 6 July 2025. 18:34:58. From pubs.rsc.org

Patrick ON (2020) Leveraging microgravity to improve medical diagnostics – one drop at a time. ISS National Lab

Perez JM, Josephson L, O'Loughlin T, Högemann D, Weissleder R (2002) Magnetic relaxation switches capable of sensing molecular interactions. Nat Biotechnol 20(8):816–820

Peshin S, Madou M, Kulinsky L (2022) Microvalves for applications in centrifugal microfluidics. Sensors (Basel) 22(22):8955. https://doi.org/10.3390/s22228955. Accessed 30 June 2025. 18:53:32. From www.mdpi.com

Pethig R (2010) Review article—dielectrophoresis: status of the theory, technology, and applications. Biomicrofluidics 4(2). https://doi.org/10.1063/1.3456626. Accessed 16 July 2025

Piccolo Xpress, Vladimir E. Ostoich, Kenneth Aron, Dennis M. Bleile (2025) Systems for the detection of short and long samples. US Patent No. 7765069. Accessed 4 Aug. 2005

Pour SRS, Calabria D, Emamiamin A, Lazzarini E, Pace A, Guardigli M, Zangheri M, Mirasoli M (2024) Microfluidic-based non-invasive wearable biosensors for real-time monitoring of sweat biomarkers. Biosensors 14(1):29

Raveendran J, Raj VS, Pradeep A, Vasu SP, Stanley J, Nair B, Thiagarajan R, Thekkedath SBG (2021) Lab on a chip device for multi-analyte detection and a method of fabrication thereof. Patent number: 11009480. Accessed 18 May 2021

Reyes DR, Iossifidis D, Auroux P-A, Manz A (2002) Micro total analysis systems. 1. Introduction, theory, and technology. Anal Chem 74(12):2623–2636

Rhee M, Burns MA (2009) Microfluidic pneumatic logic circuits and digital pneumatic microprocessors for integrated microfluidic systems. Lab Chip 9(21):3131–3143

Rich RL, Myszka DG (2001) Survey of the year 2000 commercial optical biosensor literature. J Mol Recognit 14(5):273–294. https://doi.org/10.1002/jmr.547. Accessed 15 July 2025

Sackmann EK, Fulton AL, Beebe DJ (2014) The present and future role of microfluidics in biomedical research. Nature 507(7491):181–189. https://doi.org/10.1038/nature13118

Sarah M (2023) The VitalOne diagnostics machine. Bloomberg

Sengupta J, Hussain CM (2021) Graphene-based field-effect transistor biosensors for the rapid detection and analysis of viruses: a perspective in view of COVID-19. Carbon Trends 2:100011. https://doi.org/10.1016/j.cartre.2020.100011

Seymour CW, Gesten F, Prescott HC, Friedrich ME, Iwashyna TJ, Phillips GS, Lemeshow S, Osborn T, Terry KM, Levy MM (2017) Time to treatment and mortality during mandated emergency care for sepsis. N Engl J Med 376(23):2235–2244. https://doi.org/10.1056/NEJMoa1703058. Accessed 27 June 2025. 00:49:29. From DOI.org (Crossref)

Shin A, Shiri R, Liu Y, Peshin S, George D, Madou M (2022) Burstable liquid storage package for biological materials and valve substitution. US20220331802A1. Accessed 15 April 2022

Sinkala E, Riba J (n.d.) Miniaturization and automation of a full-length single-cell RNA-seq workflow. CYTENA GmbH

Squires TM, Quake SR (2005) Microfluidics: fluid physics at the nanoliter scale. Rev Mod Phys 77(3):977–1026. https://doi.org/10.1103/RevModPhys.77.977. Accessed 7 June 2025. 20:48:22. From DOI.org (Crossref)

Srinivasan V, Pamula VK, Fair RB (2004a) Droplet-based microfluidic lab-on-a-chip for glucose detection. Anal Chim Acta 507(1):145–150. https://doi.org/10.1016/j.aca.2003.12.030

Srinivasan V, Pamula VK, Fair RB (2004b) An integrated digital microfluidic lab-on-a-chip for clinical diagnostics on human physiological fluids. Lab Chip 4(4):310–315

Stone HA, Stroock AD, Ajdari A (2004) Engineering flows in small devices: microfluidics toward a lab-on-a-Chip. Annu Rev Fluid Mech 36:381–411. https://doi.org/10.1146/annurev.fluid.36.050802.122124

Strohmeier O, Keller M, Schwemmer F, Zehnle S, Mark D, von Stetten F, Zengerle R, Paust N (2015) Centrifugal microfluidic platforms: advanced unit operations and applications. Chem Soc Rev 44(17):6187–6229. https://doi.org/10.1039/C4CS00371C

Strong EB, Knutsen C, Wells JT, Jangid AR, Mitchell ML, Martinez NW, Martinez AW (2019) Wax-printed fluidic time delays for automating multi-step assays in paper-based microfluidic devices (MicroPADs). Inventions 4(1):20. https://doi.org/10.3390/inventions4010020. Accessed 6 July 2025. 20:30:41. From www.mdpi.com

Stroock AD, Dertinger SKW, Ajdari A, Mezić I, Stone HA, Whitesides GM (2002) Chaotic mixer for microchannels. Science 295(5555):647–651. https://doi.org/10.1126/science.1066238. Accessed 15 July 2025

Tabeling P (2023) Introduction to microfluidics. Oxford University Press

Tahvildari R, Beamish E, Tabard-Cossa V, Godin M (2015) Integrating nanopore sensors within microfluidic channel arrays using controlled breakdown. Lab Chip 15(6):1407–1411. https://doi.org/10.1039/C4LC01366B

Tan W-H, Takeuchi S (2007) A trap-and-release integrated microfluidic system for dynamic microarray applications. Proc Natl Acad Sci USA 104(4):1146–1151

Tanya N, Dhananjaya D, Shashi KM (2015) Tunable electrophoretic separations using a scalable, fabric-based platform | analytical chemistry. Anal Chem 87(4):2480–2487. Accessed 6 July 2025. 22:23:57

Teng P, Tian D, Fu H, Wang S (2020) Recent progress of electrowetting for droplet manipulation: from wetting to superwetting systems. Mater Chem Front 4(1):140–154. https://doi.org/10.1039/C9QM00458K. Accessed 7 July 2025. 02:41:47. From pubs.rsc.org

Thévenot DR, Toth K, Durst RA, Wilson GS (2001) Electrochemical biosensors: recommended definitions and classification. Anal Lett 34(5):635–659

Thirumalai D, Santhamoorthy M, Kim S-C, Lim H-R (2024) Conductive polymer-based hydrogels for wearable electrochemical biosensors. Gels 10(7):459

Thorsen T, Maerkl SJ, Quake SR (2002) Microfluidic large-scale integration. Science 298(5593):580–584

Toepke MW, Beebe DJ (2006) PDMS absorption of small molecules and consequences in microfluidic applications. Lab Chip 6(12):1484–1486. https://doi.org/10.1039/B612140C

Tomimuro K, Tenda K, Ni Y, Hiruta Y, Merkx M, Citterio D (2020) Thread-based bioluminescent sensor for detecting multiple antibodies in a single drop of whole blood. ACS Sens 5(6):1786–1794. https://doi.org/10.1021/acssensors.0c00564. Accessed 27 June 2025. 00:52:53. From DOI.org (Crossref)

Tsaloglou M-N, Christodouleas DC, Milette J, Milkey K, Romine IC, Im J, Lathwal S, Selvam DT, Sikes HD, Whitesides GM (2025) Point-of-need diagnostics in a post-Covid world: an opportunity for paper-based microfluidics to serve during syndemics. Lab Chip 25(5):741–751. https://doi.org/10.1039/D4LC00699B

Turner AP (2013) Biosensors: sense and sensibility. Chem Soc Rev 42(8):3184–3196

Ulrich MP, Christensen DR, Coyne SR, Craw PD, Henchal EA, Sakai SH, Swenson D, Tholath J, Tsai J, Weir AF et al (2006) Evaluation of the Cepheid GeneXpert® system for detecting Bacillus anthracis. J Appl Microbiol 100(5):1011–1016. https://doi.org/10.1111/j.1365-2672.2006.02810.x. Accessed 16 July 2025

Ulum MF, Maylina L, Noviana D, Wicaksono DHB (2016) EDTA-treated cotton-thread microfluidic device used for one-step whole blood plasma separation and assay. Lab Chip 16(8):1492–1504. https://doi.org/10.1039/C6LC00175K. Accessed 27 June 2025. 00:58:23. From DOI.org (Crossref)

Umapathi U, Chin S, Shin P, Koutentakis D, Ishii H (2018) Scaling electrowetting with printed circuit boards for large area droplet manipulation. MRS Adv 3(26):1475–1483

Vanderpoorten O, Peter Q, Challa PK, Keyser UF, Baumberg J, Kaminski CF, Knowles TPJ (2019) Scalable integration of nano-, and microfluidics with hybrid two-photon lithography. Microsyst Nanoeng 5(1):40. https://doi.org/10.1038/s41378-019-0080-3

Vo-Dinh T, Cullum B (2000) Biosensors and biochips: advances in biological and medical diagnostics. Fresenius J Anal Chem 366(6):540–551

Wang B, Li Y, Zhou M, Han Y, Zhang M, Gao Z, Liu Z, Chen P, Du W, Zhang X et al (2023) Smartphone-based platforms implementing microfluidic detection with image-based artificial intelligence. Nat Commun 14(1):1341. https://doi.org/10.1038/s41467-023-36017-x

Wanunu M (2012) Nanopores: a journey towards DNA sequencing. Phys Life Rev 9(2):125–158

Washburn EW (1921) The dynamics of capillary flow. Phys Rev 17(3):273–283. https://doi.org/10.1103/PhysRev.17.273. Accessed 3 July 2025. 01:35:13. From Aps

Wei J, Hong H, Wang X, Lei X, Ye M, Liu Z (2024) Nanopore-based sensors for DNA sequencing: a review. Nanoscale 16(40):18732–18766. https://doi.org/10.1039/D4NR01325E

Weigl BH, Bardell RL, Cabrera CR (2003) Lab-on-a-chip for drug development. Adv Drug Deliv Rev 55(3):349–377

Wheeler AR, Moon H, Bird CA, Ogorzalek Loo RR, Kim C-JC, Loo JA, Garrell RL (2005) Digital microfluidics with in-line sample purification for proteomics analyses with MALDI-MS. Anal Chem 77(2):534–540

Xia Y, Whitesides GM (1998) Soft lithography. Angew Chem Int Ed 37(5):550–575

Xing E, Chen H, Xin X, Cui H, Dou Y, Song S (2025) Recent advances in smart phone-based biosensors for various applications. Chem 13(7):221

Yamamoto K, Takagi S, Ichikawa Y, Motosuke M (2022) Lubrication effects on droplet manipulation by electrowetting-on-dielectric (EWOD). J Appl Phys 132(20):204701. https://doi.org/10.1063/5.0118241. Accessed 7 July 2025. 02:54:12. From DOI.org (Crossref)

Yang K, Peretz-Soroka H, Liu Y, Lin F (2016) Novel developments in mobile sensing based on the integration of microfluidic devices and smartphones. Lab Chip 16(6):943–958. https://doi.org/10.1039/C5LC01524C. Accessed 27 June 2025. 00:57:04. From DOI.org (Crossref)

Yazdani F, Sadir S, Huyop FZ, Wicaksono DHB (2015) Cotton thread for size-based blood cells sorting. Adv Mater Res 1112:437–440. https://doi.org/10.4028/www.scientific.net/AMR.1112.437. Accessed 27 June 2025. 00:56:46. From DOI.org (Crossref)

Ymeti A, Greve J, Lambeck PV, Wink T, van Hövell SW, Beumer, Wijn RR, Heideman RG, Subramaniam V, Kanger JS (2007) Fast, ultrasensitive virus detection using a young interferometer sensor. Nano Lett 7(2):394–397

Yu L, Koh CG, Lee LJ, Koelling KW, Madou MJ (2002) Experimental investigation and numerical simulation of injection molding with micro-features. Polym Eng Sci 42(5):871–888. https://doi.org/10.1002/pen.10998. Accessed 30 June 2025. 18:21:20. From Wiley Online Library

Zambry NS, Obande GA, Khalid MF, Bustami Y, Hamzah HH, Awang MS, Aziah I, Manaf AA (2022) Utilizing electrochemical-based sensing approaches for the detection of SARS-CoV-2 in clinical samples: a review. Biosensors 12(7):473

Zhang G-J, Ning Y (2012) Silicon nanowire biosensor and its applications in disease diagnostics: a review. Anal Chim Acta 749:1–15. https://doi.org/10.1016/j.aca.2012.08.035

Zhang Y, Wu G, Si W, Ma J, Yuan Z, Xie X, Liu L, Sha J, Li D, Chen Y (2017) Ionic current modulation from DNA translocation through nanopores under high ionic strength and concentration gradients. Nanoscale 9(2):930–939. https://doi.org/10.1039/C6NR08123A

Zhang Y, Devendran C, Lupton C, de Marco A, Neild A (2019) Versatile platform for performing protocols on a chip utilizing surface acoustic wave (SAW) driven mixing. Lab Chip 19(2):262–271. https://doi.org/10.1039/C8LC01117F

Zhang M, Cui X, Li N (2022) Smartphone-based mobile biosensors for the point-of-care testing of human metabolites. Mater Today Bio 14:100254. https://doi.org/10.1016/j.mtbio.2022.100254

Zhang Z, Boselli E, Papautsky I (2023) Potentiometric sensor system with self-calibration for long-term, in situ measurements. Chemosensors 11(1):48

Zhong Z, He J, Li G, Xia L (2023) Recent advances in magnetic nanoparticles-assisted microfluidic bioanalysis. Chem 11(3):173

Zhou G, Mao X, Juncker D (2012) Immunochromatographic assay on thread. Anal Chem 84(18):7736–7743. https://doi.org/10.1021/ac301082d. Accessed 27 June 2025. 00:57:19. From DOI.org (Crossref)

Optical Sensors for Point-of-Care Devices

7

Johnson Dalmieda

Abstract

Since the earliest days of civilization, point-of-care testing was performed by physicians in a very rudimentary way to diagnose ailments and illnesses in patients. Although the methods used were crude, the demand for these services highlighted the great need for cheap, rapid, and reliable diagnosis methods at the patient's location. Optical sensors serve this purpose quite well due to their portability, cost efficiency, and reliability, needing seldom more than eyesight to obtain a quick diagnosis. Due to the simplicity of the sensing mechanism, this method can be translated quite easily into portable instrumentation such as smartphone-based sensing, lab-on-a-chip devices, and paper-based assays. This is very useful due to the need for affordable, rapid, on-site testing in fields such as medical diagnostics and environmental monitoring, particularly in the Global South. In this chapter, we will discuss the fundamental principles of optical response and detection, current methods used for optical sensing in point-of care applications, and innovations being made to improve the field of optical point-of-care testing. Emphasis will be placed on the different methods of detecting optical responses to stimuli, integrating these sensing methods into portable devices, novel developments in the field of optical point-of-care devices, and challenges that lie ahead.

Keywords

Absorbance · Fluorescence · Naked-eye · Photodiode · Lateral flow assay · Spectroscopy · Microfluidics

J. Dalmieda (✉)
Department of Chemistry, Columbia University, New York, NY, USA
e-mail: jd3847@columbia.edu

V. Patel et al. (eds.), *Biosensor Technology in Translating Novel Materials into Practical Devices*, https://doi.org/10.1007/978-981-95-5519-2_7

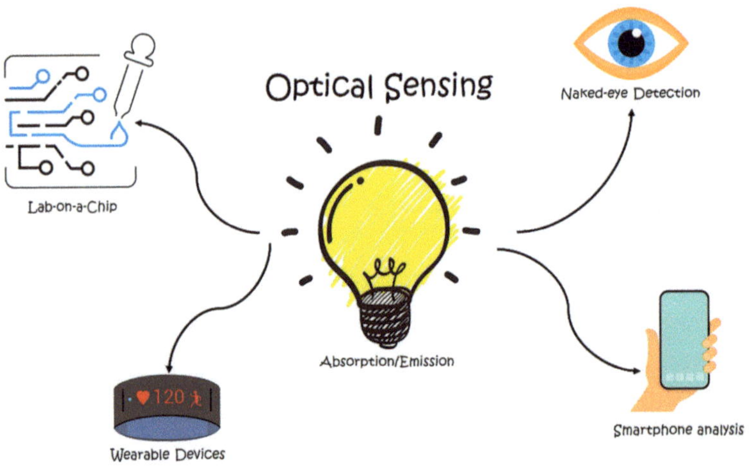

7.1 Point-of-Care Testing

7.1.1 History

The origins of Point-of-Care (POC) testing can find its roots in Ancient Babylon and Sumer, where the art of *Uroscopy* (the visual examination of urine) was regularly performed for diagnostic purposes (Fig. 7.1). Urine was decanted into a special flask known as a *matula*, and the colour of the urine was used to determine the patient's humoral balance (Connor 2001). At the time, urine was believed to be a filtrate for the four "*humours*"—blood, yellow bile, black bile, and phlegm. It was considered important to keep these humours in equilibrium, and any imbalance in these humours would cause disease, and subsequently would be reflected through the colour of the patient's urine (Armstrong 2007).

In these times, physicians provided many diagnoses based on uroscopy. Kidney problems would be apparent when redness was present in the urine. White flecks would indicate gout (Grant 1974). Post-intercourse, if an individual's urine was clear, it was thought that they were pregnant. Physicians would even go one step further and determine the sex of the child based on the cloudiness of the mother's urine (Tavormina 2020).

However, due to the high demand for uroscopic services, and the lack of trained physicians at the time, trust in the practice of uroscopy began falling off around c. 1500. Regardless, the need for rapid, cheap, on-the-spot testing for ailments was, and still is, quite prevalent (Stolberg 2007). And although uroscopy eventually became associated with snake oil salespeople looking to make a quick buck, many lessons from the time are still applied today. One might even argue that uroscopy was one of the first examples of a *POC* testing system.

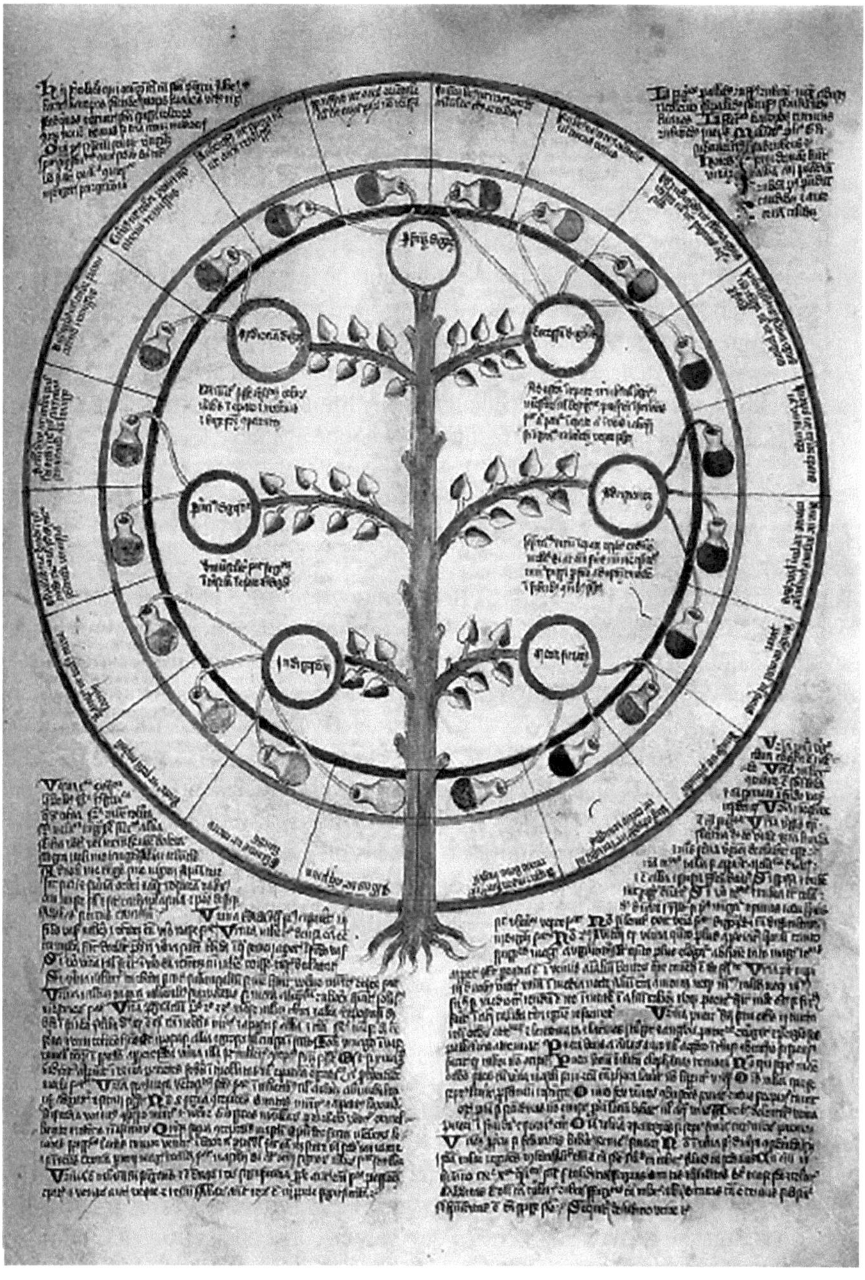

Fig. 7.1 Uroscopy chart. Apocalypsis S Johannis. Fol. 42r (c. 1420). (Reproduced with permission from Connor (2001))

7.1.2 What Is Point-of-Care Testing?

POC is defined as medical testing in situ, or at the site of care. This would mean that testing and diagnostics are done outside of a lab-based setting. Established in the 1980s, this new form of testing provided rapid testing and results within critical care areas (Kost 1995). Initially, POC testing was used in the presence of the patient within the hospital setting, leading to the advent of the *hybrid laboratory*. The rapid turnaround time for diagnosis, as well as the quick implementation of treatments (due to the patient already being present within the hospital), are characteristics of the hybrid laboratory, which emphasized improved patient outcomes (Kost 1992).

The ultimate purpose, the *raison d'etre*, of POC testing is to enable *facile, evidence-based medical decisions* such that the patient is provided with rapid yet accurate prognoses and treatments, especially during life-threatening situations in which access to a medical laboratory or facility may not be available (Kost et al. 2008).

7.1.3 Why Point-of-Care Testing?

The biggest advantage POC testing offers is its *portability*. During natural disaster events, such as hurricanes or earthquakes, medical infrastructure may either be severely damaged or destroyed. The ability to deploy POC testing in these areas makes it significantly easier to triage and to treat affected people in times of crisis, relieving the stress placed on the already-strained medical infrastructure in these areas (Kost et al. 2006).

Pre-testing at home is also a major advantage of POC testing, allowing one to administer the test themselves, providing the patient with a preliminary diagnosis as well as allowing healthcare practitioners to focus their efforts on treatment by eliminating unlikely diagnoses (Shirazi et al. 2021). One prominent example of an at-home test is a pregnancy test. These tests use a urine sample (ring a bell?) to test for human chorionic gonadotropin (hCG), a hormone produced in the placenta that is used as a biomarker for pregnancy (McCarthy and Eapen 2015).

Never did the need for POC testing become more prevalent than during the COVID-19 pandemic. Due to the global spread of COVID-19, the World Health Organization (WHO) declared COVID-19 a "Public Health Emergency of International Concern," leading to many countries effectively shutting down all non-essential services to the public (MacKinnon et al. 2020).

Due to the limitations placed on human contact, POC testing was seen as a viable pathway towards determining whether someone was infected with COVID-19. Using a simple lateral flow assay (LFA) device, one could obtain a quick COVID-19 diagnosis within 5 to 10 minutes (Fig. 7.2).

This quick turnaround allows one to take the proper precautions and obtain the proper treatments all in their own home, reducing the exposure others may encounter if they sought outpatient services for diagnosis (Farmer et al. 2022).

In this chapter, rather than simply reviewing optical POC devices, like many others have already done (Ming et al. 2024; Huang et al. 2024; Rasheed et al. 2024), I

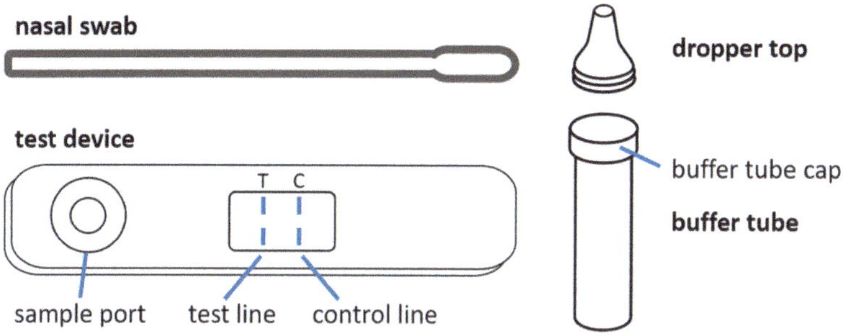

Fig. 7.2 A typical lateral flow assay (LFA) test used for the diagnosis of COVID-19. (Reproduced with permission from Farmer et al. (2022))

aim to lay out the underlying principles of optical sensing and begin a discussion on how these underlying principles can then be translated into practical devices for point-of-care applications. In this way, I aim to instil in the reader an intuition of what is fundamentally required for the feasibility of POC devices so that they may not just be able to have an idea of what is available, but potentially use what is learned herein to apply these principles to novel POC devices. I will do this by describing in detail the physical requirements needed for optical sensing, begin a discussion on how these requirements are integrated into devices, providing an overview of what has been done and what is currently in progress, and lay out the challenges and contradictions that will need to be reconciled to move forward.

7.2 Optical Sensors

7.2.1 Principles of Optical Sensing

Optical sensing is predicated on the principle that changes due to a stimulus response are reflected visually. Following this, an optical sensor can be defined as a type of sensor that converts a change in the optical properties of a material into information, whether it be a change in a material's absorption or emission of light (Moreira et al. 2017).

Absorption is characterized by a system's absorption band, which correlates with the energy required to bring the system from a ground state to its excited state. These states can either be electronic (moving an electron from a ground state to an excited state) or vibrational (a perturbation in a system's ground-state rotational-vibrational motion). Since *electronic transitions* are what are usually observed in the visible range, that will be the focus of this section (although we will revisit vibrational transitions in a bit).

When a continuous band of light is passed through a system, what is observed is that certain wavelengths of light are either missing or lower in intensity. These wavelengths correspond to the energies required to promote an electron from its

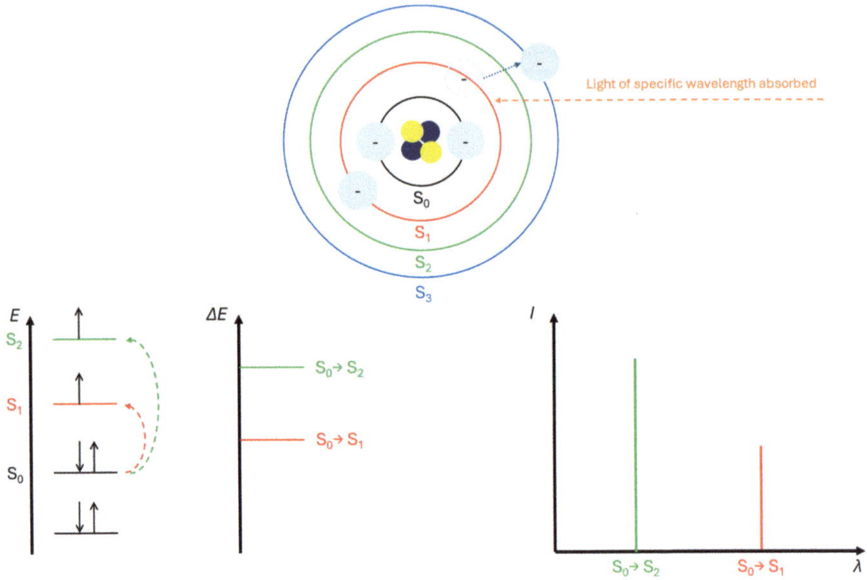

Fig. 7.3 When a system is subject to continuous light irradiation, photons with energies that correspond to specific transitions are absorbed

current occupied state to the next available unoccupied state (Fig. 7.3) (Agilent Technologies Inc. 2021).

In the example shown, the system has three states: the ground state (S_0), the first excited state (S_1), and the second excited state (S_2). Notice that each state uses the nomenclature S_n. This is because all these states are (assumed to be) singlet states, in which the total spin multiplicity of the system (taking the sum of all spins, where spin up is +1/2 and spin down is −1/2) is 0 (no unpaired electrons) (Valeur and Berberan-Santos 2012). Upon absorption of light at a specific wavelength, the electrons in the ground state move to an excited state without a change in spin multiplicity, leading to a decrease in intensity at those wavelengths. The decrease in transmission (I) is much more prominent in the $S_0 \rightarrow S_1$ transition because it is much more accessible due to the lower energy cost.

The concentration of a particular analyte system can be deduced from the absorbance via the *Beer-Lambert law*. The relation is given by (Eq. 7.1).

$$A = \varepsilon c l \tag{7.1}$$

This linear equation relates the *absorbance* observed A, with the analyte system *concentration* c, the *path length* that light must travel through the analyte system l, and the *molar extinction coefficient* ε, which is a measure of how strongly an analyte system absorbs light (Mayerhöfer et al. 2020).

Another way to optically observe changes in a system is through observing light *emission*. As previously mentioned, electrons will move from the ground state to an excited state when irradiated with light. Eventually, the excited electron will relax back to the ground state. This loss of energy is accompanied by the emission of photons with a wavelength corresponding to the energy difference between the ground state and the excited state.

One way emission is observed is through *fluorescence*. Through the act of absorption, an electron is excited from the ground state S_0 to the excited states S_1, S_2, S_3,... and so on. Fluorescence emission occurs when the electron relaxes from the excited state back to the ground state while retaining its spin multiplicity (Mallick 2023). Relaxation, however, isn't so straightforward. If an analyte system is irradiated, the electron will occupy a vibrational mode within S_1 such that the nuclear configuration of the molecule remains unchanged, in accordance with the Franck-Condon principle. Relaxation will first occur non-radiatively through the vibrational modes in S_1 so that the nuclei can realign themselves in accordance with the new electronic configuration before radiative relaxation to S_0 (this is why fluorescence emission usually occurs at a lower energy than the energy used for irradiation) (Fig. 7.4) (Ziering and Franzen n.d.).

Phosphorescence is related to fluorescence, with the key difference being that upon relaxation, spin multiplicity is not retained. This can occur due to intersystem crossing from the singlet excited states (S_1, S_2, S_3,...) to a triplet excited state (T_1, T_2, T_3,...) where the total spin multiplicity is 1 (two unpaired electrons). Phosphorescence relaxation takes much longer than fluorescence relaxation because

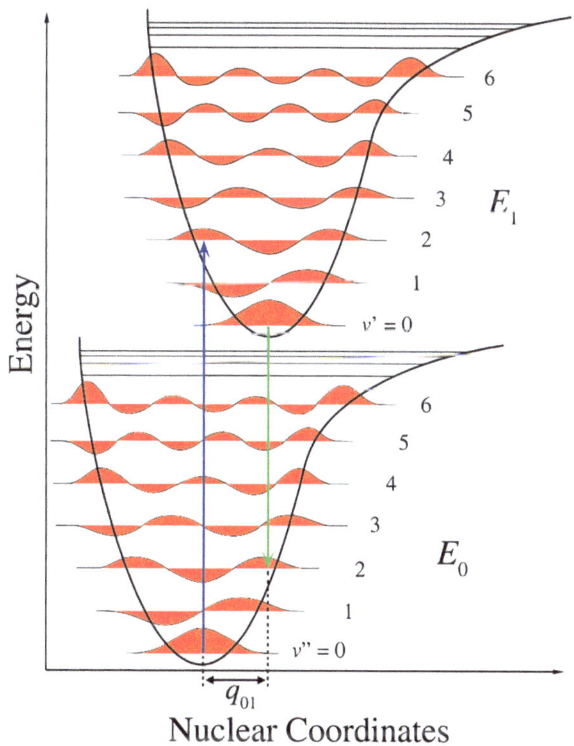

Fig. 7.4 Franck–Condon principle energy diagram, highlighting the vibrational harmonics present within each energy well. The blue arrow represents absorbance and the green arrow represents fluorescence (CC-BY-SA-3.0; Samoza)

electronic transitions between different spin states are considered "forbidden" by spin selection rules. The reason that intersystem crossing in the excited state occurs even though the transition is considered "forbidden" is because of sustained irradiation of the system ("forbidden" transitions do not mean that they don't occur, they are just far less likely to occur than "allowed" transitions (Franz et al. 2000).

Since absorption and emission occur in the visible range, the easiest way to detect these changes is through *eyesight.* Although reliance on one's eyesight is not the most reliable measure, it serves as a quick and simple way of determining the presence of an analyte. For more sensitive and quantitative measures, however, one will need to make use of *optoelectronic detectors*; that is, detectors that convert a change in a system's optical properties to an electrical signal that can then be read out (Morris and Langari 2012). For the purposes of optical sensing, *photodiodes* are the most commonly used detector devices. Photodiodes are detector devices that produce current upon irradiation of specific wavelength ranges of light. Photodiodes are what can be considered *p-n junctions*. The p-n junction is formed when a negatively doped semiconductor (which contains free electrons) is brought into contact with a positively doped semiconductor (which contains free "holes"; positive charge carriers). The region in between the n-doped and the p-doped junctions is called the "depletion zone", where there are no free carriers present. This region possesses an electric charge because there are charged ions within the region, but no counterions to neutralize them. This leads to the presence of an electric field vector pointing from the n-doped to the p-doped region. Generally, the valence band of the p-doped semiconductor and the conduction band of the n-doped semiconductor are aligned,

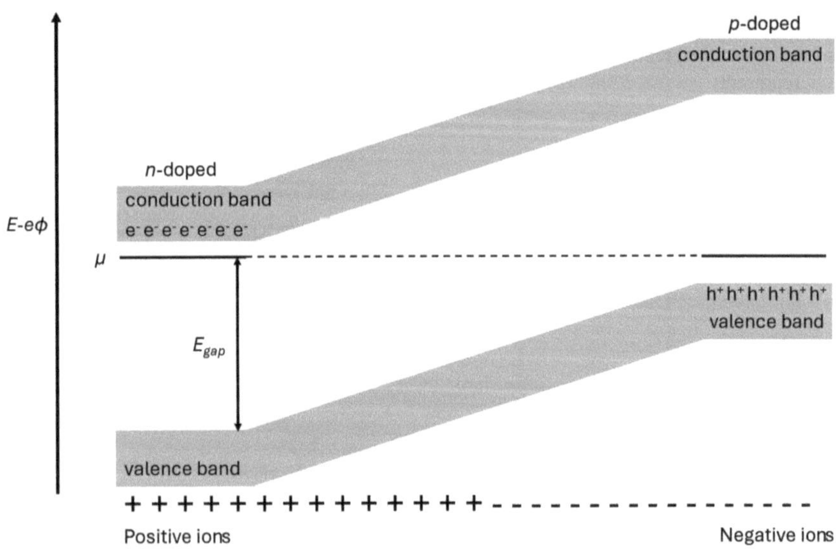

Fig. 7.5 Energy diagram of a p-n junction. If electrons in the depletion region are excited, they will move to the left while the holes generated will move to the right, which creates a current

which means that the change in electrostatic potential is compensated by the drop in band energy as electrons move toward the n-doped semiconductor (Fig. 7.5).

By applying light to this junction at energies equal to or exceeding the band gap, electrons will be excited in the entire junction. In both the n-doped and p-doped regions, the electrons quickly relax. However, in the depletion region, electrons will flow towards the left and holes will flow towards the right, thus generating current (Simon 2013).

Using the principle of p-n junctions, the metal-oxide semiconductor field effect transistor (MOSFET) was developed. An n-(p-)MOSFET consists of a p-(n-)doped semiconductor encapsulating two n-(p-) semiconductors, effectively creating two p-n junctions. Bridging the two p-n junctions is an oxide insulator along with a metal gate electrode (Fig. 7.6). At zero voltage, current cannot flow between the source and drain. However, upon application of a positive (negative) gate voltage relative to the ground (greater than a threshold voltage $V_{threshold}$), which will attract negative (positive) charge (known as a "field effect"). This effectively creates a continuous conductive channel connecting the source and the drain (Fig. 7.6).

The two most commonly found detectors for portable optical sensing are the charge-coupled device (CCD) detector and the complementary metal-oxide semiconductor (CMOS) detector. CCD detectors use p-MOSFETs as the basis of their detection platform. Upon light irradiation, electrons are excited, which allows for electron flow from the p-semiconductor to the n-semiconductor. Upon application of a negative voltage bias, the positive charges accumulated in the p-semiconductors create a conducting channel between the source and drain, resulting in an electrical signal. The charge is then transferred along neighbouring diodes until it is read out by a charge amplifier, which converts the charge into a voltage. Having a series of CCD detectors spatially separated, with a diffraction grating or filter in front, can allow for measurement of absorbance or emission spectra where intensities at particular light wavelengths can be measured. CMOS detectors are similar, with the sole exception being that CMOS detectors alternate with n-MOSFETs and p-MOSFETs. These detectors are generally less expensive since the capture and sensing elements are both on the same integrated circuit, whereas on a CCD

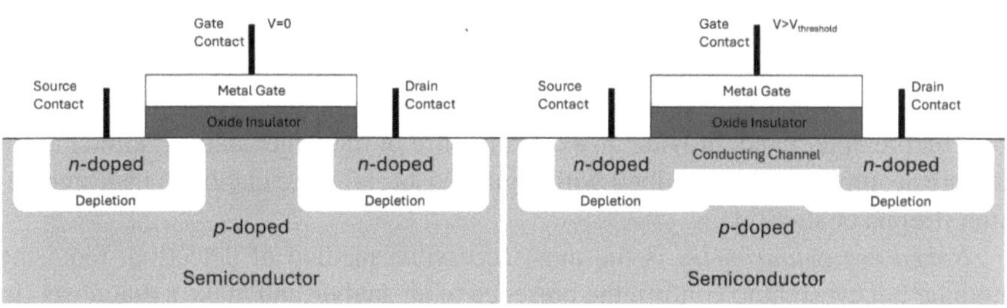

Fig. 7.6 An n-MOSFET with zero bias (left), in which there is no conductance, and with applied bias V (right), in which there is now a conducting channel connecting the source and the drain contacts

detector image sensing is done by the MOSFETs and detection is done separately by a charge amplifier (Sze and Lee 2012).

7.2.2 Why Optical Sensing?

POC has been previously defined in this chapter as a *rapid* and *portable* way to diagnose patients on-site, without requiring elaborate, complicated equipment. Optical sensors offer a *cheap*, *reliable* way to measure various biomarkers while providing a rapid *qualitative* response by way of a visual change, whether it be a change in colour or the emission of light. In addition, because light absorption and emission only happen at specific wavelengths, it is possible to have multiplexed sensing, in which different biomarkers can be identified based on the specific absorption or emission wavelength. Along with this, the intensity of the absorption or emission can provide a *quantitative* measure of the biomarker. All of these factors make optical sensing a promising method for POC testing (Mostufa et al. 2024).

One thing to note is that, due to the simplicity and robustness of the fundamental principles behind optical enhancement and detection, the principal components required for optical response and detection can easily be miniaturized and translated into point-of-care devices. The library of optical induction is practically limitless, with many well-known chemical and physical systems, such as Rhodamine B, for the detection of various biomarkers (Slate et al. 2009), or gold nanoparticles for biological assays (Karnwal et al. 2024). In addition, due to the progress of semiconductor technology, transistors are now smaller than ever, and active pixel sensors can have as many as 50 million pixels in an array that can fit into a smartphone (FE Tech Desk n.d.). This makes optical POC sensing extremely easy to import into handheld and miniature devices while still retaining the high resolution required for trace analysis.

7.2.3 Optical Sensing Methods

Optical sensing methods currently exist for POC testing. These sensors can be subdivided into qualitative methods and quantitative methods. Qualitative methods are ones that indicate the presence of a target analyte or biomarker. These methods give a quick "yes" or "no" response and are the easiest to implement for POC testing. The trade-off is that you cannot obtain a specific concentration. Quantitative methods, on the other hand, provide an exact measure of the target analyte, allowing for a more accurate prognosis, albeit with higher costs and more elaborate instrumentation (Luppa et al. 2011).

Naked-eye colourimetry is the most accessible method of detection, requiring nothing but eyesight to confirm the presence of an analyte and make a diagnosis. To that end, gold nanoparticle solutions are most commonly used because of their rapid colour change, as well as the distinct colour change from red to blue/purple upon nanoparticle aggregation. This method is very useful for rapid detection of metal

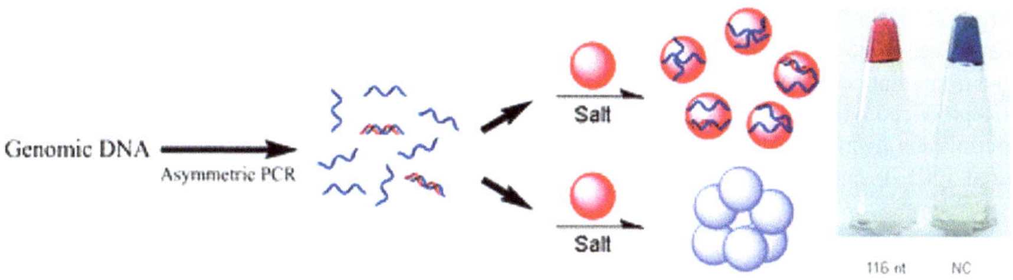

Fig. 7.7 A scheme of gold nanoparticles being dispersed when asymmetric polymerase chains are present, compared to aggregation when no polymerase chains are present (left), which can be visually seen in the sample centrifuge tubes comparing the nanoparticles with polymerase present versus without (right). (Reproduced with permission from Deng et al. (2013))

ions as well as the detection of various proteins and enzymes (Fig. 7.7) (Jazayeri et al. 2018).

One example of a naked-eye colourimetric sensor is shown in the following study by Deng et al. (2013). Here, they demonstrate a naked-eye sensor based on DNA amplicons bound to gold nanoparticles. Using an asymmetric polymerase chain reaction, specific single and double-stranded DNA sequences were amplified and bound to gold nanoparticles, preventing aggregation and facilitating the specific detection of these DNA sequences via colour change. When these nanoparticles are unbound to DNA, they will aggregate in salt solution and will appear blue. Upon binding to DNA, aggregation is prevented, and the nanoparticles will appear red. This was used in this study to detect the presence of *B. anthracis*, a bacterium that causes anthrax. Another pathway for naked-eye detection is through photoresponsive molecules and polymers, such as what was used by Jiang et al., who used polydiacetylene for the detection of H5N1, or bird flu (Jiang et al. 2015). To develop the photoresponsive polymer, 10,12-pentacosadiynoic acid and 1,2-dimyristoyl-sn-glycero-3-phosphocholine were combined in optimized ratios to form a polymeric vesicle. An anti-H5-antibody was bound to the vesicle, and bovine serum albumin was used to improve selectivity for H5N1. The polymeric vesicle on its own appears blue. After interaction with the H5N1 virus the vesicle would appear red, with the intensity of the red colour being indicative of the concentration of H5N1 copies. Naked-eye measurements can assist in the detection of concentrations as low as 1.54 copies/μL, but when paired with a UV-vis spectrophotometer, this limit is lowered to 0.53 copies/μL. Interactions with H3N2, Newcastle disease, and porcine virus did not elicit a colour change, highlighting not only the sensitivity, but also the selectivity of this method.

An extremely common qualitative naked-eye colourimetric method is the *Lateral Flow Assay* (LFA). Lateral flow assays consist of a cartridge that contains an antibody adhered to a backing paper. Upon interaction with a biomarker in the sample, the antibody will undergo a colour change (generally from colourless to red), indicating the presence of the biomarker (Fig. 7.8).

To perform the test, you introduce the sample to the sample pad. The sample may be diluted with buffer solution to facilitate flow. The sample solution then flows

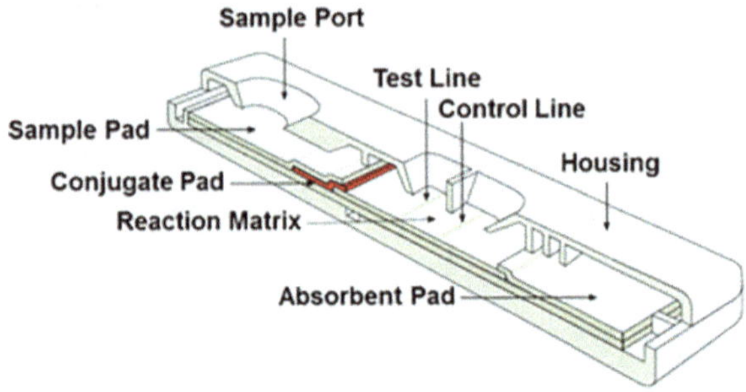

Fig. 7.8 A typical LFA cartridge, highlighting all the important components. (Reproduced with permission from Yetisen et al. (2013))

through the backing paper via capillary action and encounters the reaction matrix. The backing paper contains conjugates which also bind to the antibodies, leading to a colour change. As the solution encounters the reaction matrix, the analyte binds to the antibodies immobilized on the test line, while the conjugate binds to the antibodies on the control line. A positive result is determined if the test line changes in colour along with the control line. If only the control line changes colour, then a negative result is obtained. If the control line fails to change colour, the test is faulty, and a new cartridge may need to be used (Yetisen et al. 2013). These tests are available commercially and are used for the detection of the human chronic gonadotropin (hCG) for *pregnancy testing* (McCarthy and Eapen 2015) and more recently for the detection of COVID-19 (Farmer et al. 2022).

LFAs are generally separated into two categories: sandwich assays and competitive assays. In sandwich assays, the intensity of the test line increases with increasing biomarker concentration, with the inverse being true for competitive assays. Competitive assays can subsequently be separated into two categories: direct and indirect. In direct assays, the competing antibody is functionalized with a colourimetric reporter. At low target concentrations, the competitor binds to the test line, leading to a colour change. High target concentrations lead to preferential binding of the target, suppressing the appearance of colour. Indirect assays use a colourimetric receptor with the competitor on the test line. At low target concentrations, the bioreceptor will bind to the competitor, and the test line will be coloured. At high target concentrations, the bioreceptor binds to the target and passes over the test line, leading to no colour change (Pedreira-Rincón et al. 2025).

Recent innovations in LFA technology involve the optimization of the flow assay. One innovation was an aptamer-based assay, an example of which was developed by Alnajrani et al. for the detection of dabigatran etexilate, a blood thinner (Alnajrani et al. 2022). By using a 60-mer aptamer bound to gold nanoparticles, they were able to develop a competitive assay in which the aptamer-nanoparticle system was biotinylated to allow for interaction with the streptavidin test line. Further down, a lysosome control line was used for non-specific binding of the aptamer. Upon conjugation with the dabigatran etexilate, the aptamer-nanoparticle system would undergo a conformational change in which the biotin moiety is released, allowing for the aptamer to pass over the test line without interaction. Using this method, they were able to obtain a colourimetric response at concentrations as low as 20 nM in both buffer and blood samples. Another innovative assay method is the restrictive assay, in which size exclusion is the primary method of competition. This was demonstrated by Xiao et al. for the detection of CD4 cells, which are used to determine the immune system performance of HIV infected individuals (Xiao et al. 2019). Here, CD4 cells were bound to fluorescent antibodies, and a filter pad was placed before the test and control lines to block CD4 functionalized with the fluorophore. With no CD4 present, the fluorophore passes through the filter pad unrestricted and binds to the goat anti-mouse immunoglobulin G on the test line, which will fluoresce brightly. Binding to the CD4 restricts the passage of the fluorophore through the filter pad, leading to less fluorophore conjugation on the test line and subsequently lower fluorescence intensity. The control line contains rabbit immunoglobulin G that is already functionalized with fluorophores, so its fluorescence intensity remains unchanged. With this method, a detection limit of 44 cells/μL was obtained.

Absorbance spectroscopy is a quantitative method for the determination of various analytes that makes use of the previously mentioned characteristic absorbance bands that exist within analyte systems for detection (Liu et al. 2019). Commercial systems exist, such as the Ocean Optics HR2000+, as well as various other custom-built setups (Jesuraj and Hassan 2023). The instrumentation used for *fluorescence* is effectively the same, with the main difference being that excitation occurs not with

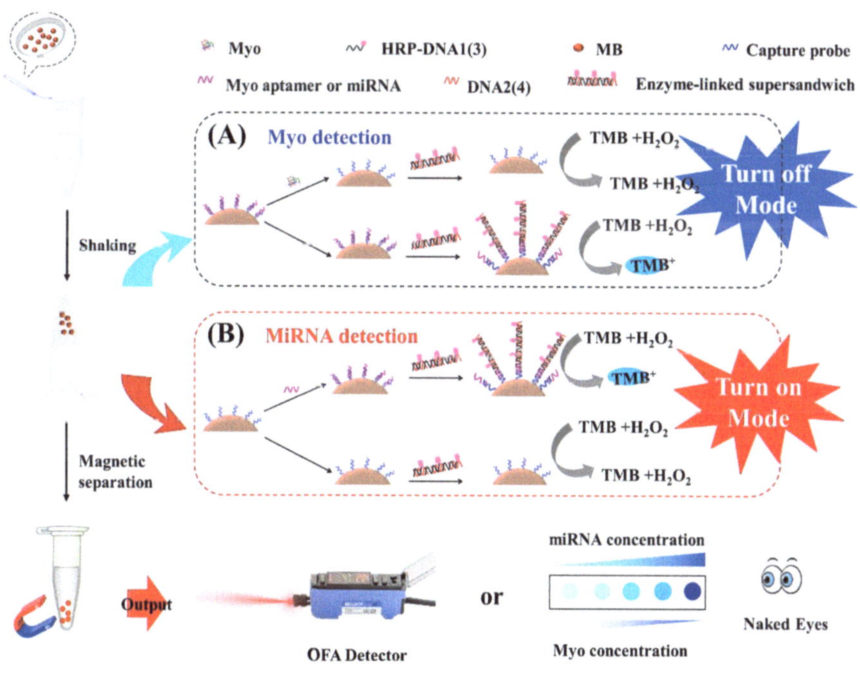

Fig. 7.9 The outline for the measurement of miRNA-141, a biomarker for prostate cancer. The detector used consists of an LED white light for irradiation and a photodiode for detection. (Reproduced with permission from Barroso et al. (2022))

white light, but with light of a wavelength that is specific to the analyte (Fig. 7.9) (Rennie et al., 2017).

A method based on visible absorption spectroscopy for the determination of white blood cells was developed by Barroso et al. (2022) All that is required for this method is a single drop of blood for determination, which is placed in a plug-in capsule and inserted into the prototype Aglo T2020 vis-SWNIR POC spectrophotometer. Concentration calibration was done using the characteristic white blood cell absorbance peak at ~600 nm for low concentrations and ~450 nm for high concentrations. Using this method, a functional range of 5.6 to 17.8×10^9 cells/L was obtained, using principal component analysis and artificial intelligence for optimization of datasets as it relates to spectral changes.

A company based out of Toronto, MolecuLight, developed a fluorescence imaging point-of-care device (i:X) for bioimaging purposes. Rennie et al. used this technology combined with the naturally present porphyrins in bacteria to determine the presence of bacteria in wounds (Rennie et al., 2017). The device utilized a 405 nm excitation light to irradiate the wound, which would lead to skin and collagen tissue to emit green and bacteria to emit red due to the porphyrins present (collected by a dual-band fluorescence emission filter in front of the detector). The benefit of this method is that no addition of chemicals or ex situ testing is required. All testing is done in situ and does not require invasive procedures for analysis, with the drawback being a lack of quantitative data.

There are many ways in which the field of optical sensing for POC is being improved by way of optimizing sensitivity, sample size/volume, accuracy, and turnaround time. One recent innovation to those ends is the incorporation of microfluidics into POC testing systems. *Microfluidics* provides an efficient way to analyse multiple analytes while dealing with small sample volumes for rapid diagnostics (Zarean Mousaabadi et al. 2023).

LFA, as mentioned before, is an example of a microfluidic system that is commercially available. However, for testing multiple analytes at once without having to use a different assay each time, microfluidic channels are needed. One example comes from Bordbar et al., where they had fabricated a paper substrate with microfluidic structures for 16 different biomarkers primarily for the determination of COVID-19, and for the determination and isolation of other comorbiditics such as diabetes, chronic kidney diseases, and liver disorders (Bordbar et al. 2022).

A fluorescence-based microfluidic optical sensor for the detection of COVID-19 was also developed by Soares et al., in which they were able to use a smartphone to measure a quantitative signal using the greyscale intensity of the image. Beads functionalized with N-benzyl-N-methylethanolamine (NBNM) agarose were packed into the microfluidic channels and centrifuged together with the patient samples. Upon interacting with full-length SARS-CoV-2 RNA, fluorescence is observed (Fig. 7.10). Using the microfluidic centrifuge method, multiple samples can be run at once, reducing turnaround time (Soares et al. 2021).

Zinc oxide arrays have been used recently for the detection of cancer cells. A zinc fluoride hydroxide (Zn(OH)F) array-based microfluidic device was developed by Zhao et al., using a substrate-induced growth strategy (Zhao et al. 2021). Using

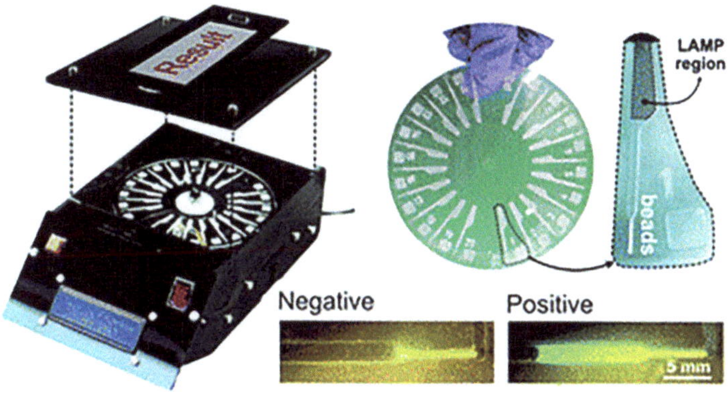

Fig. 7.10 A bead-based microfluidic device based on fluorescence for the determination of COVID-19. (Reproduced with permission from Soares et al. (2021))

glass capillaries, ZnO arrays were first fabricated to be used as the substrate. Following this, the growth of Zn(OH)F arrays was done, facilitated by the existing ZnO arrays. This effectively served as an immunoassay for the detection of labelled cancer cells. To aid in the interaction of the Zn(OH)F array with the cancer biomarkers, specifically human epididymis-specific protein 4 (HE4), the arrays were functionalized with mouse anti-HE4, and a stepwise flow method was followed, which involved the flow of the HE4 biomarker solution which the mouse anti-HE4 would capture, followed by goat anti-HE4, which would sandwich the HE4 biomarker in the array. Finally, a Cy3 fluorescent dye functionalized with immunoglobulin G would be flowed through, binding to the goat anti-HE4 and allowing for the detection of fluorescence within the array via confocal microscopy. The Zn(OH)F arrays enhance the already intense fluorescence of Cy3 due to the evanescent electric field generated by the array upon irradiation with 550 nm light, which enhances the emission intensity of the Cy3 dye. When detecting HE4, the limit of detection using the 566 nm emission line was 9.3 fM.

One type of microfluidic device is what is known as "lab-on-a-chip." These devices are characterized by the ability to perform several analyses on a single chip, ranging in size from only a few millimetres to a few centimetres across (Dkhar et al. 2023). One example of this is a silicon waveguide-based optical sensor developed by Kohler et al. for the detection of fibrinogen, a protein that contributes to blood clotting (Kohler et al. 2021). A pump laser is shone onto a series of silicon-nitrogen organic hybrid lasers (SiNOH). This allows the SiNOH laser to emit light through the waveguide towards the microfluidic chamber, in which the waveguides are functionalized with antibodies specific to certain analytes. Readout is done with a grating coupler array, which diffracts the light onto a readout camera. Using this setup to measure fibrinogen, they use the induced phase shift as an indicator of analyte presence, with a larger phase shift indicating higher concentrations. In doing this, an LOD of 2.14 nm was obtained. Microfluidic devices can also be integrated into wearable sensor technologies, such as the fluorometric patch developed by Sekine

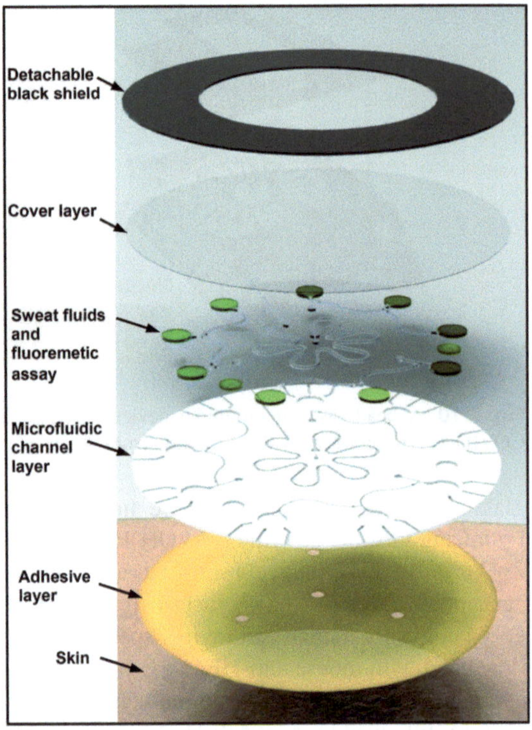

Fig. 7.11 A wearable microfluidic device for the purposes of testing ion levels in sweat. (Reproduced with permission from Sekine et al. (2018))

et al. (2018) This device is an extremely simple design in which microfluidic channels prefilled with fluorescent biomarkers can be stuck onto the patient's skin by way of an adhesive (Fig. 7.11). Sweat excreted from the patient then flows through these microfluidic channels and comes into contact with the fluorophores. Upon exposure to light, these fluorophores will emit green light, with their intensities corresponding to the concentration of the target analyte. By using a smartphone image, image processing software can be used to determine the intensity of emitted light compared to a reference. This method was used to measure the concentrations of Na, Cl, and Zn in human sweat, and was found to accurately measure concentrations of each ion down to 20 mM for Na, 5 mM for Cl, and 1 mM for Zn, which is well below the range expected in physiological systems (20–60 mM).

An important aspect that is of concern when designing POC devices is the transducing material, upon which a stimulus will elicit a response. Smart materials are a class of such materials, defined by their reliable and replicable response to stimuli, making them very attractive candidates for on-site diagnostics (Mahato et al. 2018). One example is a miniaturized five-channel assay based on electrochemiluminescence (ECL) developed by Abbasi and Wachsmann-Hogiu (2024) Here, microfluidic channels were cast directly on top of a CMOS detector for imaging and analysis (Fig. 7.12). A carrier electrolyte solution utilizing luminol was used for its emissive properties, which are intensified when voltage is applied. The microfluidic channels are placed on a conductive Indium Tin Oxide (ITO) substrate (for voltage

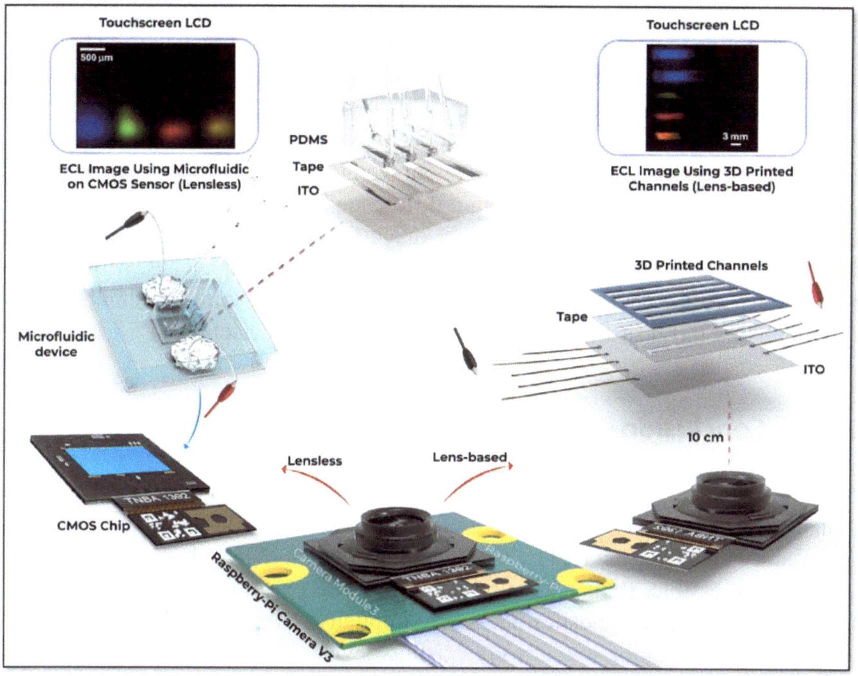

Fig. 7.12 The component parts of an electrochemiluminescence-based microfluidic device. (Reproduced with permission from Abbasi and Wachsmann-Hogiu (2024))

application), which is then placed over a CMOS detector. As an increasing AC voltage is applied across the channels, the intensity increases. When solutions of hydrogen peroxide are flowed through the channels in the presence of the electrolyte solution and a voltage bias, a blue glow is emitted, which is dependent on the concentration of hydrogen peroxide in solution. By optimizing the channel properties and the voltage, an LOD of 614.24 μM is obtained. To make visual changes in analyte concentration even clearer, a mixture of luminophores that involved Ir(III) and Ru(II) complexes was utilized. Between the range of 5 and 12 V, the luminophore solution changes colours from green to orange. To exhibit the possibility of multiplexed measurements, three different analytes were chosen to interact with the three luminophore systems: luminol, Ir(III), and Ru(II). Uric acid and glucose were chosen due to their production of hydrogen peroxide in the presence of enzymes. TPrA was chosen because it is a co-reactant of Ru(II) in ECL systems and because it is a known carcinogen, making it an important analyte for measurement. The device was able to measure both uric acid and glucose with LODs of 26.09 and 16.21 μM, respectively. There was also a marked difference in the measurement between 50 mM and 100 mM TprA, with the channels changing colour from red to pink.

A smart biosensor for the detection of Penicillin G based on a photonic hydrogel was developed by Wang et al. (2024) This was done by embedding Fe_2O_3@SiO_2

colloidal photonic crystals into a poly(N-isopropylacrylamide-co-acrylamide) hydrogel. Using the amidation reaction between the amino groups in the hydrogel and the carboxylic acid groups in the penicillinase, the hydrogel was functionalized with penicillinase so that it can react with penicillin G. This functionalization changes the colour of the hydrogel from blue to orange. The colour reverts back to blue after interaction with penicillin G, with the quantity of change being measured by reflectance spectroscopy, showing a difference in diffraction wavelength going from 663 nm to 510 nm. The functional range for penicillin G determination was found to be 2.8 μM to 2.8 mM, above which the response plateaus. Most importantly, however, the device can be reused up to 50 times by simply washing with hot water, making this a sustainable solution to penicillin G detection.

7.3 Conclusion

In this chapter, the importance of POC testing is discussed. From this need, we have managed to utilize our understanding of human physiology to improve upon existing practices for POC devices by making them smaller, more reliable, more robust, and more accessible. To that end, optical sensing was proposed as a feasible method for accurate on-site diagnostics due to its simplicity in operating principle, as well as its ease of integration into already existing devices. Two types of optical stimuli response, absorbance and emission, are discussed in detail. In addition, the common detection methods used for optical sensing are also discussed. With this knowledge in hand, many applications of optical POC devices were explored, ranging from simple, naked eye detection to disposable methods such as lateral flow assays, to new developments in microfluidics and "lab-on-a-chip" devices, to wearable and reusable optical sensors.

Although the scope is broad, particularly with the advent of artificial intelligence (AI) and its integration into POC testing (Han et al. 2025) several challenges still lie ahead:

1. There is a disconnect between what is already available commercially and what is being published.
2. There are still issues with reliability, and the specificity of these devices is still not fully controlled.
3. Although fabricating an individual proof-of-concept can be relatively cheap, scalability becomes an issue that, for many devices, has not been addressed.
4. Environmental control becomes a hurdle, especially when comparing sensor performances in varying conditions.

However, even with these challenges in mind, the outlook for these devices is positive, and there is much to be learned and to be done in advancing POC testing. To accomplish this, working together with the industry to understand scaling up these devices will be important. In addition, rather than focusing on lowering the limits of detection or improving the dynamic range of these devices, an attempt at stress-testing and ensuring standardization under different conditions may be necessary.

References

Abbasi R, Wachsmann-Hogiu S (2024) Optimization and miniaturization of SE-ECL for potential-resolved, multi-color, multi-analyte detection. Biosens Bioelectron 257:116322. https://doi.org/10.1016/j.bios.2024.116322

Agilent Technologies Inc. The Basics of UV-Vis Spectrophotometry. 2021

Alnajrani MN, Aljohani MM, Chinnappan R, Zourob M, Alsager OA (2022) Highly sensitive and selective lateral flow Aptasensor for anti-coagulant dabigatran Etexilate determination in blood. Talanta 236:122887. https://doi.org/10.1016/j.talanta.2021.122887

Armstrong JA (2007) Urinalysis in Western culture: a brief history. Kidney Int 71(5):384–387. https://doi.org/10.1038/sj.ki.5002057

Barroso TG, Ribeiro L, Gregório H, Monteiro-Silva F, Neves dos Santos F, Martins RC (2022) Point-of-care using Vis-NIR spectroscopy for white blood cell count analysis. Chemosensors 10(11):460. https://doi.org/10.3390/chemosensors10110460

Bordbar MM, Samadinia H, Sheini A, Aboonajmi J, Javid M, Sharghi H, Ghanei M, Bagheri H (2022) Non-invasive detection of COVID-19 using a microfluidic-based colorimetric sensor Array sensitive to urinary metabolites. Microchim Acta 189(9):316. https://doi.org/10.1007/s00604-022-05423-1

Connor H (2001) Medieval Uroscopy and its representation on misericords—part 1: Uroscopy. Clin Med 1(6):507–509. https://doi.org/10.7861/clinmedicine.1-6-507

Deng H, Zhang X, Kumar A, Zou G, Zhang X, Liang X-J (2013) Long genomic DNA amplicons adsorption onto unmodified gold nanoparticles for colorimetric detection of bacillus Anthracis. Chem Commun 49(1):51–53. https://doi.org/10.1039/C2CC37037A

Dkhar DS, Kumari R, Malode SJ, Shetti NP, Chandra P (2023) Integrated lab-on-a-Chip devices: fabrication methodologies, transduction system for sensing purposes. J Pharm Biomed Anal 223:115120. https://doi.org/10.1016/j.jpba.2022.115120

Farmer S, Razin V, Peagler AF, Strickler S, Fain WB, Damhorst GL, Kempker RR, Pollock NR, Brand O, Seitter B, Heilman SS, Nehl EJ, Levy JM, Gottfried DS, Martin GS, Greenleaf M, Ku DN, Waggoner JJ, Iffrig E, Mannino RG, F. Wang Y, Ortlund E, Sullivan J, Rebolledo PA, Clavería V, Roback JD, Benoit M, Stone C, Esper A, Frank F, Lam WA (2022) Don't forget about human factors: lessons learned from COVID-19 point-of-care testing. Cell Rep Methods 2(5):100222. https://doi.org/10.1016/j.crmeth.2022.100222

FE Tech Desk (n.d.) March smartphone frenzy: Nothing Phone 3a series, Xiaomi 15 Ultra, and more — 5 devices to watch out for. Financial Express

Franz KA, Kehr WG, Siggel A, Wieczoreck J, Adam W (2000) Luminescent materials. In: Ullmann's encyclopedia of industrial chemistry. Wiley-VCH Verlag GmbH & Co. KGaA, Weinheim. https://doi.org/10.1002/14356007.a15_519

Grant E (1974) A source book in medieval science. Harvard University Press, Cambridge

Han G, Goncharov A, Eryilmaz M, Ye S, Palanisamy B, Ghosh R, Lisi F, Rogers E, Guzman D, Yigci D, Tasoglu S, Di Carlo D, Goda K, McKendry RA, Ozcan A (2025) Machine learning in point-of-care testing: innovations, challenges, and opportunities. Nat Commun 16:3165. https://doi.org/10.1038/s41467-025-58527-6

Huang S-W, Wu Y-F, Ahmed T, Pan S-C, Cheng C-M (2024) Point-of-care detection devices for wound care and monitoring. Trends Biotechnol 42(1):74–90. https://doi.org/10.1016/j.tibtech.2023.07.001

Jazayeri MH, Aghaie T, Avan A, Vatankhah A, Ghaffari MRS (2018) Colorimetric detection based on gold Nano particles (GNPs): an easy, fast, inexpensive, low-cost and short time method in detection of Analytes (protein, DNA, and ion). Sens Biosensing Res 20:1–8. https://doi.org/10.1016/j.sbsr.2018.05.002

Jesuraj A, Hassan U (2023) Point-of-care portable 3D-printed multispectral sensor for real-time enzyme activity monitoring in healthcare applications. Biosensors (Basel) 13(1):120. https://doi.org/10.3390/bios13010120

Jiang L, Luo J, Dong W, Wang C, Jin W, Xia Y, Wang H, Ding H, Jiang L, He H (2015) Development and evaluation of a Polydiacetylene based biosensor for the detection of H5 influenza virus. J Virol Methods 219:38–45. https://doi.org/10.1016/j.jviromet.2015.03.013

Karnwal A, Kumar Sachan RS, Devgon I, Devgon J, Pant G, Panchpuri M, Ahmad A, Alshammari MB, Hossain K, Kumar G (2024) Gold nanoparticles in Nanobiotechnology: from synthesis to biosensing applications. ACS Omega 9(28):29966–29982. https://doi.org/10.1021/acsomega.3c10352

Kohler D, Schindler G, Hahn L, Milvich J, Hofmann A, Länge K, Freude W, Koos C (2021) Biophotonic sensors with integrated Si3N4-organic hybrid (SiNOH) lasers for point-of-care diagnostics. Light Sci Appl 10(1):64. https://doi.org/10.1038/s41377-021-00486-w

Kost GJ (1992) The hybrid laboratory. The clinical laboratory of the 1990s is a synthesis of the old and the new. Arch Pathol Lab Med 116(10):1002–1003

Kost GJ (1995) Guidelines for point-of-care testing. Improving patient outcomes. Am J Clin Pathol 104(4 Suppl 1):S111–S127

Kost GJ, Tran NK, Tuntideelert M, Kulrattanamaneeporn S, Peungposop N (2006) Katrina, the tsunami, and point-of-care testing. Am J Clin Pathol 126(4):513–520. https://doi.org/10.1309/NWU5E6T0L4PFCBD9

Kost GJ, Tran NK, Louie RF (2008) Point-of-care testing: principles, practice, and critical-emergency-disaster medicine. In: Encyclopedia of analytical chemistry. Wiley. https://doi.org/10.1002/9780470027318.a0540.pub2

Liu X, Zhang H, Qin S, Wang Q, Yang X, Wang K (2019) Optical fiber amplifier for quantitative and sensitive point-of-care testing of myoglobin and MiRNA-141. Biosens Bioelectron 129:87–92. https://doi.org/10.1016/j.bios.2018.12.056

Luppa PB, Müller C, Schlichtiger A, Schlebusch H (2011) Point-of-care testing (POCT): current techniques and future perspectives. TrAC Trends Anal Chem 30(6):887–898. https://doi.org/10.1016/j.trac.2011.01.019

MacKinnon M, Vanderklippe N, Robertson G (2020) Flattery and foot dragging: China's influence over the WHO under scrutiny. The Globe and Mail Toronto

Mahato K, Baranwal A, Srivastava A, Maurya PK, Chandra P (2018) Smart materials for biosensing applications. In: Techno-Societal 2016. Springer International Publishing, Cham, pp 421–431. https://doi.org/10.1007/978-3-319-53556-2_41

Mallick PK (2023) Fundamentals of molecular spectroscopy. Springer Nature Singapore, Singapore. https://doi.org/10.1007/978-981-99-0791-5

Mayerhöfer TG, Pahlow S, Popp J (2020) The Bouguer-beer-Lambert law: shining light on the obscure. ChemPhysChem 21(18):2029–2046. https://doi.org/10.1002/cphc.202000464

McCarthy D, Eapen S (2015) Pregnancy Test Device and Method . US20150094227A1

Ming T, Lan T, Yu M, Cheng S, Duan X, Wang H, Deng J, Kong D, Yang S, Shen Z (2024) Advancements in biosensors for point-of-care testing of nucleic acid. Crit Rev Anal Chem:1–16. https://doi.org/10.1080/10408347.2024.2366943

Moreira L, Guimarães NM, Azevedo NF (2017) Imaging strategies for bioinspired materials. In: Bioinspired materials for medical applications. Elsevier, pp 215–239. https://doi.org/10.1016/B978-0-08-100741-9.00008-5

Morris AS, Langari R (2012) Instrument types and performance characteristics. In: Measurement and instrumentation. Elsevier, pp 11–37. https://doi.org/10.1016/B978-0-12-381960-4.00002-4

Mostufa S, Rezaei B, Ciannella S, Yari P, Gómez-Pastora J, He R, Wu K (2024) Advancements and perspectives in optical biosensors. ACS Omega 9(23):24181–24202. https://doi.org/10.1021/acsomega.4c01872

Pedreira-Rincón J, Rivas L, Comenge J, Skouridou V, Comprubí-Ferrer D, Muñoz J, O'Sullivan CK, Chamorro-Garcia A, Parolo C (2025) A comprehensive review of competitive lateral flow assays over the past decade. Lab Chip 25(11):2578–2608. https://doi.org/10.1039/D4LC01075B

Rasheed S, Kanwal T, Ahmad N, Fatima B, Najam-ul-Haq M, Hussain D (2024) Advances and challenges in portable optical biosensors for onsite detection and point-of-care diagnostics. TrAC Trends Anal Chem 173:117640. https://doi.org/10.1016/j.trac.2024.117640

Rennie MY, Lindvere-Teene L, Tapang K, Linden R (2017) Point-of-care fluorescence imaging predicts the presence of pathogenic bacteria in wounds: a clinical study. J Wound Care 26(8):452–460. https://doi.org/10.12968/jowc.2017.26.8.452

Sekine Y, Kim SB, Zhang Y, Bandodkar AJ, Xu S, Choi J, Irie M, Ray TR, Kohli P, Kozai N, Sugita T, Wu Y, Lee K, Lee K-T, Ghaffari R, Rogers JA (2018) A Fluorometric skin-interfaced microfluidic device and smartphone imaging module for *in situ* quantitative analysis of sweat chemistry. Lab Chip 18(15):2178–2186. https://doi.org/10.1039/C8LC00530C

Shirazi S, Stanford CM, Cooper LF (2021) Testing for COVID-19 in dental offices. J Am Dent Assoc 152(7):514–525.e8. https://doi.org/10.1016/j.adaj.2021.04.019

Simon SH (2013) The Oxford solid state basics. Oxford University Press, Oxford, UK

Slate D, Algeo TP, Nelson KM, Chipman RB, Donovan D, Blanton JD, Niezgoda M, Rupprecht CE (2009) Oral rabies vaccination in North America: opportunities, complexities, and challenges. PLoS Negl Trop Dis 3(12):e549. https://doi.org/10.1371/journal.pntd.0000549

Soares RRG, Akhtar AS, Pinto IF, Lapins N, Barrett D, Sandh G, Yin X, Pelechano V, Russom A (2021) Sample-to-answer COVID-19 nucleic acid testing using a low-cost centrifugal microfluidic platform with bead-based signal enhancement and smartphone read-out. Lab Chip 21(15):2932–2944. https://doi.org/10.1039/D1LC00266J

Stolberg M (2007) The decline of Uroscopy in early modern learned medicine (1500–1650). Early Sci Med 12(3):313–336. https://doi.org/10.1163/157338207X205142

Sze SM, Lee M-K (2012) Semiconductor devices: physics and technology. Wiley

Tavormina MT (2020) The dome of Uryne. Oxford University Press, Oxford

Valeur B, Berberan-Santos M (2012) Molecular fluorescence: principles and applications. Wiley-VCH

Wang X, Wang Y-L, Yu H-R, Lv X-B, Liang T, Cheng C-J (2024) A Penicillinase-modified poly(N-Isopropylacrylamide-co-acrylamide) smart hydrogel biosensor with superior recyclability for sensitive and colorimetric detection of penicillin G. Biosens Bioelectron 254:116221. https://doi.org/10.1016/j.bios.2024.116221

Xiao W, Xiao M, Yao S, Cheng H, Shen H, Fu Q, Zhao J, Tang Y (2019) A rapid, simple, and low-cost CD4 cell count sensor based on blocking Immunochromatographic strip system. ACS Sens 4(6):1508–1514. https://doi.org/10.1021/acssensors.8b01628

Yetisen AK, Akram MS, Lowe CR (2013) Paper-based microfluidic point-of-care diagnostic devices. Lab Chip 13(12):2210. https://doi.org/10.1039/c3lc50169h

Zarean Mousaabadi K, Talebi Vandishi Z, Kermani M, Arab N, Ensafi AA (2023) Recent developments toward microfluidic point of care diagnostic sensors for viral infections. TrAC Trends Anal Chem 169:117361. https://doi.org/10.1016/j.trac.2023.117361

Zhao D, Wu Z, Zhang W, Yu J, Li H, Di W, Duan Y (2021) Substrate-induced growth of micro/nanostructured Zn(OH)F arrays for highly sensitive microfluidic fluorescence assays. ACS Appl Mater Interfaces 13(24):28462–28471. https://doi.org/10.1021/acsami.1c04752

Ziering M, Franzen S (n.d.) The Franck-Condon principle. LibreTexts Chemistry

Smartphone-Based Commercialized Biomedical Devices

8

Vikas Kumar Shukla, Priya Kumari, and Manish S. Sengar

Abstract

Smartphone-based biomedical devices have emerged as transformative tools at the intersection of engineering, biotechnology, and digital health. They are reshaping the delivery of diagnostic and monitoring capabilities in both clinical and nonclinical environments. The ubiquity, computational power, and connectivity of smartphones make them uniquely suited to function as diagnostic hubs. This enables the integration of microfluidics, electrochemical transducers, optical imaging systems, and artificial intelligence into compact, portable, and cost-effective platforms. This convergence has facilitated applications ranging from infectious disease detection, cancer biomarker analysis, to chronic disease management and global epidemiological surveillance. This chapter critically examines both the enabling technologies and the inherent constraints that govern smartphone-integrated biomedical devices. It explores fundamental challenges, including sensor precision, sample variability, environmental interference, and user-dependent operation, while mapping these limitations to emerging solutions in nanomaterial-based sensing, CRISPR-driven nucleic acid detection, federated learning architectures, and modular lab-on-chip platforms. Beyond technical considerations, the text analyzes the regulatory complexity of Software as a

V. K. Shukla
Department of Chemistry and Biochemistry, Worcester Polytechnic Institute, Worcester, MA, USA

P. Kumari
CL203E Core Laboratory, Department of Chemistry, Indian Institute of Technology Kanpur, Kanpur, Uttar Pradesh, India

M. S. Sengar (✉)
Laboratory for Life, Sciences and Technology (LiST), Department of Chemistry, Danube Private University (DPU), Austria, Wiener Neustadt, Austria

V. Patel et al. (eds.), *Biosensor Technology in Translating Novel Materials into Practical Devices*, https://doi.org/10.1007/978-981-95-5519-2_8

Medical Device (SaMD), the ethical implications of algorithmic transparency and informed consent, and the risks of digital inequities in global health contexts.

Emerging research directions highlight the transformative role of smartphones in next-generation diagnostic ecosystems, where multi-parametric analysis, longitudinal health tracking, and digital twins will support personalized, predictive, and preventive medicine. The integration of artificial intelligence (AI)-driven closed-loop therapeutics, blockchain-secured data infrastructures, and scalable mobile networks positions smartphones as critical agents in reshaping both individual healthcare pathways and public health systems. By uniting principles from physics, chemistry, biology, computer science, and regulatory governance, this chapter presents a comprehensive and mechanistic account of smartphone-based biomedical technologies. It underscores their novelty as adaptive, distributed, and intelligent platforms that not only democratize diagnostics but also chart a path toward globally connected, anticipatory healthcare infrastructures.

Keywords

Smartphone sensors · Nucleic acid · CRISPR · On-chip sensors · Biomedical devices

8.1 Introduction

In the twenty-first century, smartphone penetration is tremendous. Based on the World Health Organization program of Be Healthy, Be Mobile (BHBM) reported data, 7 billion people have mobile subscriptions worldwide, and 70% are from developing countries. Moreover, noncommunicable disease is a major cause of 41 million deaths each year, around 71% of all deaths. Considering the widespread availability of mobiles among people and noncommunicable diseases such as heart disease, kidney disease, and diabetes as a significant cause (https://www.who.int/initiatives/behealthy/). Therefore, developing smartphone-based biomedical devices for medical diagnostics is a prominent need in this direction. Smartphone-based biomedical devices are also known as point-of-care testing (POCT) due to easy-to-handle, rapid diagnosis, robustness, cost-effectiveness, and on-site medical diagnosis (Luppa et al. 2011; Zarei 2017; Arduini et al. 2016). POCT devices require the integration of multiple branches such as chemistry and biochemistry, electrical engineering, physics, and biology. The miniaturization of biomedical devices enhances the portability and facilitates the on-site utilization of devices (Martinez et al. 2008). The COVID-19 pandemic highlighted the need for POCT due to at-home antigen testing (Budd et al. 2023) and point-of-care nucleic acid testing (Wilner et al. 2023). The POCT devices made a paradigm shift in the portability and medical diagnosis (Daniels et al. 2023).

However, these devices added a multitude of advantages, but still suffer significant challenges across different modalities, such as lateral flow assays (LFAs) (Kakkar et al. 2024), vertical flow assays (VFAs) (Lei et al. 2022), nucleic acid amplification tests(NAATs) (Maleki and Hojati 2022), optical (Zhang et al. 2022), and electrochemical sensors (Huang et al. 2024). Achieving high sensitivity and accuracy, with a low limit of detection to detect biomarkers present at physiological levels in biofluids. Moreover, the comparable accuracy with the standard clinical laboratory test is always a significant challenge with POCT devices. The use of POCT devices by untrained users is also a major challenge due to quantifying or understanding the test results, such as in LFA, where a faint test line sometimes appears, indicating a positive or negative test; this poses a significant hurdle in the POCT devices (Mukadi et al. 2015). Additionally, the requirement of a machine learning-based algorithm to quantify the false positive or false negative results to enhance the reliability and accuracy of POCT devices will increase the widespread adoption of POCT devices. Considering all the challenges, POCT devices integrated with machine learning/artificial intelligence can overcome the limitations, causing hurdles to the advancement of point-of-care sensors (Ballard et al. 2020; Sun et al. 2023; Yang et al. 2023). There are multiple commercially available point-of-care devices overcoming the limitations using different detection mechanisms, strategies, and artificial intelligence, for better signal processing and data analysis. The commercially available devices listed in Table 8.1 are available in the market based on different biofluids.

The smartphone-based devices are based on four different transduction methodologies, such as electrical, optical, mechanical, and electrochemical. These different transduction methodologies require some additional accessories with the smartphone, which increases the accuracy and precision of medical diagnosis. Moreover, the use of multiplex biomarker detection enhances the reliability of medical diagnosis, as one biomarker may change due to other causes as well. Therefore, the integration of multiplex detection with machine learning enables POCT devices for accurate detection and monitoring of disease (Goncharov et al. 2023; Role of machine learning assisted biosensors in point-of-care-testing for clinical decisions 2025). For example, optimization of the vertical flow assay for multiplexed detection has been achieved by deep learning, which optimally identifies the immunoreaction conditions (Ballard et al. 2020). Additionally, machine learning overcomes the interference in the signal and signal drift caused by unwanted substances present in the complex biofluid, which improves the quantification accuracy and increases the reproducibility compared to classical statistical regression methods (Sun et al. 2023). In this chapter, we will concentrate on the integration of smartphones with biomedical devices, emphasizing various signal transduction methodologies. This discussion will cover the advantages of smartphones in biomedical applications, as well as the challenges related to technical and scientific constraints, regulatory affairs, and the acquisition and management of health data. Additionally, we will explore advancements in sensors utilizing nanomaterials, the role of machine learning, and future directions for the development of POCT devices.

Table 8.1 Commercially available smartphone-based POCT devices

Device name	Sensing modalities mechanism	Cost (USD)	Invasive/ noninvasive	Medical diagnosis of disease
iHealth Align	Electrochemical: test strip modified with glucose oxidase and its interaction with blood, produced an electrical signal directly proportional to glucose concentration	$16.95 to $25	Invasive	Glucometer for monitoring of blood glucose levels (https://ihealthlabs.com/)
AliveCor Kradia Mobile	Electrochemical: finger-touched recording of electrical signals of hearts	$79–$149	Noninvasive	Monitor heart rhythm to predict abnormalities such as atrial fibrillation (https://alivecor.com/).
MobiSante MobiUS	Mechanical: use of piezoelectric transducers to emit and receive ultrasonic waves and data processed using smartphone	$7000 to $10,000		Portable ultrasound device for disease like obstetrics, and cardiology.
CliniCloud	Optical and mechanical: use of stethoscope and thermometer	$99–$149		Fever diagnostics (https://www.design-industry.com.au/clinicloud)
DermLite	Optical: uses smartphone camera, using polarized light and magnifications to capture high resolution image of skin	$500–$1500		Dermatoscope for skin cancer detection such as melanoma (https://dermlite.com/)
EyeNetra	Optical: smartphone added with lenses to capture the pattern of the eye movement	$1000 to $2000		Autorefractor for the vision (https://eyenetra.com/).
Masimo MightySat	Optical: used of red and infrared light absorbed by haemoglobin is analyzed	$250–$400		Finger-clip pulse oximeter for respiratory monitoring (https://www.masimo.com/).
Nonin Onyx II model 9560	Optical: employs red and infrared light to measure SpO_2 and pulse rate	$666		Wireless pulse oximeter for SpO_2 and pulse rate (Tomlinson et al. 2018)
Mobile Assay-mReader	Optical: used image radiometry to read lateral flow assay test strip	$51 to $78		Early detection of Bortytis cinerea (fungus that damage plants) (https://mars20bysdc.com/)

8.2 Integration of Smartphones and Their Sensors in Biomedical Devices

A wide array of sensors compatible with smartphones exists, which can also interface with external sensors through specialized adapters to enhance medical diagnostics. Within this context, several built-in sensors present in smartphones include the following:

- *Accelerometer:* The sensor utilized in smartphones to detect changes in orientation and movement is integral to a variety of applications. This technology plays a crucial role in enhancing user experience in gaming, facilitating automatic screen rotation, and supporting pedometric functionalities. Its ability to accurately measure angular displacement and acceleration allows for dynamic interaction with the device, thereby advancing the capabilities of mobile technology.
- *Gyroscope:* This sensor is used in virtual reality and augmented reality by measuring the angular velocity, which facilitates the precise determination of device orientation. This capability enhances accuracy in spatial orientation, thereby contributing to a more immersive and responsive user experience in these interactive environments. It provides the orientation of devices with enhanced accuracy.
- *Global positioning system (GPS):* This module serves a critical function by providing information regarding the geolocation of a device. Such information is essential for a variety of applications, including cartography, navigation, and geographic analysis. Understanding the precise location of a device is pivotal in enhancing the accuracy and efficiency of location-based services and technological interventions.
- *Barometer:* This sensor is designed to quantify atmospheric pressure, playing a crucial role in meteorological forecasting, altitude determination, and a variety of additional applications. Its ability to accurately measure pressure variations contributes significantly to our understanding of weather patterns and environmental dynamics.

Although these sensor modules may not seem directly involved in medical diagnosis, they play an important indirect role by integrating with medical sensors to enhance services. For instance, an accelerometer helps users align their mobile phones accurately for imaging, thereby ensuring the reproducibility of lateral flow assays. Similarly, GPS and barometric sensors assist in determining patient location and assessing local weather conditions, which can be crucial for timely medical assistance (Li et al. 2016; Majumder and Deen 2019). Thus, the incorporation of these sensor modules provides a significant advantage in improving the overall experience for medically ill patients (Karim et al. 2023).

The following outlines the additional integrated sensors utilized for medical diagnostics:

- *Light sensor:* The device regulates the intensity of light emitted from the screen by measuring ambient light levels. It dynamically adjusts the screen brightness in real-time to optimize the visual experience for the user, thereby enhancing user comfort and reducing eye strain associated with mobile device usage.
- *Fingerprint sensor:* This sensor functions as a biometric authentication tool, contributing significantly to user security. Its deployment is particularly advantageous in safeguarding patient health data, thereby enhancing privacy measures within healthcare systems. This capability underscores the importance of biometric technologies in the protection of sensitive personal information, ensuring compliance with privacy regulations, and fostering trust in digital health solutions.
- *Heart-rate sensor:* The heart rate sensor typically employs photoplethysmography (PPG) as a method for measuring heart rate. This intrinsic sensor is instrumental in providing essential insights into personalized health metrics. By analyzing variations in light absorption and reflection in the vasculature, PPG technology offers valuable data for monitoring cardiovascular health and can facilitate the early detection of potential health issues (Quer et al. 2021).
- *Near-field communication (NFC):* NFC is a technology that facilitates short-range communication between devices in close proximity, commonly utilized for applications such as payments and data exchange. This technology can be effectively employed for wireless data transfer between biosensor modules and smartphones, enabling subsequent analysis and result generation. The integration of NFC in this context enhances the accessibility and efficiency of data transmission, thus supporting advanced analytical processes in various biomedical and health monitoring applications (Boonkaew et al. 2024).

Numerous in-built sensors present in smartphones can be directly or indirectly integrated into biosensor modules, significantly enhancing their role in medical diagnostics. For instance, the smartphone camera serves as a valuable tool for optical detection (Karim et al. 2023), contributing to the overall functionality of these diagnostic systems. Such integration not only expands the potential applications of smartphones in healthcare but also promotes the development of accessible and efficient diagnostic methods.

The ubiquitous availability of smartphones among a substantial segment of the population, combined with their intuitive user interfaces, significantly facilitates the integration of smartphone technology with handheld medical devices. This convergence not only augments the functionality of these devices but also makes them more economically viable and practical for routine use. External biosensor modules can be specifically designed to focus on the detection, quantification, and monitoring of disease biomarkers. These external biosensor modules are developed utilizing various sensing transduction methodologies, including electrical, optical, electrochemical, and mechanical approaches, thereby enhancing their applicability in clinical and diagnostic settings.

8.2.1 Optical Biomedical Devices

Most optical-based medical diagnostic devices necessitate the use of specialized cameras, lasers, and monochromatic wavelength light. These components provide distinct advantages, including the ability to capture high-resolution images and facilitate absorption measurements at specific wavelengths. For example, Guo *et.al* reported a smartphone-based multiplexed DNA-based detection using a lateral flow assay in remote and low-resource settings. They implemented a CNN-based model for the self-prediction of results based on the data, with more than 98% accuracy (Guo et al. 2021). Similarly, Palekar *et.al* reported detection of kidney biomarkers using a smartphone-based portable colorimetric sensor. They have used 3D printed integrated LED lights in a controlled environment and then calculated the RGB values based on the variation in the intensity of test lines. The biomarkers are uric acid, creatinine, and albumin, detectable in the physiological range (Palekar et al. 2025).

8.2.2 Electrochemical Biomedical Devices

Electrochemical medical sensors are engineered through the modification of the working electrode utilizing various nanomaterials tailored to specific requirements, such as antibody–antigen interactions or antibody-protein binding events (da Silva et al. 2017). The selection of the most suitable electrochemical technique is critical for accurately capturing the nuanced variations in analyte concentration at the working electrode, thereby enhancing the sensitivity and specificity of the sensor. The electrochemical integrated smartphone based devices have higher sensitivity and are capable of quantifying the analyte concentration in the physiological range. For example, Boonkaew et al developed a near field communication smartphone-based electrochemical microfluidic device for C-reactive protein (CRP) quantification in artificial serum, plasma, and whole blood. The electrode of the POCT device was modified by the nanobodies for higher sensitivity, and the chronocoulometric response was recorded using redox species $[K_3Fe(CN)_6]^{3-/4-}$. The CRP is known for many inflammatory diseases, and its quantitative measurement in the complex biofluid is crucial for the detection of disease (Boonkaew et al. 2024). Su et al detected the exosomes, which are potential cancer-related biomarkers. Su developed an electrochemically enabled smartphone for the quantification and analysis of exosomes in biofluids. They reported the limit of detection as low as 7.23 ng of CD63-positive exosomes in 5 μL of serum within 2 hr. (Su et al. 2022). We understood that electrochemically developed smartphone-based medical diagnostic devices need a compact biosensor module, such as a potentiostat, to work. Therefore, an affordable potentiostat is a mandatory requirement for better reach of electrochemical smartphone devices. Sun *et.al* fabricated two different power-based potentiostats, with the first prototype costing less than $30 (Sun et al. 2014).

8.2.3 Electrical Biomedical Devices

Biomedical devices equipped with electrical technology are designed to monitor and analyze bioelectrical heart rhythms, helping to identify various medical conditions. For instance, both the Apple Watch and Fitbit include ECG sensors to detect irregular heart rhythms that may indicate atrial fibrillation. Additionally, the Samsung Galaxy Watch is capable of measuring body composition, including body-fat percentage, body-water content, and skeletal muscle mass using bioelectrical impedance analysis (Vargas et al. 2023).

8.2.4 Other Biomedical Devices

There are other transduction methodologies that have introduced acoustic-based systems, which encompass both sonar and passive sensing technologies. These systems leverage integrated microphones and speakers to facilitate contactless monitoring. Specifically, active sonar systems generate tailored sound waves through the speaker while simultaneously capturing audio via the microphone, thus enabling the measurement of human physiological movements such as breathing and heartbeat through the analysis of acoustic reflections (Min et al. 2023; Ray et al. 2019).

A pertinent example of this technology is the ApneaApp (King et al. 2017), a noncontact monitoring system that utilizes a smartphone to meticulously track subtle respiratory and motion patterns in the chest and abdomen. This application is designed to detect sleep apnea and hypopnea events by continuously emitting inaudible frequency-modulated continuous wave signals, subsequently analyzing the reflections that return from the individual. There are other biomedical devices such as motion-tracking systems, color analysis pattern systems, and many more. In addition, hybrid multimodal sensors possess the capability to simultaneously monitor biomolecular activities while also measuring parameters such as pH and ion concentrations. These advanced biomedical sensors are engineered in the form of wearable devices, facilitating continuous health monitoring and promoting proactive healthcare management (Song et al. 2023; Hybrid multimodal wearable sensors for comprehensive health monitoring 2025).

8.3 Machine Learning with Biomedical Devices

The integration of smartphones with medical accessories provides a platform for developing applications capable of processing various recorded signals, including electrical, optical, mechanical, and electrochemical. A smartphone-enabled interface must be capable of running machine learning models such as CNN (including ResNet50, MobileNetV2, and Visual Transformer networks), LSTM, YOLO, SVM, and both supervised and self-supervised learning applications (Najjar 2023; Cui et al. 2020; Choi et al. 2020). The accuracy and precision of these models are critical for enhancing disease prediction. In Table 8.2, we will review the developed models and their corresponding accuracy metrics.

8.4 Advantages of Smartphone-Based Biomedical Devices

The information presented in Table 8.1 highlights the various advantages of commercially available smartphone-based POCT devices. In a similar vein, Table 8.2 focuses on detection methods that utilize invasive and noninvasive sampling through smartphone-based POCT. The benefits of POCT include the following:

- *Portability:* To enhance the accessibility of smartphone-based medical diagnostic devices, it is essential for them to be compact and user-friendly. Additionally, the positioning of related sensing accessories should be carefully considered to ensure the longevity of the devices. This approach will not only broaden the device's reach but also significantly boost testing capabilities.
- *Accessibility:* According to the WHO's BHBM program, approximately 70% of the global population has access to smartphones. What is essential now is the availability of an affordable biosensor module with enhanced analytical measurement capabilities. Additionally, the integration of machine learning models must ensure accuracy and precision for medical diagnostic tests.
- *Cost-effectiveness:* Thanks to significant advancements in the semiconductor industry, the cost of smartphones has dramatically decreased over the past few years. This reduction in price has encouraged many people to purchase smartphones, which, when integrated with diagnostic devices, have proven to be more affordable than traditional laboratory testing. However, traditional lab tests are still regarded as the gold standard for comparison with smartphone-based diagnostic devices.
- *Telemedicine:* Telemedicine services allow patients to consult with doctors regarding their medical concerns. Through this service, individuals can receive medical consultations after a diagnosis is made, utilizing smartphone-based sensors. This approach enhances personalized healthcare and supports individuals in rural areas.

The integration of smartphones with biomedical devices presents numerous advantages, particularly in the context of POCT (Guo et al. 2021; Sun et al. 2014). This technological convergence significantly reduces the size of instruments, minimizes the required sample volume, accelerates the time to results, and enhances accessibility in rural areas. However, POCT devices are often plagued by challenges related to sensitivity, selectivity, limits of detection, and the occurrence of false positive results. In the forthcoming discussion, we will explore these challenges in depth and examine strategies to mitigate these limitations, ultimately aiming to enhance the robustness and accuracy of POCT systems.

Table 8.2 Invasive- and noninvasive-based study for medical diagnosis

Biological sample	Specimen	Biomarkers	Sensing modalities	Artificial and machine learning models	Cost (per test)	Limit of detection	Time
Invasive	Serum	CRP (Ballard et al. 2020)	Colorimetric (AuNPs)	FCNN, liner regression R^2= 0.95, CV= 11.2%	\$2	LoD: 0.1 µg/mL Detection range: 0.1–1000 µg/mL	<12 min
	Serum	Myoglobin, CK-MB, h-FABP (Goncharov et al. 2023)	Fluorescent (CPN)	FCNN, linear and poly- regression R^2 = 0.92 and CV: ~12%	\$3.3	LoD: 0.52 ng/ml for myoglobin, 0.3 ng/mL for CK-MB, 0.49 ng/mL for FABP	<15 min
	Serum	Cholesterol (Jang et al. 2024)	Electrochemical (FET-based)	FCNN R^2 > 0.976 CV < 6.46%	NA	LoD: 28.5 µg/dL	<2.5 min
	Cervical brushing samples	HPV16 and HPV18 (Roh et al. 2023)	Fluorescent	Mark R-CNN Accuracy: 97.9% F1 score: 97.8%	NA	LoD: 2aM (1.2 copies/uL)	~2 h
	Whole blood	Plasmodium sp. causing malaria (Guo et al. 2021)	Colorimetric	CNN ResNet50, accuracy 97.83%	~\$20	NA	<1 h
	Plasma, whole blood	CRP (Boonkaew et al. 2024)	Electochemical	Linear calibration	~\$0.23	LoD: 7.6 pg/mL Linear range (10 ng/mL–100 µg/ml)	15 min

Noninvasive	NP swabs	SARS-CoV-2 RNA (Yang et al. 2023)	SERS	RNN, accuracy: 98.9%	NA	Detection range: 10^3–10^9	<25 min
	Urine, saliva, sweat	Tuberculosis Rv-1656 antigen, SARS-CoV-2 (Tay et al. 2023)	Colorimetric (TMB)	Computational-driven models	~$800 (reader)	LoD: (saliva) 0.1–1 nM	NA
	Sweat	Glucose, lactate, uric acid, magnesium ions, pH value (Cheng et al. 2023)	Electrochemical	Linear regression	NA	NA	10–15 min

*(abbreviation used in the table 8.2)CRP: C-reactive protein, R^2 regression square, *CV* coefficient of variation, *LoD* limit of detection, *FCNN* fully connected neural networks, *RNN* recurrent neural network, *SERS* surface enhanced Raman spectroscopy, *NA* not applicable, *NP* nasopharyngeal swab

8.5 Challenges and Limitations

8.5.1 Technical and Scientific Constraints in Smartphone-Based Biomedical Devices

The development and deployment of smartphone-based biomedical systems are fundamentally constrained by a range of factors originating from physics, chemistry, biology, engineering, and socio-technological systems. These challenges include hardware sensitivity limitations, unstable biotic interfaces, environmental variability, inconsistent regulatory coverage, and fragmented data protection strategies. Together, these obstacles hinder reproducibility, diagnostic accuracy, and the global scalability of smartphone-enabled diagnostics (Banik et al. 2021; Tyagi et al. 2024). Commercial smartphones are engineered for consumer-centric applications, photography, navigation, and communication, not biomedical precision. Core components such as CMOS image sensors, microphones, gyroscopes, and accelerometers are optimized for general performance, lacking the spectral range, noise suppression, and quantification fidelity required for diagnostic purposes. CMOS sensors, in particular, exhibit lower quantum efficiency and narrower spectral responsivity compared to scientific-grade CCD detectors (Baker et al. 2025). This shortfall is especially problematic for biosensing platforms that depend on the detection of fluorescence, chemiluminescence, or narrow-band optical signatures. To compensate, signal acquisition systems must undergo detailed algorithmic recalibration. In optical diagnostics, distortions caused by lens aberration, chromatic dispersion, or illumination asymmetry must be corrected using image transformation matrices, radiometric compensation, and denoising pipelines. In quantitative assays, whether enzyme-linked immunoassays, lateral flow tests, or molecular amplification platforms, these corrections directly impact the accuracy of threshold-based classification and analyte quantification (Madrid et al. 2022).

Smartphone microphones, typically tuned to voice frequency ranges, lack the bandwidth or sensitivity for nuanced auscultatory data such as heart murmurs or respiratory artifacts. Similarly, embedded inertial sensors often suffer from low sampling rates and cumulative integration drift, which compromise the resolution required for clinical gait analysis or tremor detection. Device-to-device variability compounds these challenges. Differences in pixel architecture, image pipeline firmware, optical focal length, and processing algorithms introduce inconsistencies in raw data acquisition. Embedded software enhancements, including white balance correction, gamma compression, and edge sharpening, may irreversibly modify biomedical signal integrity, complicating efforts toward cross-device standardization or reference calibration (Antonini et al. 2025; Kong et al. 2024; Chan et al. 2025; Ahmad et al. 2025; Biomedical devices and sensors 2025).

8.5.2 Biological and Biochemical Constraints

Biological fluids, such as blood, saliva, urine, sweat, and interstitial fluid, are chemically complex, heterogeneous, and physiologically variable. They consist of proteins, enzymes, lipids, salts, nucleic acids, and cellular components, all of which can interfere with the functionality of biosensors (Sengar et al. 2023). These interferences arise through nonspecific binding, matrix effects, pH shifts, ionic fluctuation, or enzyme degradation, each of which can degrade signal specificity or alter reaction kinetics. Electrochemical biosensors face challenges in unprocessed samples (Sengar et al. 2024). Interferents such as uric acid, glucose, or ascorbic acid generate overlapping oxidation peaks, reducing selectivity (Kumari et al. 2024). Protein adsorption onto electrodes, biofouling, degrades redox kinetics, suppresses current response, and destabilizes open circuit potential. Over time, these factors cause signal drift and compromise detection thresholds (Bui et al. 2023; Kamble et al. 2025; Sengar et al. 2025).

Optical biosensing methods are similarly constrained. The kinetics of antibody-antigen interactions, enzyme-substrate catalysis, and DNA hybridization are highly sensitive to temperature, pH, ionic strength, and reagent purity. Enzymatic assays follow Michaelis–Menten behavior and respond nonlinearly to variations in substrate concentration or environmental factors (Banik et al. 2021). Fluorescent dyes and chromophores are susceptible to photo-instability under ambient light or uncontrolled LED output, resulting in photobleaching and spectral distortion (Baker et al. 2025). Microfluidic systems embedded in smartphone-based devices introduce further instability. Fluid handling mechanisms reliant on capillary action or evaporation-driven flow can experience clogging, uneven wicking, or inconsistent reagent contact. Variability in paper porosity, hydrophilic coating, and substrate aging reduces reproducibility. In ambient conditions, degradation of stored reagents, including antibodies and enzymes, due to moisture, heat, or oxidation, remains a key limitation. Without controlled storage and rehydration protocols, degradation compromises analytical performance and test reliability (Ameku et al. 2022; Sengar et al. 2021).

8.5.3 Environmental and Operational Variability

Point-of-care and field-based smartphone diagnostics must function under uncontrolled environmental conditions. Temperature gradients, ambient light variability, humidity levels, electromagnetic noise, and barometric pressure all influence signal generation and detection. In optical systems, lighting variability alters spectral response. Smartphone sensors adapt exposure and white balance based on ambient conditions, which alters image consistency. Without internal light control or reference standards, colorimetric and fluorescence assays may yield divergent results for the same sample (Banik et al. 2021; Sengar et al. 2025; Panigrahi et al. 2025). Thermal shifts affect enzyme activity, nucleic acid hybridization, and antigen binding. Reaction rates governed by the Arrhenius equation double with each 10 °C increase in temperature. Without onboard thermal regulation, these variations shift assay timing, reaction kinetics, and calibration curves. Microfluidic flow dynamics are also temperature-sensitive, with viscosity and capillarity affected by thermal gradients. In open-channel or paper-based systems, evaporation can artificially concentrate solutes or reduce the flow rate (Vashist et al. 2014; Piaggio et al. 2021).

Humidity changes degrade reagent stability and influence substrate swelling. Paper substrates may rehydrate prematurely under high humidity or desiccate under dry conditions, affecting assay progression. In polymer-based channels, water absorption alters surface energy, modifying flow behavior. Mechanical disturbances, such as device tilt, motion, or impact, can disrupt optical alignment or fluid flow. These physical inconsistencies are magnified when used in mobile or outdoor scenarios. Human operational variability remains a critical limiting factor. Users may deviate from prescribed protocols in sample application, incubation timing, or result interpretation. Devices designed for lay use require built-in guidance mechanisms such as visual prompts, audio feedback, and user-lockout periods to enforce timing. Even with these features, consistency across users remains challenging (Kumari et al. 2024; Zhao et al. 2020).

8.5.4 Regulatory, Security, and Ethical Hurdles

Smartphone diagnostics blur traditional boundaries of device classification, introducing ambiguity across regulatory jurisdictions. Regulatory bodies must assess not only physical components but also digital logic and dynamic software systems. Algorithms that evolve via machine learning pose validation challenges, particularly when their output changes based on incoming data. Frameworks such as SaMD require validation protocols across software lifecycle stages, development, deployment, update management, and cybersecurity resilience (Hossain et al. 2024). Cross-platform variability, app-store distribution mechanisms, and external dependencies (sensor modules, data APIs) further complicate oversight. Diagnostics involving AI must also meet explainability, fairness, and reproducibility requirements under evolving international standards (Biomedical devices and sensors 2025; Cohen et al. 2020).

Cybersecurity risks are amplified by constant connectivity. Diagnostic data often passes through unsecured wireless links or resides on third-party cloud infrastructure. Improper encryption, exposed endpoints, or flawed update mechanisms create attack surfaces. AI models, in particular, are vulnerable to adversarial manipulation through subtle data perturbations. Data jurisdiction and cross-border data flows raise legal concerns. Patient data stored in remote servers may fall under foreign data protection laws. Many LMICs lack mature legal frameworks, exposing users to unregulated data mining or discriminatory profiling. Digital consent interfaces are often designed for compliance rather than comprehension, diminishing user autonomy (Tyagi et al. 2024; Madrid et al. 2022; Ross et al. 2023).

8.5.5 Data Security, Privacy, and Ethical Concerns

Smartphone-integrated diagnostics capture health-related data with high temporal resolution and potentially high granularity. This includes not only biomarker data but behavioral metadata, mobility, geolocation, and usage timing, which can be re-aggregated into predictive health models. Each of these data streams carries re-identification risk. Data flow in these systems occurs across multiple layers: device-level processing, transmission interfaces, remote computation, and long-term storage. Each layer introduces exposure to breach. Bluetooth protocols, unsecured cloud APIs, and legacy encryption schemes are frequent vulnerabilities. SDKs from third parties may introduce hidden telemetry or share data with undisclosed recipients (Hossain et al. 2024; Ross et al. 2023). Consent practices are often superficial. Lengthy privacy policies, obligatory acceptance for functionality access, and vague data-sharing statements all reduce transparency. Behavioral data, even anonymized, may be exploited in downstream applications unrelated to diagnostics. Without data dividends, feedback mechanisms, or participatory governance, patients lose visibility and control over the value extracted from their data. Bias in training datasets for AI-based systems remains a persistent risk. Unequal representation across population groups leads to skewed predictions. Misdiagnosis, underperformance in minority cohorts, or uncalibrated recommendations can amplify healthcare disparities (Tyagi et al. 2024; Krittanawong et al. 2021) (Fig. 8.1).

8.5.6 Regulatory and Legal Barriers

Regulatory frameworks struggle to accommodate the hybrid nature of smartphone-based biomedical systems. Traditional classifications based on risk and intended use do not map well to modular systems where hardware, software, and algorithms interact dynamically. The absence of clearly defined units of regulation, whether device, app, or cloud platform, complicates oversight. Agencies such as the FDA in the United States and EMA in Europe mandate different approval routes for devices, including 510(k), De Novo, and PMA. Devices using AI models or adaptive algorithms often require bespoke clinical validation. In the EU, MDR and IVDR add layers of documentation, QMS compliance, and performance benchmarking. SaMD classifications trigger further obligations across the software lifecycle, cybersecurity, and real-world evidence generation (Kumar et al. 2024).

Global deployment is hindered by a lack of harmonized standards. Country-specific regulatory pathways, India's CDSCO, China's NMPA, Japan's PMDA, demand region-specific technical dossiers, often in incompatible formats (Ali et al. 2024). This disjointed landscape inflates regulatory costs and discourages small developers. Legal liability remains unresolved in distributed diagnostic systems. Responsibility for diagnostic error in decentralized usage is unclear. Device manufacturers, app developers, platform providers, and end-users may share risk, but no unified legal model governs this division. Intellectual property complexities arise due to the use of mixed-ownership components. Patented microfluidic devices, proprietary algorithms, and open-source libraries often coexist in one product, creating friction in licensing and enforcement (Biomedical devices and sensors 2025). Addressing these barriers will require adaptive regulatory science, stakeholder engagement, and international cooperation on performance-based, flexible approval models. Without these structural reforms, innovation will remain fragmented and unevenly accessible (Banik et al. 2021; Tyagi et al. 2024).

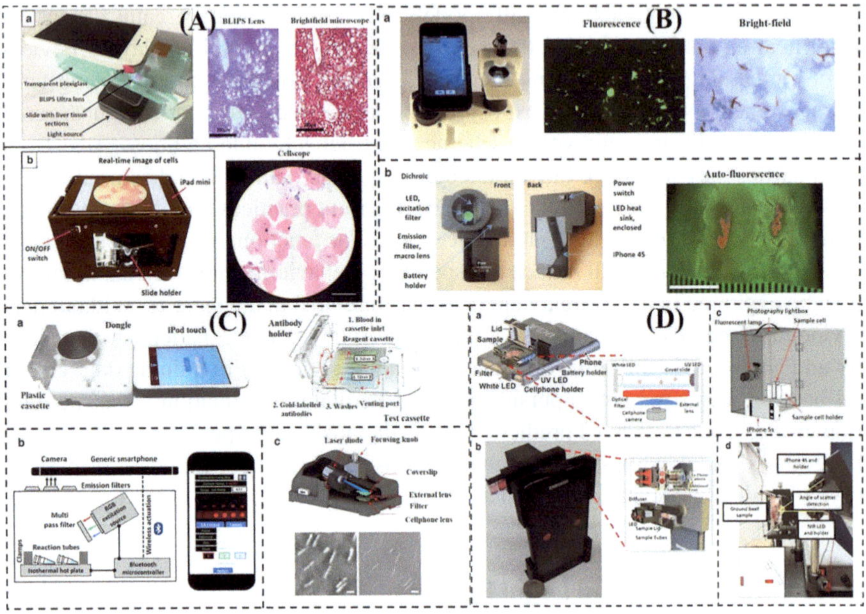

Fig. 8.1 Smartphone-based imaging and diagnostic systems. (**A**) Smartphone-based imaging platforms. (a) The BLIPS lens-based smartphone microscopy system along with acquired images of a human liver tissue section, compared to corresponding images captured by a conventional bright-field microscope. (b) Real-time image acquisition of cancer cells using a smartphone-based system. (**B**) Fluorescence-based smartphone imaging systems. (a) The CellScope system with 3D-printed components for fluorescence microscopy; representative images show Mycobacterium tuberculosis under green fluorescence and red bright-field illumination. (b) The PRODIGI system, illustrating its modular design for real-time autofluorescence imaging of wounds; green fluorescence indicates collagen, while red fluorescence denotes bacterial presence. (**C**) Smartphone-integrated nucleic acid and immunoassay detection platforms. (a) A smartphone-based immunoassay system for viral detection, integrated with a microfluidic cassette preloaded with antibodies and enzyme reagents. (b) A smartphone-operated reverse transcription loop-mediated isothermal amplification (RT-LAMP) device, featuring a mobile application for real-time reaction monitoring. (c) A smartphone-based fluorescence imaging platform for DNA visualization and fragment sizing; the device-acquired image depicts fluorescent DNA bands. (**D**) Smartphone-enabled colorimetric and scattering-based biosensing platforms. (a) A smartphone-based protein microarray detection system with a 3D-printed optical attachment and schematic illustration of the fluorescence detection module. (b) Schematic of a smartphone-assisted fluorescence colorimetric assay platform for biomolecular analysis. (c) Prototype of a near-infrared (NIR) smartphone-based device utilizing Mie scattering to detect bacterial contamination in beef; the inset highlights angular orientations used for scattering detection. (d) The iTube smartphone platform for colorimetric assay analysis; the magnified view illustrates the internal optical configuration and detection module. (Adapted from Banik et al. (2021) copyright © 2021 Springer Nature)

8.6 Emerging Trends and Research Directions

Smartphone-based biomedical diagnostics are undergoing a technological renaissance driven by the intersection of advanced scientific disciplines, including quantum-scale materials engineering, programmable molecular biology, low-power embedded computation, and human-centred cyber-physical systems (Kumar et al. 2024). These trajectories are collectively redefining the smartphone as a multifunctional biosensing device, no longer constrained by its original commercial architecture for communication and media but reimagined as a portable analytical laboratory with embedded intelligence. This transformation is underpinned by innovations that transcend the limitations of classical mobile computing (Banik et al. 2021). Recent advancements have extended smartphone capabilities beyond image and signal capture into domains that demand high analytical fidelity, such as biomolecular discrimination, electrochemical quantification, and real-time physiological pattern recognition. By incorporating synthetic biorecognition frameworks, nanoscale transduction elements, and autonomous signal interpretation, smartphones are being transformed into platforms capable of executing complex diagnostic protocols without requiring centralized laboratory infrastructure (Bui et al. 2023).

These technological developments are influencing not only the analytical modalities but also the spatiotemporal deployment of diagnostics. The traditional dependency on centralized laboratories with controlled environments is being replaced by ubiquitous testing at the site of care or user proximity, supported by cloud-based data infrastructure and edge computation. This decentralization is fostering a shift toward dynamic health surveillance, enabling smartphones to perform continuous monitoring of biological states and behavioral contexts in both clinical and ambient settings. The following subsections delineate the major axes of research that are actively reshaping the future landscape of mobile diagnostics, each rooted in distinct scientific principles yet synergistically integrated through the smartphone platform (Hossain et al. 2024; Krittanawong et al. 2021).

8.6.1 Nanotechnology-Enabled Biosensing

Nanotechnology provides a fundamental enhancement in the interaction between biological targets and transducer surfaces by exploiting material behavior at submicrometer dimensions. Nanostructured elements increase the effective surface area, enhance signal-to-noise ratios, and allow manipulation of electron transport and photonic interactions for more precise analyte detection. Metallic nanoparticles, particularly those based on noble metals such as gold and silver, support resonance phenomena where collective electron oscillations interact with incident electromagnetic fields. This localized surface plasmon resonance (LSPR) effect alters the optical properties of the nanoparticle in response to molecular binding events, which can be detected through smartphone imaging sensors with spectral filters. Functionalization of these particles with site-specific recognition ligands enables selective binding, converting molecular interactions into quantifiable shifts in absorbance or scattering (Patel et al. 2024; Dkhar et al. 2023; Nandi et al. 2024).

Carbonaceous nanomaterials, including graphene and carbon nanotubes, offer high charge carrier mobility, chemical tunability, and mechanical flexibility. When incorporated into electrochemical sensors, these materials enable field-effect transduction where the presence of charged biomolecules induces conductivity changes measurable through portable potentiostats (Sengar et al. 2022a, b). These electrical signals, digitized through smartphone-integrated circuits, provide a direct route to molecular concentration analysis without external amplification. Quantum-confined semiconductor nanocrystals, known as quantum dots, present tunable electronic band gaps that emit wavelength-specific fluorescence. This photonic behavior permits the simultaneous detection of multiple biomolecules in a single assay by coupling unique emission wavelengths to different targets. Their resistance to photobleaching and compatibility with compact light-emitting and detection hardware make them ideal for integration into mobile assay cartridges (Kumar et al. 2024; Kumari et al. 2025; Shubhangi et al. 2024; Yadav et al. 2021).

Advances in nanofabrication have also enabled the construction of hierarchical topographies such as nanowires, nanopillars, and porous films, each designed to increase ligand density, promote binding kinetics, and lower detection thresholds. These structures, when combined with surface chemistry strategies such as thiol-gold self-assembly, silanization, and covalent linker chemistries, facilitate robust biorecognition under physiological conditions. Nanotechnology is therefore expanding the analytical frontier of smartphone biosensing by bridging material science with bioanalytical chemistry, providing the necessary sensitivity and selectivity for real-world deployment (Mahapatra et al. 2025; Patel et al. 2023; Purohit et al. 2025).

8.6.2 CRISPR-Based Molecular Diagnostics

Clustered Regularly Interspaced Short Palindromic Repeats (CRISPR) systems have been adapted from bacterial immune mechanisms into versatile molecular recognition and cleavage tools. In diagnostic applications, programmable guide RNAs direct CRISPR-associated proteins (Cas) to complementary nucleic acid sequences, enabling highly specific detection of pathogens, mutations, and genetic polymorphisms (Chen et al. 2023; Azimzadeh et al. 2022).

Cas12a and Cas13a, in particular, exhibit collateral cleavage activity once activated by binding to their target. This enzymatic function enables the breakdown of reporter molecules that produce fluorescence or colorimetric readouts. The integration of this biochemical signal transduction with smartphone camera systems allows quantitative assessment without the need for thermal cycling or bulky instrumentation. These diagnostic workflows often employ isothermal amplification techniques such as loop-mediated isothermal amplification (LAMP) and recombinase polymerase amplification (RPA), which operate at a single temperature (Hu et al. 2025). These reactions are suited for energy-efficient environments and compatible with portable thermal units or chemically activated heating elements. Diagnostic platforms like SHERLOCK and DETECTR utilize the CRISPR-Cas system to detect viral genomes, bacterial DNA, and oncogenic mutations with sensitivity in the attomolar range and discrimination at the single-nucleotide level. When paired with smartphones, these systems benefit from enhanced user guidance, automated image capture, and algorithmic interpretation, enabling scalable deployment in remote or low-resource environments (Zhan et al. 2025; Chakraborty 2024; Razavi et al. 2024).

To ensure field usability, researchers have developed lyophilized CRISPR reagent pellets, microfluidic reaction cartridges, and smartphone-adaptable optical modules. These components support room-temperature storage, minimal user handling, and modular assay development. CRISPR diagnostics are positioned to extend the molecular diagnostic capabilities of smartphones into genomics, infectious disease surveillance, and personalized medicine. The precision and adaptability of CRISPR systems make them central to future diagnostic architectures that demand high specificity and modular assay reconfiguration (He et al. 2025).

8.6.3 Artificial Intelligence and Federated Learning

Artificial intelligence (AI) introduces computational models capable of interpreting high-dimensional, noisy, and nonlinear biosensor outputs. These models include convolutional neural networks (CNNs) for image data and recurrent neural networks (RNNs) for time-series signals, each optimized for extracting meaningful features from raw diagnostic inputs. CNNs enable spatially resolved analysis of biomedical imagery, such as identifying morphological changes in stained samples, classifying diagnostic strips, or quantifying colorimetric responses. These networks are embedded into smartphone applications and trained to achieve clinical-grade accuracy under variable environmental conditions, accounting for light intensity, camera resolution, and sample presentation. RNN architectures, including LSTM and gated recurrent units (GRUs), analyze biosignals captured through smartphone-connected sensors. These models detect temporal anomalies such as arrhythmias, respiratory irregularities, or neuromuscular tremors, allowing for early detection of physiological deterioration (Chato and Regentova 2023; Dandge et al. 2025).

Training high-performance models requires access to large datasets, which often include sensitive health information. Federated learning addresses this challenge by enabling collaborative model training across decentralized devices. Instead of centralizing data, each smartphone updates the model locally and shares anonymized parameter updates. These updates are aggregated to refine a global model, maintaining data sovereignty while achieving statistical robustness. Privacy-preserving techniques such as differential privacy, secure multiparty computation, and homomorphic encryption reinforce the security of federated learning, ensuring that model contributions cannot be reverse-engineered to infer individual health records. In mobile diagnostics, federated AI frameworks allow model customization to individual users while leveraging global training efficiency. This paradigm is advancing diagnostic equity, allowing models to adapt to diverse populations without compromising ethical standards (Banik et al. 2021; Hossain et al. 2024; Chakraborty 2024).

8.6.4 Bioelectronic Interfaces and Flexible Sensors

Bioelectronic interfaces establish bidirectional communication between living systems and electronic circuits by converting biochemical and biophysical events into electrical signals. These interfaces, when designed using flexible materials, can be conformally integrated with the human body for continuous data acquisition. Polymeric substrates with low Young's modulus, such as PDMS and polyurethane, form the mechanical backbone of skin-conformal devices. Conductive materials such as graphene, carbon ink, and PEDOT: PSS serve as transduction layers, interfacing with biological matrices including skin, sweat, and interstitial fluid (Tyagi et al. 2024). Epidermal electronics systems (EES) integrate arrays of miniaturized sensors onto ultrathin films that adhere to the skin surface. These sensors monitor physiological parameters such as galvanic skin response, heart rate variability, and cutaneous temperature. Signals are wirelessly transmitted to smartphones using BLE or NFC protocols (Zhang and Liu 2016; Li et al. 2022).

Sweat-based biosensors utilize microfluidic channels and ion-selective electrodes to measure electrolyte concentration, pH, and metabolic byproducts such as lactate and cortisol. These measurements provide insights into hydration status, physical exertion, and stress levels. Smartphone integration facilitates personalized feedback loops for health optimization. Microneedle arrays penetrate the outermost layer of skin to access interstitial fluid, enabling minimally invasive sampling of glucose, drug metabolites, and cytokines (Zhao et al. 2020). These arrays are designed to avoid pain receptors and can be coupled to microelectronic circuits for real-time signal acquisition and transmission. Implantable bioelectronics, including ingestible capsules and subcutaneous probes, extend the diagnostic reach into internal anatomical compartments. These systems monitor internal physiological parameters such as gastrointestinal pH, drug release kinetics, or intracranial pressure, relaying data to smartphones through body-compatible RF communication systems. Flexible electronics expand the functional envelope of smartphone diagnostics into continuous, multimodal sensing, enabling longitudinal health tracking in a nondisruptive manner (Wang et al. 2023; Zhang et al. 2024).

8.6.5 Modular and Open-Source Diagnostic Ecosystems

Modular diagnostic systems emphasize reconfigurability, enabling rapid adaptation to emerging health threats or changing clinical requirements. In these architectures, functional subsystems including sample preparation, analyte sensing, and data processing are designed as independent, swappable units. Hardware modularity is achieved through standardized electrical interfaces and mechanical docking systems that allow interchangeable attachment of microfluidic cartridges, biosensor arrays, or optical modules to smartphones. These components are fabricated using accessible techniques such as 3D printing, injection molding, and printed circuit board milling, supporting local manufacturing (Piaggio et al. 2021; Azimzadeh et al. 2022; Hunt et al. 2021).

Software modularity enables the reuse of signal acquisition and analysis code across diagnostic contexts. Open APIs and modular software development kits (SDKs) facilitate custom application development, allowing a single device to operate as a platform for multiple diseases or biomarker panels. Open-source initiatives contribute to the democratization of diagnostic innovation by publishing design blueprints, firmware code, and performance validation protocols. These resources empower local researchers to build, validate, and scale diagnostic tools independently of proprietary constraints. Community-driven development, as observed during the COVID-19 pandemic, demonstrates the scalability and responsiveness of open-source ecosystems in times of public health urgency. Crowdsourced innovation accelerates the iteration cycle, enhances transparency, and fosters global collaboration (Vashist et al. 2014; Krittanawong et al. 2021).

Standardization of performance benchmarks and quality control protocols within open-source platforms ensures consistency across independently produced diagnostic units. Centralized repositories and peer-reviewed sharing platforms serve as validation hubs for maintaining system fidelity. The modular-open source paradigm decentralizes diagnostic development, enabling equitable access and rapid innovation while reducing dependence on commercial supply chains (Hossain et al. 2024).

8.6.6 Digital Phenotyping and Cognitive Biomarkers

Digital phenotyping characterizes behavioral and cognitive health through continuous analysis of smartphone-generated data streams. Unlike traditional biomarkers that focus on static biochemical metrics, digital phenotypes are derived from temporal patterns of interaction, movement, and cognition. Smartphones are equipped with sensors that capture multimodal inputs, including accelerometry, GPS location, ambient audio, and touchscreen dynamics. These data streams are processed to infer variables such as circadian rhythm stability, social connectivity, mobility patterns, and speech modulation. Cognitive biomarkers extracted from app-based assessments include reaction time, working memory load, language complexity, and decision latency. These metrics are predictive of neurological and psychiatric conditions such as depression, schizophrenia, and Alzheimer's disease (Zhang and Liu 2016; Li et al. 2022). Continuous monitoring enables identification of subclinical deviations from personal baselines, supporting early intervention strategies. Real-time analysis enables smartphones to act as behavioral sentinel systems, providing alerts or recommendations when abnormal patterns are detected (Banik et al. 2021; Chakraborty 2024).

Studies have demonstrated the viability of using digital signals to monitor disease progression, assess treatment adherence, and predict relapse in mental health conditions. These capabilities position smartphones as tools for digital psychiatry and neurology, extending diagnostic reach into domains historically limited by subjective assessment. Implementation requires sophisticated signal de-noising, dimensionality reduction, and contextual modeling to differentiate pathological changes from benign variability. Ethical implementation mandates secure data handling, user consent, and algorithmic transparency. By integrating behavioral science, computational analytics, and mobile platforms, digital phenotyping is unlocking new frontiers in noninvasive cognitive diagnostics and personalized mental health management (Gao et al. 2024; Mishra et al. 2024) (Fig. 8.2).

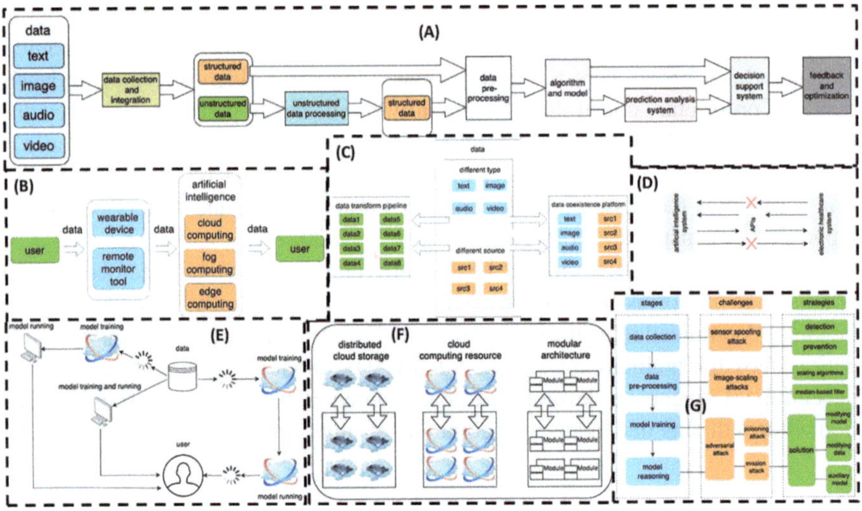

Fig. 8.2 Conceptual architecture of artificial intelligence integration in smart healthcare systems. (**a**) Workflow representation of artificial intelligence applications in healthcare, illustrating the pipeline from multi-modal data collection (text, image, audio, video) through preprocessing, *modeling, prediction* analysis, and decision support to feedback and system optimization. (**b**) Framework for remote patient monitoring, highlighting data acquisition via wearable or remote monitoring devices, followed by processing through cloud, fog, and edge computing infrastructures before returning insights to the user. (**c**) Schematic representation of data heterogeneity management, demonstrating challenges in integrating diverse data types (text, image, audio, video) and multiple data sources within a unified data coexistence platform. (**d**) Conceptual diagram of AI–EHR (Electronic Health Record) integration, showing limitations in direct interoperability and the need for advanced interface protocols. (**e**) Architecture of real-time AI processing systems, detailing continuous data acquisition, model training, inference, and user interaction within a closed-loop framework. (**f**) Scalability strategy for AI-enabled systems, showing distributed cloud storage, modular computing resources, and flexible cloud-based architecture for large-scale implementation. (**g**) Security and robustness framework of AI models in healthcare, outlining key threat vectors (such as adversarial and poisoning attacks) across different stages of the AI pipeline and corresponding mitigation strategies. (Adapted from Gao et al. (2024) © 1996–2025 MDPI (Basel, Switzerland))

8.7 Regulatory and Ethical Aspects

Smartphone-based biomedical diagnostics represent a technological class fundamentally divergent from traditional medical devices. Rather than static, single-purpose tools, these platforms operate as dynamic, adaptive, and distributed ecosystems comprising modular hardware, evolving software, remote analytical infrastructures, and decentralized user environments. Their diagnostic outputs emerge from the interplay of physical sensors, mobile applications, embedded inference engines, and user-driven interaction sequences, all of which may change independently over time. These characteristics defy the foundational assumptions of current regulatory paradigms, which are structured around the validation of discrete, predictable, and clinically-contained instruments. Consequently, both regulatory classification and ethical governance of smartphone-integrated biomedical systems remain unsettled, fragmented, and inconsistently applied across jurisdictions (Cohen et al. 2020; Azimzadeh et al. 2022; Chakraborty 2024).

8.7.1 Regulatory Classification and Oversight Frameworks

The regulatory architecture governing smartphone-based diagnostics must contend with multifactorial device identities that do not map cleanly onto legacy medical device taxonomies. Diagnostic functionalities may be dispersed across sensing hardware (optical cartridges, microneedle patches), mobile software (decision-support algorithms, user interfaces), cloud-based analytics (machine learning models), and real-time user interactions (sample collection or device positioning). Each of these domains can influence the clinical reliability of the system, yet may be regulated separately, if at all. The result is a highly fractured compliance landscape, with no clear regulatory entity assuming responsibility for system-level validation or safety certification (Biomedical devices and sensors 2025; Vashist et al. 2014).

Software-based diagnostics, either standalone or paired with smartphone-connected hardware, are increasingly governed under the category of Software as a Medical Device (SaMD), as defined by the International Medical Device Regulators Forum (IMDRF) (https://www.imdrf.org/sites/default/files/docs/imdrf/final/technical/imdrf-tech-190321-udi-sag.pdf, Cho et al. 2024). Regulatory bodies in North America, Europe, and Asia have adopted SaMD-specific guidance for validating performance claims, managing risk, and documenting the software development lifecycle. In this framework, critical parameters include intended medical purpose, risk of harm from incorrect outputs, algorithm transparency, and cybersecurity posture. For mobile diagnostic platforms incorporating physical sensor attachments, the regulatory path often depends on the novelty of the hardware and its claimed indications. Devices replicating established diagnostic principles (photoplethysmography for heart rate) may be eligible for 510(k) clearance by demonstrating substantial equivalence to a predicate [Patou et al. 2016]. In contrast, platforms introducing new biosensing modalities, molecular assay chemistries, or machine learning-based classifications often fall under De Novo or Premarket Approval (PMA) pathways. These require exhaustive demonstration of analytical and clinical performance through controlled studies, often complicated by environmental variability and uncontrolled usage patterns inherent to mobile deployment (Kumar et al. 2024).

AI integration introduces persistent ambiguity. Adaptive algorithms, those that retrain on new data or modify decision thresholds based on user behavior, violate the assumptions of static behavior central to traditional regulatory models. The US FDA's Total Product Lifecycle (TPLC) framework proposes an iterative oversight model for such systems, encompassing premarket assurance of algorithm architecture, real-time post-market monitoring, and predefined update protocols termed "predetermined change control plans." However, practical implementation remains limited, particularly outside high-income markets (Cho et al. 2024).

Standardization of development and validation practices for mobile diagnostics is anchored in international technical standards. These include ISO 13485 for quality management systems, IEC 62304 for software lifecycle processes, ISO 14971 for risk management, and ISO/IEC 27001 for information security management. Device developers must maintain comprehensive documentation of version control, traceability matrices, failure mode and effects analyses (FMEAs), and cybersecurity audits. Interactions between mobile platforms and cloud servers, including data routing, authentication protocols, and firmware patching, are increasingly scrutinized under these regimes (Hossain et al. 2024; Azimzadeh et al. 2022).

Global deployment introduces further regulatory heterogeneity. National authorities in different regions impose varying requirements for clinical trials, device labeling, software source code disclosure, and local testing. China's NMPA, Japan's PMDA, India's CDSCO, and Brazil's ANVISA each define divergent approval timelines, audit scopes, and documentation formats, often incompatible with one another. This lack of harmonization inflates compliance costs and delays time-to-market, particularly for small and mid-sized enterprises without dedicated regulatory staff. While IMDRF's harmonization efforts and WHO's prequalification mechanisms offer partial relief, widespread interoperability of regulatory pathways remains elusive. Regulatory sandboxes, defined test environments where new technologies are piloted under temporary exemptions, have emerged in several jurisdictions to accelerate the evaluation of mobile diagnostics. These programs permit early clinical deployment under conditional constraints, enabling real-world performance monitoring without full market authorization. Such frameworks require close collaboration between regulators, developers, clinicians, and legal experts, and depend on granular logging of diagnostic decisions, usage contexts, and adverse event triggers (Banik et al. 2021; Tyagi et al. 2024).

Post-market obligations in smartphone diagnostics are often underdefined. Unlike traditional medical devices housed within institutional infrastructures, mobile diagnostics may be used by laypersons in uncontrolled environments with no central record of usage events, updates, or failures. Effective post-market surveillance demands embedded telemetry, over-the-air (OTA) software patching mechanisms, usage analytics pipelines, and anomaly detection models capable of identifying performance degradation or usage anomalies. These elements are rarely codified in current regulatory checklists, leaving major gaps in lifecycle governance (Gao et al. 2024).

As smartphone diagnostics increasingly rely on software behaviors, crowd-sourced data, and personalized inference models, their regulatory oversight must shift from deterministic device validation toward dynamic system supervision. The complexity and heterogeneity of diagnostic architectures necessitate a move beyond hardware-centric scrutiny, requiring regulators to develop new tools for monitoring emergent behavior, distributed accountability, and the cumulative effect of asynchronous component updates (Piaggio et al. 2021; Chakraborty 2024).

8.7.2 Ethical Frameworks for Data-Driven Mobile Diagnostics

Ethical evaluation of smartphone-based biomedical technologies must operate at the intersection of clinical utility, digital rights, and social justice. These devices do not merely deliver diagnostic outputs; they alter how individuals engage with health data, how care is accessed, and how responsibility is distributed across sociotechnical systems. Conventional bioethical categories like autonomy, beneficence, nonmaleficence, and justice are insufficient to capture the full spectrum of ethical tensions in these digitally mediated environments. One central concern is the legitimacy of informed consent. In traditional clinical contexts, consent involves dialogue between patients and health professionals, contextualized by mutual understanding and tailored to cognitive and emotional states. In mobile diagnostics, consent is frequently embedded in scroll-through disclaimers, pre-checked boxes, or bundled application permissions. These interfaces reduce consent to a legal artifact, failing to reflect comprehension, voluntariness, or contextual appropriateness. In populations with limited digital literacy, impaired decision-making capacity, or economic vulnerability, such formats exacerbate the risk of exploitation, surveillance, or nonconsensual data extraction. Data privacy and control are similarly destabilized. Diagnostic platforms collect multimodal data streams including biometric markers, behavioral signals, environmental metrics, and device interaction patterns. These are often aggregated in opaque cloud infrastructures with limited transparency regarding retention policies, secondary uses, or cross-border transfers. Even when identifiers are stripped, linkability with publicly available demographic or behavioral datasets enables re-identification, posing latent risks to anonymity, dignity, and psychological safety (Ross et al. 2023; Chakraborty 2024).

Algorithmic opacity remains a persistent ethical dilemma. Machine learning models embedded in diagnostic applications often rely on training data drawn from specific demographic, geographic, or clinical contexts. When applied outside these domains, model behavior may degrade, yielding false negatives or false positives with uneven distribution across racial, gendered, or socioeconomic lines. The absence of model interpretability mechanisms prevents users from interrogating how or why decisions were made, eroding both accountability and recourse. Equitable access remains an unresolved tension. While smartphone penetration has increased globally, disparities persist in access to high-performance devices, network bandwidth, app compatibility, and localized language support. Systems designed for flagship phones may underperform or be entirely inaccessible on low-end models. Populations without stable electricity or internet connectivity cannot participate in cloud-reliant diagnostic infrastructures, leaving them systematically excluded from the health benefits these technologies promise to deliver (Banik et al. 2021; Pillay et al. 2025).

Behavioral implications of continuous self-monitoring raise further ethical challenges. Constant exposure to health metrics can induce anxiety, compulsive checking behaviors, or maladaptive self-regulation, particularly in individuals with health-related phobias or obsessive tendencies. Diagnostic overreach where individuals treat uncertain or false-positive results as clinical certainties can lead to unnecessary medical interventions, disrupted clinical relationships, and erosion of trust in professional judgment. Accountability in mobile diagnostics remains diffuse and fragmented. In traditional settings, liability resides within defined institutional hierarchies. In smartphone-based systems, responsibility may be shared across sensor manufacturers, app developers, third-party data processors, network providers, and end-users. Diagnostic harm resulting from software bugs, data latency, model errors, or misinterpretation lacks clear pathways for restitution, legal remedy, or systemic correction (Tyagi et al. 2024; Kumari et al. 2025).

Ethical design methodologies have been proposed to mitigate these risks. Privacy-by-design enforces minimization of data collection, local processing, and secure deletion policies. Consent traceability ensures that user permissions are auditable and revocable. Explainable AI frameworks aim to render algorithmic outputs interpretable, enabling users to understand diagnostic justifications. Value-sensitive design embeds stakeholder priorities such as cultural appropriateness, user dignity, and inclusivity into the technical development process. These approaches remain underutilized in commercial platforms, constrained by development timelines, market pressures, and misaligned incentives. Governance mechanisms that span beyond technical standards are necessary. Participatory ethics models, where affected communities co-develop use policies, deployment strategies, and oversight structures, offer a more robust alignment with local health priorities. Ethics review boards must adapt to include digital health experts, behavioral scientists, legal scholars, and community advocates, reflecting the expanded scope of ethical stakes introduced by mobile diagnostics. The long-term ethical sustainability of smartphone-based biomedical systems depends not solely on their diagnostic precision or computational elegance, but on the structures through which they are designed, evaluated, and deployed. These structures must align innovation with inclusion, autonomy with accountability, and technical possibility with human value (Kumar et al. 2024; Chakraborty 2024; Gooding and Kariotis 2021).

8.8 Future Prospects

The development of smartphone-based biomedical diagnostics is undergoing a systemic shift toward an integrated model of predictive, preventive, and precision healthcare. These platforms are becoming embedded within a broader cyber-physical architecture, where continuous data streams from biological, behavioral, and environmental domains converge within mobile systems for real-time interpretation and intervention. As sensor technologies mature and computational frameworks evolve, smartphones are transitioning from passive data acquisition interfaces into active, autonomous agents that can execute diagnostic, prognostic, and therapeutic functions across distributed care environments.

This transformation is driven by synergistic advances across edge computing, nanoscale engineering, digital biosensing, machine learning, and embedded feedback control systems. Future iterations of these diagnostic platforms will no longer operate as isolated modules but will instead form nodes within intelligent diagnostic ecosystems. These systems will possess the capacity to contextualize physiological deviations within individual baselines, behavioral rhythms, and environmental exposures, offering unprecedented spatiotemporal resolution in health surveillance. Achieving this vision necessitates not only hardware and software innovation but also progress in regulatory adaptation, data interoperability, human–machine interface design, and scalable global deployment. The following subsections delineate emerging directions where fundamental change is anticipated: next-generation diagnostic ecosystems, closed-loop therapeutic control, and global health infrastructure integration (Banik et al. 2021; Chakraborty 2024; Gao et al. 2024).

8.8.1 Next-Generation Diagnostic Ecosystems

The maturation of smartphone-based biomedical diagnostics is converging toward a distributed, multi-modal ecosystem capable of real-time, context-aware health inference. These ecosystems will be characterized by their ability to interoperate across device platforms, sensor modalities, and data domains while maintaining low-latency analytics and user-adaptive behavior. Within this paradigm, smartphones will no longer serve merely as interface terminals but will operate as central computational hubs capable of autonomously orchestrating biosensing, interpretation, and therapeutic signaling. At the structural level, these diagnostic ecosystems will integrate lab-on-chip (LOC) or lab-on-phone microfluidic platforms embedded with biosensing elements, reagent reservoirs, microvalves, and thermal controllers. These substrates will support multiplexed assays for the detection of nucleic acids, proteins, and metabolites in sub-microliter samples, all contained within single-use, disposable cartridges. The smartphone's processing unit will be responsible for controlling thermal cycling, managing fluidic actuation, and executing data acquisition protocols via attached or embedded optical and electrochemical readout systems (Tyagi et al. 2024; Ross et al. 2023; Gao et al. 2024).

Microfluidic assay outcomes will be interpreted in real-time through on-device inference models capable of deconvoluting signal-to-noise ratios, compensating for temperature fluctuations, and normalizing readouts across interindividual variability. These outputs will then be integrated with behavioral and environmental metadata collected through inertial sensors, GPS, ambient light detectors, and voice analysis tools to generate multidimensional health state representations. The emergent diagnostic profile will include biochemical markers, biophysical measurements, and behavioral signatures, enabling simultaneous characterization of immunological status, metabolic flux, cardiovascular resilience, circadian alignment, and stress physiology. Rather than providing discrete data points, these systems will deliver dynamic, trajectory-based health models calibrated to each user's physiotype. This transformation in functionality necessitates robust support for bidirectional communication with peripheral biosensors such as epidermal patches, ingestible capsules, or implantable probes via Bluetooth Low Energy (BLE), ultra-wideband (UWB), or near-field communication (NFC). Cross-device data harmonization protocols will ensure temporal alignment and data fidelity, permitting the fusion of heterogeneous signals into unified diagnostic indices (Sengar et al. 2021; Patel et al. 2023).

Temporal integration is a core attribute of next-generation diagnostic systems. Instead of episodic testing, these platforms will support longitudinal monitoring, enabling the construction of individualized baselines against which deviations are interpreted. Health anomalies will thus be contextualized not against static population norms but within dynamic personal trajectories, enhancing both specificity and early detection sensitivity. Epidemiological applications will be embedded through secure, anonymized cloud synchronization. Aggregated data will inform population-scale models for outbreak prediction, disease clustering, and environmental exposure mapping. Such functionality positions diagnostic ecosystems not only as tools for personal health inference but as infrastructure for real-time syndromic surveillance and public health intelligence. Implementation of this model demands advances in interface standardization, adherence to secure data transmission protocols, scalable edge inference models, and hardware miniaturization without loss of analytical performance. It will also require integration with national and international health data systems via FHIR (Fast Healthcare Interoperability Resources), HL7, or similar frameworks to ensure clinical interoperability (Banik et al. 2021; Tyagi et al. 2024; Kumar et al. 2024; Chakraborty 2024).

8.8.2 AI-Coupled Therapeutics and Closed-Loop Systems

The transition from static diagnostics to dynamic, autonomous therapeutic modulation is being enabled through the convergence of biosensing technologies with AI-driven decision frameworks. Closed-loop systems, characterized by their ability to monitor physiological parameters and deliver real-time, adaptive interventions without external input, represent a critical future axis of smartphone-mediated therapeutics. At the foundation of these architectures is the continuous acquisition of biometrics from wearable or implantable sensors. Signals derived from glucose levels, EEG activity, muscle contraction, heart rate variability, or neurotransmitter flux are relayed to a smartphone, where real-time AI models determine whether deviations warrant intervention. This decision is then translated into a control signal delivered to a drug-dispensing actuator, neuromodulator, or behavioral intervention interface. Model predictive control (MPC), reinforcement learning, and Bayesian adaptive control strategies will dominate the algorithmic landscape, enabling predictive modulation rather than reactive correction. In diabetes management, continuous glucose monitors will inform insulin pumps regulated by smartphone-based algorithms that learn from intra-day glycemic dynamics and contextual variables such as physical activity and meal composition (Wasilewski et al. 2024; Konnaiyan and Zhdanov 2025).

In neuropsychiatric applications, smartphones will serve as intermediary processors between brain–computer interfaces and neuromodulatory implants, executing logic based on affective state classifiers derived from speech, facial expression, and sensorimotor patterns. These systems will deliver deep-brain stimulation (DBS) pulses or pharmacological cues in response to algorithmically inferred depressive states, seizure pre-onsets, or psychomotor dysregulation. Cognitive behavioral therapy (CBT) modules will operate as digital therapeutics, activated in closed loops by AI classifiers trained to detect relapse indicators in schizophrenia, bipolar disorder, or anxiety disorders. These systems will interpret keystroke dynamics, speech inflections, and interaction latency as cognitive biomarkers, triggering dialog modules, motivational prompts, or remote clinician notifications (Tyagi et al. 2024; Honko et al. 2016).

Edge AI on-device execution of machine learning inference will become essential in this domain to minimize latency, reduce energy consumption, and avoid privacy risks associated with cloud-based processing. Algorithms will require real-time failover modes, signal validation layers, and interruptible execution protocols to prevent therapeutic misfires in cases of signal corruption or model uncertainty. The safety profile of such autonomous systems will be governed by multilevel safeguards, including manual override interfaces, biometric authentication for therapy initiation, and continuous performance logging for post-hoc auditability. Regulatory architectures must evolve to support adaptive algorithmic behavior, ensuring that clinical validation can accommodate model drift and environmental nonstationarity. These therapeutic systems blur the boundary between sensing and actuation, establishing smartphones not only as diagnostic interfaces but as cybernetic mediators of physiological regulation. Their capacity to learn, adapt, and intervene in real time signals a paradigmatic shift in healthcare from reactive management to anticipatory modulation informed by embedded intelligence (Chakraborty 2024; Wasilewski et al. 2024; Honko et al. 2016).

8.8.3 Global Health and Epidemiological Applications

The global applicability of smartphone-based biomedical platforms lies in their capacity to decentralize health services and extend precision diagnostics into infrastructure-limited environments. Their modularity, affordability, and ubiquity make them ideally suited to address disparities in healthcare access, particularly in regions where formal laboratory infrastructure and specialist personnel are limited or absent. In infectious disease control, smartphone-coupled assays incorporating isothermal amplification (RPA, LAMP), antigen detection, or CRISPR-based nucleic acid sensing offer field-deployable alternatives to polymerase chain reaction (PCR) [Azimzadeh et al. 2022, Chen et al. 2023]. These systems can operate without thermocyclers or laboratory centrifuges and can be assembled within mobile phone-compatible cartridges that deliver fluorescence, colorimetric, or electrochemical readouts within minutes (Tyagi et al. 2024).

When synchronized with geospatial data and connected via encrypted mobile networks, these diagnostics enable real-time epidemic surveillance. Confirmed pathogen identifications can be geotagged and uploaded to national dashboards, allowing public health authorities to monitor case distribution, detect emergence patterns, and implement containment protocols dynamically. This decentralized reporting mechanism provides a granular, temporal layer of epidemiological data beyond what traditional laboratory reporting infrastructures can achieve. In telehealth frameworks, smartphone diagnostics serve as front-line triage tools. Community health workers equipped with these systems can collect and transmit diagnostic data to remote clinicians, enabling specialist consultation across significant geographic barriers. This model facilitates early diagnosis and treatment of conditions, including anemia, malaria, tuberculosis, and malnutrition, directly at the point of need (Wasilewski et al. 2024; Honko et al. 2016).

Smartphone-integrated maternal and neonatal health technologies are being developed to screen for conditions including preeclampsia, gestational diabetes, fetal hypoxia, and neonatal bilirubinemia. These tools empower community-based practitioners to perform high-risk screening and immediate referral, reducing time-to-intervention and preventing complications associated with delayed care. Offline-capable software, multilingual interfaces, solar charging systems, and low-bandwidth optimization are essential enablers of these tools in remote environments. Smartphone diagnostics are being designed with ruggedized casings, embedded fail-safes, and temperature-insensitive reagents to withstand harsh environmental conditions without degradation of diagnostic integrity. From a data science perspective, these devices support longitudinal health data collection across large cohorts, enabling high-resolution health surveillance. Combined with wearable sensors and passive behavioral monitoring, this architecture permits identification of at-risk populations, characterization of disease burden, and allocation of intervention resources in a data-driven manner. For sustainability, open-source manufacturing frameworks, localized reagent production, and interoperable software architectures are being promoted to reduce dependence on proprietary supply chains and enhance local capacity building. Ethical data governance, culturally sensitive design, and community participatory research models are critical to ensuring adoption and trust in these technologies (Banik et al. 2021; Tyagi et al. 2024; Kumar et al. 2024; Chakraborty 2024).

In aggregate, smartphone-based diagnostics are redefining the frontiers of global health delivery, embedding precision, connectivity, and real-time analytics into regions where traditional systems have struggled to penetrate. Their role in population-scale surveillance, individualized diagnostics, and adaptive intervention will continue to expand as technological and infrastructural innovations converge.

8.9 Conclusion

Smartphone-based biomedical devices have redefined the interface between technology and healthcare, emerging as transformative platforms that extend diagnostic precision beyond centralized laboratories into patient-centered and resource-limited settings. Their ability to integrate biosensors, microfluidics, optical and electrochemical transduction, and artificial intelligence within a widely accessible mobile infrastructure has positioned smartphones as both diagnostic engines and data hubs. These technologies embody the paradigm of decentralized, real-time, and personalized healthcare, where biological signals can be captured, analyzed, and contextualized at the point of need. Despite their promise, the translation of smartphone-integrated diagnostics into clinical practice is hindered by challenges spanning physics, chemistry, biology, and socio-technical systems. Smartphone cameras and sensors, though optimized for consumer applications, lack the native resolution and dynamic range of laboratory instruments, necessitating extensive calibration and algorithmic compensation. Biological samples such as blood, saliva, and urine introduce variability and interferents that complicate assay reproducibility, while microfluidic components suffer from clogging, evaporation, and environmental sensitivity. User-dependent variability and environmental noise further compromise measurement fidelity, and the deployment of adaptive machine learning models raises regulatory and ethical questions regarding algorithmic drift, accountability, and inclusivity. Addressing these requires not only engineering refinement but also regulatory frameworks that treat smartphone diagnostics as adaptive, distributed systems rather than static devices.

The novelty of this chapter lies in its multidisciplinary approach, uniting perspectives from physics, chemistry, biology, data science, and regulatory governance to provide a mechanistic understanding of smartphone-based biomedical devices. Unlike conventional reviews limited to applications, this chapter critically examines the fundamental limitations—optical artifacts, fluidic inconsistencies, sensor stability, and data governance—while mapping them to cutting-edge solutions such as nanostructured sensing materials, CRISPR-based nucleic acid detection, federated learning, and modular open-source ecosystems. It also foregrounds the regulatory and ethical complexities unique to smartphone diagnostics, highlighting issues of informed consent, algorithmic transparency, and equitable access. By framing these technologies as distributed, multi-stakeholder networks rather than isolated tools, this chapter provides a novel conceptual framework for guiding both innovation and policy. Looking forward, the evolution of smartphone-based biomedical systems will be driven by advances in three converging domains. First, technological sophistication will expand through multiplexed lab-on-chip platforms, wearable and implantable biosensors, and edge AI algorithms capable of low-latency, privacy-preserving inference. The incorporation of nanomaterials such as plasmonic nanoparticles and metal–organic frameworks will extend sensitivity to femtomolar levels, opening new horizons in early cancer detection, infectious disease screening, and environmental toxin monitoring. Second, therapeutic integration will transform smartphones into components of closed-loop systems, linking biosensors with actuators for drug delivery, neuromodulation, or behavioral intervention. Coupled with digital twins and blockchain-secured records, these systems will enable adaptive, individualized care pathways that blur the boundary between diagnostics and therapy. Third, global health impact will be realized as smartphones serve as infrastructures for outbreak surveillance, syndromic monitoring, and precision public health. Their ubiquity in low- and middle-income countries positions them as critical tools for reducing disparities, enabling early epidemic response, and guiding health policy through real-time population-level data streams.

The future of smartphone-integrated diagnostics will depend on innovations in materials science, secure and interpretable AI, regulatory adaptability, and infrastructure equity. With continued interdisciplinary collaboration, these systems will advance from supplemental diagnostic tools to foundational components of a globally connected, predictive, and preventive healthcare ecosystem.

References

Ahmad RS, Khan MS, Hilal ME, Khan B, Zhang Y, Khoo BL (2025) Advancements in wearable heart sounds devices for the monitoring of cardiovascular diseases. SmartMat 6(1). https://doi.org/10.1002/smm2.1311

Ali F, Neha K, Ilyas A, Ali H (2024) Introduction, challenges, and overview of regulatory affairs. In: Global regulations of medicinal, pharmaceutical, and food products. CRC Press

Ameku WA et al (2022) Laser-scribed graphene-based electrochemical sensors: a review. Chemosensors 10(12):505. https://doi.org/10.3390/chemosensors10120505

Antonini A et al (2025) Smartphone as a sensor in mHealth: narrative overview, SWOT analysis, and proposal of mobile biomarkers. Sensors (Basel) 25(12):12. https://doi.org/10.3390/s25123655

Arduini F et al (2016) Electrochemical biosensors based on nanomodified screen-printed electrodes: recent applications in clinical analysis. TrAC Trends Anal Chem 79:114–126. https://doi.org/10.1016/j.trac.2016.01.032

Azimzadeh M, Mousazadeh M, Jahangiri-Manesh A, Khashayar P, Khashayar P (2022) CRISPR-powered microfluidics in diagnostics: a review of main applications. Chem 10(1):3. https://doi.org/10.3390/chemosensors10010003

Baker DV et al (2025) Smartphones as a platform for molecular analysis: concepts, methods, devices and future potential. Lab Chip 25(5):884–955. https://doi.org/10.1039/D4LC00966E

Ballard ZS et al (2020) Deep learning-enabled point-of-care sensing using multiplexed paper-based sensors. Npj Digit Med 3(1):66. https://doi.org/10.1038/s41746-020-0274-y

Banik S et al (2021) Recent trends in smartphone-based detection for biomedical applications: a review. Anal Bioanal Chem 413(9):2389–2406. https://doi.org/10.1007/s00216-021-03184-z

Biomedical devices and sensors. Wiley. Wileycom. Accessed 28 July 2025. [Online]. Available: https://www.wiley.com/en-us/Biomedical+Devices+and+Sensors-p-9781394317165

Boonkaew S, Szot-Karpińska K, Niedziółka-Jönsson J, De Marco A, Jönsson-Niedziółka M (2024) NFC smartphone-based electrochemical microfluidic device integrated with nanobody recognition for C-reactive protein. ACS Sens 9(6):3066–3074. https://doi.org/10.1021/acssensors.4c00249

Budd J et al (2023) Lateral flow test engineering and lessons learned from COVID-19. Nat Rev Bioeng 1(1):13–31. https://doi.org/10.1038/s44222-022-00007-3

Bui TH, Thangavel B, Sharipov M, Chen K, Shin JH (2023) Smartphone-based portable bio-chemical sensors: exploring recent advancements. Chemosensors 11(9):9. https://doi.org/10.3390/chemosensors11090468

Chakraborty S (2024) Democratizing nucleic acid-based molecular diagnostic tests for infectious diseases at resource-limited settings—from point of care to extreme point of care. Sens Diagn 3(4):536–561. https://doi.org/10.1039/D3SD00304C

Chan J, Goel M, Gollakota S, Nandakumar R (2025) Mobile medical systems for equitable healthcare. Nat Rev Bioeng:1–20. https://doi.org/10.1038/s44222-025-00330-5

Chato L, Regentova E (2023) Survey of transfer learning approaches in the machine learning of digital health sensing data. J Pers Med 13(12):1703. https://doi.org/10.3390/jpm13121703

Chen H, Zhou X, Wang M, Ren L (2023) Towards point of care CRISPR-based diagnostics: from method to device. J Funct Biomater 14(2):97. https://doi.org/10.3390/jfb14020097

Cheng Y et al (2023) Dual-signal readout paper-based wearable biosensor with a 3D origami structure for multiplexed analyte detection in sweat. Microsyst Nanoeng 9(1):36. https://doi.org/10.1038/s41378-023-00514-2

Cho T, Gowda V, Schulzrinne H, Miller BJ (2024) Integrated Devices: A New Regulatory Pathway to Promote Revolutionary Innovation. The Milbank Quarterly 102(2):367–382. https://doi.org/10.1111/1468-0009.12692

Choi RY, Coyner AS, Kalpathy-Cramer J, Chiang MF, Campbell JP (2020) Introduction to machine learning, neural networks, and deep learning. Transl Vis Sci Technol 9(2):14. https://doi.org/10.1167/tvst.9.2.14

Cohen IG, Gerke S, Kramer DB (2020) Ethical and legal implications of remote monitoring of medical devices. Milbank Q 98(4):1257–1289. https://doi.org/10.1111/1468-0009.12481

Cui F, Yue Y, Zhang Y, Zhang Z, Zhou HS (2020) Advancing biosensors with machine learning. ACS Sens 5(11):3346–3364. https://doi.org/10.1021/acssensors.0c01424

da Silva ETSG, Souto DEP, Barragan JTC, de F. Giarola J, de Moraes ACM, Kubota LT (2017) Electrochemical biosensors in point-of-care devices: recent advances and future trends. ChemElectroChem 4(4):778–794. https://doi.org/10.1002/celc.201600758

Dandge K, Kumawat DM, Jadhav DP (2025) Leveraging artificial intelligence and wearable technologies in glucose management: a comprehensive scoping review of current trends and future directions. Int J Environ Sci:856–886. https://doi.org/10.64252/a6fbg258

Daniels R, Cottin J, Khanafer N (2023) Point-of-care testing for SARS-CoV-2: a prospective study in a primary health Centre. Diagnostics 13(11):1888. https://doi.org/10.3390/diagnostics13111888

Dkhar DS, Kumari R, Malode SJ, Shetti NP, Chandra P (2023) Integrated lab-on-a-chip devices: fabrication methodologies, transduction system for sensing purposes. J Pharm Biomed Anal 223:115120. https://doi.org/10.1016/j.jpba.2022.115120

Gao X, He P, Zhou Y, Qin X (2024) Artificial intelligence applications in smart healthcare: a survey. Future Internet 16(9):308. https://doi.org/10.3390/fi16090308

Goncharov A et al (2023) Deep learning-enabled multiplexed point-of-care sensor using a paper-based fluorescence vertical flow assay. Small Weinh Bergstr Ger 19(51):e2300617. https://doi.org/10.1002/smll.202300617

Gooding P, Kariotis T (2021) Ethics and law in research on algorithmic and data-driven technology in mental health care: scoping review. JMIR Ment Health 8(6):e24668. https://doi.org/10.2196/24668

Guo X et al (2021) Smartphone-based DNA diagnostics for malaria detection using deep learning for local decision support and blockchain technology for security. Nat Electron 4(8):615–624. https://doi.org/10.1038/s41928-021-00612-x

He C et al (2025) Application of CRISPR-Cas system in human papillomavirus detection using biosensor devices and point-of-care technologies. BME Front 6:0114. https://doi.org/10.34133/bmef.0114

Honko H, Andalibi V, Aaltonen T, Parak J, Saaranen M, Viik J, Korhonen I (2016) W2E--Wellness Warehouse Engine for Semantic Interoperability of Consumer Health Data. IEEE J Biomed Health Inform, 20(6):1632–1639. https://doi.org/10.1109/JBHI.2015.2469718

Hossain B et al (2024) Machine learning for cardiovascular healthcare: opportunities, challenges, and the path forward. J Angiother 8(12):1–11. https://doi.org/10.25163/angiotherapy.81210205

Hu F et al (2025) A rapid and ultrasensitive RPA-assisted CRISPR–Cas12a/Cas13a nucleic acid diagnostic platform with a smartphone-based portable device. Biosens Bioelectron 280:117428. https://doi.org/10.1016/j.bios.2025.117428

Huang Z et al (2024) Electrochemical biosensor for point-of-care testing of low-abundance biomarkers of neurological diseases. Anal Chem 96(25):10332–10340. https://doi.org/10.1021/acs.analchem.4c01278

Hunt B, Ruiz A, Pogue B (2021) Smartphone-based imaging systems for medical applications: a critical review. J Biomed Opt 26(4):040902. https://doi.org/10.1117/1.JBO.26.4.040902

Hybrid multimodal wearable sensors for comprehensive health monitoring. Nat Electron. Accessed 27 July 2025. [Online]. Available: https://www.nature.com/articles/s41928-024-01247-4

Jang H-J et al (2024) Deep learning-based kinetic analysis in paper-based analytical cartridges integrated with field-effect transistors. ACS Nano 18(36):24792–24802. https://doi.org/10.1021/acsnano.4c02897

Kakkar S et al (2024) Lateral flow assays: Progress and evolution of recent trends in point-of-care applications. Mater Today Bio 28:101188. https://doi.org/10.1016/j.mtbio.2024.101188

Kamble PR, Sengar MS, Kumari P, Kadu AK (2025) Development of a simple electrochemical sensor for antipsychotic medication perphenazine based on Mn3O4 nanomaterial modified glassy carbon electrode. J Electrochem Soc 172(4):047516. https://doi.org/10.1149/1945-7111/adcbda

Karim K, Lamaoui A, Amine A (2023) Paper-based optical sensors paired with smartphones for biomedical analysis. J Pharm Biomed Anal 225:115207. https://doi.org/10.1016/j.jpba.2022.115207

King RC, Villeneuve E, White RJ, Sherratt RS, Holderbaum W, Harwin WS (2017) Application of data fusion techniques and technologies for wearable health monitoring. Med Eng Phys 42:1–12. https://doi.org/10.1016/j.medengphy.2016.12.011

Kong F, Zou Y, Li Z, Deng Y (2024) Advances in portable and wearable acoustic sensing devices for human health monitoring. Sensors 24(16):16. https://doi.org/10.3390/s24165354

Konnaiyan KR, Zhdanov A (2025) 17 - smartphone-based devices for healthcare monitoring and management. In: Nguyen TA (ed) Blockchain and digital twin for smart healthcare. Elsevier, pp 329–344. https://doi.org/10.1016/B978-0-443-30300-5.00019-1

Krittanawong C et al (2021) Integration of novel monitoring devices with machine learning technology for scalable cardiovascular management. Nat Rev Cardiol 18(2):75–91. https://doi.org/10.1038/s41569-020-00445-9

Kumar U, Kesharwani RK, Pal MK (2024) The most recent developments and applications of smartphone-based devices in biomedical and mHealth. In: Advanced research in electronic devices for biomedical and mHealth. Apple Academic Press

Kumari P, Sengar MS, Sengar N (2024) A mini review on lactic acidosis effect, cause, symptoms, complications, metabolism, and Pathodology with its diagnosis, treatment, and preventions. J Chem Rev 6(1):27–38. https://doi.org/10.48309/jcr.2024.407092.1230

Kumari P et al (2025) Elucidating the binding mechanism of 1,4-bis[(3-Piperidino)propanamido]anthracen-9,10-dione (1,4-BPAQ) to human telomeric G-quadruplexes: a multi-technique approach including spectroscopic, calorimetric and molecular docking insights. J Comput Aided Mol Des 39(1):37. https://doi.org/10.1007/s10822-025-00615-2

Lei R, Wang D, Arain H, Mohan C (2022) Design of gold nanoparticle vertical flow assays for point-of-care testing. Diagnostics 12(5):1107. https://doi.org/10.3390/diagnostics12051107

Li F, Bao Y, Wang D, Wang W, Niu L (2016) Smartphones for sensing. Sci Bull 61(3):190–201. https://doi.org/10.1007/s11434-015-0954-1

Li S et al (2022) Biosensors and bioelectronics on smartphone. In: Handbook of cell biosensors. Springer, Cham, pp 627–655. https://doi.org/10.1007/978-3-030-23217-7_157

Luppa PB, Müller C, Schlichtiger A, Schlebusch H (2011) Point-of-care testing (POCT): current techniques and future perspectives. Trends Anal Chem TRAC 30(6):887–898. https://doi.org/10.1016/j.trac.2011.01.019

Madrid RE, Ashur Ramallo F, Barraza DE, Chaile RE (2022) Smartphone-based biosensor devices for healthcare: technologies, trends, and adoption by end-users. Bioengineering 9(3):101. https://doi.org/10.3390/bioengineering9030101

Mahapatra S, Singh A, Paul R, Chandra P (2025) A dual-mode on-chip 3d-printed nanoengineered platform for extraction and electrochemical detection of enrofloxacin. Small 21(33):e2502880. https://doi.org/10.1002/smll.202502880

Majumder S, Deen MJ (2019) Smartphone sensors for health monitoring and diagnosis. Sensors 19(9):2164. https://doi.org/10.3390/s19092164

Maleki B, Hojati Z (2022) A precise review on NAATs-based diagnostic assays for COVID-19: a motion in fast POC molecular tests. Eur J Clin Investig 52(11):e13853. https://doi.org/10.1111/eci.13853

Martinez AW, Phillips ST, Carrilho E, Thomas SWI, Sindi H, Whitesides GM (2008) Simple telemedicine for developing regions: camera phones and paper-based microfluidic devices for real-time, off-site diagnosis. Anal Chem 80(10):3699–3707. https://doi.org/10.1021/ac800112r

Min J et al (2023) An autonomous wearable biosensor powered by a perovskite solar cell. Nat Electron 6(8):630–641. https://doi.org/10.1038/s41928-023-00996-y

Mishra A et al (2024) Emergence of integrated biosensing-enabled digital healthcare devices. Sens Diagn 3(5):718–744. https://doi.org/10.1039/D4SD00017J

Mukadi P et al (2015) SMS photograph-based external quality assessment of reading and interpretation of malaria rapid diagnostic tests in The Democratic Republic of the Congo. Malar J 14:26. https://doi.org/10.1186/s12936-014-0535-9

Najjar R (2023) Redefining radiology: a review of artificial intelligence integration in medical imaging. Diagn Basel Switz 13(17):2760. https://doi.org/10.3390/diagnostics13172760

Nandi I, Patel V, Srivastava R, Chandra P (2024) Opto-electrochemical transducers for molecular sensing utilizing nanozyme-based sensing technologies. Microchem J 205:111360. https://doi.org/10.1016/j.microc.2024.111360

Palekar S, Kalambe S, Kalambe J, Kulkarni MB, Bhaiyya M (2025) A portable smartphone-based 3D-printed biosensing platform for kidney function biomarker quantification. Biosensors 15(3):3. https://doi.org/10.3390/bios15030192

Panigrahi DR et al (2025) Π-electron and pH-regulated photochemical detection of trinitrophenol using nanoconfined graphene quantum dots. ACS Appl Nano Mater 8(5):2614–2622. https://doi.org/10.1021/acsanm.5c00141

Patel V, Bhargava A, Puri A, Ghosh A, Srivastava R (2023) A pretreated electrodeposited nickel oxide film on gold PCB electrode for solid-state lactate sensing. 2023 IEEE BioSensors Conference (BioSensors):1–3. https://doi.org/10.1109/BioSensors58001.2023.10281096

Patel V et al (2024) Evolution of materials, geometries, and fabrication of sweat patches and their use in high-throughput point-of-care/onsite sensing. Microchem J 204:111165. https://doi.org/10.1016/j.microc.2024.111165

Patou F, AlZahra'a Alatraktchi F, Kjægaard C, Dimaki M, Madsen J, Svendsen WE (2016) Evolvable Smartphone-Based Platforms for Point-of-Care In-Vitro Diagnostics Applications. Diagnostics 6(3):33. https://doi.org/10.3390/diagnostics6030033

Piaggio D, Namm G, Melillo P, Simonelli F, Iadanza E, Pecchia L (2021) Pupillometry via smartphone for low-resource settings. Biocybern Biomed Eng 41(3):891–902. https://doi.org/10.1016/j.bbe.2021.05.012

Pillay TS, Khan AI, Yenice S (2025) Artificial intelligence (AI) in point-of-care testing. Clin Chim Acta 574:120341. https://doi.org/10.1016/j.cca.2025.120341

Purohit B, Kumari R, Srivastava A, Chandra P (2025) A bioelectronic immunosensing platform comprising a gold dendritic 3D architecture sandwiched between graphene sheets for Oral cancer detection. ACS Appl Bio Mater 8(6):5015–5023. https://doi.org/10.1021/acsabm.5c00368

Quer G et al (2021) Wearable sensor data and self-reported symptoms for COVID-19 detection. Nat Med 27(1):73–77. https://doi.org/10.1038/s41591-020-1123-x

Ray TR et al (2019) Bio-integrated wearable systems: a comprehensive review. Chem Rev 119(8):5461–5533. https://doi.org/10.1021/acs.chemrev.8b00573

Razavi Z, Soltani M, Souri M, Pazoki-Toroudi H (2024) CRISPR-driven biosensors: a new frontier in rapid and accurate disease detection. Crit Rev Anal Chem:1–25. https://doi.org/10.1080/10408347.2024.2400267

Roh YH et al (2023) CRISPR-enhanced hydrogel microparticles for multiplexed detection of nucleic acids. Adv Sci 10(10):2206872. https://doi.org/10.1002/advs.202206872

Role of machine learning assisted biosensors in point-of-care-testing for clinical decisions. ACS Sensors. Accessed 27 July 2025. [Online]. Available: https://pubs.acs.org/doi/10.1021/acssensors.4c01582

Ross GMS et al (2023) Best practices and current implementation of emerging smartphone-based (bio)sensors—part 1: data handling and ethics. TrAC Trends Anal Chem 158:116863. https://doi.org/10.1016/j.trac.2022.116863

Sengar MS, Saxena S, Satsangee SP, Jain R (2021) Silver nanoparticles decorated functionalized multiwalled carbon nanotubes modified screen printed sensor for the voltammetric determination of butorphanol. J Appl Organomet Chem 1(2):95–108. https://doi.org/10.22034/jaoc.2021.289344.1023

Sengar MS, Saxena S, Satsangee SP, Jain R (2022a) CuO decorated polyaniline nanocomposite-based sensor for the electrochemical determination of an opioid analgesic. Ionics 28(2):903–918. https://doi.org/10.1007/s11581-021-04333-1

Sengar MS, Saxena S, Satsangee SP, Jain R (2022b) Graphene Oxide/1-butyl-3-Methylimidazolium Tetrafluoroborate Nanocomposite: Synthesis Characterization and its Application for the Electrochemical Determination of an Antihistamine and Anticholinergic Embramine. J Electrochem Soc 169(9):096506. https://doi.org/10.1149/1945-7111/ac8cb5

Sengar MS, Kumari P, Sengar N (2023) Theoretical and computational approaches and strategies in molecularly imprinted polymer development. In: Molecularly imprinted polymers for environmental monitoring: fundamentals and applications. IOP Publishing. https://doi.org/10.1088/978-0-7503-4962-8ch3

Sengar MS, Kumari P, Sengar N (2024) Challenges in the development of nanobiosensors in the diagnosis of cancer. In: Nano biosensors for non-invasive diagnosis of cancer. IOP Publishing. https://doi.org/10.1088/978-0-7503-6234-4ch13

Sengar MS, Kumari P, Sengar N, Satsangee SP, Jain R (2025) Co3O4/fluoro-copolymer nanocomposite modified boron-doped diamond electrode non-enzymatic sensor for the determination of skeletal muscle relaxant drug cyclobenzaprine in biological fluids. Talanta 287:127636. https://doi.org/10.1016/j.talanta.2025.127636

Shubhangi R, Kumari K, Kachhawaha SK, Singh SK, Rai, Chandra P (2024) Pristine NiMOF sandwiched between 1D and 3D engineered au particles and dendrites for Ultraswift folic acid sensing in cellular microenvironment. Anal Chem 96(50):19898–19907. https://doi.org/10.1021/acs.analchem.4c03564

Song Y et al (2023) 3D-printed epifluidic electronic skin for machine learning-powered multimodal health surveillance. Sci Adv 9(37):eadi6492. https://doi.org/10.1126/sciadv.adi6492

Su J et al (2022) Smartphone-based electrochemical biosensors for directly detecting serum-derived exosomes and monitoring their secretion. Anal Chem 94(7):3235–3244. https://doi.org/10.1021/acs.analchem.1c04910

Sun A, Wambach T, Venkatesh AG, Hall DA (2014) A low-cost smartphone-based electrochemical biosensor for point-of-care diagnostics. IEEE Biomed Circuits Syst Conf Healthc Technol Proc 2014:312–315. https://doi.org/10.1109/BioCAS.2014.6981725

Sun H et al (2023) Paper microfluidics with deep learning for portable intelligent nucleic acid amplification tests. Talanta 258:124470. https://doi.org/10.1016/j.talanta.2023.124470

Tay DMY et al (2023) Accelerating the optimization of vertical flow assay performance guided by a rational systematic model-based approach. Biosens Bioelectron 222:114977. https://doi.org/10.1016/j.bios.2022.114977

Tomlinson S, Behrmann S, Cranford J, Louie M, Hashikawa A (2018) Accuracy of smartphone-based pulse oximetry compared with hospital-grade pulse oximetry in healthy children. Telemed J E-Health Off J Am Telemed Assoc 24(7):527–535. https://doi.org/10.1089/tmj.2017.0166

Tyagi AK, Richa, Kumari S (2024) Smartphone-based sensors for biomedical applications. In: Artificial intelligence-enabled blockchain technology and digital twin for smart hospitals. Wiley, pp 327–345. https://doi.org/10.1002/9781394287420.ch17

Vargas E, Nandhakumar P, Ding S, Saha T, Wang J (2023) Insulin detection in diabetes mellitus: challenges and new prospects. Nat Rev Endocrinol 19(8):487–495. https://doi.org/10.1038/s41574-023-00842-3

Vashist SK, Schneider EM, Luong JHT (2014) Commercial smartphone-based devices and smart applications for personalized healthcare monitoring and management. Diagn Basel Switz 4(3):104–128. https://doi.org/10.3390/diagnostics4030104

Wang J et al (2023) Microneedle-based transdermal detection and sensing devices. Lab Chip 23(5):869–887. https://doi.org/10.1039/D2LC00790H

Wasilewski T, Kamysz W, Gębicki J (2024) AI-assisted detection of biomarkers by sensors and biosensors for early diagnosis and monitoring. Biosensors 14(7):356. https://doi.org/10.3390/bios14070356

Wilner OI, Yesodi D, Weizmann Y (2023) Point-of-care nucleic acid tests: assays and devices. Nanoscale 15(3):942–952. https://doi.org/10.1039/D2NR05385C

Yadav M, Kumari P, Kumar S (2021) Spectroscopic and molecular docking studies on the interaction of aloe. Chemistry and Biology Interface 11(4):112–123

Yang Y et al (2023) Rapid detection of SARS-CoV-2 RNA in human nasopharyngeal specimens using surface-enhanced Raman spectroscopy and deep learning algorithms. ACS Sens 8(1):297–307. https://doi.org/10.1021/acssensors.2c02194

Zarei M (2017) Portable biosensing devices for point-of-care diagnostics: recent developments and applications. TrAC Trends Anal Chem 91:26–41. https://doi.org/10.1016/j.trac.2017.04.001

Zhan J, Wang S, Li X, Zhang J (2025) Molecular engineering of functional DNA molecules toward point-of-care diagnostic devices. Chem Commun 61(22):4316–4338. https://doi.org/10.1039/D5CC00338E

Zhang D, Liu Q (2016) Biosensors and bioelectronics on smartphone for portable biochemical detection. Biosens Bioelectron 75:273–284. https://doi.org/10.1016/j.bios.2015.08.037

Zhang M, Cui X, Li N (2022) Smartphone-based mobile biosensors for the point-of-care testing of human metabolites. Mater Today Bio 14:100254. https://doi.org/10.1016/j.mtbio.2022.100254

Zhang X, Wang Y, He X, Yang Y, Chen X, Li J (2024) Advances in microneedle technology for biomedical detection. Biomater Sci 12(20):5134–5149. https://doi.org/10.1039/D4BM00794H

Zhao W, Tian S, Huang L, Liu K, Dong L, Guo J (2020) A smartphone-based biomedical sensory system. Analyst 145(8):2873–2891. https://doi.org/10.1039/C9AN02294E

Development of Continuous Glucose Monitoring Systems for Better Diabetes Management

9

Sushant Sharma, Rohit Mohite, Paras J. Keyravan, Archita Jha, Kishor Deshmukh, Dilnawaz Ansari, Hussain Valikarimwala, Amey Khatavkar, Buddhadev Purohit, and Rohit Srivastava

Abstract

Diabetes is a major global health concern affecting millions worldwide, where frequent blood glucose monitoring is critical to prevent further complications. The development of point-of-care self-monitoring of blood glucose (SMBG) devices revolutionized diabetes management. However, limitations, including their invasive nature and isolated glucose level determination, led to the development of continuous glucose monitoring (CGM) devices. The use of minimally invasive sensors and a longer period of measurement contributes to higher adherence in diabetes patients, which further leads to better glycaemic performances. This chapter describes the evolution of CGM devices as a case study for continuous monitoring of diabetes, the sensing mechanism of the devices, and the electronic components for real-time data acquisition and transmission. A comparison of different commercially available CGMs is discussed here. Finally, this chapter addresses the future of CGM and highlights the potential of artificial intelligence

S. Sharma · R. Mohite · P. J. Keyravan · B. Purohit (✉)
Department of Biosciences and Bioengineering, Indian Institute of Technology Bombay, Powai, Mumbai, India

A. Jha
MKSSS's Cummins College of Engineering for Women, Pune, Maharashtra, India

K. Deshmukh · D. Ansari
MGM University, Chhatrapati Sambhajinagar, Maharashtra, India

H. Valikarimwala · A. Khatavkar
MIT-ADT University, Pune, Maharashtra, India

R. Srivastava
Biosciences and Bioengineering, Indian Institute of Technology Bombay, Mumbai, Maharashtra, India

V. Patel et al. (eds.), *Biosensor Technology in Translating Novel Materials into Practical Devices*, https://doi.org/10.1007/978-981-95-5519-2_9

and machine learning in these systems. These advancements make CGM a breakthrough in diabetes care and a model system for personalized medicine.

Keywords
Continuous monitoring · Glucose · Machine learning · Blood glucose monitoring

9.1 Introduction

Biosensors are progressively being used for the detection and monitoring of various diseases alongside conventional laboratory-based diagnosis. The International Union of Pure and Applied Chemistry (IUPAC) defines a biosensor as: "A device that uses specific biochemical reactions mediated by isolated enzymes, immune systems, tissues, organelles or whole cells to detect chemical compounds usually by electrical, thermal or optical signals" (Nagel et al. 1992). Biosensors offer fast detection, ease of operation, analysis at the site of detection, cost-effectiveness, portability to remote locations, and can be operated by someone without any extensive training. Biosensors are especially important for critical care settings to reduce the time gap between treatment and diagnosis (Purohit et al. 2020). The next generation of biosensors is equipped with machine learning algorithms for enhanced data analysis required for multiplexing and to answer complex biological phenomena (Mahato et al. 2024; Mahato and Wang 2021; Saha et al. 2023; Tehrani et al. 2022). The most commercially successful biosensor is the development of the glucose biosensor, which contributes to more than 85% of the revenue of the total biosensor market worldwide (Kumar et al. 2022). The development of the glucose biosensor forever changed the global approach to diabetes management. Diabetes is a rapidly increasing disease with a prevalence of 830 million people in 2022. It is one of the top 10 causes of death worldwide, accounting for an enormous 12% of global healthcare spending going to care for diabetes and diabetes related complications (Yu et al. 2024). A group of disorders in the metabolism of carbohydrate, arising from insufficient insulin production, insulin response, or both, resulting in chronic hyperglycaemia, is referred to as diabetes mellitus (Poznyak et al. 2020).

High blood sugar levels (>80–120 mg/dL) also contribute to vision loss, nerve damage, diabetic foot ulcer, cardiovascular diseases, and ultimately death (Purohit et al. 2022). Sedentary lifestyles, high intake of processed food, and genetic predisposition contribute to this widespread prevalence of diabetes (www.diabetesatlas.org). According to the WHO, 8.5% of adults over age 18 were affected by diabetes in 2014. Moreover, 1.5 million deaths in 2019 were caused due to diabetes, and 48% of these deaths happened before 70 years of age (Antar et al. 2023). Hence, a frequent monitoring of glucose levels is crucial for diabetes management, and within the systems available for measuring glucose levels, self-monitoring of blood glucose (SMBG) devices have been critical in the management of diabetes. For the last 20 years, SMBG has aided in tracking glucose levels of the blood, and has also helped to prescribe doses and frequency of insulin, and food intake timings. Patients who undergo a minimum of three insulin injections daily are prescribed SMBG

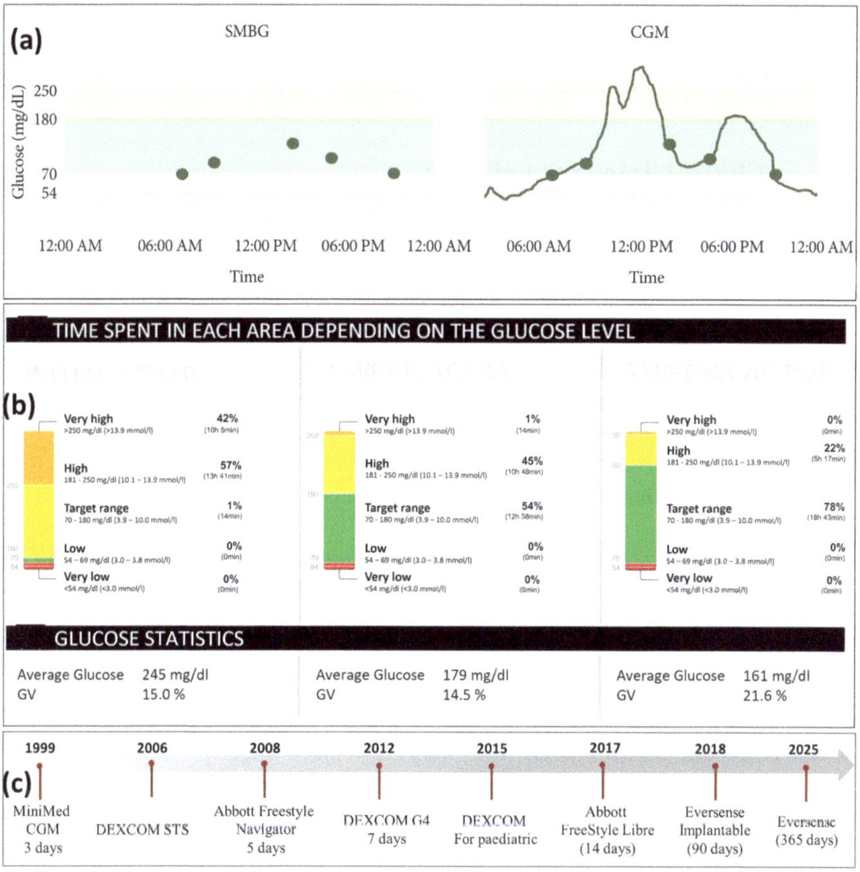

Fig. 9.1 The relevance of CGM in diabetes management. (**a**) The higher resolution of glucose in CGM devices over SMBG devices. (Reused with permission from et al. Yoo and Kim 2020). (**b**) Possibilities of using CGM for long-term glucose monitoring. Ambulatory glucose profile and glucose statistics of a 53-year-old patient's initial, middle, and five weeks of physical activity. (Reused with permission from Schubert-Olesen et al. 2022). (**c**) Timeline of development of different CGM devices

(Rodbard 2007). Although SMBG devices have been clinically indispensable, they are known to be painful (invasive devices with needles), provide isolated glucose levels, and are time-intensive. Continuous glucose monitoring (CGM) devices are minimally invasive and can accurately calculate the glucose level throughout the day (Girardin et al. 2009; Klonoff 2005; Vazeou 2011). A comparison shown in Fig. 9.1a highlights the difference between SBGM and CGM devices for the resolution of glucose spikes during a longer period of time (Yoo and Kim 2020). CGM devices offer high accuracy, a smaller sample size, monitor the instantaneous fluctuation of sugar level, as well as detect hypoglycaemic conditions when a user undergoes a prolonged hyperglycaemic state. Usually, CGMs alert the extreme cases of hyperglycaemia and hypoglycaemia when the alarm is enabled, and these early interventions contribute to reduced risk of life-threatening conditions (Patton and Clements 2012). Major commercial CGM devices, such as Freestyle Libre, Dexcom, Eversense, and Guardian Sensor, are used extensively for diabetes management.

9.2 Clinical Relevance of CGM

International consensus of CGM monitoring on blood sugar level (percentage of time in the various glycaemic ranges) in Type 1 Diabetes/Type 2 Diabetes (T1D/T2D) provided recommendations which are summarized in Table 9.1.

In one of the studies, 322 individuals (≥8 years of age) with HbA1c 7.0–10.0% (53–86 mmol/mol) used one of the CGM devices (Dexcom SEVEN, Medtronic MiniMed Paradigm REAL-Time Insulin Pump and Continuous Glucose-Monitoring System, Abbott FreeStyle Navigator), and post 26 weeks, a significant improvement in HbA1c was observed. The report suggests a strong correlation between improvement in glucose management with wearing the devices for 6 or more days per week (Beck et al. 2010).

In another study, termed as (Multiple Daily Injections and Continuous Glucose Monitoring in Diabetes-DIAMOND), the individuals using CGM (Dexcom G4) showed higher glycaemic control and higher adherence than usual care (D. S. Group et al. 2017). An open-label randomized trial of 226 adults, REPLACE-BG, found that there is no additional benefit of using CGMs with SBMG, in comparison to CGMs only. This study highlighted the efficacy of CGMs, and FDA-approved CGM device (Dexcom G5 Mobile CGM System) to replace finger-prick glucose testing (R.-B. S. Group et al. 2017). In Type 2 diabetes, CGMs have also been proven to reduce the time under hypoglycaemic and hyperglycaemic conditions better than SBGM devices (Vigersky et al. 2012). A study on 556 Indian patients revealed a reduction of 0.85% HbA1c levels upon use of CGM device for diabetes management (Dey et al. 2024; Kumar et al. 2025).

Table 9.1 International consensus-recommended CGM parameters

Glycaemic range	T1D/T2D recommendation	Pregnancy recommendation
Time in range (TIR)	>70% of time in range [70–180 mg/dl (3.9–10.0 mmol/L)]	>70% of time in range [63–140 mg/dl (3.5–7.8 mmol/L)]
Time below range (TBR 1)	<4% [<70 mg/dl (<3.9 mmol/L)]	<4% [<63 mg/dl (<3.5 mmol/L)]
Time below range (TBR 2–severe hypoglycaemia)	<1% [<54 mg/dl (<3.0 mmol/L)]	<1% [<54 mg/dl (<3.0 mmol/L)]
Time above range (TAR 1–hyperglycaemia)	<25% [>180 mg/dl (>10 mmol/L)]	<25% time above range [>140 mg/dl (>7.8 mmol/L)]
Time above range (TAR 2–severe hyperglycaemia)	<5% [>250 mg/dl (>13.9 mmol/dl)]	–

Figure 9.1b shows the further possibilities of CGMs for diabetes management, where a 53-year-old T2D patient was treated with oral anti-diabetes medicines, and wore a CGM for 7 days trial period. The ambulatory glucose profile (AGP) was used for visualization of glycaemic variability throughout the observation period. The graph shows the improvement in glycaemic control of person at the initial stage, during, and after regular physical activity (Brinkmann et al. 2021; Schubert-Olesen et al. 2022).

9.3 Working Principle

All glucose-sensing devices can be classified into three different generations based on the transfer of charge species from the glucose oxidase (GOx) enzyme to the electrode surface, and the subsequent generation of measurable electrical signals proportional to glucose concentration (Clark and Lyons 1962; Wijayanti et al. 2023). The first-generation GOx sensor uses oxygen as the electron acceptor, which gets reduced by GOx to hydrogen peroxide in the presence of glucose. Glucose concentration is determined by electrochemically monitoring the hydrogen peroxide level (Campbell et al. 2017). The major limitation of the first-generation GOx sensor is that its sensor signal can be easily affected by the dissolved oxygen concentration of the sample (Lee et al. 2019). To counter this issue, the second-generation GOx sensor uses a soluble electron transfer mediator to overcome the oxygen limitation observed in the first-generation GOx sensor. Mediators like ferrocene derivatives, organic salts, and quinones have the ability to perform rapid, reversible redox reactions. This progress also enabled the invention of a true miniature device and the use of disposable electrodes in terms of glucose sensing. The third generation of glucose sensor relies on the idea of direct electron transfer between the enzyme reaction centre and the electrode. Flavin adenine dinucleotide (FAD)-glucose dehydrogenase, a three-subunit enzyme, is involved, which has a catalytic subunit, an electron transfer subunit, and a small subunit (Lee et al. 2021). The oxidation of glucose at the reaction centre produces electrons, which are transferred to the electron transfer subunit and then finally via FAD, 3Fe-4S cluster, and haeme-subunits to the sensing electrode. Since very little sample volume is required, no external chemical or mediators are needed, and the signal can be generated at very low potential without interferences from other molecules, the third-generation biosensors are ideal for monitoring glucose levels in different body fluids. Based on the operational procedure, the commercial CGMs operating on electrochemical biosensing principles can be grouped into non-invasive reverse iontophoresis (RI) based CGMs (such as GlucoWatch), minimally invasive transdermal sensors, and implanted optical EverSense CGM sensor. RI-based CGMs called GlucoWatch® G2 Biographer by Cygnus Inc. was first developed in 2001 using sweat samples for the glucose monitoring, where a current density is applied on skin to extract sweat and analytes onto the electrode surface (as shown in Fig. 9.2a, b). In 2007, the GlucoWatch® G2 Biographer was discontinued from the market (Zheng et al. 2023; Zhu et al. 2023).

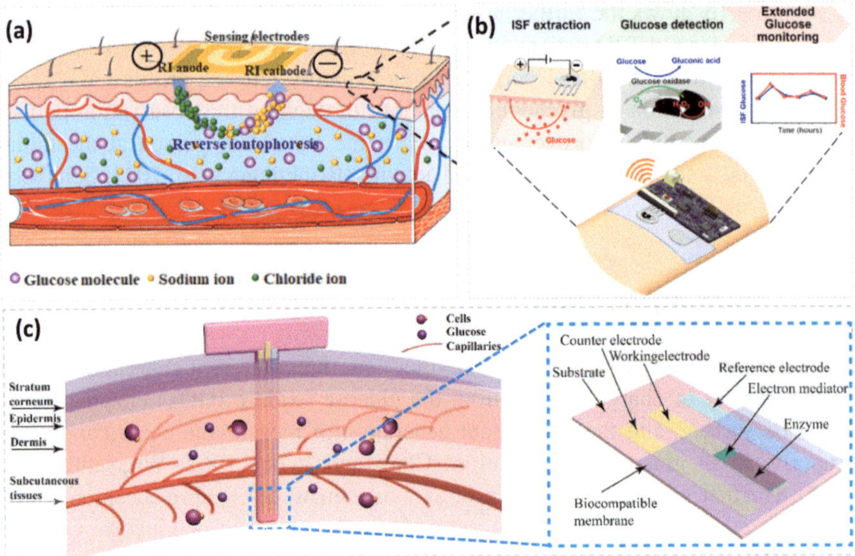

Fig. 9.2 Reverse iontophoresis-based CGM. (**a**) A graphical representation of transdermal extraction of glucose on a glucose sensor, and (**b**) skin-worn electrochemical biosensor for the noninvasive monitoring of glucose in the ISF. (Reused with permission from Zhu et al. 2023, De la Paz et al. 2023); (**c**) A scheme for a common transdermal glucose biosensor. (Reused with permission from Liu et al. 2023)

The most commercially successful CGMs are based on amperometric transdermal sensor, where the sensor is inserted up to the subcutaneous layer, and the glucose is measured by the reaction of GOx. As shown in Fig. 9.2c, the sensor is composed of three electrodes, with an electron mediator layer in between the electrode and the enzymes to reduce the electroactive interferences caused by high detection voltage (Liu et al. 2023). Nafion® (perfluorosulfonated ionomer) is used to decrease the interference from other electroactive substrates, and biocompatible membranes are used to minimize body response (Purohit et al. 2022). Eversense 365 CGM by Senseonics Inc., which got FDA approval in 2025, is a third-generation CGM device operated based on optical sensing is capable of 365 days of glucose monitoring (Kumar et al. 2025). Its predecessors were capable of 14 days and 90 days of continuous monitoring. In this chapter, we primarily focuse on commercially successful transdermal electrochemical sensors.

9.4 Components of CGMs

9.4.1 Electrodes

The first FDA-approved CGM device Medtronic MiniMed and its subsequent versions are based on a first-generation three-electrode system. The working (Pt), counter (Pt), and reference (Ag/AgCl) were developed over a ceramic Al_2O_3 base, and the enzyme GOx was crosslinked on the Pt electrode with either bovine serum albumin or human serum albumin. The most commonly used cross-linker, glutaraldehyde, is now increasingly replaced due to its toxicity and substituted with UV-cross-linker. To overcome the oxygen deficiency at GOx catalysis, it uses a polyurea polyurethane polymer to enhance the permeability of oxygen and hinder the glucose movement. The final layer used was an amphiphilic membrane with its hydrophobic unit (such as siloxane polymer) facilitating oxygen permeability and its hydrophilic unit (such as diisocyanate) facilitating glucose diffusion. A ratio was maintained between these two polymers for optimal glucose and oxygen permeability, and even a second layer of branched acrylate was used to nullify the effect of temperature on the amphiphilic layer (Kumar Das et al. 2022). The design and different layers of the Medtronic CGM sensor are shown in Fig. 9.3a. Dexcom electrodes, as shown in Fig. 9.3b, are based on a two-electrode system with a helically wound counter/reference electrode. The working electrode (Pt) and reference (Ag/AgCl) were made from fine wire, and a layer of polymerized para-xylylene was used as an insulator between them. An additional electrolyte domain with a buffer solution for ion transport was present to protect the electrodes from a pH gradient. An anti-interference layer was used, and the enzyme layer was developed in a colloidal polyurethane polymer. An amphiphilic layer composed of a hydrophobic domain (such as polyurethane and polyamides polysiloxane), and a hydrophilic domain (such as polyvinyl alcohol, poly (ethylene glycol), etc.) provided a balanced permeability of oxygen and glucose (Das et al. 2022). Abbott CGM sensors used a carbon working and counter electrode, and an Ag/AgCl reference electrode, with an electron transfer mediator between the catalytic site and electrode. The sensing layer of GOx is formed by a polymer backbone, a cross-linker, and a metal

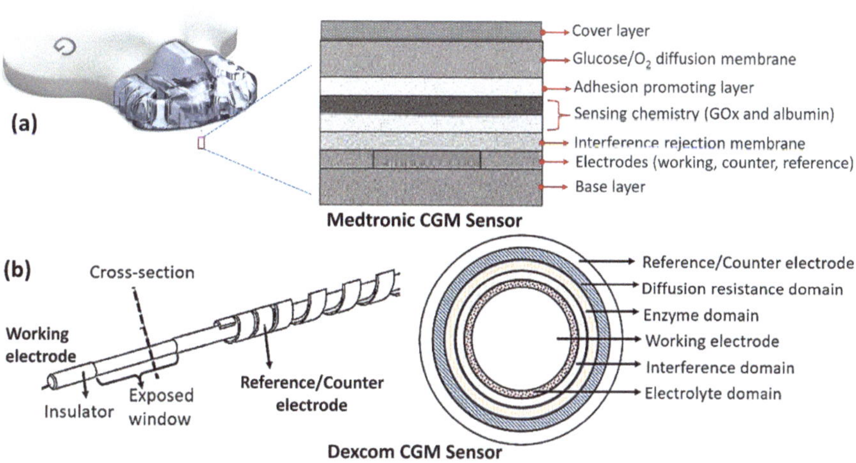

Fig. 9.3 (**a**) Medtronic and (**b**) Dexcom CGM sensors and different layers of their working electrodes. (Reused with permission from Das et al. 2022)

transition complex for efficient glucose sensing. This CGM was based on the second generation of glucose sensor and was not affected by fluctuations in oxygen level. A poly(vinylpyridine-co-styrene) layer was used to control the movement of glucose, and another layer of poly(ethylene glycol) or polyhydroxyl was used for biocompatibility (Henning 2009).

9.4.2 Electron Transfer Mediators

One significant challenge in enzymatic glucose sensors is achieving efficient electron transfer between the enzyme active site and the electrode surface. Direct electron transfer is often hindered by the enzyme's protein structure, which can insulate the active site from the electrode. Mediator-based systems solve this problem by incorporating redox mediators that shuttle electrons between the enzyme and electrode. In the second generation of biosensors, an electron transfer molecule is used to bridge the redox-enzymatic reactions with the electrode (Adachi et al. 2020). Common mediators include ferrocene derivatives, osmium complexes, and conducting polymers. These compounds have redox potentials that allow them to accept electrons from the enzyme and transfer them to the electrode at relatively low operating potentials. This reduces interference from other electroactive species and improves sensor selectivity. Osmium-based redox polymers (Abbott CGM sensor) have gained particular attention in recent years due to their excellent biocompatibility and stability. These polymers can be covalently attached to glucose oxidase, creating a three-dimensional network that promotes rapid electron transfer while maintaining enzyme activity over extended periods. This approach has been successfully implemented in several commercial CGM devices. Nanomaterial-mediated electron transfer is also tested using (Ru (III) + PD), which performed better than ferrocene monosulfate (Quan et al. 2025). Silver nanowires are used as mediators in catechol biosensors, increasing the efficiency and being better than traditional methods (Salvo-Comino et al. 2021).

9.4.3 Anti-Biofouling Layer

The electrochemical measurement of the glucose concentration in the subcutaneous ISF is influenced by the presence of various endogenous, drug, and food molecules (Heinemann 2022). Dexcom G6 uses a permselective membrane to reduce the effect of acetaminophen and related components. The Dexcom G6 is still susceptible to signal drift to hydroxyurea, an antineoplastic drug used during chemotherapy, which might show an elevated glucose level. Abbott FreeStyle Libre 2 suggests to intake less than 500 mg of ascorbic acid (vitamin C) per day to minimize the interference. Medtronic CGM systems exhibit similar problems to acetaminophen and hydroxyurea. Nafion® is most commonly used anti-interference layer to repel negatively charged interferents. Cellulose acetate and other electropolymerized membranes, such as poly(phenylenediamine), polyphenol, poly(aminophenol), and various substituted naphthalenes, help improve the CGM signal (Purohit et al. 2022).

9.4.4 Electronic Components

Once the glucose sensor detects a signal (an amperometric signal in the form of a small current produced by the redox reaction of glucose oxidase), a set of electronic subsystems work together to process the signal in a form that can be easily recognized. The power source, analogue front end (AFE), and microcontroller are the main electronic parts that accomplish this (Mansour et al. 2024). These components work together to filter, amplify, process, and wirelessly transmit the signal to external devices such as smartphones and smartwatches for further monitoring.

Analog Front End: AFE digitizes the signal that comes from the biosensor and prepares it for further processing. Since most glucose sensors are amperometric, their output is a current signal, often in the microampere or even nanoampere range. The current signal is amplified using a transimpedance amplifier (Lin et al. 2022). The signal is further filtered to remove any high-frequency noise and improve the signal-to-noise ratio. The next step is to pass the signal through an analogue-to-digital converter (ADC), which converts the signal to a digital format that the microcontroller can further process ("Crucial role of analog front ends, creating bridge to digital world," n.d.; Falconi and Mandal 2019). Recent technological advancements have led AFEs to become more multipurpose, and they contain many other components, such as temperature sensors.

Microcontroller: In modern CGM architectures, an electrochemical AFE interfaces to a microcontroller over standard serial buses such as I^2C, SPI, or UART, while the MCU/SoC manages control logic, local processing, storage, and wireless connectivity (Cappon et al. 2019). Real-time systems commonly use Bluetooth Low Energy is commonly used for data transmission (Funtanilla et al. 2019), whereas FreeStyle Libre employs NFC for scan-to-read functionality. Several research prototypes and some implantable devices demonstrate RFID for both power and telemetry (Xiao et al. 2015).

Power Source: Commercially, the most commonly used power sources for wearable biosensors are lithium batteries, and research is primarily aimed at how to make these lithium batteries smaller, lighter, and more power efficient (Al-Daraghmeh and Stone 2023). However, these batteries have a short lifespan and are not environmentally friendly, and hence, research has started into more viable alternatives. Self-powered devices have been a common area of interest amongst researchers for the past few years, so that the need for traditional batteries can be eliminated altogether. Thermoelectric generators, triboelectric nanogenerators, piezoelectric nanogenerators, biofuels, and solar cells are technologies that are currently being researched, all showing great promise for the future of self-powered CGM systems. Thermoelectric generators work on the Seebeck effect and convert the temperature difference between the body and the surroundings into electrical energy. Since human skin is usually warmer than ambient air, wearable TEGs can produce a small but continuous current to power the various electronic components of CGM devices (Yeo et al. 2022). Recently, Yuan and team reported a fully integrated, self-powered CGM system in the form of a multisensory bracelet that utilizes flexible thermoelectric generators as its power source (Yuan and Zhu 2020). Triboelectric nanogenerators (TENGs) are another emerging technology that converts mechanical energy to electricity by using the triboelectric effect, which is the generation of static electricity through friction (Zhou et al. 2023). A study by Zhao and team successfully developed a wearable biosensor for sweat analysis using fibre-based triboelectric nanogenerators (Zhao et al. 2022). Photovoltaic cells were utilized as power sources to make a self-powered smartwatch for sweat glucose monitoring in a recent study (Zhao et al. 2019). Meanwhile, Valdez-Ramirez and team integrated a biofuel cell into minimally invasive microneedles to detect glucose from interstitial fluid (Valdés-Ramírez et al. 2014). These advancements in energy-harvesting technologies offer an alternative to traditional batteries but have not seen widespread commercial use due to problems in scalability and unstable power supply. Thus, research on this topic is essential to make self-powered CGM devices more commercially viable in the near future.

Flexible electronics**:** One of the key factors contributing to CGM systems is the development of flexible printed circuit boards (FPCBs). The FPCBs can be placed or attached to the skin, making them ideal for continuous monitoring (Huang et al. 2025). This design improves comfort and ensures reliable glucose readings during daily activities. Miniaturization continues to be a critical advancement in continuous glucose monitors. Surface-mount technology (SMT) enables dense integration of essential electronics such as analogue front-end (AFE) ICs, microcontrollers, temperature sensors, and wireless radios onto highly compact boards, as seen in modern CGM modules (Moeinfard et al. 2024). Moreover, integration of microelectromechanical systems (MEMS) sensors with advanced AFE and IoT connectivity, exemplified by ultralow-power platforms like BioGAP-enables low-latency and energy-efficient biosignal processing in a small form factor (Frey et al. 2023; Irrera et al. 2024). These miniaturized, highly integrated systems contribute substantially to improved usability and everyday wearability of CGMs.

9.4.5 Wireless Communication

Bluetooth Low Energy (BLE): BLE is designed for low-power devices, making it most suitable for wearable sensors like CGM. BLE should not be confused with classic Bluetooth, both of which have different protocols and differ in data throughput ("Bluetooth Low Energy (BLE): A Complete Guide," n.d.). BLE spends most of its time in sleep mode and only transmits data in short bursts called data packets ("What is BLE? How does BLE work? | Litum," n.d.). This feature allows BLE to have a much longer battery life compared to classic Bluetooth. BLE operates in the 2.4 GHz ISM band, with data rates of 1 Mbps under LE 1 M and up to 2 Mbps in Bluetooth 5.0's LE 2 M PHY (Koulouras et al. 2025). Although optimal conditions can yield ranges of 50–100 m, practical indoor ranges are generally limited to approximately 10–20 m due to obstructions and environmental interference (Collotta et al. 2017). Commonly used BLE modules for biomedical applications include the Nordic Semiconductor nRF52 series and Silicon Labs BG22. Gia et al. used an nRF52 series BLE to develop an IoT-based CGM system (Gia et al. 2017).

Near-Field Communication (NFC)**:** NFC is a wireless communication method operating in a frequency range of 13.56 MHz that builds on the technology of radio frequency ID tags (RFID) (Mareli et al. 2013). NFC technology is extremely short-range and enables two-way communication only when devices touch each other or are a few centimetres apart, making NFC extremely secure. The main advantage that NFC poses is that it does not require an external battery. This is because an NCF is powered by the electromagnetic field produced by the NFC reader (for example, a smartphone) when it comes in close contact with the NFC tag's antenna (Olenik et al. 2021). An NFC-enabled CGM monitor was successfully developed by Anabtawi et al. (2016).

9.5 Commercial CGM Devices

Minimed iPro introduced the first wearable CGM device towards the end of the 1990s, whose ability to replace the SMBG strips was doubted by consumers (Garg and Akturk 2018). GlucoWatch® G2™ Biographer, a wristwatch-based CGM, was approved in 1999 by the FDA for providing ISF glucose readings. This product was later retracted from the market in 2007. The limited accuracy of the devices, their requirement of blood glucose calibration, and sensor-pump integration were some of the key challenges of the first CGM platforms that were sought to improve. This led to competition within the medical technology industries to produce dependable CGM products, causing breakthroughs in this field (Min et al. 2021). The first CGM device was commercialized by Medtronic (USA) in 2005, which was marketed as Guardian TM. Later in 2006, Dexicom (USA) released the STS System, which, over the past decade, led to many other major advancements in the functionality, design and cost-effective CGM devices, improving the quality of life for diabetic patients (Teymourian et al. 2020). Currently, major CGMs in the market include Abbot's Freestyle Libre 2 (USA), and Dexcom G6 (Dexcom, USA) which the user can wear for up to 14 and 10 days respectively. These devices are calibration-free, provide CGM data and trends and alarm the user about hyperglycaemic and hypoglycaemic conditions ("Dexcom G6 CGM System | No Fingersticks, No Scanning | Dexcom," n.d.; "FDA clears Abbott Freestyle Libre 2 for sale as integrated continuous glucose monitor | 2020-06-15 | BioWorld," n.d.). In 2017, Guardian Sensor 3 of Medtronic received approval from the FDA. This device had 7 days of wear time and could be paired with Medtronic Minimed 670G insulin pump to form the first ever hybrid closed-loop system that could adjust the basal insulin delivery automatically based on glucose levels of the body ("MiniMed™ 670G System Support | Medtronic," n.d.). CGM systems as such have the capability to compete with SMBG strips by obtaining a mean absolute relative difference (MARD) of $\leq 10\%$, as they rely on a thin needle-mounted enzyme-based sensors (Min et al. 2021). In 2020,

Senseonics (USA) received the FDA approval for Eversense which has a wear time of 90 days ("Eversense Continuous Glucose Monitoring (CGM) Device | Glucose Monitoring System Devices for Diabetes Management," n.d.). Eclipse 3 ICGM is a CGM device being developed by Glysense (San Diego, USA), which aims at making an implantable CGM system that can be worn for a maximum of 2 years (Min et al. 2021). Biolinq (USA) is another company exploring the possibilities of using microneedles, which reach the ISF at the epidermis, i.e., at around 500 μm depth from the skin surface, rather than conventional CGMs that penetrate at least 5–11 nm into the subcutaneous layer of the skin. These microneedle-based CGM patches allow painless blood glucose monitoring ("Biolinq | Wearable Biosensors," n.d.). Recently, Eversense365, for its implantable optical sensor, got approval for 365 days of continuous monitoring (Bailey et al. 2025; Garg et al. 2022). Table 9.2 summarizes the properties of commercially available CGM devices.

9.6 Limitations

There has been a significant improvement in the design of the majority of the commercial CGM devices (Purohit and Chandra 2023). This was partly due to the FDA and other regulatory bodies requiring human factor studies for the devices before being approved, including improvements in the accuracy of glucose measurement, hypoglycaemic alarm, and user-friendly displays ("Applying Human Factors and Usability Engineering to Medical Devices | FDA," n.d.). However, there are several limitations still persisting with the CGM devices. A standard SMBG is still required for the initial calibration and regular periodic calibration of the CGM devices by measuring the capillary blood glucose levels, with the exception of isCGM. Sensors have approval for only a certain period of time, with implantable sensors having the longest life. Some of the common issues associated with CGMs include development of skin rashes and reactions on site, biofouling, transmission issues of the devices (specifically at night), functional defect of the device, peeling, falling, and sweating off. Minor problems that can be potentially hazardous are also reported, such as when smartphones are connected to devices that are in silent or vibration mode, the alarm of the sensor is also silenced. For an even wider reach of CGM can be achieved by making the devices and its components cost-effective (Petrie et al. 2017).

9.7 Future Prospective and Conclusion

The future of CGM devices for diabetes management is a global necessity for improving the lives of close to half a billion people. The CGM devices need to be more accurate, resistant to biofouling and interference molecules, and integrated or connected with other devices for a holistic approach to improve healthcare (Campos-Náñez and Breton 2017). Moreover, for more Type I and Type II diabetes patients to adopt CGM devices, it should ideally be non-invasive and should not require any

Table 9.2 Comparison of commercially available CGM devices

Device	Calibration	Age of use	Warm up	Wear length	Alarm	Data display	Accuracy (MARD)
Freestyle libre 2	Not required, factory calibrated	4+ years	1 hour	14 days	Yes	Reader, freestyle LibreLink app	9.2% in adults, 9.7% in paediatrics
Freestyle libre 3	Not required, factory calibrated	4+ years	1 hour	14 days	Yes	Reader, freestyle LibreLink app	9.2% in adults, 9.7% in paediatrics
Dexcom G6	Not required, factory calibrated	2+ years	2 hours	10 days	Yes	Dexcom clarity app	10.0%
Dexcom G7	Not required, factory calibrated	2+ years	27 minutes	10.5 days	Yes (can delay by 6 hours)	Dexcom clarity app	8.2% in arm, 9.1% in abdomen
Eversense	2 times/ day	18+ years	24 hours	90 days	Yes, on-body vibration	Eversense app	9.8%
Eversense E3	2 times/ day for 21 days, followed by 1 time per day after 21 days	18+ years	24 hours	180 days	Yes, on-body vibration	Eversense app	8.5%
Eversense 365	1 time/day for 13 days followed by 1 time/ week for the next 351 days	18+ years	24 hours	365 days	Yes, on-body vibration	Eversense 365 app	8.5%
Guardian sensor 3	2 times/ day minimum	2+ years	2 hours	7 days	Yes	Guardian connect app	8.7% in arm, 9.1% in abdomen
Guardian sensor 4	Not required, factory calibrated	14+ years	2 hours	7 days	Yes	Guardian connect app	10.6%

kind of insertion into the skin. Hence, there is a need for the implantation of a sensor and its removal without professional surgical procedures (Lee et al. 2021). Recently, the development of Artificial Intelligence (AI) in the field of healthcare has illuminated possibilities of improved long-term management of diabetes (Subramanian

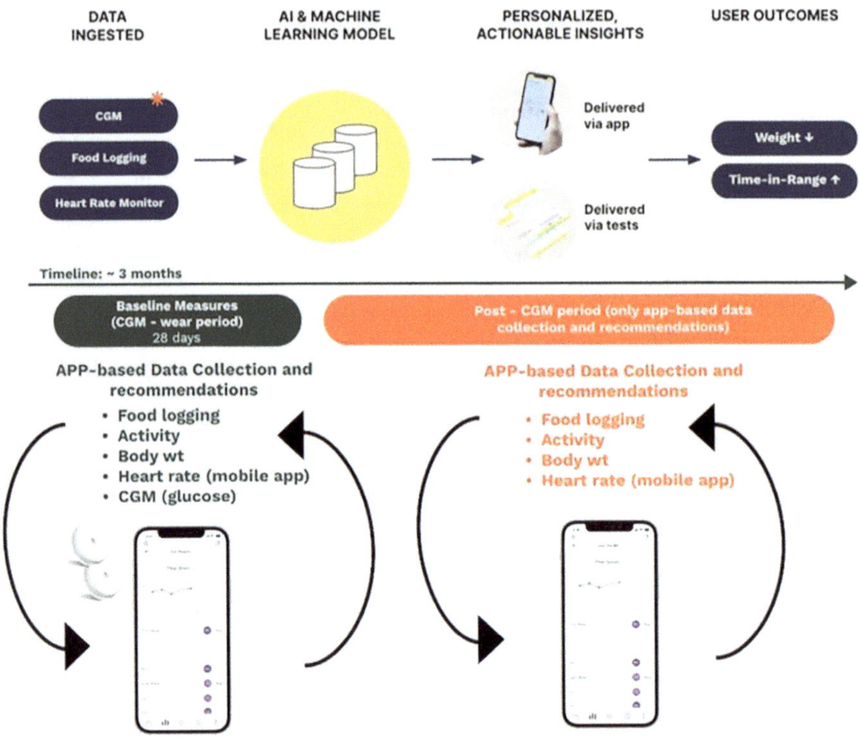

Fig. 9.4 A scheme for effective and personalized lifestyle recommendation for using wearable CGM and a machine learning approach. Here, the participants used the January AI app, Abbott Freestyle Libre, and an HR monitor by Apple Watch for 28 days. (Reused with permission from Zahedani et al. 2023)

et al. 2020). AI can analyse the large amounts of data generated by CGM using its powerful algorithm and predict blood glucose trends in the future, identify patterns and also detect early signs of disease risk (Shen and Kleinberg 2025). Zahedani et al. conducted a study where they monitored the lifestyle of 2217 participants, integrating food habits, physical activity, and body weight with CGM data. After two months, they found an increase in healthy eating, and reduced body weights in overweight or obese participants. The associated application was based on a machine learning approach, and was designed to suggest lifestyle recommendations based on personal goals and user preferences. This is one glimpse at a future with CGMs integration for everyday lifestyle, even for non-diabetic individuals (Zahedani et al. 2023). Figure 9.4 shows the pathway of personalized lifestyle recommendation using wearable CGM.

The CGM devices can resolve the glucose concentration in blood better than any other devices for multiple-day analysis. In the last 25 years, the CGM devices have become more sensitive and capable of tracking glucose for a longer period of time compared to their predecessors. EverSense 365, the latest CGM, can monitor glucose for an astonishing one year. The developments reported from academic and state-of-the-art devices show an increasing trend in self-powered sensors, integration with nonenzymatic elements, wireless data transmission, machine learning based data analysis, and complete automation of the systems. The CGM devices need to overcome the challenges such as the requirement of periodic calibration, maintaining higher accuracy in the presence of interfering drugs, and being cost-effective for wider adaptation in the developing world. Machine learning methods can be used to monitor the glucose level post-therapy and medication, and it can be used further for dose adjustment. In the near future, this CGM data will be trained by machine learning algorithms for food intake and physical activity recommendation for population-level healthcare initiatives.

References

Adachi T, Kitazumi Y, Shirai O, Kano K (2020) Development perspective of bioelectrocatalysis based biosensors. Sensors (Switzerland). https://doi.org/10.3390/s20174826

Al-Daraghmeh MY, Stone RT (2023) A review of medical wearables: materials, power sources, sensors, and manufacturing aspects of human wearable technologies. J Med Eng Technol 47:67–81. https://doi.org/10.1080/03091902.2022.2097743

Anabtawi N, Freeman S, Ferzli R (2016) A fully implantable, NFC enabled, continuous interstitial glucose monitor. In: 3rd IEEE EMBS international conference on biomedical and health informatics, BHI 2016, pp 612–615. https://doi.org/10.1109/BHI.2016.7455973

Antar SA, Ashour NA, Sharaky M, Khattab M, Ashour NA, Zaid RT, Roh EJ, Elkamhawy A, Al-Karmalawy AA (2023) Diabetes mellitus: classification, mediators, and complications; A gate to identify potential targets for the development of new effective treatments. Biomed Pharmacother 168:115734. https://doi.org/10.1016/J.BIOPHA.2023.115734

Applying Human Factors and Usability Engineering to Medical Devices | FDA [WWW Document] (n.d.). https://www.fda.gov/regulatory-information/search-fda-guidance-documents/applying-human-factors-and-usability-engineering-medical-devices. Accessed 8.26.25

Bailey TS, Liljenquist DR, Denham DS, Brazg RL, Ioacara S, Masciotti J, Ghosh-Dastidar S, Tweden KS, Kaufman FR (2025) Evaluation of accuracy and safety of the 365-day implantable Eversense continuous glucose monitoring system: the ENHANCE study. Diabetes Technol Ther 27:407–411. https://doi.org/10.1089/DIA.2024.0592

Beck RW, Weinzimer S, Miller K, Beck R, Xing D, Fiallo-Scharer R, Gilliam LK, Kollman C, Laffel L, Mauras N, Ruedy K, Tamborlane W, Tsalikian E (2010) Effectiveness of continuous glucose monitoring in a clinical care environment: evidence from the Juvenile Diabetes Research Foundation Continuous Glucose Monitoring (JDRF-CGM) trial. Diabetes Care 33:17–22. https://doi.org/10.2337/DC09-1502

Biolinq | Wearable Biosensors [WWW Document] (n.d.). https://www.biolinq.com/. Accessed 8.18.25

Bluetooth Low Energy (BLE): A Complete Guide [WWW Document] (n.d.). https://novelbits.io/bluetooth-low-energy-ble-complete-guide/. Accessed 8.12.25

Brinkmann C, Kröger J, Siegmund T, Thurm U, Halle M (2021) AGP-Fibel Bewegung: mit CGM Glukoseverläufe bei Bewegung analysieren: mit Beispielen und Übungen

Campbell AS, Islam MF, Russell AJ (2017) Intramolecular electron transfer through poly-Ferrocenyl glucose oxidase conjugates to carbon electrodes: 1. Sensor sensitivity, Selectivity and Longevity. Electrochim Acta 248:578–584. https://doi.org/10.1016/J.ELECTACTA.2017.07.150

Campos-Náñez E, Breton MD (2017) Effect of BGM accuracy on the clinical performance of CGM: an in-Silico study. J Diabetes Sci Technol 11:1196–1206. https://doi.org/10.1177/1932296817710476

Cappon G, Vettoretti M, Sparacino G, Facchinetti A (2019) Continuous glucose monitoring sensors for diabetes management: a review of technologies and applications. Diabetes Metab J 43:383–397. https://doi.org/10.4093/DMJ.2019.0121

Clark LC, Lyons C (1962) Electrode systems for continuous monitoring in cardiovascular surgery. Ann N Y Acad Sci 102:29–45. https://doi.org/10.1111/J.1749-6632.1962.TB13623.X

Collotta M, Pau G, Talty T, Member S, Tonguz OK (2017) Bluetooth 5: a concrete step forward towards the IoT

Crucial role of analog front ends, creating bridge to digital world [WWW Document] (n.d.). https://www.avnet.com/americas/resources/article/crucial-role-of-analog-front-ends-creating-bridge-to-digital-world/. Accessed 8.12.25

Das SK, Nayak KK, Krishnaswamy PR, Kumar V, Bhat N (2022) Review—electrochemistry and other emerging technologies for continuous glucose monitoring devices. ECS Sens Plus 1:031601

Dexcom G6 CGM System | No Fingersticks, No Scanning | Dexcom [WWW Document] (n.d.). https://www.dexcom.com/g6-cgm-system. Accessed 8.18.25

Dey AK, Gupta M, Gokalani R (2024) Impact of continuous glucose monitoring on glycemic control and lifestyle changes among diabetes patients: evidence from a diverse Indian cohort. Int J Diabetes Technol 3:119–127. https://doi.org/10.4103/ijdt.ijdt_36_24

Eversense Continuous Glucose Monitoring (CGM) Device | Glucose Monitoring System Devices for Diabetes Management [WWW Document] (n.d.). https://www.eversensecgm.com/. Accessed 8.18.25

Falconi C, Mandal S (2019) Interface electronics: state-of-the-art, opportunities and needs. Sens Actuators A Phys 296:24–30. https://doi.org/10.1016/J.SNA.2019.07.002

FDA clears Abbott Freestyle Libre 2 for sale as integrated continuous glucose monitor | 2020-06-15 | BioWorld [WWW Document] (n.d.). https://www.bioworld.com/articles/435809-fda-clears-abbott-freestyle-libre-2-for-sale-as-integrated-continuous-glucose-monitor?v=preview. Accessed 8.18.25

Frey S, Guermandi M, Benatti S, Kartsch V, Cossettini A, Benini L (2023) BioGAP: a 10-Core FP-capable ultra-low power IoT processor, with medical-grade AFE and BLE connectivity for wearable biosignal processing. https://doi.org/10.1109/COINS57856.2023.10189286

Funtanilla VD, Caliendo T, Hilas O (2019) Continuous glucose monitoring: a review of available systems. Pharm Therap 44:550

Garg SK, Akturk HK (2018) A new era in continuous glucose monitoring: food and drug administration creates a new category of factory-calibrated nonadjunctive, interoperable class ii medical devices. Diabetes Technol Ther 20:391–394. https://doi.org/10.1089/DIA.2018.0142

Garg SK, Liljenquist D, Bode B, Christiansen MP, Bailey TS, Brazg RL, Denham DS, Chang AR, Akturk HK, Dehennis A, Tweden KS, Kaufman FR (2022) Evaluation of accuracy and safety of the next-generation up to 180-day long-term implantable Eversense continuous glucose monitoring system: the PROMISE study. Diabetes Technol Ther 24:84–92. https://doi.org/10.1089/DIA.2021.0182

Gia TN, Ali M, Dhaou IB, Rahmani AM, Westerlund T, Liljeberg P, Tenhunen H (2017) IoT-based continuous glucose monitoring system: a feasibility study. Proc Comput Sci 109:327–334. https://doi.org/10.1016/J.PROCS.2017.05.359

Girardin CM, Huot C, Gonthier M, Delvin E (2009) Continuous glucose monitoring: A review of biochemical perspectives and clinical use in type 1 diabetes. Clin Biochem 42:136–142. https://doi.org/10.1016/J.CLINBIOCHEM.2008.09.112

Group DS, Beck RW, Riddlesworth T, Ruedy K et al (2017) Effect of continuous glucose monitoring on glycemic control in adults with type 1 diabetes using insulin injections: the DIAMOND randomized clinical trial. JAMA 317:371–378

Group R-BS, Aleppo G, Ruedy KJ, Riddlesworth TD et al (2017) REPLACE-BG: a randomized trial comparing continuous glucose monitoring with and without routine blood glucose monitoring in adults with well-controlled type 1 diabetes. Diabetes Care 40:538–545

Heinemann L (2022) Interferences with CGM systems: practical relevance? J Diabetes Sci Technol 16:271–274. https://doi.org/10.1177/19322968211065065

Henning T (2009) Commercially available continuous glucose monitoring systems. In: In vivo glucose sensing, pp 113–156. https://doi.org/10.1002/9780470567319

Huang W, Yang Y, Xu Y, Xiao F, Wang L (2025) Sweat wearable sensor based on confined Pt nanoparticles in 2D conductive metal–organic frameworks for continuous glucose monitoring. Adv Sci:e07212. https://doi.org/10.1002/ADVS.202507212

Irrera F, Gumiero A, Zampogna A, Boscari F, Avogaro A, Gazzanti Pugliese di Cotrone MA, Patera M, Della Torre L, Picozzi N, Suppa A (2024) Multisensor integrated platform based on MEMS charge variation sensing technology for biopotential acquisition. Sensors 24. https://doi.org/10.3390/S24051554

Klonoff D (2005) A review of continuous glucose monitoring technology. Diabetes Technol Ther 7:770–775. https://doi.org/10.1089/DIA.2005.7.770

Koulouras G, Katsoulis S, Zantalis F (2025) Evolution of Bluetooth technology: BLE in the IoT ecosystem. Sensors 25:996. https://doi.org/10.3390/S25040996

Kumar Das S, Nayak KK, Krishnaswamy PR, Kumar V, Bhat N (2022) Review—electrochemistry and other emerging technologies for continuous glucose monitoring devices. ECS Sens Plus 1:031601. https://doi.org/10.1149/2754-2726

Kumar A, Mahato K, Purohit B, Chandra P (2022) Commercial aspects and market pull of biosensors in diagnostic industries. In: Miniaturized biosensing devices. Springer Nature Singapore, Singapore, pp 351–368. https://doi.org/10.1007/978-981-16-9897-2_15

Kumar KV, Yerraguntla KR, Jenne MP, Gadi A, Sepoori A, Gunda A, Gudivada MS (2025) Advancements in continuous glucose monitoring: a revolution in diabetes management. Biomed Mater Devices:1–10. https://doi.org/10.1007/S44174-025-00396-0

Lee I, Loew N, Tsugawa W, Ikebukuro K, Sode K (2019) Development of a third-generation glucose sensor based on the open circuit potential for continuous glucose monitoring. Biosens Bioelectron 124–125:216–223. https://doi.org/10.1016/J.BIOS.2018.09.099

Lee I, Probst D, Klonoff D, Sode K (2021) Continuous glucose monitoring systems – current status and future perspectives of the flagship technologies in biosensor research. Biosens Bioelectron 181:113054. https://doi.org/10.1016/J.BIOS.2021.113054

Lin SH, Lefeuvre E, Tai CH, Wang HY (2022) Fabrication of high-performance non-enzymatic sensor by direct electrodeposition of nanomaterials on porous screen-printed electrodes. J Taiwan Inst Chem Eng 137:104386. https://doi.org/10.1016/J.JTICE.2022.104386

Liu Y, Yang L, Cui Y (2023) Transdermal amperometric biosensors for continuous glucose monitoring in diabetes. Talanta 253:124033. https://doi.org/10.1016/J.TALANTA.2022.124033

Mahato K, Wang J (2021) Electrochemical sensors: from the bench to the skin. Sens Actuators B Chem 344:130178. https://doi.org/10.1016/J.SNB.2021.130178

Mahato K, Saha T, Ding S, Sandhu SS, Chang AY, Wang J (2024) Hybrid multimodal wearable sensors for comprehensive health monitoring. Nat Electron 7:735–750. https://doi.org/10.1038/s41928-024-01247-4

Mansour M, Saeed Darweesh M, Soltan A (2024) Wearable devices for glucose monitoring: a review of state-of-the-art technologies and emerging trends. Alex Eng J 89:224–243. https://doi.org/10.1016/J.AEJ.2024.01.021

Mareli M, Rimer S, Paul BS, Ouahada K, Pitsillides A (2013) Experimental evaluation of NFC reliability between an RFID tag and a smartphone. IEEE AFRICON Conf. https://doi.org/10.1109/AFRCON.2013.6757740

Min J, Sempionatto JR, Teymourian H, Wang J, Gao W (2021) Wearable electrochemical biosensors in North America. Biosens Bioelectron 172:956–5663. https://doi.org/10.1016/j.bios.2020.112750

MiniMed™ 670G System Support | Medtronic [WWW Document] (n.d.). https://www.medtronic-diabetes.com/customer-support/minimed-670g-system-support. Accessed 8.18.25

Moeinfard T, Ghafar-Zadeh E, Magierowski S (2024) CMOS point-of-care diagnostics technologies: recent advances and future prospects. Micromachines 15:1320. https://doi.org/10.3390/MI15111320

Nagel B, Dellweg H, Gierasch LM (1992) Glossary for chemists of terms used in biotechnology. Pure Appl Chem 64:143–168. https://doi.org/10.1351/PAC199264010143

Olenik S, Lee HS, Güder F (2021) The future of near-field communication-based wireless sensing. Nat Rev Mater 6:286–288. https://doi.org/10.1038/S41578-021-00299-8

Patton SR, Clements MA (2012) Continuous glucose monitoring versus self-monitoring of blood glucose in children with type 1 diabetes- are there pros and cons for both? US Endocrinol 8:27

Petrie JR, Peters AL, Bergenstal RM, Holl RW, Fleming GA, Heinemann L (2017) Improving the clinical value and utility of CGM systems: issues and recommendations: A joint statement of the European Association for the Study of diabetes and the American Diabetes Association Diabetes Technology Working Group. Diabetologia 60:2319–2328. https://doi.org/10.1007/S00125-017-4463-4

Poznyak A, Grechko AV, Poggio P, Myasoedova VA, Alfieri V, Orekhov AN (2020) The diabetes mellitus–atherosclerosis connection: the role of lipid and glucose metabolism and chronic inflammation. Int J Mol Sci 21:1835. https://doi.org/10.3390/IJMS21051835

Purohit B, Chandra P (2023) Surface engineering and functional nanomaterials for point-of-care analytical devices. Springer Nature Singapore, Singapore. https://doi.org/10.1007/978-981-99-3025-8

Purohit B, Vernekar PR, Shetti NP, Chandra P (2020) Biosensor nanoengineering: design, operation, and implementation for biomolecular analysis. Sens Int 1:100040. https://doi.org/10.1016/j.sintl.2020.100040

Purohit B, Kumar A, Mahato K, Chandra P (2022) Continuous glucose monitoring for diabetes management based on miniaturized biosensors. In: Pranjal C, Mahato K (eds) Miniaturized biosensing devices. Springer Nature Singapore, Singapore, pp 149–175. https://doi.org/10.1007/978-981-16-9897-2_7

Quan C, Zhang Y, Liu Y, Wen L, Yang H, Huang X, Yang M, Xu B (2025) Electrochemical glucose sensor based on dual redox mediators. Biosensors (Basel) 15. https://doi.org/10.3390/bios15010009

Rodbard D (2007) Optimizing display, analysis, interpretation and utility of Self-Monitoring of Blood Glucose (SMBG) data for Management of Patients with diabetes. J Diab Sci Technol (Online) 1:62. https://doi.org/10.1177/193229680700100111

Saha T, Del Caño R, Mahato K, De la Paz E, Chen C, Ding S, Yin L, Wang J (2023) Wearable electrochemical glucose sensors in diabetes management: a comprehensive review. Chem Rev 123:7854–7889. https://doi.org/10.1021/ACS.CHEMREV.3C00078

Salvo-Comino C, Martin-Pedrosa F, Garcia-Cabezon C, Rodriguez-Mendez ML (2021) Silver nanowires as electron transfer mediators in electrochemical catechol biosensors. Sensors (Switzerland) 21:1–13. https://doi.org/10.3390/s21030899

Schubert-Olesen O, Kröger J, Siegmund T, Thurm U, Halle M (2022) Continuous glucose monitoring and physical activity. Int J Environ Res Public Health 19:12296. https://doi.org/10.3390/IJERPH191912296

Shen Y, Kleinberg S (2025) Personalized blood glucose forecasting from limited CGM data using incrementally retrained LSTM. IEEE Trans Biomed Eng 72:1266–1277. https://doi.org/10.1109/TBME.2024.3494732

Subramanian M, Wojtusciszyn A, Favre L, Boughorbel S, Shan J, Letaief KB, Pitteloud N, Chouchane L (2020) Precision medicine in the era of artificial intelligence: implications in chronic disease management. J Transl Med 18. https://doi.org/10.1186/S12967-020-02658-5

Tehrani F, Teymourian H, Wuerstle B, Kavner J, Patel R, Furmidge A, Aghavali R, Hosseini-Toudeshki H, Brown C, Zhang F, Mahato K, Li Z, Barfidokht A, Yin L, Warren P, Huang N, Patel Z, Mercier PP, Wang J (2022) An integrated wearable microneedle array for the continuous monitoring of multiple biomarkers in interstitial fluid. Nat Biomed Eng 6:1214–1224. https://doi.org/10.1038/S41551-022-00887-1

Teymourian H, Barfidokht A, Wang J (2020) Electrochemical glucose sensors in diabetes management: an updated review (2010–2020). Chem Soc Rev 49:7671–7709. https://doi.org/10.1039/D0CS00304B

Valdés-Ramírez G, Li YC, Kim J, Jia W, Bandodkar AJ, Nuñez-Flores R, Miller PR, Wu SY, Narayan R, Windmiller JR, Polsky R, Wang J (2014) Microneedle-based self-powered glucose sensor. Electrochem Commun 47:58–62. https://doi.org/10.1016/J.ELECOM.2014.07.014

Vazeou A (2011) Continuous blood glucose monitoring in diabetes treatment. Diabetes Res Clin Pract 93:S125–S130. https://doi.org/10.1016/S0168-8227(11)70028-6

Vigersky RA, Fonda SJ, Chellappa M, Walker MS, Ehrhardt NM (2012) Short- and long-term effects of real-time continuous glucose monitoring in patients with type 2 diabetes. Diabetes Care 35:32–38. https://doi.org/10.2337/DC11-1438

What is BLE? How does BLE work? | Litum [WWW Document] (n.d.). https://litum.com/what-is-ble-how-does-ble-work/. Accessed 8.12.25

Wijayanti SD, Tsvik L, Haltrich D (2023) Recent advances in electrochemical enzyme-based biosensors for food and beverage analysis. Foods. https://doi.org/10.3390/foods12183355

Xiao Z, Tan X, Chen X, Chen S, Zhang Z, Zhang H, Wang J, Huang Y, Zhang P, Zheng L, Min H (2015) An implantable RFID sensor tag toward continuous glucose monitoring. IEEE J Biomed Health Inform 19:910–919. https://doi.org/10.1109/JBHI.2015.2415836

Yeo M, Sattar M, Yeo W-H, Woodruff GW (2022) Recent advances in materials for wearable thermoelectric generators and biosensing devices. Materials 15:4315. https://doi.org/10.3390/MA15124315

Yoo JH, Kim JH (2020) Time in range from continuous glucose monitoring: a novel metric for glycemic control. Diabetes Metab J 44:828–839. https://doi.org/10.4093/DMJ.2020.0257

Yu TS, Song S, Yea J, Jang K (2024) Diabetes management in transition: market insights and technological advancements in CGM and insulin delivery. Adv Sensor Res 3. https://doi.org/10.1002/ADSR.202400048

Yuan J, Zhu R (2020) A fully self-powered wearable monitoring system with systematically optimized flexible thermoelectric generator. Appl Energy 271:115250. https://doi.org/10.1016/J.APENERGY.2020.115250

Zahedani AD, Veluvali A, McLaughlin T, Aghaeepour N, Hosseinian A, Agarwal S, Ruan J, Tripathi S, Woodward M, Hashemi N, Snyder M (2023) Digital health application integrating wearable data and behavioral patterns improves metabolic health. NPJ Digit Med 6:1–15. https://doi.org/10.1038/S41746

Zhao J, Lin Y, Wu J, Nyein HYY, Bariya M, Tai LC, Chao M, Ji W, Zhang G, Fan Z, Javey A (2019) A fully integrated and self-powered smartwatch for continuous sweat glucose monitoring. ACS Sens 4:1925–1933. https://doi.org/10.1021/ACSSENSORS.9B00891

Zhao T, Fu Y, Sun C, Zhao X, Jiao C, Du A, Wang Q, Mao Y, Liu B (2022) Wearable biosensors for real-time sweat analysis and body motion capture based on stretchable fiber-based triboelectric nanogenerators. Biosens Bioelectron 205:114115. https://doi.org/10.1016/J.BIOS.2022.114115

Zheng H, Pu Z, Wu H, Li C, Zhang X, Li D (2023) Reverse iontophoresis with the development of flexible electronics: a review. Biosens Bioelectron 223:115036. https://doi.org/10.1016/J.BIOS.2022.115036

Zhou Y, Zhang P, Li J, Mao X (2023) Recent progress of triboelectric nanogenerator-based power management and information processing circuit. Mater Today Sustain 23:100426. https://doi.org/10.1016/J.MTSUST.2023.100426

Zhu W, Yu H, Pu Z, Guo Z, Zheng H, Li C, Zhang X, Li J, Li D (2023) Effect of interstitial fluid pH on transdermal glucose extraction by reverse iontophoresis. Biosens Bioelectron 235:115406. https://doi.org/10.1016/J.BIOS.2023.115406

Wearable Devices for Healthcare Monitoring

10

Krishna Prasad Aryal, Dhruvi Kakadiya, Sutirtha Roy, Moshfiq-Us-Saleheen Chowdhury, Aditya Shekhar Nittala, and Richa Pandey

Abstract

Wearable healthcare sensing devices have become significant in upgrading continuous, real-time health monitoring, offering personalized and cautious healthcare solutions. This chapter mainly scans the key applications of wearable devices, including vital sign monitoring (e.g. heart rate, respiration rate, blood pressure), chronic disease handling (e.g. blood glucose, cardiovascular diseases), and mental health monitoring (e.g. stress and anxiety). The incorporation of advanced sensors, such as capacitive, piezoelectric, and optical sensors, and wearable devices, provides non-invasive, continuous tracking of physiological parameters. Advancements and improvements in materials utilized, including flexible substrates, carbon-based nanomaterials, and self-powered systems, resulted in the enhancement of device comfort, performance, and durability. This chapter emphasizes the potential of wearable biosensors in real-time health monitoring and the transformative impact they have on managing chronic conditions. Furthermore, the role of these devices in addressing mental health issues, such as

K. P. Aryal (✉) · D. Kakadiya
Department of Biomedical Engineering, University of Calgary, Calgary, AB, Canada
e-mail: krishna.aryal1@ucalgary.ca

S. Roy · Moshfiq-Us-Saleheen Chowdhury
Department of Electrical and Software Engineering, University of Calgary, Calgary, AB, Canada

A. S. Nittala
Department of Computer Science, University of Calgary, Calgary, AB, Canada

R. Pandey (✉)
Department of Biomedical Engineering, University of Calgary, Calgary, AB, Canada

Hotchkiss Brain Institute, University of Calgary, Calgary, AB, Canada
e-mail: richa.pandey@ucalgary.ca

V. Patel et al. (eds.), *Biosensor Technology in Translating Novel Materials into Practical Devices*, https://doi.org/10.1007/978-981-95-5519-2_10

stress and anxiety, through biomarkers like heart rate variability and cortisol levels, is also discussed. The continuing evolution of these technologies offers promising avenues for improving overall healthcare delivery and outcomes.

Keywords

Healthcare monitoring · Personalized monitoring · Wearables · Continuous glucose monitoring

10.1 Introduction

Wearable healthcare monitoring devices (WHMDs) have become critical instruments in modern healthcare, allowing for continuous, real-time tracking of crucial health indicators. These gadgets combine advanced sensor technology and data analytics to enable health monitoring outside of typical clinical settings, resulting in multiple benefits for patients, healthcare professionals, and the healthcare system in general. The growing use of WHMDs is promoting the integration of digital health and patient care, strengthening disease management, enabling early intervention, and improving health outcomes. This study examines the importance of continuous and real-time health monitoring, the integration of wearable devices into digital health ecosystems, and the consequences for patient care.

Wearable healthcare devices include a variety of technologies for monitoring physiological characteristics such as heart rate, blood pressure, blood glucose levels, oxygen saturation, physical activity, and sleep patterns. Smartwatches, fitness trackers, wearable electrocardiogram (ECG) monitors, glucose monitoring devices, and continuous glucose monitors (CGMs) are popular diabetes care tools. Wearable technology has grown as a result of developments in sensor downsizing, battery life, wireless connectivity, and data analytics capabilities (Piwek et al. 2016).

The fundamental benefit of WHMDs is their capacity to give continuous, real-time data about a user's health, allowing for more proactive, data-driven approaches to healthcare. Traditional healthcare approaches sometimes rely on infrequent testing during scheduled appointments or emergency visits, resulting in missed opportunities for early detection of health concerns. In contrast, wearable devices provide continuous monitoring, enabling quicker treatments and improved management of chronic illnesses such as cardiovascular disease, diabetes, and hypertension.

Continuous health monitoring is essential for a variety of reasons, most notably the management of chronic illnesses. Monitoring health data over time for patients with illnesses such as hypertension or diabetes enables healthcare providers to discover patterns, track treatment success, and alter management tactics as needed. Wearable blood glucose monitors, for example, can continually track blood sugar levels throughout the day, notifying users and healthcare practitioners when levels are abnormally high or low. This information allows patients to make appropriate modifications in real-time, minimizing serious problems like diabetic ketoacidosis or hypoglycaemia (Dagli et al. 2021).

Similarly, continuous heart rate and ECG monitoring via wearables can provide vital information for individuals with cardiovascular diseases. Early detection of abnormal heart rhythms, such as atrial fibrillation (AFib), allows for earlier intervention and reduces the risk of strokes or other major heart-related events (Almeida et al. 2020). Wearables can also monitor the body's response to physical exercise and stress, allowing for a better knowledge of a person's general health and wellness.

The value of continuous monitoring goes beyond chronic disease treatment. Wearables can provide real-time insights into a person's well-being, allowing for the early diagnosis of failing health in the elderly and vulnerable groups. For example, wearable fall detection systems can automatically warn caretakers or healthcare experts if a fall happens, allowing timely aid and potentially lowering the severity of harm (Piwek et al. 2016). Similarly, wearables can monitor vital signs such as body temperature, heart rate, and oxygen saturation, enabling the early detection of infections or serious medical disorders. The capacity to monitor health in real time allows people to take greater control of their health, resulting in more informed decisions and better health outcomes. Real-time feedback also boosts patient engagement, which is essential for boosting adherence to treatment plans and lifestyle changes. Wearables that track physical activity or sleep can motivate individuals to adopt healthier behaviours, such as increasing physical activity or improving sleep hygiene (Choi et al. 2021).

Wearable healthcare devices are an essential component of the larger digital health ecosystem, which includes the use of technology to monitor, manage, and enhance health. Wearables collect and transmit enormous volumes of health data that can be incorporated into digital health platforms, where artificial intelligence (AI), machine learning (ML), and cloud computing can be used to evaluate and understand this data (Choi ct al. 2021). This integration allows healthcare practitioners to extract actionable insights from data, resulting in more tailored and effective care.

Remote patient monitoring (RPM), which is an important part of modern healthcare, is enabled by digital health systems. RPM enables healthcare providers to track patient data outside of the clinic, allowing for ongoing management of chronic illnesses and eliminating the need for in-person visits. Wearable ECG monitors, for example, can convey real-time heart data to a healthcare physician, allowing them to analyse the patient's status and provide recommendations remotely. This is especially crucial for people in rural or underdeveloped areas, where access to healthcare services may be restricted. RPM also lessens the pressure on healthcare facilities, allowing professionals to devote more time to urgent situations.

The link between wearable gadgets and digital health extends to telemedicine. With the development of virtual consultations, healthcare professionals can increasingly integrate wearable data into telemedicine systems to give more informed, data-driven consultations. During a telemedicine consultation, a healthcare provider can evaluate real-time health data, such as blood pressure, heart rate, or blood glucose levels, to inform their diagnosis and treatment suggestions (Bansal et al. 2020). This combination of wearables, digital health platforms, and telemedicine improves care quality while increasing convenience and accessibility. Wearable devices also offer individualized medicine by providing detailed information about a person's health status over time. This information can be used by healthcare experts to create treatment regimens that are tailored to an individual's personal needs, preferences, and lifestyle. Personalized care is especially useful in the management of chronic illnesses, where long-term monitoring and fine-tuning of treatments are critical for improving health outcomes.

Furthermore, the integration of wearables into digital health systems allows for predictive analytics. Machine learning algorithms can detect trends in real-time health data and anticipate prospective health concerns, such as the possibility of a heart attack or stroke. Using this predictive power, healthcare providers can intervene sooner, lowering the need for emergency interventions and increasing patient outcomes (Almeida et al. 2020).

Wearable healthcare monitoring devices are revolutionizing patient care by providing continuous, real-time monitoring of vital health metrics. These devices facilitate early detection, personalized treatment, and proactive disease management, all of which contribute to better health outcomes. Through their integration with digital health platforms, wearables enable more efficient, accessible, and data-driven healthcare, empowering both patients and healthcare providers. As technology continues to evolve, wearable devices will play an increasingly critical role in transforming the healthcare landscape, supporting preventive care, and fostering a shift toward more patient-centred, proactive healthcare systems.

This chapter outlines the evolution, design, and applications of wearable healthcare devices. It covers early developments in wearable technology, the integration of advanced sensors and biosensors for specific applications, and the role of flexible electronics in enhancing comfort. It also explores the types of wearable sensors, material selection (including flexible and stretchable electronics), data transmission, and storage methods. Additionally, it discusses fabrication strategies and the diverse applications of wearable healthcare devices. The final section highlights recent advancements in the field, emphasizing innovation in biosensing technologies and their integration into wearable platforms for improved healthcare monitoring.

10.2 Evolution of Wearable Healthcare Devices

The rapid development of wearable healthcare monitoring devices represents both technological innovation and the growing demand for personalized, continuous healthcare solutions. This section focuses on the historical route of wearables, the significant advancements that shaped their functionality, and the integration of various biosensing platforms that have resulted in the revolution in healthcare monitoring.

10.2.1 Early Developments in Wearable Technology

The sequence of development and evolution of this technology can be summarized in a step-by-step manner as shown in Fig. 10.1, including key milestones in its history (Afyf et al. 2016; Salehi et al. 2022). Before the 1980s, devices like the Pulsar calculator watch and digital hearing aid were utilized. However, these devices were entirely mechanical and with a low degree of precision. Later, the concept of tracking physical activity was introduced. In the early 2000s, devices like wrist-worn watches and Fitbit were introduced, offering fitness tracking features. These electronics were mainly utilized for athletes and fitness purposes. Later, in the 2010s, devices such as Jawbone Up and Digital Eyeglasses were introduced. Meanwhile, the presence of wireless connectivity via Bluetooth and Wi-Fi enables real-time data synchronization with smartphones and other devices (Jin et al. 2020). The noticeable development of multifunctional smartwatches in the 2015 resulted in the transformation of wearables into very applicable and versatile devices capable of monitoring health metrics, providing notifications, and running applications. During this period, features such as sleep tracking, ECG monitoring, and SpO2 measurement were major milestones developed.

Later in the 2000s, biosensing wearable devices were developed significantly, and these devices were utilized to detect various biochemical markers, exploring applications for monitoring chronic diseases and stress. Recently, the integration of flexible electronics and materials has been a growing topic, improving its comfort

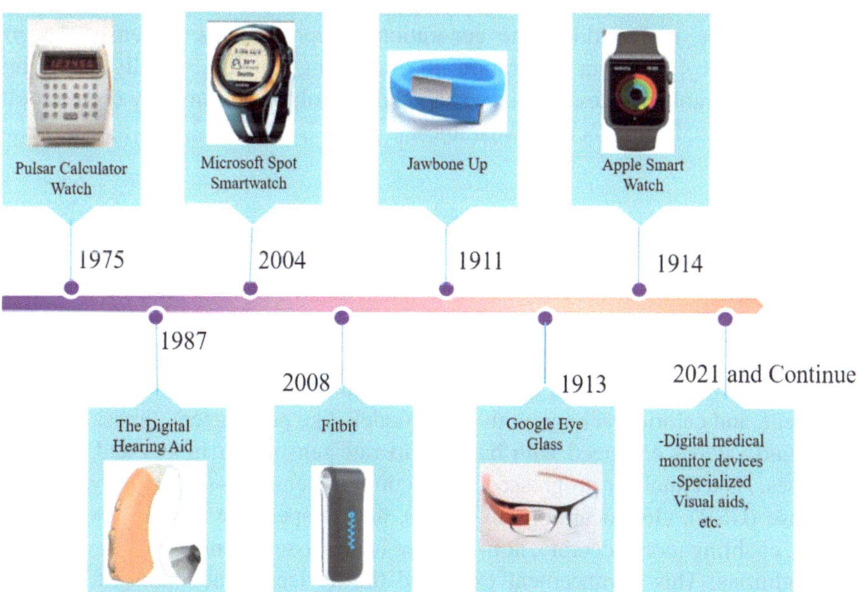

Fig. 10.1 A brief literature review from the 1970s to 2000s on wearable technologies. (Reproduced from Salehi et al. (2022). Licensed under CC BY 4.0)

Table 10.1 Generational improvements in wearables

Generation	Device examples	Sensor design	Power Efficiency	Data Integration
Ist Gen (1970s–1980s)	Pulsar calculator watch, digital hearing aid	Basic analogue sensors or mechanical switches	Low, disposable, or short-life batteries	No integration, isolated functionalities
2nd Gen (2000–2010)	Microsoft Spot Watch, Fitbit, Jawbone Up	Basic digital sensors (e.g. accelerometers, pedometers)	Moderate, lithium-based rechargeable batteries	USB or early wireless sync with computers or mobile devices
3rd Gen (2010–2020)	Apple Watch, Google Glass	Multi-modal sensors (e.g. HR, SpO_2, motion, EEG)	Optimized battery life, low-power processors	Real-time syncing with mobile apps and cloud-based storage
4th Gen (2020–Now)	Smart textiles, digital medical monitors	Flexible/stretchable biosensors (e.g. graphene, MXene)	High, self-powered via motion or body heat (TENGs, PENGs)	AI-enabled analytics, EHR integration, and telemedicine support

and integration. Similarly, recent advancements are also focused on the integration of sensors into textiles and hybrid designs. For example, reduced graphene oxide (rGO), its derivatives, and MXenes, which possess excellent flexibility, are making wearable devices more comfortable and multifunctional (Amani et al. 2025).

While Table 10.1 outlines the generational improvements in sensor design, power efficiency, and data integration, the following timeline visually highlights landmark wearable devices that have shaped this evolution-from early digital tools to today's smart, health-focused wearables.

10.2.2 Key Advancements and Functionality Improvements

Due to the growing demands for real-time health monitoring, wearable devices have significantly evolved over the years, driven by rapid technological advancements (de-la-Fuente-Robles et al. 2022). Initially, these devices were primarily designed for basic activity and lifestyle monitoring, including step counting, heart rate measurement, and calorie tracking, with early models like pedometers, fitness trackers, and smartwatches equipped with basic heart rate sensors for fitness and wellness purposes. As technology progressed, more complex sensors—such as galvanic skin response (GSR), electrocardiogram (ECG), and temperature sensors—were integrated, enabling more accurate, non-invasive health assessments for early detection of conditions. This advancement expanded the devices' functionality to include ECG monitoring for cardiac health, blood oxygen (SpO_2) monitoring for respiratory conditions, and stress and sleep tracking using GSR. The next phase of development emphasized data integration and the use of artificial intelligence (AI) and machine learning to analyse multimodal data, offering real-time health assessments, predictive health monitoring, and personalized feedback (Guk et al. 2019). Furthermore, the integration with mobile applications and cloud-based platforms has enhanced the user experience, allowing for remote monitoring, cloud data storage, and user-friendly interfaces. A major leap occurred with the development of wearable biosensors tailored for specific health conditions, including glucose monitoring for diabetes, mental health tracking (e.g. stress, anxiety, and depression), and monitoring of neurological conditions like Parkinson's disease through real-time tracking of motor functions and tremors. Finally, innovations in materials science have introduced flexible electronics, conductive fabrics, stretchable and thin-film sensors, and skin-compatible materials, making wearable devices more lightweight, comfortable, and adaptable for continuous wear, further enhancing their practicality and effectiveness in real-world health monitoring scenarios (Ometov et al. 2021).

10.2.3 Rise of Bio Wearables

The incorporation of biosensing technologies into wearables has elevated their application from fitness and lifestyle gadgets to tools for healthcare monitoring. These devices now offer comprehensive insights into a user's physiological condition, which can be significant for coping with diseases, improving well-being, and easing personalized medicine. Several sorts of biosensors can be integrated into wearable platforms to detect different analytes, enabling diverse applications in healthcare.

Among the various sensors in the application, electrochemical sensors are the ones that have been widely used for monitoring biomarkers (Duan et al. 2025). It can be utilized for the detection of body fluids such as sweat, saliva, and interstitial fluid. For example, electrochemical sensors embedded in wearable patches can also measure the composition of sweat, including glucose, lactate, and sodium concentrations. These types of embedded sensors are very useful and necessary for athletes or individuals with chronic disease conditions, such as diabetes, offering real-time data on hydration, metabolic rate, and other health indicators. Similarly, optical sensors are helpful for monitoring oxygen saturation (SpO_2) and heart rate using light. Recently, wearable devices like smartwatches integrating with optical sensors have been used to continuously monitor a user's heart rate and oxygen saturation levels (Niknejad et al. 2020).

In recent times, the combination of different sensor modalities into a single wearable device platform is a growing trend in biosensing technology. These types of multimodal sensors can simultaneously monitor several health indicators-such as temperature, heart rate, electrical activity, and biochemical markers, offering a wide view of an individual's health (Zhang et al. 2023).

10.3 Components and Functional Design of Wearable Healthcare Devices

The effectiveness of wearable healthcare devices mainly depends on the functioning of their core components. Each component, from sensors to materials, plays a significant role in ensuring reliable and consistent performance, flexibility, user comfort, and long-term usability. This section provides detailed information on major components and their impact on the design and functionality of wearables.

10.3.1 Types of Wearable Sensors

Wearable sensors can be categorized into the following types based on the methodology and functionality (Bandodkar and Wang 2014; Abowd and Mynatt 2000). It is summarized in Table 10.2.

Table 10.2 Different categories of wearable sensors

Category	Type	Description	Example/applications
1. Invasive sensors	–	Require injection or incision to collect fluids like blood	Glucose/cholesterol testing (finger prick); less suitable for continuous use
2. Non-invasive Sensors	–	Use external body fluids (sweat, saliva, tears, etc.); comfortable and safe	Suitable for real-time and continuous monitoring
	a. Electrochemical	Detect chemical species via redox reactions in sweat and saliva	Glucose monitors (e.g. Abbott Freestyle Libre)
	b. Optical	Use light interaction (e.g. PPG, NIRS) for physiological signal detection	Apple Watch (heart rate, blood oxygen), fitness bands
	c. Inertial	Measure movement, acceleration, posture	Accelerometers, gyroscopes in smartwatches or smart textiles
	d. Electrical	Detect electrical signals like ECG, EMG, and EEG from the body	Wearable ECG patches, brainwave monitors
	e. Pressure	Sense applied pressure (external/internal); detect physical force	Smart insoles, posture-correcting wearables, and flexible pressure mats
	f. Piezoelectric	Generate an electrical signal in response to mechanical deformation	Pulse sensors, respiration monitors, and motion trackers in stretchable substrates

10.3.2 Design of Wearables

Based on their functionality, two main types of designs are reported. Compact and flexible designs, in which wearability and user comfort are paramount. Compact, lightweight, and flexible sensor designs minimize obtrusiveness, enabling seamless integration into daily life. For example, WHOOP straps are designed to be non-intrusive, offering continuous health monitoring without compromising user experience. On the other hand, multi-functional sensor arrays, in which integration of multi-functional sensor arrays allows simultaneous tracking of diverse health parameters, enhancing diagnostic capabilities and reducing the need for multiple devices. The Hexoskin bright shirt exemplifies this approach by incorporating sensors to measure heart rate, respiration, and activity in a single wearable garment.

10.3.3 Materials

The performance, comfort, and long-term usability of wearable sensors heavily depend on the materials used in their construction. As wearable devices are designed for close and continuous contact with the human body, the selection of appropriate materials is critical for ensuring user safety, functionality, and durability. Materials used in wearable technologies must not only provide reliable signal transmission and sensing capabilities but also maintain comfort, flexibility, and compatibility with human skin. Based on their functional roles and application needs, these materials can be broadly categorized into flexible/stretchable electronics and biocompatible/skin-friendly materials.

10.3.3.1 Flexible and Stretchable Electronics

Advancements in material science have revolutionized wearable electronics. Those materials that offer both excellent conductivity and mechanical flexibility, such as graphene, MXene, and conductive polymers, have been utilized extensively (Mukhopadhyay 2015). These types of advanced materials facilitate seamless integration into fabrics and various other substrates. For example, graphene oxide and its derivatives, coated with different fabrics, are being utilized for real-time health assessment in deformation sensing and galvanic skin response (GSR) sensing applications.

10.3.3.2 Biocompatible and Skin-Friendly Materials

The fundamental basis of wearable material design is biocompatibility, which plays a crucial role in wearables designed for prolonged skin contact. Additionally, various types of materials, such as medical-grade silicones, thermoplastic elastomers, and breathable textiles, are commonly utilized to reduce irritation and enhance comfort. While using continuous glucose monitors, for example, hypoallergenic adhesives are used to ensure compatibility with sensitive skin.

10.3.3.3 Metal Electrodes

Metal-based electrodes are widely used in wearable devices due to their high electrical conductivity, stability, and well-established performance in bioelectronic interfaces (Wang 2013). Common metals such as gold (Au), silver (Ag), platinum (Pt), and copper (Cu) are frequently employed in various forms—including thin films, nanowires, and nanoparticles—as sensing elements or conductive tracks. These electrodes are especially useful in applications like ECG, EMG, and EEG monitoring, where accurate and stable signal acquisition is essential. However, for long-term wear, efforts are often made to combine or coat metal electrodes with soft, flexible, and biocompatible substrates to enhance comfort and reduce skin irritation.

10.3.4 Data Transmission and Storage

10.3.4.1 Wireless Communication

Recently, there have been different sources for wireless communication protocols such as Bluetooth Low Energy (BLE), Wi-Fi, and Near-Field Communication (NFC) to transmit data seamlessly from the wearable sensing device to smartphones, tablets, or cloud platforms (Alpár et al. 2011). BLE is a power-efficient version of traditional Bluetooth, designed specifically for low-power devices such as fitness trackers and smartwatches. Wi-Fi provides high-speed data transmission over longer distances compared to BLE. It is suitable for wearables that require large data transfers or need to connect to cloud-based platforms without the mediation of a smartphone. Similarly, NFC enables very short-range (typically less than 10 cm) communication between devices, and it is commonly used for secure data transfers, authentication, and contactless payments (Otto et al. 2006). These protocols ensure the reliable connectivity while optimizing power consumption. Fitbit devices, for example, synchronize data with smartphones via BLE, providing real-time updates on activity and health metrics (Hwang and Gope 2015).

10.3.4.2 Cloud Integration and Data Security

Cloud-based systems play a pivotal role in the storage, processing, and analysis of the vast datasets generated by wearable health devices (Rodgers et al. 2015). Through seamless integration with the cloud, users and healthcare providers gain convenient access to health data anytime and anywhere, enabling advanced analytics for timely and personalized health insights. Popular platforms like Google Fit and Apple Health exemplify how cloud connectivity promotes interoperability between different devices and systems, thereby fostering a more integrated and connected healthcare ecosystem. To ensure the protection of sensitive health information, robust data encryption methods, secure access controls, and decentralized storage frameworks are employed. These measures help mitigate privacy risks and strengthen overall data security. However, despite these advancements, several challenges remain. One of the major concerns is data privacy and ownership—users often lack clarity over who owns their health data and how it is being used.

Additionally, cybersecurity threats such as unauthorized access, data breaches, and ransomware attacks pose significant risks, particularly when health data is transmitted over open networks or stored on third-party cloud servers (Kumar and Lee 2012). Another challenge is data interoperability, as not all wearable devices and platforms follow the same data standards, making integration and consistent analysis across systems more difficult. Finally, internet dependency may also limit access to cloud services in remote or low-connectivity areas, potentially affecting the continuity of health monitoring.

10.4 Fabrication and Design Strategies

Fabricating wearable biomedical sensors requires a multidisciplinary approach that integrates materials science, electrical engineering, and biomedical engineering. The goal is to develop sensors that are not only highly sensitive and reliable but also comfortable for long-term wear. This section outlines the key fabrication methods for different sensor types, detailing their construction, integration into wearable devices, and optimization for continuous disease monitoring.

10.4.1 Electrochemical Sensor Fabrication

The fabrication of electrochemical sensors, particularly for applications such as glucose biosensing, involves a combination of material selection, structural design, and surface functionalization to ensure optimal functionality, stability, and biocompatibility. Electrochemical sensors typically consist of three electrodes: a working electrode (WE) where the electrochemical reaction occurs, a reference electrode (RE) that provides a stable reference potential, and a counter electrode (CE) that facilitates current flow without directly participating in the reaction. The placement of these electrodes is carefully designed to maintain an accurate electrochemical potential at the working electrode (Westbroek et al. 2005). The counter electrode is generally larger than the working electrode to ensure a stable potential difference during measurements.

The choice of materials for electrodes significantly influences sensor performance. Conductive substrates such as gold, platinum, and carbon-based materials, including glassy carbon or carbon nanotubes, are commonly used due to their excellent electrochemical properties (Rastogi et al. 2014). Nanomaterials, including graphene, metal nanoparticles, and carbon nanotubes, are often incorporated to increase the electrode surface area, thereby enhancing sensitivity and electron transfer efficiency (Shu et al. 2021). Various fabrication techniques are employed to construct electrodes, including physical vapor deposition (PVD) for precise metal film deposition (Bahri et al. 2023), screen printing for flexible substrates (Bounegru and Apetrei 2020), laser ablation for intricate patterning, and electrochemical deposition for controlled thickness (Tonelli et al. 2019).

Surface modifications further enhance sensor performance. Functionalization with enzymes like glucose oxidase (GOx) or glucose dehydrogenase (GDH) enables selective sensing, while nanostructured coatings increase the effective surface area, improving electrochemical signal strength (Xu et al. 2020). Polymer coatings such as Nafion are used to prevent interference from non-target substances (Beitollahi et al. 2020). The integration of sensor components includes multi-electrode arrays for simultaneous measurements, microfluidic channels for efficient sample delivery, and flexible substrates for wearable applications. Signal readout and data acquisition are handled using microcontrollers like Arduino or STM32, while wireless communication modules, including Bluetooth and Wi-Fi, enable real-time health monitoring (Windmiller and Wang 2013). Calibration using electrochemical techniques such as cyclic voltammetry (CV) and differential pulse voltammetry (DPV) ensures accurate and reliable measurements. Ensuring biocompatibility and durability is essential, as wearable electrochemical sensors must maintain performance while being exposed to sweat, body movement, and environmental conditions.

10.4.2 Strain Sensor Fabrication

Strain sensors, used for detecting deformations or body movements, require materials with high flexibility and conductivity. Conductive materials such as metals (gold, silver, platinum), carbon-based nanomaterials (carbon nanotubes, graphene) (Yan et al. 2018), and conductive polymers (polypyrrole, polyaniline) (Liu et al. 2018) are widely used to develop stretchable and responsive strain sensors. Metallic nanostructures such as nanowires and nanorods further enhance conductivity and mechanical properties (Lee et al. 2014).

The fabrication of strain sensors relies on techniques such as screen printing, which deposits conductive inks onto flexible substrates (Anderson et al. 2019), and laser etching, which enables the creation of precise microstructures. Chemical vapour deposition (CVD) is used for depositing thin metallic films (Chhetry et al. 2021), while electrospinning produces nanofiber networks that enhance mechanical flexibility and sensitivity (Zhou et al. 2024). Inkjet printing provides a scalable approach for high-resolution patterning of conductive materials onto flexible substrates (Kao et al. 2020). The design of strain sensors is critical for optimizing performance. Grid patterns and microstructures maximize the surface area, allowing greater resistance to changes in response to strain. Serpentine or zigzag designs enhance mechanical flexibility while maintaining conductivity during stretching.

To improve sensitivity, strain sensors incorporate nanomaterials to increase electron mobility and responsiveness. Composite materials composed of conductive fillers embedded in stretchable matrices enhance both mechanical and electrical properties. Porous structures further amplify strain sensitivity by introducing deformable pathways that respond to mechanical stress. Piezoresistive materials, which exhibit resistance changes under strain, are commonly integrated for their stability and precision (Li et al. 2021). Calibration is essential to establish a correlation between resistance changes and applied strain, ensuring reliable measurements.

Signal conditioning circuits, including Wheatstone bridge configurations and amplification modules, convert small resistance variations into measurable electrical signals. Wireless communication modules enable real-time data transmission, making these sensors suitable for wearable health monitoring applications.

10.4.3 Optical Sensor Fabrication

Optical sensors operate based on principles such as absorption (Lei et al. 2024), reflectance (Espiau 1985), fluorescence (Wolfbeis 2005), surface plasmon resonance (SPR) (Prabowo et al. 2018), and Raman spectroscopy (Đuričković et al. 2010). Absorption and transmission-based sensors detect changes in light intensity as it passes through an analyte, while reflectance sensors measure variations in reflected light to infer surface properties. Fluorescence-based sensors utilize molecules that emit light upon excitation, providing high sensitivity for biochemical detection. Surface plasmon resonance sensors detect molecular interactions by measuring shifts in the propagation of plasmon waves, while Raman spectroscopy enables chemical identification through the vibrational analysis of molecular bonds.

Miniaturization is a crucial aspect of optical sensor fabrication. Lab-on-a-chip (LOC) devices integrate optical sensors with microfluidic systems for real-time, small-scale analysis. Photonic integrated circuits (PICs) incorporate multiple optical components onto a single chip, reducing device size while improving efficiency. Flexible optical sensors, fabricated using thin-film deposition techniques, enable seamless integration into wearable systems. Sensitivity enhancements are achieved through the use of nanostructured materials such as gold nanoparticles, quantum dots, and carbon nanotubes, which enhance light interaction and signal amplification. Optical resonance effects, including micro-ring resonators, further improve sensor responsiveness. Calibration methods such as wavelength shift correction and advanced signal processing techniques ensure precision. To improve durability, optical sensors are encapsulated using protective coatings such as silicone or epoxy, shielding them from environmental influences.

10.4.4 Methods for Integrating Sensors into Wearable Devices

Integrating sensors into wearable devices requires a combination of flexible electronics, material innovation, and ergonomic design. Flexible printed circuits (FPCs) provide a lightweight and adaptable platform for embedding sensors directly into garments and accessories (Cai et al. 2017). These circuits maintain functionality even under continuous mechanical stress, making them ideal for fitness trackers and health-monitoring wearables. Conductive textiles offer another integration strategy, wherein sensor elements are woven, printed, or coated onto fabric substrates, ensuring flexibility without compromising durability.

On-skin patches and epidermal sensors represent an emerging category of wearable devices designed for continuous physiological monitoring. These ultrathin, biocompatible patches adhere directly to the skin, enabling non-invasive glucose monitoring and sweat-based biosensing. Wireless communication modules, including Bluetooth Low Energy (BLE), Wi-Fi, and Near Field Communication (NFC), facilitate real-time data transfer to external devices. Despite their advantages, wearable sensors must address challenges related to power efficiency, as continuous data transmission requires energy-efficient designs.

10.4.5 Ensuring Comfort and Usability for Long-Term Wear

Wearable sensors must be designed for prolonged use without causing discomfort or irritation. Skin-friendly materials such as medical-grade silicones, hydrogels, and biocompatible polyurethanes ensure that sensors remain comfortable for extended periods. Lightweight and flexible designs, utilizing soft electronics fabricated from stretchable substrates such as PDMS and polyimide, enable sensors to conform to body movements without compromising wearability. Power management strategies, including Bluetooth Low Energy and energy harvesting techniques such as piezoelectric generators and solar cells, extend battery life and reduce dependency on frequent charging. Aesthetic considerations also play a significant role, with smart fabrics and discreet sensor placement enabling seamless integration into everyday clothing. By prioritizing these factors, wearable sensors can achieve widespread adoption in continuous health monitoring applications.

10.4.6 Scalability and Regulatory Considerations for Clinical Deployment

For wearable sensors to transition from laboratory prototypes to clinically or commercially viable products, scalability and regulatory compliance are essential. Fabrication methods must support mass production using cost-effective, reproducible techniques such as screen printing, roll-to-roll processing, and inkjet printing on flexible substrates. Materials must be biocompatible and meet safety standards outlined by regulatory agencies like the FDA or EMA. Additionally, clinical-grade sensors require rigorous validation through standardized testing protocols, including ISO and IEC guidelines, to ensure consistent performance, safety, and durability under real-world conditions. Addressing these factors early in the design and fabrication process is critical for successful translation to healthcare markets.

10.4.7 Power Management for Continuous Operation

Efficient power management is crucial for the continuous functionality of wearable health devices, especially those requiring real-time data acquisition and wireless transmission. Advanced power management circuits are integrated to regulate voltage, minimize energy loss, and extend battery life. Low-dropout regulators (LDOs), power gating, and dynamic voltage scaling are commonly employed to optimize energy consumption. Additionally, energy harvesting technologies-such as thermoelectric, piezoelectric, and photovoltaic systems-can be incorporated to supplement power supply from body heat, motion, or ambient light. Coupled with energy-efficient communication protocols like Bluetooth Low Energy (BLE), these strategies collectively enhance device autonomy and user convenience in long-term monitoring applications.

10.4.8 Matching Fabrication Methods to Sensor Materials

The appropriate fabrication method is critical for optimizing sensor performance, reliability, and scalability. For instance, screen printing is highly suitable for carbon-based and conductive polymer inks on flexible substrates, offering scalability and low cost. Spin coating is particularly effective for producing uniform thin films of conductive polymers and nanomaterials, commonly used in electrochemical and pressure sensors. Laser ablation is ideal for metals and graphene-based materials, enabling precise patterning and rapid prototyping. Chemical vapor deposition (CVD) is commonly used for depositing high-quality thin films of materials like graphene and metal oxides, while electrospinning is preferred for producing nanofiber networks using polymers or hybrid composites with excellent mechanical flexibility. For noble metals such as gold or platinum, physical vapor deposition (PVD) provides uniform coatings critical for electrochemical sensors. Tailoring fabrication techniques to specific material properties, such as using screen printing for carbon-based inks, spin coating for polymer films, or laser ablation for graphene-ensures optimized sensor design and facilitates commercial or clinical deployment.

10.5 Applications of Wearable Healthcare Devices

Wearable healthcare devices have revolutionized the way health parameters are monitored, providing continuous, real-time data that supports both preventive and diagnostic healthcare. These devices cater to a wide range of medical needs, from tracking vital signs to managing chronic diseases, and offer significant benefits in enhancing patient care and promoting proactive health management. This section examines the primary applications of wearable devices across various healthcare domains.

10.5.1 Vital Sign Monitoring

10.5.1.1 Heart Rate

Heart rate monitors are wearable devices that continuously track heart or pulse rates using either electrical or optical detection methods. They are commonly used for monitoring heart rate during exercise, tracking stress and sleep, and checking vital signs at home. While generally accurate, particularly chest-band monitors, they are not as precise as FDA-approved medical devices and should not be used as a substitute for medical care. These devices offer valuable insights for personal health management but should be complemented by regular consultations with healthcare providers for comprehensive care (Khan et al. 2016).

Heart rate monitoring devices utilize flexible and conformal electronics, which provide improved skin integration and signal fidelity. Traditional silicon-based electronics, though unparalleled in data processing, are often bulky and rigid, limiting their suitability for epidermal and implantable applications. By integrating flexible materials such as plastic and elastomeric substrates, wearable sensors achieve lightweight, conformal interfaces that enhance comfort and data accuracy.

The ideal heart rate monitoring device employs a hybrid design, combining advanced, flexible materials with silicon-integrated circuits (ICs). This approach ensures high performance in data processing while maintaining flexibility to achieve a better user fit and signal quality. Moreover, the flexibility of these devices reduces noise and improves the accuracy of heart rate measurements, making them highly effective for both fitness tracking and medical diagnostics.

10.5.1.2 Respiration Rate

The respiratory rate is a vital indicator of health, as abnormal rates can signal conditions such as sleep apnoea, asthma, and chronic obstructive pulmonary disease. Inadequate oxygen intake or carbon dioxide expulsion can lead to severe health risks such as:

(a) Measuring Respiration Rate: Various sensors measure respiration rate by detecting the flow of breath or the expansion and contraction of the chest and abdomen. Impedance plethysmography, for example, utilizes electrodes on the body to measure changes in impedance, which reflect changes in lung volume during breathing. Most wearable respiration sensors expand and contract with the lungs, employing strain or pressure sensing to detect volume changes.

    To achieve accurate respiration monitoring, various sensing mechanisms are employed, each using distinct physical principles. These include (1) strain gauges, (2) inductive loops, (3) pressure sensors, (4) optical fibres, and (5) piezoelectric/triboelectric sensors. Strain gauges exploit the Poisson effect, where tensile stress increases length and resistance in conductive materials or capacitance in dielectric materials. Inductive loops utilize conductive materials that form loops around the body, with changes in inductance corresponding to variations in body circumference. Pressure sensors rely on compressible materials sandwiched between stiffer materials to detect pressure fluctuations during chest expansion. Optical fibres measure respiration through variations in light transmittance as the fibres stretch. Lastly, piezoelectric and triboelectric sensors generate electrical signals directly from applied pressure, providing an additional means of respiration monitoring.

(b) Breath Flow Detection: Sensors near the nose or mouth measure changes in air temperature, humidity, pressure, or CO_2 concentration. Acoustic sensors on the neck can also track respiration rates, accurately detecting conditions like respiratory obstructions. These sensors are less susceptible to motion artefacts compared to chest-based sensors, but they may be less comfortable and more conspicuous. Various technologies have been developed to enhance the accuracy and practicality of breath flow detection, including textile-based respiration sensors, patch-type sensors, and self-powered sensors, each offering distinct advantages based on their sensing principles and application requirements.

1. Textile-Based Respiration Sensors: Textile-integrated respiration sensors have gained attention for their ability to seamlessly incorporate sensing elements into garments, providing a non-invasive approach to continuous monitoring. These textiles use various mechanisms to detect respiratory activity. Knitted conductive fibres form resistive strain-sensing textiles, where stretching reduces the contact area and increases resistance. Inductive loops, constructed from knitted copper wires, change inductance in response to lung expansion, while pressure sensors use compressible textiles between conductive electrodes to increase capacitance upon compression. Additionally, capacitive sensors, embedded as textile electrodes in garments, measure capacitance variations resulting from respiratory movements. Another emerging approach involves printing carbon-filled silicone directly onto fabrics, forming resistive respiration-sensing elements.

   While textile-based sensors offer an effective means of monitoring respiration, they require a careful balance between comfort and sensitivity. A tight fit is often necessary to maintain signal accuracy, yet this can lead to discomfort during prolonged wear. Moreover, these sensors must be durable, capable of with standing repeated use, and washable to ensure practicality in everyday applications.
2. Patch-Type Sensors: Patch-type respiration sensors offer an alternative solution, resembling adhesive bandages that adhere to the skin. These sensors are typically smaller, more cost-effective, and disposable, making them suitable for temporary or single-use applications. Many patch-based sensors employ composites of carbon nanomaterials, such as carbon nanotubes or graphene, embedded in elastomers. These materials provide a combination of flexibility, mechanical strength, and high sensitivity to strain. For instance, aligned carbon nanotubes, when attached to a polydimethylsiloxane (PDMS) support, exhibit resistance variations in response to respiratory strain. Similarly, graphene-woven fabrics incorporated into stretchable substrates detect respiration by measuring resistance changes associated with breathing-induced deformation.
3. Self-Powered Sensors: Recent advancements in wearable technology have introduced self-powered sensors that utilize piezoelectric and triboelectric mechanisms to generate signals without an external power source. Polyvinylidene fluoride (PVDF) films, for example, generate a voltage in response to mechanical deformation, with enhanced designs—such as curved PVDF structures—improving signal amplitude. Triboelectric sensors function based on electron

transfer between materials, such as stretchable rubber and aluminium foil, and are often integrated into abdominal bands for respiration monitoring (Bayoumy et al. 2021).

By reducing the overall power requirements, self-powered sensors enable the use of smaller-capacity power sources, which is particularly beneficial for wearable applications. However, despite their ability to generate electrical signals from respiration-induced motion, additional power may still be necessary for data processing and communication, requiring further innovations in energy-efficient system integration.

10.5.1.3 Blood Pressure

Blood pressure is a crucial indicator of general health, reflecting the force of blood against artery walls during heartbeats (systolic) and between beats (diastolic). The traditional device for measuring blood pressure is the sphygmomanometer, which includes an inflatable cuff, a pump, and a manometer. The cuff inflates to stop blood flow, then slowly deflates. The systolic pressure is noted when blood starts flowing again, and the diastolic pressure is noted when the flow becomes smooth.

Despite their clinical ubiquity, sphygmomanometers have limitations. They are stationary, costly, and unable to provide continuous monitoring, which is critical for detecting asymptomatic conditions. They also cannot measure the constant pressure changes in pulse waveforms (arterial tonometry), which is useful in diagnosing heart conditions. Additionally, incorrect cuff sizing can result in inaccurate readings.

Advancements in material science have led to the development of sensitive strain sensors capable of measuring pulse pressure waveforms. These sensors are commonly capacitive, utilizing compressible dielectrics to alter capacitance or piezoelectric materials to generate voltage under pressure. Early designs also utilized strain-dependent resistors, but their higher power demands have made them less common.

Capacitive strain sensors typically feature a compressible dielectric, like PDMS, known for its biocompatibility, affordability, and flexibility. Enhancements in sensor design, such as microstructured PDMS, have significantly increased sensitivity and response time, enabling precise blood pressure measurements suitable for arterial tonometry. For instance, microstructured PDMS moulded into pyramidal shapes improves sensitivity and reduces relaxation time significantly. Piezoelectric materials are also prominent in pressure sensing. When strained, they generate voltage, which can be harnessed to create highly sensitive devices for monitoring pulse pressure at various body locations. These materials can be integrated with flexible substrates and textiles, offering isotropic pressure sensing. The integration of these sensors with thin film transistors (TFTs) for signal amplification is critical, as the sensors must distinguish the subtle pulse pressure from the larger background pressure. Some designs incorporate the sensor's dielectric directly into the TFT, simplifying the system and enhancing signal clarity (González Ramírez et al. 2023).

Addressable sensor arrays offer another advancement, enabling the localization of the strongest pulse signal and allowing for measurements of pulse delay between different body locations, a crucial diagnostic tool for cardiac health. While many pulse pressure sensors have been developed, few have been rigorously correlated with traditional blood pressure readings. More comprehensive studies are needed to establish the reliability and variability of these methods across different users.

10.5.2 Chronic Disease Management

10.5.2.1 Blood Glucose

According to the World Health Organization, 14% of adults worldwide have diabetes (World Health Organization 2024). Glucose monitoring is vital for maintaining the health and quality of life of diabetics, requiring frequent daily measurements. Traditionally, even the most non-invasive glucose monitors require blood samples. However, new electronics fabrication techniques on flexible substrates have enabled the development of non-invasive wearable glucose sensors that monitor glucose concentration without drawing blood.

Diabetes management has seen significant advancements with the introduction of Continuous Glucose Monitoring (CGM) systems. CGMs provide real-time tracking of glucose levels by measuring interstitial fluid glucose concentrations, offering a non-invasive alternative to traditional blood glucose monitoring methods. CGMs operate through a tiny sensor inserted under the skin, which continuously measures glucose levels and transmits the data to a monitor or smartphone (Reddy et al. 2023). This real-time data allows patients to track trends and make informed decisions about their diet, exercise, and insulin usage. Unlike traditional finger-prick methods, CGMs provide a comprehensive glucose profile, capturing fluctuations throughout the day and night. Studies have demonstrated that CGMs improve glycaemic control by helping patients maintain glucose levels within the target range, reducing the risk of hyperglycaemia and hypoglycaemia. The frequent, real-time feedback enables timely adjustments to lifestyle and medication, significantly enhancing overall diabetes management. Furthermore, CGMs contribute to better long-term outcomes by reducing HbA1c levels, minimizing complications, and improving the quality of life for individuals with diabetes.

Incorporating CGM technology has shifted diabetes care towards a more proactive approach, enabling both patients and healthcare providers to respond swiftly to changes in glucose levels. This continuous feedback loop empowers patients, leading to better adherence to treatment plans and improved health outcomes.

10.5.2.2 Cardiovascular Diseases

Wearable devices have become integral in cardiovascular care, offering continuous monitoring and early detection of cardiac events, thereby enhancing remote patient management. These devices, such as smartwatches and patches, are equipped with sensors that monitor physiological parameters, notably electrocardiograms (ECGs) (De Zambotti et al. 2019). By leveraging advanced sensing technologies, wearables contribute to three key areas of cardiovascular monitoring: (1) ECG-based tracking, and (2) Early detection of cardiac events, and (3) Remote patient monitoring.

1. ECG Monitoring: Wearable ECG monitors, like the Zio patch, provide continuous, single-lead ECG monitoring, enabling the detection of transient arrhythmias and improving patient health by facilitating timely medical interventions. Similarly, devices like the AliveCor KardiaMobile, an FDA-cleared, single-channel ECG recorder, detect conditions such as atrial fibrillation, aiding in early diagnosis and management.
2. Early Detection of Cardiac Events: The integration of photoplethysmography (PPG) sensors in wearables enables continuous heart rhythm monitoring, which, when combined with ECG data, enhances the early detection of cardiac anomalies. For instance, the Apple Watch has been utilized in studies to monitor heart rate and rhythm, contributing to the identification of conditions like atrial fibrillation.
3. Remote Patient Monitoring: Wearable devices facilitate remote monitoring by transmitting real-time data to healthcare providers, enabling continuous oversight of patients' cardiovascular health without the need for frequent in-person visits. This approach has been particularly beneficial during the COVID-19 pandemic, promoting decentralized and personalized care for patients.

Despite their advantages, challenges such as device accuracy, data privacy concerns, and the need for standardized regulatory policies persist. Addressing these issues is crucial for the broader adoption of wearable technology in clinical practice.

10.5.3 Mental Health Monitoring

10.5.3.1 Stress and Anxiety

Wearable devices have emerged as valuable tools in monitoring and managing mental health, particularly stress and anxiety. These devices track physiological markers that indicate stress levels, providing real-time feedback to users and healthcare providers. By leveraging biometric data, wearable technology contributes to two primary areas of stress monitoring: heart rate variability (HRV) and cortisol level tracking (Rodgers et al. 2019).

Heart Rate Variability (HRV): Heart rate variability (HRV) is a widely recognized indicator of autonomic nervous system activity and stress levels. Wearables such as the Apple Watch and Fitbit incorporate HRV monitoring through photoplethysmography (PPG) sensors. These sensors detect variations in the time intervals between heartbeats, which can reflect stress responses. A lower HRV is often associated with higher stress levels, while a higher HRV indicates a more relaxed state. By providing continuous HRV data, these devices help users understand their stress patterns and make informed decisions about stress management techniques.

Cortisol Levels: Advancements in wearable biosensors have also enabled the non-invasive measurement of cortisol, a hormone released in response to stress.

Devices equipped with sweat analysis capabilities can monitor cortisol levels, offering a direct measure of the body's stress response. For example, emerging wearable patches utilize microfluidic technology to collect and analyse sweat, providing insights into cortisol fluctuations throughout the day. This information can be critical in identifying stress triggers and evaluating the effectiveness of stress-reduction interventions.

Wearable devices that track HRV and cortisol levels represent a transformative approach to mental health monitoring. By providing actionable insights into stress and anxiety, these technologies facilitate early intervention, improve mental health outcomes, and promote overall well-being. The continued development and integration of such wearables into mental healthcare hold promise for advancing the field and supporting individuals in managing their mental health more effectively.

10.5.3.2 Sleep Patterns

Monitoring sleep patterns is a crucial aspect of wearable healthcare devices, as sleep quality is closely tied to mental health. Wearable devices, including smartwatches, rings, and headbands, are now equipped with sensors that track vital indicators such as heart rate, motion, and respiratory patterns throughout the night. These devices can offer a detailed analysis of an individual's sleep stages, which include light sleep, deep sleep, and rapid eye movement (REM) sleep. Understanding these stages is essential because disruptions in these stages have been linked to various mental health issues, including anxiety and depression (Ahmed et al. 2024).

Furthermore, sleep disorders like sleep apnoea can be detected using wearables that monitor oxygen levels and breathing patterns. Devices with pulse oximetry and respiratory sensors can track fluctuations in oxygen saturation and the frequency of apnoeic events, allowing users to identify potential sleep apnoea early. Sleep apnoea, in particular, is known to exacerbate mental health conditions, as the intermittent lack of oxygen can lead to mood disturbances, cognitive decline, and other psychological symptoms (Alfirevic et al. 2017). These wearable devices also provide valuable insights into sleep quality, a key factor in mental health. By continuously tracking sleep duration, consistency, and disturbances, these devices help individuals identify trends that might indicate the need for intervention. For example, poor sleep hygiene or undiagnosed sleep disorders can negatively affect mental well-being, and by tracking sleep quality over time, users can gain a deeper understanding of their sleep health. Additionally, the integration of sleep data with other mental health indicators, such as stress and anxiety levels, allows for a more holistic view of a person's mental health status.

As wearable technologies continue to advance, their potential for improving mental health monitoring and management becomes more apparent. These devices provide a convenient, non-invasive method for collecting essential data that can inform both personal lifestyle adjustments and clinical interventions.

10.5.4 Physical Activity and Rehabilitation

Wearable activity trackers, such as fitness bands and smartwatches, have revolutionized the way individuals engage in physical activity. These devices are designed to track key metrics, including steps taken, calories burned, and overall fitness levels. The primary goal of these devices is to promote physical activity by encouraging users to stay active and meet personalized fitness goals. Many trackers provide real-time feedback and set challenges to motivate users, fostering a sense of accomplishment as they achieve set targets. The continuous monitoring of these metrics also helps users understand their activity patterns, identify areas of improvement, and adjust their lifestyle to improve overall health.

In rehabilitation, wearable movement sensors have become a vital tool for monitoring joint movement, posture, and progress in recovery. These sensors, typically embedded in devices such as smartwatches or specialized rehabilitation devices, collect data on the patient's physical performance. They help clinicians monitor how well the patient is performing rehabilitation exercises and whether the movement aligns with prescribed recovery protocols. By tracking joint angles, muscle engagement, and posture, these sensors offer crucial insights into the patient's physical condition. For example, in cases of musculoskeletal injury or neurological conditions, precise tracking of joint movement can help identify mobility deficits or compensatory movements that could lead to further injury. Additionally, movement sensors provide real-time feedback, guiding patients through corrective exercises and ensuring they perform them correctly to avoid improper movement that could hinder recovery.

Moreover, these devices have proven beneficial for patients who are undergoing physiotherapy at home or remotely. Movement sensors can provide continuous data about the patient's progress, enabling healthcare providers to adjust treatment plans as needed. Remote monitoring via wearables also reduces the need for frequent in-person visits, allowing patients to manage their rehabilitation more independently. By collecting data over time, these wearables enable clinicians to track subtle improvements or declines in the patient's condition, adjusting the rehabilitation process to be timelier and more personalized. Thus, wearable movement sensors not only track recovery but actively guide patients toward optimal rehabilitation outcomes, offering both physical and emotional support as they progress through the healing process.

In summary, wearable devices, such as activity trackers and movement sensors, play a crucial role in promoting physical activity and supporting rehabilitation. These devices help users track physical performance and receive feedback, which encourages engagement and progress. For rehabilitation, wearables enable clinicians to monitor and guide patients' recovery, ensuring that exercises are performed correctly and effectively. Through real-time data collection, wearables offer personalized insights, enhancing both recovery outcomes and long-term health.

10.5.5 Perinatal Health Monitoring

Wearable technology has become pivotal in perinatal health, enabling continuous and non-invasive monitoring of both maternal and foetal health parameters. These advancements facilitate the early detection of complications, improving outcomes for both mother and child.

10.5.5.1 Monitoring Foetal Health

Wearable foetal monitors have revolutionized prenatal care by offering continuous tracking of fetal heart rate, movements, and overall well-being. These devices, typically attached to the maternal abdomen, employ non-invasive sensors to gather vital data. Continuous foetal heart rate monitoring is crucial for detecting signs of foetal distress, arrhythmias, or other abnormalities that may require immediate medical attention. The ability to remotely monitor foetal activity enables healthcare providers to closely track foetal health, thereby reducing the need for frequent in-person visits.

10.5.5.2 Monitoring Maternal Contractions and Health

Maternal health monitoring devices track vital signs, including heart rate, blood pressure, and contractions. Wearables, such as smartwatches, biosensor patches, and smart clothing, provide real-time data on these parameters, which are crucial for detecting hypertensive disorders, gestational diabetes, and other pregnancy-related conditions. Monitoring uterine contractions helps predict and manage labour, as well as detect preterm labour signs, facilitating timely intervention.

10.5.5.3 Importance of Early Detection

The primary advantage of these wearable devices lies in their ability to offer continuous, real-time monitoring, enabling the early detection of potential complications. Conditions such as preeclampsia, gestational diabetes, and foetal growth restrictions can be identified and managed promptly, reducing the risks associated with these complications. Early detection not only improves maternal and foetal outcomes but also enhances the overall pregnancy experience by reducing anxiety and providing reassurance through constant health tracking. Wearable devices improve remote patient monitoring, enabling healthcare providers to monitor the health of both mother and baby remotely, eliminating the need for frequent hospital visits. This is particularly beneficial for women in remote or underserved areas, as it improves access to quality prenatal care. Remote monitoring ensures timely interventions and facilitates regular health assessments, thereby contributing to safer pregnancies.

10.6 Recent Advancements in Wearable Healthcare Devices

The rapid evolution of wearable healthcare devices has revolutionized the way health parameters are monitored, managed, and interpreted. These devices have evolved significantly beyond their origins as simple activity trackers, now addressing a wide range of healthcare challenges through advanced sensing technologies, artificial intelligence (AI), and sustainable designs. By enabling real-time health monitoring and predictive analytics, wearable devices are not only improving individual healthcare outcomes but also reshaping global healthcare systems. What sets modern wearables apart is their ability to merge cutting-edge innovations with practical healthcare applications. These devices are no longer confined to fitness tracking; they have become essential tools in chronic disease management, mental health support, and preventive healthcare. By leveraging AI-driven analytics, multimodal sensors, and eco-friendly designs, wearable technologies are redefining healthcare by empowering individuals with actionable insights and enabling healthcare providers to deliver proactive, personalized care. This section examines the most significant advancements in wearable healthcare technologies, with a focus on their role in addressing complex healthcare needs, enhancing accessibility, and promoting sustainability.

10.6.1 Incorporation of Artificial Intelligence, Machine Learning, and Generative AI for Health Analytics and Fabrication

Artificial intelligence (AI) and machine learning (ML) have emerged as transformative forces in wearable healthcare, revolutionizing the capabilities of these devices and enabling them to evolve from passive data collection tools into dynamic health management systems capable of advanced analysis and decision-making (Reddy 2024; Phatak et al. 2021; Nittala et al. 2020). AI algorithms are particularly adept at processing vast amounts of physiological data to detect subtle anomalies that might otherwise go unnoticed. For example, deep learning architectures such as convolutional neural networks (CNNs) and recurrent neural networks (RNNs) are used to analyse complex ECG waveforms, enabling accurate detection of arrhythmias and cardiac abnormalities beyond traditional threshold-based methods (May et al. 2024). Similarly, ensemble learning methods like random forests and gradient boosting are applied to multi-sensor data streams to predict events such as hypoglycaemia in diabetics or early signs of atrial fibrillation, providing highly specific and actionable insights. Unsupervised learning approaches, including clustering algorithms, help uncover hidden patterns in sleep or stress data, revealing new correlations between physiological signals and health outcomes. For instance, advanced wearables equipped with ECG sensors leverage AI to identify arrhythmias, predict potential cardiac arrest, and monitor chronic conditions such as hypertension and diabetes (May et al. 2024). By continuously analysing physiological signals, these devices deliver early warnings and tailored feedback, facilitating timely medical intervention and potentially preventing life-threatening events. In addition to diagnostics, ML algorithms enable wearables to provide highly personalized health recommendations by learning from user-specific data (Baihan et al. 2025). These recommendations encompass a range of tailored suggestions, from optimizing exercise regimens and improving dietary habits to implementing effective stress-reduction techniques (Li et al. 2024). This level of customization fosters a deeper connection between users and their health goals, resulting in improved adherence to health plans and enhanced outcomes. Generative AI is now augmenting these advancements by transforming the design and fabrication processes for wearable healthcare devices (Turakhia 2024). Using generative AI models, researchers and engineers can optimize the structural and functional aspects of wearable sensors, ensuring they are lightweight and shaped for comfortable wear across diverse user needs. Generative models analyse existing designs and user data to propose innovative and efficient configurations, thereby reducing material usage and enhancing sensor performance. For example, AI-driven computational fabrication enables the creation of flexible biosensors with improved accuracy in detecting biomarkers such as glucose and cortisol while simultaneously minimizing production costs and environmental impact. Moreover, AI and ML have opened new frontiers in mental health management. Wearables integrated with AI-driven analytics measure physiological indicators such as skin conductance, heart rate variability, and sleep patterns to assess stress and anxiety levels. These insights are delivered through personalized feedback, helping users better understand and manage their mental well-being. For example, a wearable might alert a user to elevated stress levels and suggest mindfulness exercises or relaxation techniques, empowering proactive mental healthcare. The adoption of computational fabrication further accelerates the accessibility of advanced wearables by enabling scalable, customized production. By utilizing generative AI alongside computational fabrication tools, researchers can simulate and prototype complex, multimodal sensing systems for wearable devices, reducing development time while ensuring robust and sustainable designs. This approach is instrumental in creating devices that fit naturally into daily life, improving usability and user satisfaction. By bringing together AI, ML, generative AI, and computational fabrication, wearable healthcare devices are evolving beyond passive monitoring to actively enhance diagnostic accuracy, design efficiency, and user engagement. They are transforming health management into a proactive, personalized, and accessible process, ensuring that users receive timely, targeted support for both physical and mental well-being. This convergence of advanced analytics, innovative fabrication techniques, and user-centric design is reshaping healthcare delivery and empowering individuals to take greater control of their health.

10.6.2 Development of Multimodal Sensing Devices for Comprehensive Health Assessment

Modern wearable healthcare devices are revolutionizing the way multiple health parameters are monitored, driven by remarkable advancements in multimodal sensing technologies (Khan et al. 2024). By integrating various sensors into a single system, these devices provide a comprehensive, real-time assessment of an individual's health, enabling more accurate and holistic monitoring than ever before (Nittala et al. 2021). Multimodal sensors combine capabilities that were once limited to standalone devices, offering an all-in-one solution for both personal and clinical use. One of the most promising developments is in sweat sensors (Yu et al. 2025), which harness the rich biomarker content of sweat to enable non-invasive health monitoring (Garg et al. 2024). Advanced electrochemical sensors can now detect and measure biomarkers such as glucose (Cho et al. 2024), cortisol (Wankhade et al. 2024), and lactate (Yang et al. 2024) with exceptional precision, offering critical insights into metabolic and stress levels. Holographic sweat sensors further enhance accessibility by providing visual colorimetric feedback, allowing users to interpret health data without specialized equipment (Roy et al. 2024). These technologies are particularly impactful for managing conditions like diabetes, monitoring stress, and optimizing athletic performance, making them invaluable in both medical and fitness contexts. Another ground-breaking innovation is the development of on-skin and tattoo sensors, which represent the next frontier in wearable healthcare (Nittala et al. 2021). These ultra-thin, flexible sensors, fabricated from biocompatible materials (Nicolae et al. 2024) such as alginate and silk fibroin, adhere seamlessly to the skin. They provide continuous, non-invasive monitoring of hydration levels, electrolyte balance, and metabolic activity without causing discomfort, making them suitable for long-term use. Their unobtrusive design makes them ideal for individuals who require consistent health tracking in daily life, bridging the gap between convenience and functionality. Fabric-based sensors are also redefining wearable technology by seamlessly integrating it into everyday clothing. Conductive fabrics embedded with sensors monitor vital signs such as respiration, body temperature, and joint movements, offering unobtrusive and continuous monitoring. These garments are particularly beneficial for remote health monitoring, rehabilitation, and sports performance analysis, where real-time data is essential for making informed decisions (Chowdhury et al. 2024). Their ability to integrate seamlessly into daily wear ensures that health tracking becomes an effortless part of everyday life, removing barriers to adoption. By incorporating multiple sensing modalities, these advanced wearable devices provide a detailed, real-time overview of an individual's health. Their versatility and ability to offer comprehensive health assessments make them indispensable tools for personalized health management and clinical decision-making. These innovations not only expand the functionality of wearable devices but also pave the way for a more integrated and proactive approach to healthcare.

10.6.3 Advances in Real-Time Data Processing and Feedback Mechanisms

The ability of wearable devices to process data in real-time has dramatically enhanced their efficiency, responsiveness, and overall user experience. Recent innovations in data transmission, local processing, and feedback mechanisms have addressed common challenges, such as latency and privacy concerns, while delivering actionable insights to users at critical moments (Kos et al. 2019). These advancements have transformed wearables from simple data collectors into dynamic tools that actively support health management. One of the most significant developments is the integration of edge computing, which enables wearable devices to process data locally rather than relying on cloud servers. By handling computation directly on the device, edge computing minimizes latency, enabling faster responses and real-time feedback (Uddin 2019). This approach not only improves the speed of data analysis but also enhances user privacy by reducing the amount of sensitive information transmitted to external servers. Additionally, wearables equipped with edge computing remain operational in areas with limited connectivity, ensuring uninterrupted functionality even in remote settings. Complementing this is the advancement in wireless communication technologies, including Bluetooth Low Energy (BLE), 5G, and Internet of Things (IoT) frameworks. These technologies facilitate seamless, low-latency data exchange between wearables, smartphones, and cloud systems (Custodio et al. 2012). Such real-time connectivity is crucial for issuing immediate alerts about potential health risks, such as irregular heartbeats or abnormal glucose levels. The reliability and speed of these communication systems ensure that users and healthcare providers are informed of critical health events instantly, enabling timely interventions. Modern wearables are also equipped with sophisticated feedback mechanisms designed to deliver immediate, user-friendly notifications. Devices use haptic vibrations, visual indicators, or auditory signals to alert users to abnormal health metrics. For instance, a glucose-monitoring wearable might vibrate to warn a user of high or low glucose levels, while a companion app provides detailed explanations, recommendations, and actionable advice. These feedback systems are not only informative but also empower users to take control of their health in real-time. Together, these advancements ensure that wearable devices are no longer passive monitors but active participants in the healthcare ecosystem. By combining real-time data processing, seamless connectivity, and intuitive feedback, wearables now play a pivotal role in enabling timely health interventions, fostering user engagement, and improving health outcomes. These innovations are redefining the role of wearables in personalized, proactive healthcare.

10.6.4 Sustainable Sensors and Eco-Friendly Materials

With the increasing adoption of wearable devices, sustainability has emerged as a critical consideration in their design and development. As wearable technologies become integral to everyday healthcare, researchers are addressing environmental concerns by focusing on eco-friendly materials, energy-efficient designs, and waste-reducing innovations. These advancements are not only minimizing the environmental footprint of wearables but also aligning their production and use with global sustainability goals. A key innovation in this area is the development of biodegradable materials for wearable sensors. Temporary sensors made from materials like alginate, agarose, cellulose, and silk fibroin (Roy et al. 2024; Chen et al. 2022) are designed to decompose naturally after use, significantly reducing electronic waste. These biodegradable components are particularly suitable for short-term applications, such as wound healing or diagnostic testing, where single-use devices are common (Hosseini et al. 2020). By integrating these materials, wearable technology is moving toward a more environmentally responsible future. Fabric-based sensors are another sustainable breakthrough, enabling wearables to blend seamlessly with everyday clothing. Conductive textiles enhanced with reduced graphene oxide (rGO) coatings or metallic nanowires are lightweight, washable, and highly durable, making them ideal for long-term use. These sensors provide continuous health monitoring while being reusable and eco-friendly. Their integration into garments ensures unobtrusive, sustainable health tracking without sacrificing functionality or comfort (Maji et al. 2024). Perhaps the most transformative development in sustainable wearables is the advent of self-powered devices. Energy harvesting technologies, such as piezoelectricity (which converts motion into electricity) and thermoelectricity (which utilizes body heat), are eliminating the need for traditional batteries. These innovations not only reduce waste associated with battery disposal but also enhance user convenience by extending device lifespans and eliminating the need for frequent charging. Self-powered wearables exemplify how sustainability and practicality can coexist in advanced healthcare technology (Parrilla and De Wael 2021). By adopting these sustainable materials and designs, wearable devices are evolving to meet the demands of environmentally conscious users while addressing the global challenge of electronic waste. These innovations underscore a shift toward greener healthcare solutions, ensuring that wearable technologies are as beneficial for the planet as they are for human health. This integration of sustainability into wearable healthcare marks a significant step forward in creating devices that serve both individuals and the environment.

10.6.5 Innovations from Research to Commercialization

The gap between ground-breaking research in wearable healthcare technologies and their commercial availability is rapidly closing, making advanced solutions increasingly accessible to everyday users. This transition is driven by a concerted effort to transform experimental innovations into practical, market-ready devices that meet real-world needs. By focusing on user-centric designs, energy efficiency, and strategic collaborations, wearable technologies are now empowering individuals to take control of their health like never before. One of the most impactful advancements is the development of flexible biosensors, particularly for non-invasive glucose monitoring (Salim and Lim 2019). Initially confined to research laboratories, these sensors are now commercially available, enabling diabetic patients to monitor their glucose levels with unprecedented ease and convenience. Unlike traditional monitoring methods, these wearable devices provide continuous feedback without the discomfort of finger pricks, significantly enhancing the quality of life for users. This commercialization highlights the potential of research-driven innovations to solve complex healthcare challenges. Energy-efficient designs are also playing a pivotal role in the widespread adoption of wearable healthcare devices. Manufacturers are increasingly integrating low-power electronics to extend battery life and improve user experiences. These advancements not only reduce the frequency of charging but also enhance the reliability and usability of wearables, making them more appealing to a broader audience. As a result, energy-efficient wearables are becoming essential tools for long-term health monitoring. Collaborative efforts between academic institutions and industry leaders have largely facilitated the acceleration of wearable technology from research to market. Universities and research centres drive innovation by developing novel materials, sensors, and analytical techniques, while industry partners leverage their expertise in manufacturing, marketing, and distribution. These partnerships ensure that cutting-edge solutions are not only technically advanced but also scalable and user-friendly. The synergy between research and commercialization is making wearable technologies more accessible and impactful. The successful commercialization of wearable healthcare devices is democratizing healthcare by putting advanced monitoring and diagnostic tools into the hands of millions of users. These devices are not just enhancing individual health outcomes but also contributing to a larger shift toward proactive, data-driven healthcare systems. By bridging the gap between innovation and accessibility, the wearable healthcare industry is fostering a future where advanced technologies are available to a broad and diverse audience, transforming healthcare delivery on a global scale.

However, despite the rapid progress, several barriers continue to hinder the seamless transition from research to commercialization. Regulatory approval remains a major hurdle, as wearable healthcare devices must meet stringent safety, efficacy, and compliance standards before entering the market. Intellectual property (IP) challenges, including patent disputes and protection of proprietary technologies, can delay or complicate product development. Additionally, achieving cost-effective scalability without compromising quality is critical for mass production. Clinical validation is another essential step, requiring rigorous testing in real-world settings to establish reliability, accuracy, and acceptance among healthcare providers and patients. Addressing these challenges is key to sustaining the momentum in wearable health innovation.

10.6.6 Real-World Impact on Healthcare Outcomes

The widespread adoption of wearable healthcare devices has profoundly transformed healthcare delivery, enabling more proactive, personalized, and accessible care. These devices are revolutionizing the management of chronic conditions, the implementation of preventive measures, and the delivery of healthcare in underserved regions, thereby significantly improving health outcomes and patient experiences. One of the most notable impacts is in chronic disease management, where wearable devices facilitate continuous monitoring of conditions such as diabetes, hypertension, and asthma. By providing real-time data on vital signs and health metrics, wearables enable early detection of potential complications and timely interventions. This constant vigilance reduces the frequency of hospitalizations and improves adherence to treatment regimens, empowering patients to manage their conditions with greater confidence and ease. In preventive healthcare, wearable devices equipped with advanced sensors, such as those for detecting sweat, saliva, and tears, are capable of detecting early signs of health risks before they develop into serious issues (Tseng et al. 2021). For instance, these sensors can monitor biomarkers that indicate stress, dehydration, or glucose imbalances, allowing users to take preventive actions. By facilitating early detection, these technologies help reduce the overall burden of chronic diseases and promote healthier lifestyles. Rehabilitation support is another area where wearable devices are making a significant impact. Fabric-based sensors integrated into wearable systems provide real-time feedback to patients recovering from injuries or surgeries. These devices track movement, posture, and muscle activity, enabling physical therapists and patients to monitor progress and adjust rehabilitation exercises as needed. This real-time guidance accelerates recovery, enhances therapy outcomes, and ensures adherence to prescribed rehabilitation protocols (Sardini et al. 2014). Wearables also play a critical role in telemedicine integration, particularly in underserved or remote areas where access to healthcare facilities is limited. By enabling real-time data sharing between patients and healthcare providers, wearables bridge gaps in care delivery (Scheffler and Hirt 2005). For example, remote monitoring devices allow doctors to track a patient's vital signs and intervene promptly when necessary, reducing the need for in-person visits and expanding access to care for geographically isolated populations. By seamlessly integrating into everyday life, wearable healthcare devices are fostering a shift toward a more proactive, inclusive, and effective approach to healthcare. These technologies are not only enhancing individual health outcomes but also contributing to the transformation of healthcare systems, making them more efficient, patient-centric, and accessible on a global scale.

10.7 Challenges and Limitations

Wearable health monitoring devices have significantly transformed the healthcare field. As discussed, they have proven effective in monitoring a variety of physiological parameters. However, there is still considerable room for improvement in these devices due to their limitations, which include issues related to stability, sensitivity, privacy, power sources, and a limited range of applications for psychological disorders. We highlight some of the challenges and opportunities for further development in this area across five major areas:

1. *Flexibility, Connections, Durability, and Long-Term Monitoring*: The human body and its internal organs are naturally elastic and flexible. Since most wearables interact with the skin, the data collected by these wearable health monitoring devices can sometimes be distorted or noisy. Factors contributing to this noise include constant body movement and body hair, which can reduce adhesion between the skin and the wearable device. Secondly, while the wearable

health monitoring devices are soft and slim, the connections and interfacing mechanisms that connect them to the hardware circuitry still rely on rigid electronic components. Currently, commercial wearable devices incorporate more robust interfacing mechanisms, but this comes at the cost of reduced flexibility and stretchability. While wearable health monitoring devices are widely used for monitoring, more efforts are needed to make them suitable for diagnostic purposes. Traditional diagnostic techniques typically require samples like blood, urine, and saliva, and there is limited integration of HWDs with these biological samples. Enhanced integration of HWDs with platforms that support biological sample use is essential for effective end-user applications.

2. *Integration of AI, Machine, and Adaptive Learning*: Artificial intelligence (AI) algorithms, such as supervised learning regression algorithms, can be employed to track multiple parameters over time for prognosis. Currently, many machine learning-enhanced wearable sensors lack adaptive learning capabilities. Ideally, biosensors should be able to learn from their environment through adaptive learning rather than solely relying on manually input training sets. An adaptive model continuously improves and optimizes itself by learning from its surroundings, unlike a non-adaptive system. This ability could reduce the risk of significant errors and incorrect results, which can occur with a static model.
3. *Power Consumption*: One significant limitation that impedes the utility of wearable devices is the need for a continuous power supply. Batteries used in wearables have limited space and must align with the device's design. To overcome this challenge, further advances in power management and energy harvesting technologies are required. To address this limitation, there is a need for efficient energy harvesters with improved power management. Self-powered sensors, such as piezoelectric nanogenerators (PENG) and triboelectric nanogenerators (TENG), are compact energy harvesters. These devices convert one form of energy—such as mechanical energy—into electrical energy, ensuring both comfort and miniaturization in wearable health devices.
4. *Security and Privacy*: The close integration of wearable health monitoring devices with the body raises important concerns regarding security, privacy, and ethics. Firstly, these devices have the capability to capture sensitive biological data about a user's body and health status. Currently, there are no security or privacy features included in their design. Unlike mobile devices that use security measures such as fingerprint authentication, patterns, PINs, or passwords, the body offers a more advanced method for authentication. Biological signatures, including bio-signals and bioimpedance, can be utilized for authentication, providing an additional layer of security for wearable health monitoring devices. Furthermore, because these devices are worn on the body, they are already situated within the user's personal space, which heightens privacy concerns. Data breaches involving wearable health devices could expose deeply personal health information, leading to identity theft, insurance discrimination, or unauthorized surveillance. These risks are amplified by the continuous and intimate nature of the data collected. As such, robust encryption, secure transmission protocols, and edge-computing strategies are necessary to protect data integrity and confi-

dentiality. Moreover, global data governance frameworks are needed to ensure uniform standards across countries, especially as wearable data is often stored or processed on international cloud servers. Regulations like GDPR (General Data Protection Regulation) and HIPAA (Health Insurance Portability and Accountability Act) provide important guidelines, but broader international cooperation is required to handle cross-border data flows and jurisdictional ambiguities.

Equally important is user education. Many users are unaware of what data is being collected, how it is used, or who has access to it. Educating users about consent, data sharing policies, and personal data rights is essential to empower them to make informed decisions. Developers and manufacturers must prioritize transparent privacy settings, clear data usage disclosures, and user-friendly controls to foster trust in wearable health technologies. Future efforts should focus on these areas and identify pragmatic security and privacy mechanisms for wearable health monitoring devices.

5. *Regulatory and Clinical Validation Challenges*: The transition of wearable health technologies from research to market is often hindered by stringent regulatory requirements and the need for extensive clinical validation. Devices like the Dexcom Continuous Glucose Monitor (CGM) and the Apple Watch ECG have received FDA clearance, demonstrating the rigorous validation processes required to ensure safety, efficacy, and reliability. However, many emerging technologies face significant hurdles such as securing large-scale clinical trial data, meeting regulatory standards for diverse user populations, and addressing concerns related to device accuracy under varying physiological conditions. Navigating these challenges is critical to gaining regulatory approval and widespread clinical acceptance, which remain major bottlenecks in the commercialization pipeline.

10.8 Future Perspectives

The continuous ground-breaking advancements have led to a bright future of wearable healthcare technology. It is driven by novel innovations in areas such as materials science, energy systems, and digital health platforms. These advancements aim to improve the functionality, integration, and impact of wearables on personalized healthcare and beyond.

10.8.1 Emerging Trends in Wearable Technology

One of the significant trends in the development of fully integrated smart clothing. It is comprised of both sensors and electronic components embedded into textiles. This integration of wearables with electronics transforms them into highly functional digital health devices, offering convenience, and usability (LaBoone and Marques 2024). Furthermore, the research and development of energy storage technologies such as triboelectric nanogenerators and piezoelectric materials further enhances the advancement and practicability of wearables, enabling them to function as a self-powered device. These technologies utilize sources like motion or body heat to store energy and contribute to the sustainability of wearable devices. Furthermore, flexible and stretchable batteries consisting of materials like graphene oxide and MXenes, which are being very useful to complement wearable electronics, ensuring a flexibility, consistency, and reliable power supply while maintaining user comfort. All of these advancements from different compartments pave the way for a new era of wearable technology that is not only functional but also biocompatible.

10.8.2 Integrating Wearables with Telemedicine

Particularly for underserved and remote populations, the incorporation of wearables with a telemedicine platform has revolutionized the healthcare delivery pattern (Vaghasiya et al. 2023). Real-time data sharing capabilities, as one of the significant features, of wearable devices allow continuous monitoring of critical health parameters. It bridges the gap between patients and healthcare providers, offering a lower risk. Additionally, it also reduces the burden on the healthcare system and minimizes the need for hospital visits. Utilization of wearables, embedded within a telemedicine framework, enables remote diagnosis, personalized treatment planning, and long-term management of chronic conditions. For example, cardiovascular or respiratory parameters can be monitored with wearables and also alert the healthcare providers to potential issues before they escalate, offering a proactive approach to health management.

10.8.3 Broadening the Scope of Wearable Applications

Wearable technology is one of the fastest-growing research sectors and is evolving to address broader health challenges and emerging applications. The detection of various critical diseases, such as cancer or Alzheimer's, at an early stage using specific biomarkers by wearable sensors, represents a shift towards preventive medicine. Not only for personal health management, but wearables are also being developed and utilized for environmental monitoring, such as air quality indicators, UV exposure, and allergens, offering additional insights into environmental health impacts. Overall, the advancement of wearable devices has the potential to revolutionize the way of rehabilitation and therapy, where both real-time data and feedback enhances the way of rehabilitation and therapy, where both real-time data and feedback enhance therapeutic outcomes and engagement. Such advancements in wearable technology and devices are not limited to medical applications but impact lifestyle and environmental domains, reinforcing the multifunctional nature of modern wearables.

10.9 Conclusion

Wearable healthcare technology has evolved from simple fitness trackers to intelligent, multifunctional platforms that deliver real-time, personalized, and predictive care. By integrating advanced biosensing, novel materials, and AI, these devices empower individuals and improve healthcare outcomes. Moving forward, addressing key challenges such as comfort, affordability, and data privacy is crucial for broader adoption. Ultimately, wearables are poised to play a transformative role in creating accessible, connected, and patient-centred healthcare systems worldwide.

References

Abowd GD, Mynatt ED (2000) Charting past, present, and future research in ubiquitous computing. ACM Trans Comput-Hum Interact 7(1):29–58

Afyf A, Larbi B, Riouch F, Sennouni MA, Nourdin Y (2016) Flexible antennas for wearable technologies. Handbook of research on recent developments in intelligent communication application

Ahmed MR, Newby S, Potluri P, Mirihanage W, Fernando A (2024) Emerging paradigms in fetal heart rate monitoring: evaluating the efficacy and application of innovative textile-based wearables. Sensors 24(18):6066

Alfirevic Z, Gyte GM, Cuthbert A, Devane D (2017) Continuous cardiotocography (CTG) as a form of electronic fetal monitoring (EFM) for fetal assessment during labour. Cochrane Database Syst Rev (2)

Almeida JP, Gomes DM, Santos AR (2020) Wearable electrocardiogram devices: a review of current technologies and future directions. J Med Syst 44(6):109

Alpár G, Hoepman J-H, Siljee J (2011) The identity crisis: security, privacy and usability issues in identity management. arXiv Preprint:arXiv:1101.0427

Amani AM, Kamyab H, Vafa E, Jahanbin A, Abbasi M, Vaez A, Munuswamy-Ramanujam G, Ravindran B, Gnanasekaran L, Rocchio D, Yusuf M (2025) Multifunctional MXenes nanocomposite platforms for biosensing and wearable sensor technologies. Adv Compos Hybrid Mater 8(63):1–26

Anderson N, Szorc N, Gunasekaran V, Joshi S, Jursich G (2019) Highly sensitive screen-printed strain sensors on flexible substrates via ink composition optimization. Sensors Actuators A Phys 290:1–7

Bahri M, Gebre SH, Elaguech MA, Dajan FT, Sendeku MG, Tlili C, Wang D (2023) Recent advances in chemical vapour deposition techniques for graphene-based nanoarchitectures: from synthesis to contemporary applications. Coord Chem Rev 475:214910

Baihan A, Amoon M, Altameem T, Hashem M (2025) Pioneering wearable sensor-driven health monitoring system for contagious disease prevention with intelligent crowd-counting models. IEEE Sensors J. Advance online publication

Bandodkar AJ, Wang J (2014) Non-invasive wearable electrochemical sensors: A review. Trends Biotechnol 32(7):363–371

Bansal S, Thakur M, Pandey S (2020) Privacy and security concerns in wearable healthcare devices: a systematic review. J Healthc Eng 2020:8817341

Bayoumy K, Gaber M, Elshafeey A, Mhaimeed O, Dineen EH, Marvel, Elshazly MB (2021) Smart wearable devices in cardiovascular care: where we are and how to move forward. Nat Rev Cardiol 18(8):581–599

Beitollahi H, Tajik S, Nejad FG, Safaei M (2020) Recent advances in ZnO nanostructure-based electrochemical sensors and biosensors. J Mater Chem B 8(27):5826–5844

Bounegru AV, Apetrei C (2020) Carbonaceous nanomaterials employed in the development of electrochemical sensors based on screen-printing technique-a review. Catalysts 10(6):680
Cai Z, Luo K, Liu C, Li J (2017) Design of a smart ECG garment based on conductive textile electrode and flexible printed circuit board. Technol Health Care 25(4):815–821
Chen Q, Liu Y, Gu K, Yao J, Shao Z, Chen X (2022) Silk-based electrochemical sensor for the detection of glucose in sweat. Biomacromolecules 23(9):3928–3935
Chhetry A, Sharma S, Barman SC, Yoon H, Ko S, Park C, Park JY (2021) Black phosphorus@ laser-engraved graphene heterostructure-based temperature–strain hybridized sensor for electronic-skin applications. Adv Funct Mater 31(10):2007661
Cho J, Jang Y, Kim J, Lee IS, Lee W (2024) Recent advancements in flexible biosensors for continuous glucose monitoring. J Flexible Printed Electron 3(1):47–64
Choi JH, Park SY, Kim Y (2021) Artificial intelligence and wearable health monitoring devices: integration for personalized care. Healthcare 9(8):993
Chowdhury MU, Roy S, Aryal KP, Leung H, Pandey R (2024) FabSense—A DIY approach for development of electrochemical sweat glucose sensor. In: Proceedings of the 2024 IEEE 20th International Conference on Body Sensor Networks (BSN). IEEE, pp 1–4
Custodio V, Herrera FJ, López G, Moreno JI (2012) A review on architectures and communications technologies for wearable health-monitoring systems. Sensors 12(10):13907–13946. https://doi.org/10.3390/s121013907
Dagli SM, Sharma S, Prabhu S (2021) Wearable glucose monitors: technological advancements and challenges. J Diabetes Sci Technol 15(3):532–540
De Zambotti M, Cellini N, Goldstone A, Colrain IM, Baker FC (2019) Wearable sleep technology in clinical and research settings. Med Sci Sports Exerc 51(7):1538
de-la-Fuente-Robles Y-M, Ricoy-Cano A-J, Albín-Rodríguez A-P, López-Ruiz JL, Espinilla-Estévez M (2022) Past, present and future of research on wearable technologies for healthcare: a bibliometric analysis using Scopus. Sensors (Basel) 22:8599
Duan H, Peng S, He S, Tang S-Y, Goda K, Wang CH, Li M (2025) Wearable electrochemical biosensors for advanced healthcare monitoring. Adv Sci 12:2411433
Đuričković I, Marchetti M, Claverie R, Bourson P, Chassot JM, Fontana MD (2010) Experimental study of NaCl aqueous solutions by Raman spectroscopy: towards a new optical sensor. Appl Spectrosc 64(8):853–857
Espiau B (1985) Use of optical reflectance sensors. In: Recent advances in robotics, pp 313–357
Garg M, Guo H, Maclam E, Zhanov E, Samudrala S, Pavlov A, Rahman MS, Namkoong M, Moreno JP, Tian L (2024) Molecularly imprinted wearable sensor with paper microfluidics for real-time sweat biomarker analysis. ACS Appl Mater Interfaces 16(35):46113–46122
González Ramírez ML, García Vázquez JP, Rodríguez MD, Padilla-López LA, Galindo-Aldana GM, Cuevas-González D (2023) Wearables for stress management: a scoping review. Healthcare 11(17):2369
Guk K, Han G, Lim J, Jeong K, Kang T, Lim E K, Jung J (2019) Evolution of wearable devices with real-time disease monitoring for personalized healthcare. Nano 9:813
Hosseini ES, Dervin S, Ganguly P, Dahiya R (2020) Biodegradable materials for sustainable health monitoring devices. ACS Appl Bio Mater 4(1):163–194. https://doi.org/10.1021/acsabm.0c01084
Hwang T, Gope P (2015) Robust stream-cipher mode of authenticated encryption for secure communication in wireless sensor network. Secur Commun Netw 9(6):667–679
Jin X, Liu C, Xu T, Su L, Zhang X (2020) Artificial intelligence biosensors: challenges and prospects. Biosens Bioelectron 165:112412
Kao HL, Cho CL, Chang LC, Chen CB, Chung WH, Tsai YC (2020) A fully inkjet-printed strain sensor based on carbon nanotubes. Coatings 10(8):792
Khan Y, Ostfeld AE, Lochner CM, Pierre A, Arias AC (2016) Monitoring of vital signs with flexible and wearable medical devices. Adv Mater 28(22):4373–4395. https://doi.org/10.1002/adma.201504366

Khan AR, Manzoor HU, Ayaz F, Imran MA, Zoha A (2024) Hybrid neuromorphic-federated learning for activity recognition using multi-modal wearable sensors. In: Multimodal intelligent sensing in modern applications, pp 133–164

Kos A, Milutinović V, Umek A (2019) Challenges in wireless communication for connected sensors and wearable devices used in sport biofeedback applications. Future Gener Comput Syst 92:582–592. https://doi.org/10.1016/j.future.2018.10.014

Kumar P, Lee H-J (2012) Security issues in healthcare applications using wireless medical sensor networks: A survey. Sensors 12(1):55–91

LaBoone PA, Marques O (2024) Overview of the future impact of wearable and artificial intelligence in healthcare workflows and technology. Int J Inf Manage Data Insights 4:100294. https://doi.org/10.1016/j.jjimei.2024.100294

Lee J, Kim S, Lee J, Yang D, Park BC, Ryu S, Park I (2014) A stretchable strain sensor based on a metal nanoparticle thin film for human motion detection. Nanoscale 6(20):11932–11939

Lei L, Li X, Zhang H (2024) Multi-frequency asymmetric absorption–transmission metastructures-photonic crystals and their application as a refractive index sensor. Sensors (Basel) 24(19):6281

Li W, Jin X, Han X, Li Y, Wang W, Lin T, Zhu Z (2021) Synergy of porous structure and microstructure in piezoresistive material for high-performance and flexible pressure sensors. ACS Appl Mater Interfaces 13(16):19211–19220

Li Q, Zou K, Zhang Y (2024) Artificial-intelligence-reinforced multimodal electronic skin for psychological stress assessment. Sci Bull 69(9):1173–1175

Liu H, Li Q, Zhang S, Yin R, Liu X, He Y, Guo Z (2018) Electrically conductive polymer composites for smart flexible strain sensors: a critical review. J Mater Chem C 6(45):12121–12141

Maji A, Kuila C, Phadikar U, Murmu NC, Kuila T (2024) Sustainable engineering of the wearable sensor for noninvasive health monitoring using exfoliated layered double hydroxide/reduced graphene oxide/poly (vinyl alcohol) electrospun fiber composites. ACS Appl Polym Mater 6(21):13002–13014. https://doi.org/10.1021/acsapm.4c01656

May AM, Katbamna BB, Shaikh PA, LoCoco S, Deych E, Zhou R, Liu L, Mikhova KM, Ghadban R, Cuculich PS, Cooper DH (2024) Automated differentiation of wide QRS complex tachycardia using QRS complex polarity. Commun Med 4(1):282

Mukhopadhyay SC (2015) Wearable sensors for human activity monitoring: a review. IEEE Sensors J 15(3):1321–1330

Nicolae M, Roussel V, Koelle M, Lefez C, Roudaut A, Nittala AS, Huron S, Teyssier M, Steimle J (2024) Biomaterials for prototyping in HCI. In: Mensch und Computer 2024-Workshopband, pp 10–18420

Niknejad N, Ismail WB, Mardani A, Liao H, Ghani I (2020) A comprehensive overview of smart wearables: the state-of-the-art literature, recent advances, and future challenges. Eng Appl Artif Intel 90:103529

Nittala AS, Khan A, Kruttwig K, Kraus T, Steimle J (2020) PhysioSkin: rapid fabrication of skin-conformal physiological interfaces. Proceedings of the 2020 CHI conference on human factors in computing systems, pp. 1–10

Nittala AS, Karrenbauer A, Khan A, Kraus T, Steimle J (2021) Computational design and optimization of electro-physiological sensors. Nat Commun 12(1):6351

Ometov A, Shubina V, Klus L, Skibińska J, Saafi S, Pascacio P, Flueratoru L, Gaibor DQ, Chukhno N, Chukhno O, Ali A, Channa A, Svertoka E, Qaim WB, Casanova-Marques R, Holcer S, Torres-Sospedra J, Casteleyn S, Ruggeri G, Araniti G, Burget R, Hosek J, Lohan ES (2021) A survey on wearable technology: history, state-of-the-art and current challenges. Comput Netw 193:108074

Otto C, Milenkovic A, Sanders C, Jovanov E (2006) System architecture of a wireless body area sensor network for ubiquitous health monitoring. J Mobile Multimedia 1(4):307–326

Parrilla M, De Wael K (2021) Wearable self-powered electrochemical devices for continuous health management. Adv Funct Mater 31(50):2107042. https://doi.org/10.1002/adfm.202107042

Phatak AA, Wieland FG, Vempala K, Volkmar F, Memmert D (2021) Artificial intelligence-based body sensor network framework-narrative review: proposing an end-to-end framework using wearable sensors, real-time location systems and artificial intelligence/machine learning algorithms for data collection, data mining and knowledge discovery in sports and healthcare. Sports Medicine - Open 7(1):79

Piwek L, Ellis DA, Andrews S, Joinson AN (2016) The rise of wearable technology and its impact on society. Comput Hum Behav 65:11–17

Prabowo BA, Purwidyantri A, Liu KC (2018) Surface plasmon resonance optical sensor: a review on light source technology. Biosensors 8(3):80

Rastogi PK, Ganesan V, Krishnamoorthi S (2014) A promising electrochemical sensing platform based on a silver nanoparticle decorated copolymer for sensitive nitrite determination. J Mater Chem A 2(4):933–943

Reddy S (2024) Generative AI in healthcare: an implementation science informed translational path on application, integration and governance. Implement Sci 19(1):27

Reddy N, Verma N, Dungan K (2023) Monitoring technologies-continuous glucose monitoring, mobile technology, biomarkers of glycemic control

Rodgers MM, Pai V, Conroy RS (2015) Recent advances in wearable sensors for health monitoring. IEEE Sensors J 15(6):3119–3126

Rodgers MM, Alon G, Pai VM, Conroy RS (2019) Wearable technologies for active living and rehabilitation: current research challenges and future opportunities. J Rehabil Assistive Technol Eng 6:2055668319839607

Roy S, Chowdhury MU, Noim JO, Pandey R, Nittala AS (2024) HoloChemie-sustainable fabrication of soft biochemical holographic devices for ubiquitous sensing. Proceedings of the 37th annual ACM symposium on user interface software and technology, pp. 1–19

Salehi W, Gupta G, Bhatia S, Koundal D, Mashat A, Belay A (2022) IoT-based wearable devices for patients suffering from Alzheimer disease. Contrast Media Mol Imaging 2022:3224939

Salim A, Lim S (2019) Recent advances in noninvasive flexible and wearable wireless biosensors. Biosens Bioelectron 141:111422. https://doi.org/10.1016/j.bios.2019.111422

Sardini E, Serpelloni M, Pasqui V (2014) Wireless wearable T-shirt for posture monitoring during rehabilitation exercises. IEEE Trans Instrum Meas 64(2):439–448. https://doi.org/10.1109/TIM.2014.2360994

Scheffler M, Hirt E (2005) Wearable devices for telemedicine applications. J Telemed Telecare 11(1_suppl):11–14. https://doi.org/10.1258/1357633305774447937

Shu Y, Su T, Lu Q, Shang Z, Xu Q, Hu X (2021) Highly stretchable wearable electrochemical sensor based on Ni-Co MOF nanosheet-decorated Ag/rGO/PU fiber for continuous sweat glucose detection. Anal Chem 93(48):16222–16230

Tonelli D, Scavetta E, Gualandi I (2019) Electrochemical deposition of nanomaterials for electrochemical sensing. Sensors 19(5):1186

Tseng CC, Kung CT, Chen RF, Tsai MH, Chao HR, Wang YN, Fu LM (2021) Recent advances in microfluidic paper-based assay devices for diagnosis of human diseases using saliva, tears and sweat samples. Sens Actuators B 342:130078. https://doi.org/10.1016/j.snb.2021.130078

Turakhia DG (2024) Designing learner-centric tools for physical skill-learning. Doctoral dissertation, Massachusetts Institute of Technology. MIT Libraries. https://dspace.mit.edu/handle/1721.1/156557

Uddin MZ (2019) A wearable sensor-based activity prediction system to facilitate edge computing in smart healthcare system. J Parallel Distrib Comput 123:46–53. https://doi.org/10.1016/j.jpdc.2018.10.007

Vaghasiya JV, Mayorga-Martinez CC, Pumera M (2023) Wearable sensors for telehealth based on emerging materials and nanoarchitectonics. Flex Electron 26. https://doi.org/10.1016/j.flexel.2023.100026

Wang ZL (2013) Metal and semiconductor nanowires: nanowires and nanobelts: materials, properties and devices, vol 1. Springer, Berlin

Wankhade UA, Thakare YN, Hardas BM, Pande RS (2024) Cortisol detection methods for stress monitoring: current insight and future prospect: a review. IEEE Sensors J 24:23389

Westbroek P, Priniotakis G, Kiekens P (2005) Analytical electrochemistry in textiles. Elsevier

Windmiller JR, Wang J (2013) Wearable electrochemical sensors and biosensors: a review. Electroanalysis 25(1):29–46

Wolfbeis OS (2005) Materials for fluorescence-based optical chemical sensors. J Mater Chem 15(27–28):2657–2669

World Health Organization (2024). Diabetes. 14 Nov. https://www.who.int/news-room/fact-sheets/detail/diabetes

Xu J, Xu K, Han Y, Wang D, Li X, Hu T, Ni Z (2020) A 3D porous graphene aerogel@ GOx based microfluidic biosensor for electrochemical glucose detection. Analyst 145(15):5141–5147

Yan T, Wang Z, Pan ZJ (2018) Flexible strain sensors fabricated using carbon-based nanomaterials: A review. Curr Opin Solid State Mater Sci 22(6):213–228

Yang G, Hong J, Park SB (2024) Wearable device for continuous sweat lactate monitoring in sports: a narrative review. Front Physiol 15:1376801

Yu Q, Wu J, Xiao W, Zhao C, Zhang W, Chen Y, Liu Y, Liu H, Zhou J, Ding L, Ju H (2025) An integrated, wearable paper microfluidic array device for multicomponent electrochemical sweat sensing. Cell Rep Phys Sci 6(1):102389

Zhang Y, Hu Y, Jiang N, Yetisen AK (2023) Wearable artificial intelligence biosensor networks. Biosens Bioelectron 219:114825

Zhou Z, Tang W, Xu T, Zhao W, Zhang J, Bai C (2024) Flexible strain sensors based on thermoplastic polyurethane fabricated by electrospinning: a review. Sensors 24(15):4793

Wearable Devices for Sports Monitoring 11

Gizem Baysan, Fatemeh Sharifi, Cihangir Turemis, and Volkan Cecen

Abstract

Recent advancements in materials science and device fabrication have led to the development of a new generation of biosensing devices that are portable and capable of non-invasive or minimally invasive detection. These devices enable long-term monitoring of various physiological parameters and biomarkers associated with multiple diseases. Wearable technology allows doctors, sports teams, and endurance athletes to track physiological markers, workloads, and functional movements, optimizing performance and reducing the risk of injury. As a result, both the general and sports teams can increasingly benefit from wearable performance gadgets and sensors. This chapter discusses the applications of nanotheranostics in medicine, regenerative medicine, personalized medicine, sensor fabrication, and fabric construction, as well as the challenges and future directions in sports wearable technology. By integrating wearable healthcare devices with the latest innovations in point-of-care diagnostics, these developments will revolutionize health monitoring and management, creating a more empowered and connected experience for everyone.

G. Baysan
Department of Biomechanics, Institute of Health Science, Dokuz Eylul University, Izmir, Turkey

F. Sharifi
Department of Chemical Engineering, University of Michigan, Ann Arbor, MI, USA

C. Turemis
Department of Orthopedics and Traumatology, Dokuz Eylul University, Faculty of Medicine, Izmir, Turkey

V. Cecen (✉)
Department of Biomedical Engineering, Newark College of Engineering, New Jersey Institute of Technology, Newark, NJ, USA
e-mail: volkan.cecen@njit.edu

V. Patel et al. (eds.), *Biosensor Technology in Translating Novel Materials into Practical Devices*, https://doi.org/10.1007/978-981-95-5519-2_11

Keywords

AI/ML · Sensor · Wearable devices · Nanotheranostics

11.1 Introduction

Recent technological advances in device fabrication and materials science have led to the development of a new generation of biosensing devices with advanced, portable, non-invasive, or minimally invasive detection capabilities, aiming to facilitate long-term monitoring of various biomarkers or physiological parameters related to multiple diseases (Mohan et al. 2017). Such devices can also be mounted in wearable devices. They can continuously monitor and collect multiple biological and physiological data that can be evaluated and processed using artificial intelligence (AI) for future intelligent applications or prognoses (He et al. 2023; Zhang et al. 2023). Integrating machine Learning (ML) and wearable devices will facilitate the real-time monitoring of physiological factors, biomarkers, and specific parameters to enhance disease prediction and environmental conditions (Sharifi et al. 2020). Various data related to blood pressure, heart rate, activity levels, and environmental conditions can be obtained through biosensors embedded in wearable technologies and analyzed using ML technologies (Sharifi et al. 2020). Such devices may utilize inertial movement units to capture the movement of the skin induced by respiration, cardiac activity, coughing, and other body movements, thereby enabling advanced patient care and health monitoring. The obtained data can be transferred via flash memory or a cloud-based system for further analysis (Zhang et al. 2023).

It is worth mentioning that AI-integrated wearable sensing devices can be incorporated with smartphones to monitor health and physiological-related parameters, resulting in enhanced personalized tele-healthcare systems. Therefore, various AI-embedded biosensing devices will emerge shortly to provide a new intelligent detection and diagnosis mode (Manickam et al. 2022; Yammouri and Ait Lahcen 2024).

Such intelligent methods have their limitations. The data interpretation, integration, and standardization processes, as well as the power consumption, cost-effectiveness, lifetime, and regulatory compliance of these innovative biosensors, need to be improved to enhance performance metrics, reliability, and longevity (Huang et al. 2016). For example, the Amrita IoT Medical Smart-edge system features a biosensor with decent detection precision and optimized performance metrics, making it suitable for medical wearable applications, especially in remote areas (Huang et al. 2016). A potential solution for improving energy consumption and latency is the application of fog computing technologies in bio-sensing platforms. Fog computing technologies have shown great promise in improving the efficiency of data analysis and enhancing overall functionality (Aledhari et al. 2022; Parihar et al. 2023).

Recent developments in microfabrication techniques, intelligent signal processing, and data analysis will result in the creation of miniaturized biosensing platforms integrated into wearable devices. These platforms have the potential to screen various biological and physiological markers in the long term and have numerous applications, including personalized medicine and point-of-care devices (Rodrigues et al. 2020; Tricoli et al. 2017).

Biosensor wearable devices can be applied for clinical purposes and used as an integrated network containing multiple biosensing devices and personal detectors equipped with AI technologies, cloud systems, and servers, where pathological and physiological data are collected, processed, and analyzed using various AI algorithms (Aminizadeh et al. 2023; Monteiro et al. 2021). In this regard, ultrathin interactive textile patches were developed to record physiological data similar to that obtained from electrocardiograms (ECG), electrodermal activity (EDA), and surface electromyography (sEMG) (Chaulagain et al. 2022). One of the great merits of intelligent patches is their skin-conforming characteristics, enabling them to be used long term and integrated with AI technologies. Similarly, a wearable biosensing device was developed to evaluate metabolites and nutritional levels in sweat under both physical and resting conditions (Shi et al. 2022; Wang et al. 2022).

Recent advances in machine learning algorithms have improved biosensors, enabling them to learn from their experiences and adapt to new datasets, resulting in higher performance from biosensing devices. The learning process can be unsupervised, semi-supervised, supervised, or reinforcement learning (Qureshi et al. 2023). In a similar application, a wearable biosensor was developed to provide real-time evaluation of the glucose concentration. The electrochemical biosensor measured the glucose level in the interstitial fluid, producing a related signal that was sent wirelessly to a device connected to the wearable biosensor. The AI algorithms then analyzed the data and provided the real-time glucose level (Kadian et al. 2021). Intelligent algorithms can learn and modify parameters based on individual variances, metabolism, and ambient conditions (Nayyar et al. 2021).

11.2 Applications in Regenerative Medicine, Personalized Medicine

Trends toward biosensing devices impose several fabrication characteristics. Commercial biosensor trends require small, portable, and wearable sensors that can be customized for various biomarkers and individuals, and continuously monitor specific biomarkers without requiring the involvement of experienced technicians (Singh and Singh 2020). Additionally, these sensors must be biocompatible and exhibit the highest sensitivity and usability while consuming the lowest possible power. It is also essential to obtain various biomarkers through invasive or semi-invasive methods from components such as saliva, sweat, and urea (Kumari and Toshniwal 2020). Therefore, advances in personalized usage, fabrication methods, filtering technologies, data transmission, processing, and storage must be considered to achieve the parameters above in biosensors (Lei and Guo 2022; Sharma et al. 2021).

Wearable devices are defined as electronic devices that incorporate computer functions and can be worn, carried by, or attached to the human body. As developments in regenerative medicine have accelerated in recent years, athletes constantly seek ways to push their boundaries, optimize performance, and stay ahead of the competition. Wearable technology devices are a game-changer, revolutionizing the landscape of training, performance monitoring, and injury prevention, and have become indispensable tools for both ordinary and professional athletes to enhance their athletic performances by unlocking their true potential. The current technology can detect signs of fatigue, muscle strain, and improper posture, allowing trainers to make adjustments in time before an injury occurs (Mohd Ramsi et al. 2025).

Various sports and biomedical communities have developed a range of technologies, including drones, smart shoes, smart shirts, belts, patches, and smart eyewear. While some of these devices are inexpensive and widely available, others are more costly and designed for use in controlled laboratory environments, allowing for the monitoring of movement and signals from different parts of the body. Kato Jumba K. conducted a review of wearable technology in modern athletic training and performance monitoring, utilizing real-time data on biomechanical, physiological, and environmental parameters. Various wearable devices, including smartwatches, heart rate monitors, GPS trackers, and fitness bands, were examined in elite and recreational sports, with an emphasis on their applications in injury prevention, performance enhancement, and health management, particularly in high-stakes environments (Kato Jumba 2025). Li RT, et al. also published a review that includes wearable technologies consisting of movement sensors, such as pedometers, accelerometers, and gyroscopes, as well as global positioning satellite (GPS) devices, and physiologic sensors, including heart rate monitors, sleep monitors, temperature sensors, and integrated sensors. The aforementioned wearable technologies can be used to detect position-specific patterns in movement, design more efficient sports-specific training programs for performance optimization, and screen for potential causes of injury, such as concussions and fatigue (Li et al. 2016). Since there is a wide range of usage areas for these wearable technology devices, some innovative studies are presented below.

Deglutition disorders, commonly known as dysphagia, can stem from a variety of diseases, profoundly impacting a patient's quality of life. In response to this challenge, Natta et al. developed an innovative piezoelectric sensor designed to meticulously monitor key swallowing parameters: spontaneous swallowing frequency, the duration of individual swallows, and latency time. This cutting-edge sensor is set to revolutionize the assessment of swallowing quality as a non-invasive medical device that provides clinically significant insights. It features an ultrathin and flexible architecture crafted from lightweight aluminum nitride, utilizing traditional microfabrication techniques on a delicate layer of Kapton. To ensure comfort and stability during use, a tactile coating of sticky polydimethylsiloxane–polyethylenimine polymer is applied, establishing a seamless connection with the skin (Fig. 11.1). The sensor's output voltage is efficiently transmitted to a smartphone, following amplification and filtration through a dedicated conditioning system by bluetooth technology. This streamlined process facilitates its practical application in

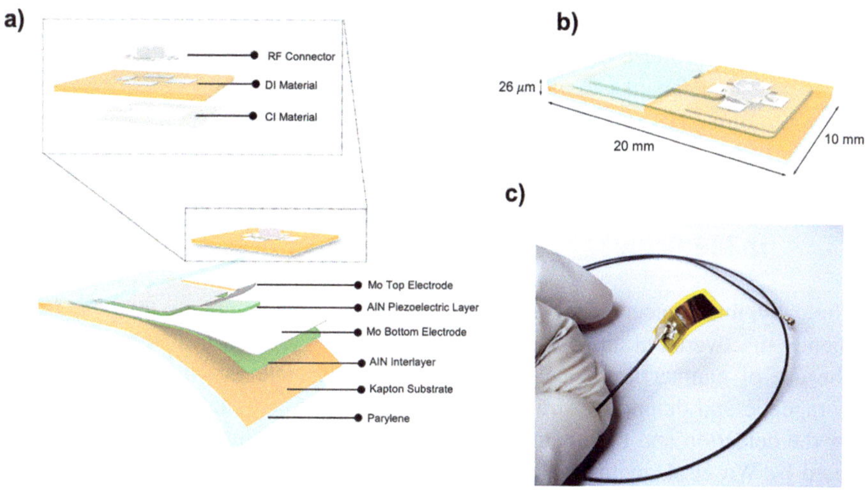

Fig. 11.1 The structure of the flexible piezoelectric sensor is illustrated through an exploded schematic of the multilayer flexible transducer (**a**), accompanied by a detailed 3D view of the layers that form the external package, shown in the inset. The design and dimensions of the final sensor (**b**) are presented, along with a picture of the fully assembled sensor (**c**) (Natta et al. 2021)

therapeutic settings. By harnessing the data collected, healthcare professionals can gain an objective measure of an individual's swallowing capabilities, paving the way for the early identification of pathological disorders and ultimately enhancing patient care (Natta et al. 2021).

Over the past 20 years, the use of nanoparticles in medicine has increased dramatically, resulting in the development of numerous novel nanobased therapeutic and diagnostic imaging techniques for a range of diseases and organs. The simplest definition of a "theranostic" nanoparticle is one that combines both diagnostic and therapeutic functionalities on a single platform. The term "theranostics" can also refer to efforts in the clinic to design personalized therapies for each patient through diagnostic testing, which may involve image-guided surgery and post-surgery evaluation. Specifically designed for use with one or more imaging modalities, these "theranostic" nanoparticles have been created for nuclear imaging, which encompasses both single-photon computed tomography and positron emission tomography, as well as optical imaging, magnetic resonance imaging, ultrasound, and computed tomography (Zavaleta et al. 2018).

To diagnose and treat physiological abnormalities, the field of interventional nanotheranostics combines the application of nanotechnology with interventional methods. Interventional techniques employ minimally invasive methods to diagnose and treat medical conditions, such as the use of endoscopes or catheters. By utilizing nanotechnology, it is possible to improve the accuracy and effectiveness of these methods. Using therapeutic delivery systems or nanoscale probes, it is possible to visualize and target specific regions of the body, such as tumors or blocked blood vessels. In addition to providing focused, minimally invasive therapies that can improve patient outcomes and minimize adverse effects, interventional nanotheranostics holds promise for transforming the treatment of many medical conditions (Sharma 2023). Thanks to all these technological developments, it is possible to benefit from nanotheranostics in the field of sports monitoring.

11.3 Examples of Different Applications of Nanotheranostics in Medicine

Clinically, lung cancer with brain metastases is still challenging to treat and is frequently discovered at an advanced stage when there are few available treatments. The use of nanotechnological technologies has become essential for improving therapeutic and diagnostic strategies. The theranostic potential of nanotechnology for the detection and treatment of brain metastases from lung cancer was investigated by Wu et al., with particular attention to nanomaterials such as liposomes, polymeric nanoparticles, quantum dots, and magnetic nanoparticles, as well as their applications in imaging methods including CT, MRI, PET, and fluorescence imaging. There is also a discussion of how nanotechnology can help bypass the blood-brain barrier and enable the administration of tailored medicine via both passive and active targeting. As important developments in immunotherapy, particular emphasis was paid to immune-modulating nanoparticles, such as checkpoint inhibitors and nanovaccines. Theranostic nanoparticles hold significant potential for real-time monitoring of treatment. These nanotechnological advancements could revolutionize cancer treatment by enhancing patient survival outcomes, enabling targeted therapies, and improving diagnostic capabilities (Wu et al. 2025).

Li et al. suggested a new method for the early diagnosis of osteoarthritis. By conjugating folic acid (FA) and near-infrared (NIR) dye onto hyaluronic acid (HA) particles, the researchers created folate receptor (FR)-targeting probes for the investigation. HA is a naturally occurring polymer that has been utilized extensively as an imaging probe and medication carrier due to its inherent biocompatible and biodegradable qualities. The probes' biological, chemical, and physical compatibility were described. In vitro research was conducted on the capacity of the FA-HA probes to identify and quantify activated macrophages. Lastly, they evaluated the efficacy of FA-HA probes in locating osteoarthritic tissue and determining the degree of osteoarthritic degeneration in human osteoarthritic explants utilizing leftover human cartilage tissue. They concluded that FA-HA probes can be used in NIR imaging to identify active macrophages. Furthermore, the quantity of activated macrophages in culture can be determined by measuring the fluorescence intensities associated with the probe. They visualized the amount of inflammatory responses in cartilage tissue within 30 minutes of applying FA-HA probes (100 μg/mL) in the presence of free probes (Li et al. 2018).

Extracellular vesicles (EVs) are diverse lipid bilayer-enclosed particles secreted by various cell types into the extracellular environment. Their release occurs across all life forms, serving as important bioactive carriers rather than mere cellular debris. EVs facilitate cellular communication and biological processes by

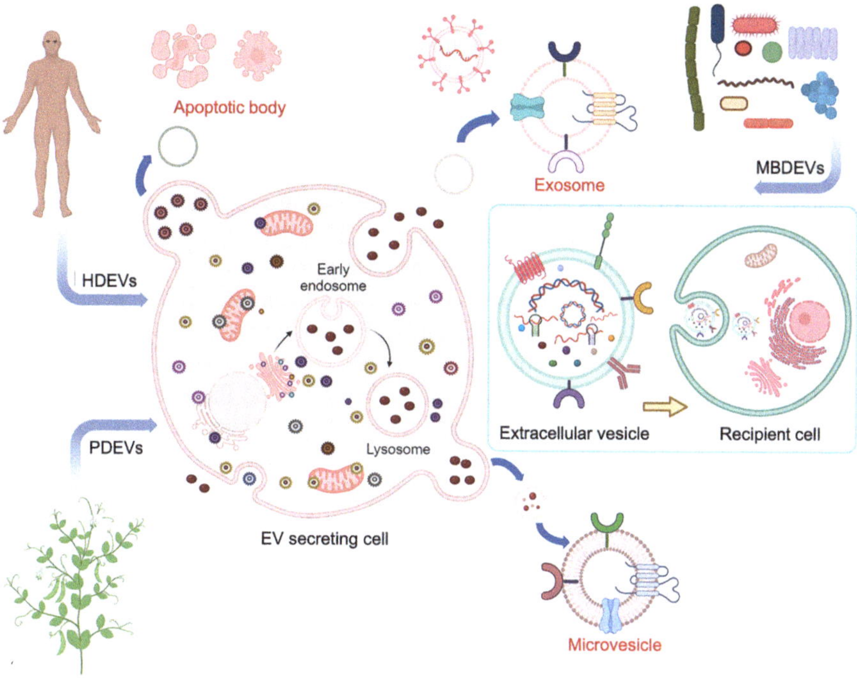

Fig. 11.2 EVs encompass a variety of bioactive components, including proteins, nucleic acids, and lipids, serving as structural elements and cellular signatures. Cells from different tissues release EVs for intercellular communication in surrounding fluids. A significant number of EVs in humans originate from stem cells, while organisms ranging from plants to bacteria also produce and release EVs into their environment (Kumar et al. 2024)

transporting proteins (such as receptors and enzymes), lipids, and nucleic acids (including miRNA, mRNA, and DNA). They are implicated in diseases such as heart disease, neurodegeneration, and cancer. EVs are classified into subtypes—such as exosomes, microvesicles, and apoptotic bodies—based on their synthesis and the originating cell type, with emerging types including large oncosomes and migrasomes (Fig. 11.2) (Kumar et al. 2024). Zhyvolozhnyi et al. claimed that sweat-derived EVs provide a rich source of potential biomarkers of human and bacterial origin. Although only a few pertinent analytes are currently employed in clinical practice, sweat contains indicators for real-time, non-invasive health monitoring. The study examined extracellular vesicles (EVs) in sweat samples from eight volunteers who performed strenuous exercise. Utilizing the ExoView platform, electron microscopy, nanoparticle tracking analysis, and Western blotting, the researchers compared the general protein composition of sweat samples obtained from alginate skin patches, whole sweat, and EV-enriched sweat, with a focus on the presence of EV markers. Approximately 20% of the 1209 distinct human proteins identified in EV-enriched sweat were detected in each of the individual samples examined (Zhyvolozhnyi et al. 2024).

Although traditional ultrasonographic imaging has proven to be a dependable diagnostic tool for muscle and tendon injuries, it has been challenging to diagnose minor musculoskeletal ailments accurately. Since a significant quantity of hydrogen peroxide (H_2O_2) is known to be produced during tissue damage, including mechanical injury, H_2O_2 has a lot of promise as a marker for both diagnosis and treatment of mechanical injuries in the musculoskeletal system. Kim et al. created poly(vanillyl alcohol-co-oxalate) (PVAX), which has anti-inflammatory and antioxidant properties and quickly scavenges H_2O_2. PVAX nanoparticles are currently in the preclinical experimental stage and have not yet received approval for clinical use in humans. However, studies using animal models indicate significant therapeutic potential for treating conditions related to oxidative stress, inflammation, and ischemia. PVAX nanoparticles produce CO_2 bubbles by hydrolysis in response to H_2O_2. Using a rat model of musculoskeletal contusion injury, they assessed the potential of H_2O_2-triggered bubble-generating anti-inflammatory PVAX nanoparticles as nanotheranostic agents for musculoskeletal injuries. In addition to having notable anti-inflammatory and anti-apoptotic properties, PVAX nanoparticles injected intramuscularly and peritendinously into the mechanical injury lesions significantly improved the ultrasonographic contrast. These results suggest that H_2O_2-triggered bubble-forming PVAX nanoparticles have significant potential as therapeutic agents for various musculoskeletal conditions and as ultrasound contrast agents (Kim et al. 2017).

11.4 Sensor Fabrication

Frequent exercise plays an essential role in revitalizing the body's health and alleviating the stresses of daily life. In a remarkable innovation, Li et al. have developed a bioinspired, sweat-resistant wearable triboelectric nanogenerator (TENG) known as the BSRW-TENG, specifically designed to monitor physical movement during exercise (Fig. 11.3) (Li et al. 2022). This cutting-edge device draws inspiration from the lotus leaf, renowned for its unique hierarchical micro- and nanostructures that exhibit superhydrophobic and self-cleaning properties. To replicate this natural phenomenon, the researchers crafted two innovative triboelectric layers: the bioinspired hierarchical resin (BH-resin) and bioinspired hierarchical polydimethylsiloxane (BH-PDMS). The TENG's intricate layers work in harmony to enhance its efficacy. A comprehensive evaluation compared the electrical performance and sweat resistance of TENGs with various surface designs: flat surfaces (flat-TENG), flat resin combined with BH-PDMS (BHP-TENG), BH-resin paired with flat PDMS (BHR-TENG), and the BSRW-TENG, which integrates both BH-resin and BH-PDMS. Notably, the BSRW-TENG achieved a remarkable twofold increase in energy output compared to the flat-TENG, attributed to the enhanced effective contact area created by its engineered micro/nanostructures. Even when saline droplets trickled down and evaporated from its surface, the BSRW-TENG consistently maintained its output, demonstrating its resilience. In contrast, the flat-TENG experienced a 41% performance decline due to the presence of lingering salt residues.

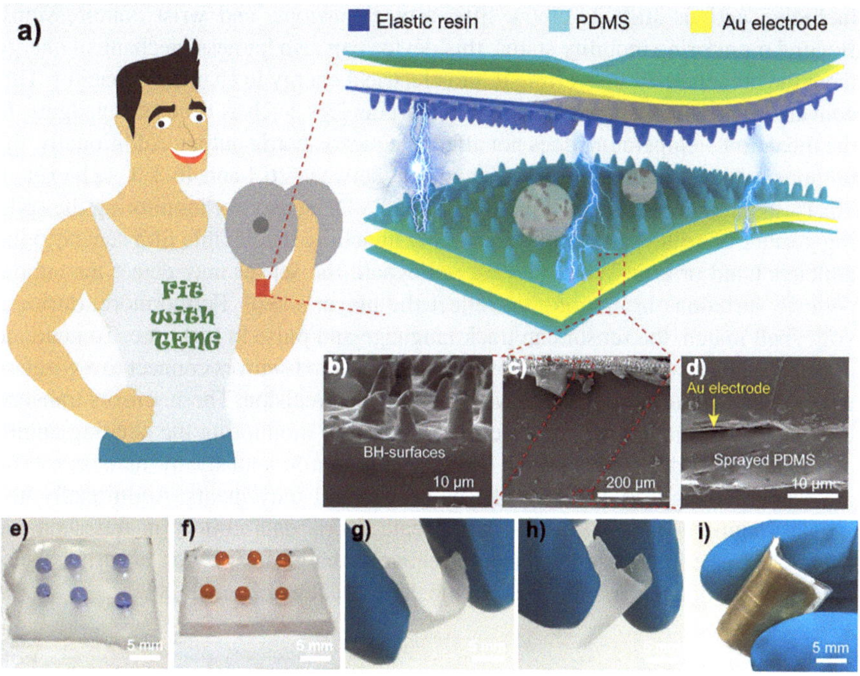

Fig. 11.3 (**a**) Schematic representation of the BSRW-TENG. (**b–d**) Scanning electron microscopy (SEM) images illustrate the interlayer structure among the triboelectric layer, electrode, and protective layer. (**e**) Superhydrophobic characteristics of the BH-resin. (**f**) Superhydrophobic characteristics of the BH-PDMS. (**g**) Visual of the BH-resin triboelectric layer. (**h**) Visual of the BH-PDMS triboelectric layer. (**i**) Visual of the fully assembled BSRW-TENG (Li et al. 2022)

Moreover, as humidity levels soared from a mere 10% to a robust 80%, the BSRW-TENG experienced a decline in output of only 11%, demonstrating an extraordinary ability to withstand moisture. In contrast, the flat-TENG TENG experienced a dramatic 54% drop in performance. The BSRW-TENG's exceptional sweat-resistance was further validated under extreme conditions, including complete surface contamination and a highly humid environment. Ultimately, this innovative wearable demonstrated its capability to deliver stable and sustained performance, remaining reliable throughout various exercise movements, such as running, leg curls, and dumbbell biceps curls, even amid the sweat and exertion typical of an intense workout (Lockie et al. 2019).

Self-powered piezoelectric sensors, which are powered by mechanical energy and can be affixed to the skin or joints of the body to detect human motion, can accomplish safe, real-time motion process monitoring without the need for an external power source. Zhao et al. designed a sensor that uses piezoelectric output as the sensing signal and PVDF (polyvinylidene fluoride) as the active material to track emergent motion. The sensor features a multi-point control capability that tracks force order, angle changes, and motion frequency during basketball shooting, including actions such as elbow lifts, arm extensions, and wrist compressions. Beyond monitoring mobility status, this device can also harness mechanical energy from the human body, converting it into electrical energy to charge a capacitor. This conversion provides a power source for smart devices, such as Bluetooth gadgets. In the meantime, temperature does not affect the piezoelectric output. Additionally, the output piezoelectric voltage remains constant between 26.1 and 46.3 °C (Zhao et al. 2021). In another study, Liu et al. designed a PVDF sensor for monitoring the spiking gesture of volleyball athletes by simply attaching the flexible film sensor to the athlete's hand or arm. When playing volleyball, the sensor may detect the subtle, delicate variations in motion that reflect the player's skill. Furthermore, during a volleyball match, the sensor can track language and pulse in real time. To generate extensive datasets seamlessly, innovative self-powered sensors connect to a wireless transmitter, capturing sports data with remarkable precision. These sensors translate the nuances of movement into electrical signals by monitoring the bending angles of the elbow and knuckle joints. They operate autonomously by harnessing the mechanical energy produced by the body's natural movements. Additionally, the wireless equipment designed for large-scale sports data collection relies on the energy harvested by these sensors to effectively charge a capacitor, ensuring a sustainable flow of data from the field to the digital realm (Liu et al. 2022).

11.5 Fabric Construction

Chen et al. pioneered an innovative approach to fabricating wearable sensors by ingeniously integrating cotton fabric as a fundamental component. This method involves intricately coating cotton fibers with conductive materials, resulting in a seamless, interconnected network that exhibits exceptional electrical conductivity (Chen et al. 2020). The incorporation of topological genus structures is essential for strategically trapping metallic seeds on substrate surfaces. To enhance both the conductivity and durability of these conductive coatings, a refined topographical modification strategy has been developed, utilizing genus-3 and genus-5 configurations. Notably, researchers have employed an effective thermally induced radical polymerization technique to capture catalyst-based nickel seed crystals. By infusing ammonia-containing polymers into soft cotton fabric, researchers have developed a sophisticated molecular topological cage characterized by covalent and hydrogen bonding. This intricate system enhances the electronic properties of wearable sensors, ensuring their longevity and reliability, and marking a significant advancement in textile-based technology. Nickel nanoparticles were subsequently grown on the surface of the catalyst-based fabric using modified electroless deposition (ELD). Recent research has showcased the remarkable qualities of a textile-based capacitive sensor, which combines durability, flexibility, and an exceptional level of comfort. This innovative sensor boasts outstanding electrical conductivity, enabling it to achieve high sensitivity and collect signals effortlessly. In-depth studies have revealed that the sensitivity of this capacitive technology is intricately influenced by the angles and distances between two conductive fabrics, creating a nuanced interplay that enhances performance. Remarkably, this textile-based sensor has successfully facilitated real-time monitoring of various human activities, including breathing, speaking, blinking, and joint movements during physical rehabilitation exercises. The integration of this technology not only offers a seamless user experience but also opens up avenues for advanced health monitoring and rehabilitation solutions (Marques et al. 2019).

11.6 Challenges and Future Directions

The processing of accumulated data is notably constrained, especially in invasion sports where unpredictable movements are commonplace (Rico-González et al. 2020). The dynamic and chaotic nature of these sports, far more complex than controlled experiments, swiftly reveals the limitations of wearable technology. In fast-paced games like basketball and ice hockey, swift body contact and rapid changes in direction create a whirlwind of activity. This raises a critical question: can current technologies accurately detect and quantify these movements? Additionally, the challenge is compounded by inconsistencies across different wearable devices, which arise from varying methodologies and algorithms (Vijayan et al. 2021). This inconsistency creates a suboptimal landscape for practitioners who rely on precise measurements to differentiate between genuine performance improvements and mere measurement errors. The scientific community often overlooks a crucial issue: wearables tend to lose data accuracy in real-time scenarios compared to post-game analysis. Additionally, these devices impact not only the players but also the coaching staff who analyze the data. This influence extends to entire sports organizations, which must adapt to leverage innovative marketing opportunities and refine their administrative processes (Slack and Parent 2006). Additionally, data availability during competition is confined to one's team, facilitating tactical analysis but failing to supplant the inherent biases and subjective observations of the coaching staff. Consequently, it remains uncertain to what degree the current generation of wearables truly aids coaches in making critical game-time decisions.

11.7 Conclusion

The fusion of AI and ML with next-generation biosensing devices represents a transformative leap into a realm of unprecedented innovation across diverse fields, including healthcare, drug discovery, and environmental monitoring (Hemdan et al. 2024). These cutting-edge biosensors significantly enhance the traditional capabilities of biosensing technologies, improving their sensitivity, specificity, and accuracy (Thirugnanasambandan et al. 2024). This enhancement enables precise and instantaneous monitoring of biomarkers, paving the way for patients to receive timely and personalized diagnostic and therapeutic insights tailored to their unique biomarker profiles. As these innovative biosensors integrate into everyday technology, such as smartphones and wearable devices, they promise to democratize health monitoring

(Nur 2024). By making diagnostics and predictive healthcare more accessible and affordable, they are particularly poised to benefit underserved or remote communities. Looking ahead, the potential for future advancements lies in the creation of comprehensive AI-driven biosensor networks. These networks will seamlessly integrate with wearable healthcare technologies and the latest innovations in point-of-care diagnostics, transforming the landscape of health monitoring and management into a more connected and empowered experience for all.

References

Aledhari M et al (2022) Biomedical IoT: enabling technologies, architectural elements, challenges, and future directions. IEEE Access 10:31306–31339

Aminizadeh S et al (2023) The applications of machine learning techniques in medical data processing based on distributed computing and the Internet of Things. Comput Methods Prog Biomed 241:107745

Chaulagain N et al (2022) Synergistic enhancement of the photoelectrochemical performance of TiO2 nanorod arrays through embedded plasmon and surface carbon nitride co-sensitization. ACS Appl Mater Interfaces 14(21):24309–24320

Chen L et al (2020) Textile-based capacitive sensor for physical rehabilitation via surface topological modification. ACS Nano 14(7):8191–8201

He L et al (2023) Smart chemical sensor and biosensor networks for healthcare 4.0. Sensors 23(12):5754

Hemdan M et al (2024) Innovations in biosensor technologies for healthcare diagnostics and therapeutic drug monitoring: applications, recent progress, and future research challenges. Sensors (Basel, Switzerland) 24(16):5143

Huang X et al (2016) A convolutional neural network based single-frame super-resolution for lensless blood cell counting. In: 2016 IEEE biomedical circuits and systems conference (BioCAS). IEEE

Kadian S et al (2021) Effect of sulfur-doped graphene quantum dots incorporation on morphological, optical and electron transport properties of CH3NH3PbBr3 perovskite thin films. J Mater Sci Mater Electron 32(13):17406–17417

Kato Jumba K (2025) Wearable technology for performance monitoring in athletes. Eurasian Exp J Sci Appl Res 7(2):71–77

Kim G-W et al (2017) Ultrasonographic imaging and anti-inflammatory therapy of muscle and tendon injuries using polymer nanoparticles. Theranostics 7(9):2463

Kumar MA et al (2024) Extracellular vesicles as tools and targets in therapy for diseases. Signal Transduct Target Ther 9(1):27

Kumari P, Toshniwal D (2020) Impact of lockdown on air quality over major cities across the globe during COVID-19 pandemic. Urban Clim 34:100719

Lei ZL, Guo B (2022) 2D material-based optical biosensor: status and prospect. Adv Sci 9(4):2102924

Li RT et al (2016) Wearable performance devices in sports medicine. Sports Health 8(1):74–78

Li S et al (2018) Hyaluronic acid-based optical probe for the diagnosis of human osteoarthritic cartilage. Nanotheranostics 2(4):347

Li W et al (2022) Bioinspired sweat-resistant wearable triboelectric nanogenerator for movement monitoring during exercise. Nano Energy 95:107018

Liu W et al (2022) A self-powered wearable motion sensor for monitoring volleyball skill and building big sports data. Biosensors 12(2):60

Lockie RG et al (2019) Relationships between training load demands measured by surface EMG wearable technology and the military drag. In: 39th Annual meeting of the southwest regional chapter of the American College of Sports Medicine
Manickam P et al (2022) Artificial intelligence (AI) and internet of medical things (IoMT) assisted biomedical systems for intelligent healthcare. Biosensors 12(8):562
Marques G et al (2019) Internet of things architectures, technologies, applications, challenges, and future directions for enhanced living environments and healthcare systems: a review. Electronics 8(10):1081
Mohan AV et al (2017) Continuous minimally-invasive alcohol monitoring using microneedle sensor arrays. Biosens Bioelectron 91:574–579
Mohd Ramsi MF, Idris SRA, Nordin SK (2025) Unleashing athletic potential: the role of wearable technology devices in sports. APB Rembau e-Bulletin
Monteiro ACB et al (2021) An overview of medical Internet of Things, artificial intelligence, and cloud computing employed in health care from a modern panorama. In: The fusion of Internet of Things, artificial intelligence, and cloud computing in health care. Springer Nature, pp 3–23
Natta L et al (2021) Conformable AlN piezoelectric sensors as a non-invasive approach for swallowing disorder assessment. ACS Sens 6(5):1761–1769
Nayyar A, Gadhavi L, Zaman N (2021) Machine learning in healthcare: review, opportunities and challenges. In: Machine learning and the Internet of Medical Things in healthcare. Academic Press, pp 23–45
Nur S (2024) The role of digital health technologies and sensors in revolutionizing wearable health monitoring systems. Int J Innov Res Comput Sci Technol 12(6):69–80
Parihar A et al (2023) Internet-of-medical-things integrated point-of-care biosensing devices for infectious diseases: toward better preparedness for futuristic pandemics. Bioeng Transl Med 8(3):e10481
Qureshi R et al (2023) Artificial intelligence and biosensors in healthcare and its clinical relevance: a review. IEEE Access 11:61600–61620
Rico-González M et al (2020) Identification, computational examination, critical assessment and future considerations of distance variables to assess collective tactical behaviour in team invasion sports by positional data: a systematic review. Int J Environ Res Public Health 17(6):1952
Rodrigues D et al (2020) Skin-integrated wearable systems and implantable biosensors: a comprehensive review. Biosensors 10(7):79
Sharifi F, Sedighi A, Rehman M (2020) Design and simulation of a point-of-care microfluidic device for acoustic blood cell separation. Eng Proc 2(1):76
Sharma AK (2023) Current trends in nanotheranostics: a concise review on bioimaging and smart wearable technology. Nanotheranostics 7(3):258
Sharma A et al (2021) Wearable biosensors: an alternative and practical approach in healthcare and disease monitoring. Molecules 26(3):748
Shi Z et al (2022) The development of wearable technologies and their potential for measuring nutrient intake: towards precision nutrition. Nutr Bull 47(4):388–406
Singh D, Singh B (2020) Investigating the impact of data normalization on classification performance. Appl Soft Comput 97:105524
Slack T, Parent MM (2006) Understanding sport organizations: the application of organization theory. Human Kinetics
Thirugnanasambandan T, Ramanathan S, Gopinath SC (2024) Revolutionizing biosensing through cutting-edge nanomaterials: an in-depth exploration of recent technological advances. Nano-Struct Nano-Objects 38:101128
Tricoli A, Nasiri N, De S (2017) Wearable and miniaturized sensor technologies for personalized and preventive medicine. Adv Funct Mater 27(15):1605271
Vijayan V et al (2021) Review of wearable devices and data collection considerations for connected health. Sensors 21(16):5589
Wang M et al (2022) A wearable electrochemical biosensor for the monitoring of metabolites and nutrients. Nat Biomed Eng 6(11):1225–1235

Wu Y et al (2025) Theranostic role of advanced nanotechnological tools in early brain metastases in lung cancer: an updated review. Int J Nanomedicine 20:7215–7232

Yammouri G, Ait Lahcen A (2024) AI-reinforced wearable sensors and intelligent point-of-care tests. J Pers Med 14(11):1088

Zavaleta C, Ho D, Chung EJ (2018) Theranostic nanoparticles for tracking and monitoring disease state. SLAS Technol Transl Life Sci Innov 23(3):281–293

Zhang Y et al (2023) Wearable artificial intelligence biosensor networks. Biosens Bioelectron 219:114825

Zhao C et al (2021) An effective self-powered piezoelectric sensor for monitoring basketball skills. Sensors 21(15):5144

Zhyvolozhnyi A et al (2024) Enrichment of sweat-derived extracellular vesicles of human and bacterial origin for biomarker identification. Nanotheranostics 8(1):48

Medical Approaches in Early-Stage Cancer Detection

12

Geetha Satya Sainaga Jyothi Vaskuri

Abstract

Early cancer detection is critical for improving treatment outcomes and patient survival rates. Advances in medical imaging technologies, liquid biopsy, biosensors, microfluidic devices, CRISPR-based diagnostics, and artificial intelligence (AI) have revolutionized early cancer detection by offering more accurate, sensitive, and non-invasive methods. The function of imaging technologies, including positron emission tomography (PET), computed tomography (CT), magnetic resonance imaging (MRI), and ultrasound in identifying cancer in its early stages, is highlighted in this chapter. Furthermore, as a viable substitute for conventional tissue biopsies, the possibility of a liquid biopsy, which incorporates circulating tumour cells (CTCs) and circulating cell-free DNA (cfDNA) as biomarkers, is explored. The sensitivity and applicability of cancer detection have increased with the development of biosensors and microfluidic technologies. CRISPR-based diagnostic tools have emerged as a potential approach in detecting mutations related to cancer. The advancement of AI has enabled significant improvement in screening for cancer with the aid of machine learning and deep learning. By combining these advanced technologies, early cancer detection is becoming more accessible and reliable, leading to the improvement in earlier screening, treatment success, and improved survival rates.

Keywords

Early cancer detection · Imaging technologies · Liquid biopsy · CRISPR · Microfluidic devices · Artificial intelligence

G. S. S. J. Vaskuri (✉)
Department of Pharmaceutical Sciences, University of Tennessee Health Science Center (UTHSC), Memphis, TN, USA

V. Patel et al. (eds.), *Biosensor Technology in Translating Novel Materials into Practical Devices*, https://doi.org/10.1007/978-981-95-5519-2_12

12.1 Introduction

Early cancer detection increases survival rates and improves treatment results. Nevertheless, about 50% of cancers are still discovered at advanced stages, which severely reduces the number of available treatment options and lowers survival rates, even with efforts and the possibility of identifying cancer at an earlier stage (Crosby et al. 2022). In addition to the potential for more effective treatments, early detection is crucial since it allows for treatment when the condition is more curable stage. Because treatment at an earlier stage may help prevent the cancer from progressing to stages where treatment becomes more difficult, improved early diagnosis could result in significant increases in survival (Loud and Murphy 2017).

Recent advancements in cancer detection have saved many lives, underscoring the critical role of early detection in improving outcomes. Better and more effective methods of early cancer diagnosis still need to be developed. Technological advancements and improvements in our biological understanding of cancer contribute to the rapid transformation of the field (Pulumati et al. 2023). Despite the advancements, there are still significant challenges that must be overcome in order to fully realize the potential of early cancer detection (Barrios 2022).

A better understanding of the biology of cancer and early-stage behaviour is essential for early detection. The goal of the research is to distinguish between benign lesions that pose minimal threat and malignant tumours that require rapid medical attention (Bland et al. 2025). This information is essential for improving treatment outcomes and lowering the risks of overtreatment, which can be harmful. Studies in human samples and enhanced disease models are revealing early tumour signals and the ways in which the immune system and tumour microenvironment promote the growth of cancer (Lawrence et al. 2023).

Developing precise risk models presents still more challenges. These models integrate a number of factors, such as genetic susceptibility, family history, environmental exposures, and demographic and behavioural data, to estimate the risk of cancer (Wang et al. 2014). As knowledge of cancer genomes and integrated risk factors advances, more extensive population cohorts need to be developed and verified in order to enhance these models (Berger and Mardis 2018).

One of the most challenging aspects of early detection is identifying reliable biomarkers, or molecular indicators that detect the existence of cancer. Cancer symptoms are typically present in very small amounts and are frequently overwhelmed by regular physiological functions. However, circulating tumour DNA, circulating tumour cells, proteins, and cancer-related metabolites are beginning to appear as promising markers (Bittla et al. 2023). The identification and confirmation of these biomarkers has been accelerated by advances in data analysis, such as machine learning, and multimodal testing that combines multiple biomarkers shows tremendous promise for enhancing detection.

Technological advances are necessary to provide detection techniques that are more precise and sensitive. New technologies, ranging from genomic analysis methods to sophisticated imaging and histology, are being investigated to identify cancer early on when tumours are still in their early stages and treatable. Furthermore, artificial markers that intensify biological indicators may greatly improve the ability to identify cancer early on (Prasanth et al. 2023; Bi et al. 2019).

Lastly, a major obstacle to converting biological findings into practical diagnostic tools is the clinical evaluation of early detection technologies, which necessitates extensive clinical trials that need a large time and commitment of resources. Translating laboratory discoveries into clinical applications requires increasing the efficacy and efficiency of these assessment procedures.

One of the most important methods for detecting cancer early is screening. Early cancer detection through screening programs, particularly those aimed at high-risk groups, can improve treatment outcomes and increase survival. The advantages of screening, however, are sometimes negligible in comparison to the possible drawbacks, such as overdiagnosis and overtreatment, and not all malignancies have established screening techniques (Moleyar-Narayana et al. 2024). The identification of lesions that might not have progressed to malignant tumours is known as overdiagnosis and often results in unnecessary, risky treatments.

Current screening initiatives have shown significant advantages in detecting cancer early, which is a crucial factor in determining patient survival. For instance, mammography has helped detect breast cancer earlier, Pap tests have significantly decreased the incidence and mortality of cervical cancer, and low-dose computed tomography (CT) has improved lung cancer outcomes (Galeş et al. 2024; Cancer screening tests 2025). The sensitivity and specificity of screening tests for other cancer types are still severely limited despite the recent advancements. For instance, indirect detection approaches like biomarker measurement or imaging techniques frequently result in false positives or false negatives, which can complicate patient management and even lead to unnecessary processes.

Significant issues are revealed by even well-established screening programs. For example, screening for prostate cancer has shown that not all early-stage cancers are aggressive or need to be treated promptly, highlighting the need for personalized and risk-stratified screening methods (Safaeian et al. 2007). In the same way, screening for colon cancer has increased survival rates, but screening for other cancers, such as some types of breast cancer, has not always been successful. These drawbacks highlight serious flaws in the methods used for early detection today, such as the difficulties of using consistent screening techniques across a range of demographics and the inability to accurately differentiate between aggressive and indolent tumours (Kotwal and Walter 2020).

In order to overcome these obstacles, interdisciplinary cooperation is needed, combining knowledge from clinicians, data science, chemistry, biology, engineering, and physics. Developments in imaging technology, computational techniques, biomarker discoveries, and molecular biology are helping the field get closer to its objective of early, highly accurate cancer detection (Berardi et al. 2020). Emerging technologies, including liquid biopsies, biosensors, microfluidic devices, and AI-driven diagnostics, are overcoming the drawbacks of traditional screening and potentially providing non-invasive, accurate, and personalized techniques for detection (Fig. 12.1). Despite these developments, substantial barriers remain, including enhancing diagnostic accuracy, reducing invasiveness and cost, and converting

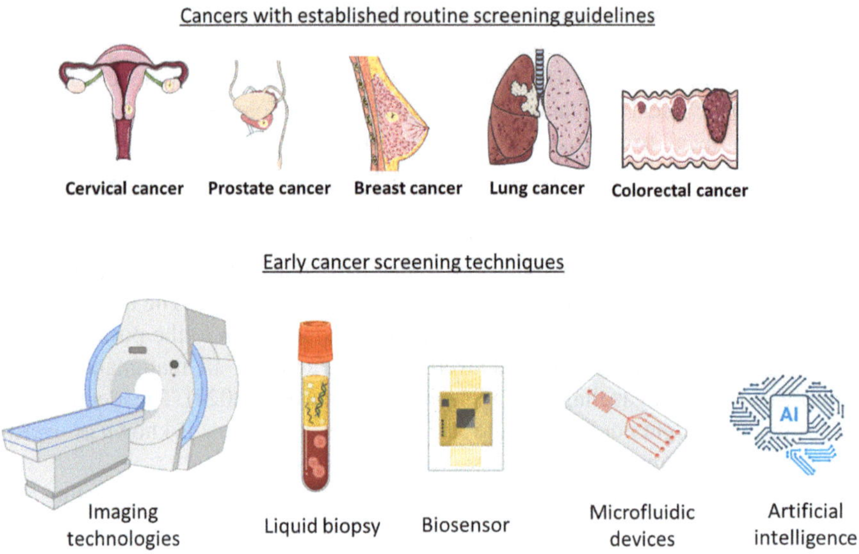

Fig. 12.1 Overview of screenable cancers and the transition from conventional to advanced early cancer detection techniques

technical innovations into scalable clinical applications. To completely achieve the potential of early cancer detection and to significantly enhance treatment efficacy and survival rates, these obstacles must be overcome (Schiffman et al. 2015).

12.2 Imaging Technologies

Imaging technologies are critical tools in the early detection of cancer (Frangioni 2008). These technologies allow for the non-invasive visualization of internal structures, enabling the identification of tumours at earlier, more treatable stages. Several imaging modalities, such as CT, MRI (Magnetic Resonance Imaging), PET (Positron Emission Tomography), ultrasound, and mammography, are commonly used in cancer screening, diagnosis, and staging (Hussain et al. 2022; Ming et al. 2020; Iranmakani et al. 2020). Each imaging technique has unique advantages and limitations, making them reliable for detecting specific types of cancer. Recent studies highlighted the effectiveness of abdominal non-contrast computed tomography (NCCT), brain CT, and PSMA PET-CT scans in identifying cancers at early stages, underscoring the potential of these tools in improving early cancer diagnosis (Griffeth 2005; PSMA PET-CT 2025).

A study named Yorkshire Kidney Screening Trial (YKST) assessed the feasibility of adding abdominal NCCT to lung cancer screening for detecting kidney cancer and other abdominal pathologies. This study aimed to explore whether abdominal NCCT could reveal accompanying observations, such as kidney cancer, during the screening process for lung cancer, particularly in high-risk groups such as smokers.

Of 4438 participants, 93% accepted abdominal NCCT, and 97% were eligible to participate; 64% of participants had a normal NCCT, while 15% required further evaluation, which resulted in serious findings in 5.3% of participants. This included 25 individuals with renal masses or complex cysts; 10 had histologically confirmed kidney cancer. The study highlighted a number needed to screen (NNS) of 402 to detect one histologically confirmed renal cancer, illustrating the feasibility of incorporating abdominal CT in lung cancer screening programs. The integration of abdominal NCCT with lung cancer screening offers the opportunity to detect kidney cancer and other abdominal pathologies early. This could be a promising method for multi-organ screening in at-risk populations. Although the study has limitations, such as a fixed age range and being limited to prior lung cancer screening attendees, it supports the potential for cost-effective early detection of serious abdominal conditions, including kidney cancer (Stewart et al. 2024).

Another study examined the use of brain CT scans in the initial staging of human epidermal growth factor receptor 2 (HER2)-positive breast cancer. It is a subtype of breast cancer with aggressiveness and risk of brain metastasis. However, brain imaging is not currently included in routine staging for early HER2-positive breast cancer; this study aimed to evaluate its utility in detecting brain metastases at the time of diagnosis. Fifty-eight patients were enrolled in the study, with no brain metastases were detected in early-stage cases. However, brain CT identified brain metastasis in one advanced-stage patient who had clinical suspicion. The findings suggest that brain CT may have limited utility in early-stage breast cancer, but it could be useful in advanced cases, particularly when brain metastasis is suspected based on clinical symptoms. Although brain CT might not be required for HER2-positive breast cancer in its early stages, it could be a useful technique for identifying brain metastases in more advanced cases, where it helps in future treatment. In order to improve early diagnosis and treatment for metastases, this study urges more research into identifying high-risk patients who might benefit from brain imaging as part of their initial staging process (Fortuna et al. 2024).

The proPSMA study assessed the prognostic value of 68Ga-PSMA-11 PET-CT scans in prostate cancer patients with intermediate- to high-risk disease. PSMA (prostate-specific membrane antigen) PET-CT scans are known for their ability to detect regional lymph node involvement and distant metastasis. This study aimed to explore their role in early detection and treatment planning. Patients with PSMA PET-CT scans showed significant differences in freedom from treatment failure (FFTF) based on whether their scan was positive or negative for regional nodal involvement (N1 vs. N0). PSMA PET-CT-defined nodal status was prognostic for medium-term oncological outcomes, indicating that men with regional nodal involvement (N1) had poorer outcomes compared to those without regional nodal involvement (N0). This suggests that PSMA PET-CT can offer useful data for early prostate cancer staging, assisting healthcare providers in identifying patients with more likely to experience distant metastases and treatment failure. Incorporating PSMA PET-CT staging into the therapy of prostate cancer could help direct treatment choices and provide early insights into the extent of disease. By ensuring that patients with high-risk characteristics receive more assertive personalized therapy, this imaging technology could have an enormous effect on treatment planning and enhance long-term survival rates (Hofman et al. 2024).

Another study compared the diagnostic accuracy of CT and combined PET with CT (PET/CT) for detecting high-grade neuroendocrine carcinoma of the cervix. CT scans showed good sensitivity (85%) for detecting primary disease in the cervix and for liver metastasis (80%), but lower specificity for lung metastasis (68%). When compared to PET/CT scans (used as the gold standard), CT alone missed important metastasis findings, leading to incorrect treatment decisions for several patients. PET/CT scans identified changes in treatment plans for 29% of patients, potentially preventing under- or overtreatment. PET/CT proved superior to CT scans in detecting metastatic disease, suggesting that it is the preferred imaging modality for both initial staging and ongoing surveillance in neuroendocrine cervical cancer. This finding underscores the importance of using PET/CT in high-grade cancers to improve the accuracy of early cancer detection and to guide appropriate treatment planning (Frumovitz et al. 2023).

In colorectal cancer (CRC), PET/CT imaging has been increasingly used for pre-treatment staging, especially with the introduction of neoadjuvant therapies. A study compared the accuracy of PET/CT versus CT alone for detecting nodal and distant metastasis in CRC patients. PET/CT was significantly more sensitive than CT for detecting nodal involvement (67% vs. 55%) and metastases (83% vs. 54%). For nodal staging, PET/CT had higher sensitivity (66.7%) and accuracy than CT (55.2%). The study revealed that PET/CT could improve the accuracy of staging, potentially leading to more tailored treatments for CRC patients, ultimately affecting their overall survival. PET/CT can significantly improve early cancer detection and staging accuracy in CRC, providing critical information for treatment planning. These findings support the integration of PET/CT into standard CRC management protocols for patients with advanced disease or those undergoing neoadjuvant treatments (Engel et al. 2024).

A generative adversarial network (GAN) pipeline has been developed to synthesize FDG-PET images from standard CT scans. This bridges the gap between high-cost, low-access PET imaging and the more widely available CT imaging. The synthetic PET images were validated for imaging quality, tumour contrast, and radiogenomic analysis, with results confirming that synthetic PET is comparable to actual PET scans in terms of tumour detection and pathway consistency. Synthetic PET was found to improve lung cancer diagnosis, staging, and prognosis in clinical settings, demonstrating its potential to enhance early detection with existing CT technology. The development of synthetic PET could offer a cost-effective alternative to traditional PET scans, making early cancer detection more accessible. This technology has the ability to improve the diagnosis and treatment planning for lung cancer patients, ultimately enhancing patient outcomes through earlier and more accurate assessments (Salehjahromi et al. 2024).

Computer-assisted diagnosis (CAD) system was used for early detection of prostate cancer using multiparametric MRI (mpMRI). Traditional transrectal ultrasound-guided biopsy has limitations, such as being invasive and having high false-negative results. The proposed method uses machine learning algorithms to analyse mpMRI images and differentiate between benign and malignant prostate tissues. By analysing 433 mpMRI images and extracting texture-based and statistical features, the study evaluated three machine learning algorithms, such as Support Vector Machine (SVM), K-Nearest Neighbour (KNN), and Ensemble Learning (EL) to classify malignant and benign prostate tissues. The results showed that diffusion-weighted imaging (DWI) combined with ensemble learning achieved the highest accuracy (75.1%) and AUC (0.82), followed by dynamic contrast-enhanced (DCE) imaging with SVM (72.2% accuracy, 0.77 AUC). The combined use of all mpMRI sequences resulted in an accuracy of 66.4% using SVM. These results highlight the potential of CAD systems to improve early prostate cancer diagnosis, reducing the workload of radiologists and enhance patient outcomes through a non-invasive imaging-based approach (Mehta et al. 2021).

In another study, the role of ultrasound in detecting early-stage epithelial ovarian cancer was evaluated in high-risk women as part of the national ovarian cancer early detection program. Despite its usefulness in identifying ovarian abnormalities, the study concluded that ultrasound alone has limited value in detecting early-stage epithelial ovarian cancer in asymptomatic women at high risk. Among 4526 participants, 98 women with persistent adnexal masses were identified, leading to 49 invasive surgical procedures. Of these, 12 gynaecologic malignancies, including fallopian tube carcinoma, primary peritoneal carcinoma, and epithelial ovarian cancer, were detected. Markedly, women who had normal ultrasound and physical examinations 6–12 months earlier have developed the cancer, which underscores the challenges of relying solely on ultrasound for early detection (Fishman et al. 2005).

Advancements in artificial intelligence (AI) have improved early breast cancer detection, particularly in assessing axillary lymph node metastasis (ALNM), which is crucial for staging and treatment strategies. The study introduced a deep learning framework, DAMF-former, designed to assist radiologists in evaluating ALNM using dual-modal ultrasound elastography (UE) images. The AI model significantly enhanced the diagnostic performance of less-experienced radiologists, increasing their AUC from 0.807 to 0.883. Furthermore, the AI-assisted approach resulted in greater agreement among radiologists of varying experience levels, with kappa values ranging from 0.805 to 0.895. These findings highlight the potential of human-AI collaboration in improving diagnostic accuracy, reducing variability among radiologists, and ultimately leading to more precise early detection of breast cancer (Gong et al. 2025).

12.3 Liquid Biopsy

Liquid biopsy is emerging as a revolutionary approach for early cancer detection. It offers a minimally invasive method to analyse tumour-derived biomarkers from biofluids such as blood and urine (Table 12.1). This technique enables molecular characterization of cancers, patient stratification for treatment, and monitoring the progression of disease (Adhit et al. 2023; Batool et al. 2023). The liquid biopsy

Table 12.1 Liquid biopsy-based early detection of various types of cancers

Type of sample	Assessment	Detection limit/ sensitivity	Cost	Limitation	Cancer	References
Blood and urine	Tissue, plasma, and urine proteome	92.6–96.3%	Medium	Technical variability	Clear cell renal cell carcinoma	Liu et al. (2023)
Blood plasma	Methylprobe, for DNA methylation-based liquid biopsy of metastasis	Up to 93%	High	Technological constraints and tumour heterogeneity	Breast, lung, and colorectal cancer	Ganesh et al. (2024)
Blood	Next-generation sequencing	95%	High	Expensive, requires bioinformatics support	Non-small cell lung cancer	Parisi et al. (2024)
Blood	Blood-based long noncoding RNA (LR) signature	86.31%	Medium	Biomarker variability	Gastric cancer	Guo et al. (2023)
Blood	Extracellular vesicles (EVs) containing lung-derived proteins (thyroid transcription factor-1 [TTF-1] and surfactant protein B [SFTPB]), along with the cancer-associated protein CD151þ EVs	70.0–87.2%	Medium	Isolation and quantification of EVs is technically challenging	Non-small cell lung cancer	Zhang et al. (2024a)
Blood	Multi-targeted nanoarrays (EGFR, EpCAM, HER2, MET, and VEGF)	88%	Medium to high	Cross-reactivity requires multiplex analysis	Lung cancer	Lian et al. (2024a)

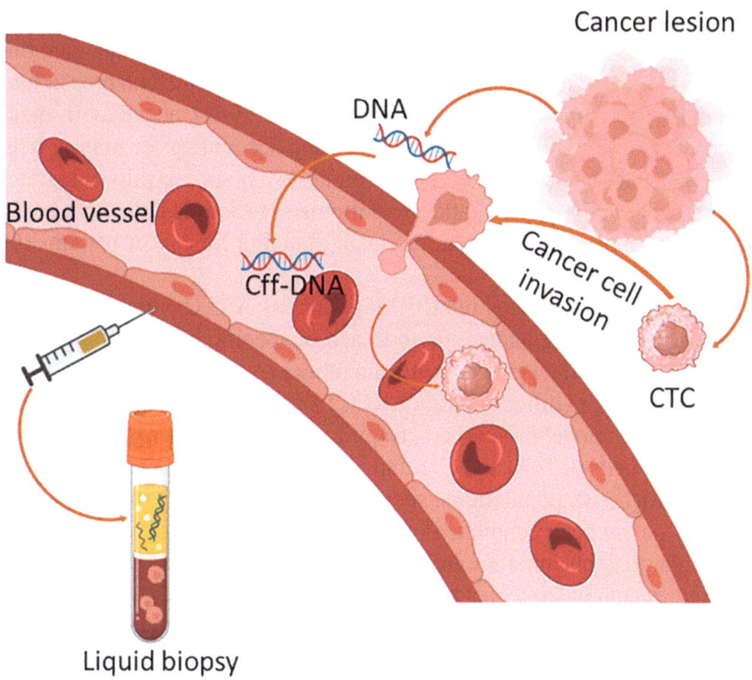

Fig. 12.2 Overview of liquid biopsy: circulating tumour DNA (cfDNA) and circulating tumour cells (CTCs)

consortium, established by the National Cancer Institute, has played a crucial role in refining biomarker detection methods, addressing technical challenges, and improving assay validation (Liquid Biopsy Consortium 2025). Liquid biopsy offers a real-time window into tumour biology by obtaining circulating tumour cells, cell-free DNA, and extracellular vesicles (Fig. 12.2). This makes it a potentially useful tool for early diagnosis and personalized treatments (Connal et al. 2023).

A study on early-stage clear cell renal cell carcinoma (ccRCC) further highlighted the potential of liquid biopsy in cancer detection. Using liquid chromatography–mass spectrometry (LC–MS), tumour tissue, plasma, and urine samples were analysed from 27 patients and healthy controls. The findings revealed that both plasma and urine proteins reflected functional tumour changes, with plasma proteins linked to cytoskeletal and metabolic activity, while urine proteins indicated immune response alterations. The study demonstrated that these biofluid-based biomarkers can distinguish RCC patients from healthy individuals with high specificity (92.6%) and sensitivity (96.3% in plasma and 92.6% in urine). These results emphasize the ability of liquid biopsy to detect cancer-related molecular changes in biofluids, paving the way for non-invasive diagnostic alternatives (Liu et al. 2023).

Beyond primary tumour detection, liquid biopsy holds great promise for identifying metastasis at an early stage, a critical factor in improving patient survival. DNA methylation, a stable and early indicator of tumour progression, has been integrated into a novel liquid biopsy assay known as methylprobe. This ultrasensitive nanosensor technology amplifies methylation signals in plasma, enabling precise detection of metastasis-associated DNA patterns. Validated on breast, lung, and CRC samples, methylprobe achieved an impressive 99.8% accuracy in metastasis detection. By incorporating machine learning and accounting for tumour heterogeneity, this approach enhances diagnostic reliability. If successfully integrated into clinical practice, methylprobe could revolutionize metastasis detection, facilitating early intervention and personalized treatment planning for cancer patients (Ganesh et al. 2024).

Early detection of asbestos-related lung cancer (ARLC) remains a significant challenge due to the long latency period, lack of specific histopathologic markers, and the confounding effects of smoking and other carcinogens. Traditional diagnostic methods suffer from differentiating ARLC from other lung cancers, necessitating the development of novel biomarkers. Liquid biopsy, particularly analysing the circulating tumour cells (CTCs) and circulating DNA, has emerged as a promising tool for screening high-risk populations, such as those exposed to asbestos. While CTC studies have not yet been conducted in ARLC patients, their ability to provide real-time molecular insights into tumour biology could revolutionize early diagnosis and personalized treatment strategies for ARLC (Ke et al. 2024).

In the realm of breast cancer detection, a newly designed colorimetric biosensor offers a highly sensitive and enzyme-free method for detecting CTCs. This biosensor employs ladder-branch hybridization chain reaction (HCR) and DNA flowers/gold nanoclusters (DFs/AuNCs) to enhance detection sensitivity, achieving a detection limit of just 3 cells/mL. The system effectively captures and quantifies breast cancer CTCs, providing a broad linear detection range from 10 to 10,000 cells/mL. By utilizing this biosensor technology, breast cancer detection could become more accessible and precise, potentially enabling earlier interventions and improving patient outcomes (Ren et al. 2024).

Further research into CTC detection for early-stage luminal A breast cancer (LABC) has demonstrated its reliability as a follow-up tool. A study in China involving 135 postoperative patients compared CTC detection with routine imaging re-examinations. The results showed no significant differences in survival rates or disease-free progression between the two groups. However, the study found that using CTC detection significantly reduced healthcare costs and hospitalization times, making it a cost-effective alternative to routine imaging follow-ups. These findings suggest that CTC detection could serve as a practical and efficient method for monitoring LABC patients, particularly in regions with limited healthcare resources (Zhang et al. 2020).

Promising biomarkers in liquid biopsy for differentiated thyroid carcinoma (DTC) are CTCs and tumour-derived extracellular vesicles (tEVs). These two biomarkers have complimentary diagnostic benefits because of their different sizes and release patterns. Both approaches are combined in the Combined DTC CTC/tEV Assay, which uses click chemistry for enhanced detection and enrichment. Compared to using each biomarker alone, this method greatly improves diagnosis accuracy, achieving an area under the receiver operating characteristic curve

Table 12.2 Various studies reported on circulating tumour cells and circulating DNA for early cancer detection

Type of sample	Assessment	Cancer	References
Blood	Circulating tumour DNA	Non-small cell lung cancer	Driussi et al. (2025)
Blood	Methylation-based circulating tumour DNA	Non-small cell lung cancer	Bossé et al. (2024)
Blood	NSG-circulating tumour DNA	Non-small cell lung cancer	Martin et al. (2024)
Blood	Circulating DNA genome-wide fragmentation	Hepatocellular carcinoma	Lian et al. (2024b)
Blood	NSG-circulating tumour DNA	Breast cancer	Wang et al. (2024a)
Blood	Circulating cell-free DNA	Nasopharyngeal carcinoma	Qiu et al. (2024)
Blood	Circulating tumour cells and tumour-derived extracellular vesicles	Thyroid cancer	Feng et al. (2024)
Blood	Circulating tumour DNA-Sanger sequencing	Breast cancer	Wahab et al. (2024)
Blood	Circulating tumour cell	Asbestos-related lung cancer	Ke et al. (2024)
Blood	Colorimetric detection of circulating tumour cells based on ladder-branch hybridization chain reaction and DFs/AuNCs nanozyme	Breast cancer	Ren et al. (2024)
Blood	Circulating tumour cell	Luminal A breast cancer	Zhang et al. (2020)

(AUROC) of 0.99. This cutting-edge assay marks a significant breakthrough in non-invasive cancer detection and personalized patient care by optimizing the diagnostic results from a single blood sample (Feng et al. 2024).

Multiple biomarkers used for liquid biopsy are summarized in Table 12.2. Circulating tumour DNA (ctDNA) analysis has greatly improved the early diagnosis of lung cancer, especially in stage I non-small cell lung cancer (NSCLC). Analysis of ctDNA methylation patterns has made blood-based assays, including the multi-cancer early detection (MCED) test, non-invasive methods for identifying cancers. A study involving 180 patients with adenocarcinomas (LUAD) and 80 with squamous cell carcinomas (LUSC) showed that pathological parameters such as tumour grade, volume, and histological pattern composition affect the detection of ctDNA. Necrosis and acute inflammation were linked to greater ctDNA shedding, and LUSC was associated with higher ctDNA levels than LUAD. These results improve the identification of patients eligible for ctDNA-based early detection and follow-up techniques and offers useful knowledge about the molecular mechanisms influencing ctDNA levels (Driussi et al. 2025).

Investigations on the predictive value of preoperative ctDNA detection in early-stage NSCLC have also shown possible histology-specific correlations with patient outcomes. However, no apparent connection between preoperative ctDNA detection and relapse within 5 years following surgery was observed in 260 NSCLC patients in the clinical stage. Nonetheless, ctDNA positivity was associated with a higher risk of pathological progression from clinical stage I to stages II–III and recurrence within 2 years in individuals with lung adenocarcinoma. These findings imply that the prognosis of lung cancer may be influenced by ctDNA analysis in a time-dependent and histology-specific manner. Although the MCED test showed promise in detecting early recurrence in patients of adenocarcinoma, additional research is necessary to confirm its clinical relevance (Bossé et al. 2024).

In order to identify and treat lung cancer recurrence, postoperative ctDNA monitoring has shown promising results. According to a study that included 108 patients with NSCLC having curative-intent resection, ctDNA positivity after surgery was associated with disease recurrence in 66.7% of cases. Since all ctDNA-positive patients received additional imaging, such as CT and positron emission tomography (PET) scans, early treatment was made possible by routine ctDNA monitoring at 3-month intervals. Clinical care was modified because 66.6% of these showed malignant characteristics. These results demonstrated the importance of ctDNA detection for post-operative follow-up, enhanced risk assessment, and enabled timely treatment to improve patient outcomes (Martin et al. 2024).

Fragmentation patterns of circulating cell-free DNA (ccfDNA) have demonstrated potential as a diagnostic for hepatocellular carcinoma (HCC) early diagnosis. In a study that examined 427 samples, 270 of which were taken prior to diagnosis, a model was developed that demonstrated exceptional accuracy in differentiating between HCC patients and healthy controls (AUC = 0.999). The detection sensitivity rose as the period to diagnosis decreased, from 8.3% for samples obtained more than four years prior to diagnosis to 36.4% for those taken within a year. These results imply that ccfDNA fragmentation analysis could be a useful method for HCC screening, possibly enabling earlier treatment prior to the onset of clinical symptoms (Lian et al. 2024b).

In stage II–III breast cancer patients receiving primary systemic therapy (PST), treatment response was evaluated using ctDNA analysis. 51.4% of the 72 individuals had significant ctDNA variations at baseline. Patients who responded well to treatment showed a considerable decrease in ctDNA levels; those who achieved complete remission showed a median decrease of 97.4%. Early change in ctDNA levels is linked highly with treatment efficacy and long-term results. Recurrence-free survival was noticeably longer in patients with an early decline in variable allele fraction (VAF). These results imply that ctDNA monitoring may be essential for directing the treatment of breast cancer and enhancing perioperative care (Wang et al. 2024a). Although there are currently no very sensitive markers for nasopharyngeal carcinoma (NPC), early diagnosis of the disease is difficult. To develop a non-invasive diagnostic paradigm, a study that used next-generation sequencing (NGS) of cfDNA examined fragmentation patterns, 5′-end motifs, and genome-wide nucleosome footprints. Based on these metrics, the NPC score showed remarkable accuracy in differentiating between NPC patients and healthy people (AUC as 99.9%, Sensitivity as 98.15%, Specificity as 100%). Even after treatment, this model continued to work better than conventional plasma Epstein-Barr virus (EBV)

DNA testing. Its promise as a better early detection technique for NPC was further highlighted by the fact that its diagnostic power was unaffected by age, sex, or TNM staging (Qiu et al. 2024).

In early-stage NSCLC, it is still difficult to predict survival and relapse outcomes with any degree of accuracy. According to a study that examined 366 plasma samples from 85 patients, a significantly worse prognosis was found to be linked to the presence of ctDNA at baseline, before treatment, or its persistence after treatment. By combining ctDNA analysis with radiographic tumour volume measurements, it increases the risk assessment, leading to better prognostication and treatment options. This combination approach implies that ctDNA monitoring and imaging methods may be essential in directing follow-up treatment for individuals with early-stage non-small cell lung cancer (Tran et al. 2024).

CtDNA analysis has demonstrated promise in evaluating therapy response and forecasting disease recurrence in individuals with locally progressed and early-stage rectal cancer. Before starting treatment, 69% of patients had ctDNA detected; however, following neoadjuvant therapy, the detection rate decreased to 15%, suggesting a successful response to treatment. Interestingly, ctDNA was found in 31% of patients with positive lymph node disease (ypN+) but not in patients with a full clinical response or those with no lymph node involvement (ypN0). All ctDNA-positive patients experienced recurrent malignancy, and ctDNA detection was linked to disease recurrence after surgery. These results demonstrate the importance of ctDNA in directing post-treatment monitoring and improving treatment plans for patients with rectal cancer (Hofste et al. 2023).

These studies highlight the potential role of liquid biopsy techniques, including ccfDNA and ctDNA analysis, in the early detection of various cancers. By identifying unique fragmentation patterns and genetic alterations, these methods provide non-invasive, highly sensitive, and specific tools for cancer screening. Their application could lead to earlier diagnosis, improved treatment monitoring, and better patient outcomes, marking a significant advancement in oncology diagnostics.

12.4 Biosensors

Biosensors offer a promising tool for cancer detection due to their affordability, portability, and ability to provide rapid results. By detecting cancer biomarkers with high specificity, biosensors enable early diagnosis and timely treatment (Sarkar et al. 2024). Electrochemical biosensors have demonstrated excellent sensitivity in the femtomolar range, rivalling PCR-based methods for detecting nucleic acids and proteins. Optical biosensors, particularly those based on surface plasmon resonance (SPR) and fluorescence, offer real-time and label-free detection but often require more sophisticated sample preparation (Table 12.3).

Biosensors are classified according to their methods of detection, and each has unique advantages for detecting cancer. Electrochemical biosensors are extremely sensitive and economical because they measure electrical signals produced by biomolecular interactions to identify cancer biomarkers (Fu et al. 2024). Optical

Table 12.3 Various types of biosensors and the target analytes for early cancer detection

Type of biosensor	Detection principle	Target analytes	Detection range
Electrochemical detector	Specific binding of target analytes to receptor molecules immobilized on the sensor surface, which generates detectable electrical signals	Circulating tumour cells, cell-free nucleic acids, exosomes, proteins, and metabolites	Femtomolar to nanomolar level based on the analyte
Optical detector (SPR, fluorescence)	Changes in light interaction with tissue or biomarkers, which differ between healthy and cancerous cells based on properties like refractive index, light scattering, and fluorescence to detect cancerous cells or disease-related molecules in a variety of fluid and tissue samples	Nucleic acids, exosomes, proteins	Pico to nano level
Piezoelectric detector	Analyse the change in the resonant frequency of a piezoelectric crystal	Nucleic acids, cell, and exosomes	Till nano level
Photoelectrochemical detector	Convert biochemical reactions into electrical signals using a photoactive material under light irradiation	Nucleic acids, cells, and antigens	Pico to nano level

biosensors use light-based detection techniques, including surface plasmon resonance (SPR) or fluorescence, to accurately identify chemicals specific to cancer (Das et al. 2023). Mass-based biosensors, such as quartz crystal microbalance (QCM) sensors, assess changes in mass by interactions between biomolecules (Ogi 2013). They are especially helpful in identifying extracellular vesicles and CTCs (Słomka et al. 2022). Biosensor capabilities have been further improved by the integration of nanotechnology and biosensors based on nanomaterials have improved detection sensitivity and specificity.

The most recent developments in biosensor technology focus on enhancing their accessibility and efficiency. Electrochemical sensors based on nanotechnology offer improved sensitivity and signal stability, which makes them appropriate for identifying genetic mutations linked to cancer (Jalalvand and Karami 2025). By combining lab-on-a-chip technologies, microfluidic biosensors enable quick, on-site cancer detection with smaller sample sizes (García-Hernández et al. 2023). Furthermore, machine learning algorithms are used by AI-enhanced biosensors to evaluate complex biomarker data, increasing the accuracy of diagnosis and lowering false positives (Wasilewski et al. 2024).

Despite their promise, biosensors still have issues that need to be resolved before they can be used extensively in medical applications. The reduction of false positives and negatives, which might influence treatment choices, depends on maintaining high sensitivity and specificity. Furthermore, for long-term usage in medical diagnostics, biosensor durability, stability, and repeatability need to be increased (Liu et al. 2024; Bohunicky and Mousa 2010). Standardizing biosensor platforms is also essential to improve their clinical usefulness and reliability in identifying a variety of cancer biomarkers.

Biosensors have the potential to completely transform early cancer diagnosis with additional advances in molecular diagnostics, artificial intelligence, and nanotechnology (Ahmed Taha et al. 2024). Biosensors could revolutionize cancer diagnosis and greatly enhance patient outcomes globally by offering an affordable, quick, and non-invasive option (Sarkar et al. 2024).

Electrochemical techniques are highly sensitive with fast response times, and can be easily customized, making them suitable for the design of point-of-care medical devices. Nevertheless, a significant obstacle in the development of such instruments is the non-specific adsorption (NSA) phenomenon, which arises from the fouling of non-target blood molecules on the recognition surface of the device. Using medical-grade stainless steel electrodes and a novel silane-based interfacial chemistry approach, an affinity-based electrochemical biosensor has been developed to address this problem. With a detection limit of 0.7 μM in goat serum, this biosensor detects lysophosphatidic acid (LPA), a biomarker that is increased in 90% of patients with stage I ovarian cancer (Ahmadi et al. 2023).

Surface plasmon resonance (SPR) technology is an excellent technique that enables the detection of bioanalytes without the labels. A hybrid layer of graphene, aurum, and titanium oxide has been used as a new SPR-based biosensor. The performance of sensors was improved by using a hexagonal lattice fibre construction with perforated air holes. A maximal sensitivity of 5714.29 nm/RIU for MCF7 cancer cells was shown by numerical studies applying the COMSOL Multiphysics Simulation tool. The biosensor is a promising tool for cancer diagnosis because it has also reached a detection resolution of 4.0×10^{-5} RIU for basal cells (Ibrahimi et al. 2023).

A novel composite magnetic nanomaterial functionalized with the aptamer Apt7 was developed for detecting HSP70, a biomarker associated with cancer progression. Au-coated FeO_4 nanoparticles with strong electrical conductivity are included in this material, which has been generated by chemical reduction. The biosensor demonstrated a detection range of 10 pg/mL to 200 ng/mL, with a detection limit of 0.525 pg/mL. Electrochemical optimization generated a dissociation constant (Kd) of 72.49 pM. The performance of this sensor was better than that of traditional ELISA techniques (Liu et al. 2025).

The neurotrophic growth factor midkine (MDK) is linked to the development of cancer. Using Au@Pt nanorods as multifunctional probes and biosynthesized quantum dots (BQDs) for antibody orientation, a triple-mode biosensor was developed to detect MDK. The detection limit of the biosensor was 1.620 fg/mL, and its detection range was 5 fg/mL to 100 ng/mL. This sensor offers an exciting approach for early cancer diagnosis and performs better than standard ELISA kits (Jiao et al. 2025).

A study examined the potential of graphene structures doped with metal atoms (Pt, Pd, Ni, Ir, and Cu) to identify lung cancer biomarkers, including benzene, aniline, toluene, and styrene gases. Significant charge transfer interactions were found through the use of density functional theory (DFT) computations. According to the results, graphene doped with copper and platinum has a lot of promise for electrical and function-based detection of lung cancer biomarkers (Korucu et al. 2024).

The probability of pancreatic cancer is determined by the biomarker known as carbohydrate antigen 125 (CA125). Zn-PTC, a very stable electrochemiluminescence (ECL) luminophore, was developed to enable the detection of CA125. A detection limit of 0.24 μU/mL was attained by the biosensor by combining an ECL resonance energy transfer (ECL-RET) device with Au-Ag bimetallic nanoclusters. This study presents a novel approach for low-potential ECL luminophores with clinical applications in pancreatic cancer diagnostics (Chen et al. 2025).

A D-shaped fibre was employed in the development of a fibre laser-based biosensor to identify biomarkers for prostate cancer. The fibre was coated with gold using a sputter coater to generate the biosensor probe, and layer-by-layer immobilization was used to carry out the antibody-antigen interaction. The biosensor is a promising tool for the detection and monitoring of prostate cancer because it showed a sensitivity of 0.2171 nm/(μg/mL) for detecting human chorionic gonadotropin (hCG) (Zamri et al. 2024).

12.5 Advanced Technologies

12.5.1 CRISPR

A gene-editing technique called the CRISPR-Cas system was first developed from bacterial immune defence systems to identify and amplify nucleic acids associated with cancer (Loureiro and Da Silva 2019). Researchers have developed quick, non-invasive, and portable diagnostic tools for early cancer detection by combining CRISPR technology with biosensors. CRISPR-associated proteins (Cas enzymes) provide the target detection and cleavage mechanism that powers CRISPR-based biosensors (Sornambikai et al. 2023). Various Cas proteins (Cas9, Cas12a, Cas13a, etc.) are used, depending on the kind of cancer biomarker identified. Cas9 is frequently employed for DNA-based detection, especially for identifying genetic alterations unique to cancer (Gong et al. 2021; Huang et al. 2018). It works by binding to a target DNA sequence with great specificity after recognizing it as complementary to its guide RNA (sgRNA) (Mengstie and Wondimu 2021). Cas9-based biosensors are appropriate for point-of-care applications since they can be employed with nucleic acid test strips.

In addition to cutting its target DNA, Cas12a also breaks down nearby single-stranded DNA (ssDNA) because of its collateral cleavage activity (Li et al. 2018). This characteristic allows for extremely sensitive signal amplification, which is helpful in identifying low-abundance cancer biomarkers such as microRNAs (miRNAs) and ctDNA. For the accurate detection of miRNAs specific to cancer, Cas12a biosensors have been combined with electrochemical sensors and strand displacement amplification (SDA) (Peng et al. 2024).

Cas13a is appropriate to identify RNA-based mutations and oncogenic miRNAs because it is primarily utilized for RNA detection. Because of its collateral RNA breakdown, RNA biomarkers can be detected quickly, sensitively, and with a low false-positive rate. For the diagnosis of colorectal and lung cancer, Cas13a biosensors have been combined with electrochemical and fluorescence-based diagnostic tools (Saini et al. 2025; Rahimi et al. 2024).

miRNAs serve as vital biomarkers for cancer diagnostics due to their differential expression patterns in cancerous and healthy cells. However, because of their great sequence homology and limited abundance, they are difficult to identify. This has led to the development of a novel CRISPR-Cas12a-based biosensor for the detection of miRNA-21 in breast cancer cells. This biosensor gets beyond sequence-dependent restrictions and expands detection to several miRNAs by combining the SDA technique with structural "Lock" nucleic acids ("Lock" DNA), enabling ultra-sensitive detection of miRNA-21 down to 28.8 aM in 90 min. The platform exhibits high specificity, minimizing off-target effects against non-target RNAs, and operates at a constant temperature of 37 °C with simple isothermal steps, making it compatible with point-of-care applications. Additionally, it can detect multiple miRNAs without redesigning crRNAs, overcoming the sequence-dependence limitation of standard CRISPR assays. This makes it a viable tool for intracellular imaging and early diagnosis (Peng et al. 2024).

Traditionally, serum prostate-specific antigen (PSA) testing has been used in prostate cancer screening. However, this method suffers from low specificity and numerous misdiagnoses resulting from benign diseases, including prostatitis or benign prostatic hyperplasia (BPH). A CRISPR-Cas9-based nucleic acid test strip that incorporates reverse transcriptase-recombinase aided amplification (RT-RAA) has been developed to improve diagnostic accuracy. This biosensor eliminates reciprocal interference and greatly increases specificity by simultaneously detecting the genes for kallikrein-related peptidase 3 (KLK3) and prostate cancer antigen 3 (PCA3). The platform achieves detection limits of 500 fg/μL for PCA3 and 50 fg/μL for KLK3 within ~30–45 min of amplification and strip analysis, offering rapid results without complex instrumentation. Clinical validation demonstrated that the PCA3/KLK3 ratio reliably distinguishes prostate cancer from benign disease, minimizing PSA-related misdiagnoses. Operating with isothermal amplification and portable test strips, this system is well-suited for point-of-care screening, particularly in resource-limited settings, and represents a practical improvement over conventional PSA testing (Chen et al. 2023).

While CRC continues to be one of the top causes of cancer-related death globally, highly sensitive and less invasive diagnostic methods must be established. By combining a nicking-induced DNA cascade reaction (DP-bridged Cas13a/NDCR) with dumbbell probe-mediated CRISPR-Cas13a, a new biosensor, uses an electrochemical signal readout to identify miRNAs. Activated Cas13a cleaves the dumbbell probe upon binding target miRNA-21, releasing an intermediate strand that causes probe cleavage on the electrode surface, resulting in enhanced electrochemical changes. With excellent stability and specificity in plasma, this technique reaches a detection limit of 8.26 fM. Crucially, diagnostic accuracy for distinguishing CRC from benign diseases and healthy controls approached 100% when applied to patient cohorts and integrated with machine learning models that analyse various CRC-related miRNAs. These results demonstrate that CRISPR-based biosensors and AI can be used to provide highly sensitive, reliable, and clinically meaningful CRC diagnosis (Pei et al. 2025).

For non-invasive cancer diagnostics, ctDNA is a promising biomarker, especially for NSCLC. However, because CRISPR-based assays require protospacer adjacent motifs (PAMs), current ctDNA detection techniques are frequently time-consuming, expensive, and limited. A novel approach combining CRISPR-Cas12a and recombinase polymerase amplification (RPA) has been developed to overcome these limitations. This approach detects mutations with a 0.02% variant allele frequency in 50 min and reaches a detection limit of 100 aM by inserting artificially inserted PAMs and altering CRISPR RNA to minimize off-target effects. This approach has demonstrated its promise for real-time cancer detection, therapeutic guidance, and prognosis prediction through its successful application to clinical NSCLC samples (Wang et al. 2023).

12.5.2 Microfluidic Devices

Microfluidic technology offers a transformative approach to cancer diagnostics, enabling highly sensitive and specific biomarker detection at low concentrations. Because microfluidics can be included in point-of-care devices, it makes routine cancer screening more accessible by enabling minimally invasive clinical diagnosis (Zhang and Nagrath 2013).

Because exosomes transmit molecular information from their source cells, they are useful markers of disease development in bodily fluids, especially in cancer. However, accurate detection is hampered by their low concentration and significant background noise in biofluids. In order to improve the effectiveness of exosome capture, a microfluidic nanochip was developed containing three-dimensional nanostructures organized in a herringbone pattern. While micromixing enhanced mass transfer, silica nanoparticle stacking enhanced interaction with exosomes. With a high capture efficiency of 97.7%, this platform was used to detect exosomes that were positive for HER2. Moreover, the simultaneous isolation of several exosome subtypes has been rendered feasible by a dual nanochip configuration, demonstrating its potential for personalized disease monitoring and multi-cancer diagnostics (Mun et al. 2024).

Since certain early symptoms are absent, ovarian cancer is often detected at an advanced stage. A new microfluidic platform that combines a gas-driven visual amplification chip (VAC) with platinum nanozyme-induced cascade signal amplification was developed to detect ovarian cancer biomarkers CA125 and HE4 with remarkable sensitivity. This technique promoted dopamine polymerization to improve the detection signal using a sandwich complex of platinum nanoparticles and antibody-functionalized magnetic silica. The sensitivity of the VAC was higher than that of traditional techniques, with detection limits of 0.1 pg/mL for HE4 and 0.001 U/mL for CA125. Its potential for point-of-care ovarian cancer detection is demonstrated by its high association with ECL evaluation (Wang et al. 2025).

One of the biggest causes of cancer-related death is HCC, and it is still difficult to diagnose in its early stages. Laboratory-based analysis and sophisticated equipment are necessary for traditional antigen detection techniques. An electrowetting-on-dielectric digital microfluidic (EWOD-DMF) technology was developed to overcome those limitations to detect HCC biomarkers rapidly, portably, and with limited expertise. Alpha-Fetoprotein (AFP), AFP-L3%, and Des-Gamma-Carboxy Prothrombin (DCP) are all measured by this technique using only 2.4 μL of serum per biomarker. With simultaneous multi-sample testing and a detection limit of 0.24 ng/mL for AFP and AFP-L3 and 1.89 ng/mL for DCP, this platform greatly improves diagnostic efficiency while requiring less processing time. It is the perfect option for early-stage HCC screening due to its affordability and portability, especially in environments with limited resources (Zhu et al. 2025).

Although miRNAs are important biomarkers for lung cancer, their low abundance makes it difficult to detect them in biofluids. MiR-92a and miR-339-3p, both associated with NSCLC, can be detected simultaneously and effectively with a new microfluidic chip that uses surface-enhanced Raman scattering. The sample flow is guided into a reaction zone by the chip's comb-like structured microchannel, where target miRNAs hybridize with hairpin DNA on Au-Ag nanobowl arrays. Highly sensitive detection was made possible by this amplification method in just 8 min, with limits of 44.36 aM for miR-92a and 63.58 aM for miR-339-3p. The technique proved to be a promising tool for NSCLC diagnosis and prognosis monitoring because of its high specificity, repeatability, and correlation with qRT-PCR data (Gu et al. 2022).

For ovarian cancer and other cancers, methylated cfDNA is an essential epigenetic marker. For rapid detection and measurement of methylated tumour suppressor genes, BRCA1 and BRCA2, in patients with ovarian cancer, a novel microfluidic chip incorporating a recently screened methylation-specific aptamer has been developed. There was no need for a lot of sample preparation because the experiment was carried out in physiological conditions that mimicked the tumour microenvironment. This technique demonstrated its usefulness for non-invasive ovarian cancer screening by successfully detecting methylation cfDNA at concentrations as low as 1 pM. This technology could be used for treatment monitoring and multi-cancer epigenetic diagnostics, in addition to ovarian cancer (Wang et al. 2024b).

12.5.3 Artificial Intelligence

Artificial intelligence (AI) has emerged as a powerful tool in oncology, enhancing risk assessment, early diagnosis, prognosis estimation, and treatment planning. A subset of AI called machine learning (ML) has shown remarkable accuracy in predicting a variety of malignancies, sometimes outperforming conventional diagnostic techniques. Deep learning (DL) and AI combined with cancer detection technologies have a bright future for enhancing patient outcomes, lowering diagnostic errors, and facilitating personalized therapies (Zhang et al. 2023).

Lung cancer is still one of the deadliest cancers, and successful treatment depends on early detection. Although CT scans are frequently utilized for early diagnosis, radiologists may misdiagnose early-stage lung cancer due to small abnormalities that are difficult to detect. To solve this, a deep learning system was designed to automatically diagnose lung cancer from chest CT scans using an ensemble of convolutional neural networks (CNNs). This model demonstrated exceptional accuracy (98.17%), sensitivity (98.21%), and specificity (98.13%) in differentiating between malignant and non-cancerous scans after being trained on a very small dataset (IQ_OTH/NCCD). Additionally, it performed better than previously proposed models, with 95.43% accuracy in classifying scans as normal, benign, or malignant. These findings demonstrate the degree to which AI-assisted diagnostic tools improve assessments of radiologists and lower diagnostic uncertainty (Abe et al. 2025).

Liquid biopsies, which examine biomarkers in plasma, offer a less intrusive option for early cancer detection. Extracellular vesicles called exosomes, which are present in plasma, are promising markers for the diagnosis of lung cancer. In order to distinguish cases of cancer-free (HC), adenocarcinoma in situ (AIS), and early-stage invasive adenocarcinoma (IAC), a recent study presented a label-free detection approach that combines surface-enhanced Raman spectroscopy (SERS) with machine learning. Using SERS spectra of exosomes and plasma to train machine learning models, the study suggested a "Combined Spectrum" method that combined spectral data from both sources into a new training dataset. The robustness of this method was demonstrated by the generated ML models, which had an accuracy of over 97% and an AUC value of over 0.9500. This methodology not only enhances early lung cancer detection but also holds potential for diagnosing other diseases using AI-powered liquid biopsy analysis (Zhang et al. 2024b).

Despite these encouraging outcomes, a number of obstacles need to be taken into account before clinical AI is used for cancer detection. Deep learning models trained on small or non-representative datasets are especially vulnerable to overfitting, which might prevent them from generalizing to larger populations (Goetz et al. 2024). Predictive accuracy and fairness may be further diminished by dataset bias, which results from unequal representation of demographics, tumour subtypes, or disease stages. Also, a lot of AI systems function as "black boxes," which makes it hard for clinicians to comprehend the logic behind predictions and may cause them to lose faith in automated results (Yang et al. 2022). Apart from the necessity of handling patient data securely, following privacy laws, and having clear clinical accountability for decisions made with AI, ethical considerations are also very important. Comparative analysis indicates that AI-augmented human interpretation, in which clinicians employ AI as a supplementary tool rather than a substitute, frequently enhances diagnostic performance by striking a balance between algorithmic efficiency and expert oversight, improving early cancer detection's sensitivity and specificity.

12.6 Conclusion

Early cancer detection has evolved as a result of advances in imaging technologies, liquid biopsies, biosensors, CRISPR-based diagnostics, microfluidic devices, and artificial intelligence. While non-invasive tumour visualization still requires imaging methods like PET, CT, MRI, and ultrasound, liquid biopsy and biosensors provide viable options for highly sensitive cancer biomarker detection. The detection capabilities are further improved by microfluidic devices and CRISPR-based techniques, while AI-driven models offer a drastic improvement in cancer diagnosis and prognosis. Improving early cancer diagnosis, decreasing diagnostic delays, and improving patient outcomes are all possible with the incorporation of these state-of-the-art technologies into clinical practice. Future studies should focus on enhancing cost-effectiveness, ensuring smooth integration into healthcare systems, and optimizing these technologies for widespread implementation. By employing these advancements, early cancer detection can become more accurate, available, and effective, which will ultimately result in better treatment plans and higher cancer patient survival rates.

References

Abe AA, Nyathi M, Okunade AA, Pilloy W, Kgole B, Nyakale N (2025) A robust deep learning algorithm for lung cancer detection from computed tomography images. Intell Med 11:100203. https://doi.org/10.1016/J.IBMED.2025.100203

Adhit KK, Wanjari A, Menon S, Siddhaarth K (2023) Liquid biopsy: an evolving paradigm for non-invasive disease diagnosis and monitoring in medicine. Cureus 15:e50176. https://doi.org/10.7759/CUREUS.50176

Ahmadi S, Lotay N, Thompson M (2023) Affinity-based electrochemical biosensor with antifouling properties for detection of lysophosphatidic acid, a promising early-stage ovarian cancer biomarker. Bioelectrochemistry 153. https://doi.org/10.1016/J.BIOELECHEM.2023.108466

Ahmed Taha B, Kadhim AC, Addie AJ, Haider AJ, Azzahrani AS, Raizada P, Rustagi S, Chaudhary V, Arsad N (2024) Advancing cancer diagnostics through multifaceted optical biosensors supported by nanomaterials and artificial intelligence: a panoramic outlook. Microchem J 205:111307. https://doi.org/10.1016/J.MICROC.2024.111307

Barrios CH (2022) Global challenges in breast cancer detection and treatment. Breast 62:S3. https://doi.org/10.1016/J.BREAST.2022.02.003

Batool SM, Yekula A, Khanna P, Hsia T, Gamblin AS, Ekanayake E, Escobedo AK, You DG, Castro CM, Im H et al (2023) The liquid biopsy consortium: challenges and opportunities for early cancer detection and monitoring. Cell Rep Med 4:101198. https://doi.org/10.1016/J.XCRM.2023.101198

Berardi R, Morgese F, Rinaldi S, Torniai M, Mentrasti G, Scortichini L, Giampieri R (2020) Benefits and limitations of a multidisciplinary approach in cancer patient management. Cancer Manag Res 12:9363. https://doi.org/10.2147/CMAR.S220976

Berger MF, Mardis ER (2018) The emerging clinical relevance of genomics in cancer medicine. Nat Rev Clin Oncol 15:353–365. https://doi.org/10.1038/s41571-018-0002-6

Bi WL, Hosny A, Schabath MB, Giger ML, Birkbak NJ, Mehrtash A, Allison T, Arnaout O, Abbosh C, Dunn IF et al (2019) Artificial intelligence in cancer imaging: clinical challenges and applications. CA Cancer J Clin 69:127. https://doi.org/10.3322/CAAC.21552

Bittla P, Kaur S, Sojitra V, Zahra A, Hutchinson J, Adefokun O, Khan S (2023) Exploring circulating tumor DNA (CtDNA) and its role in early detection of cancer: a systematic review. Cureus 15:e45784. https://doi.org/10.7759/CUREUS.45784

Bland KI, Copeland EM, Klimberg VS, Gradishar WJ (2025) The breast: comprehensive management of benign and malignant diseases. E-Book. Google Books. Available online: https://books.google.co.in/books?hl=en&lr=&id=HWy1EAAAQBAJ&oi=fnd&pg=PP1&dq=The+goal+of+the+research+is+to+distinguish+between+benign+lesions+that+pose+minimal+threat+and+malignant+tumors+that+require+rapid+medical+attention&ots=HyI2SV3uCE&sig=kbWZs9h4bmxYEAUVhf1SzsbpgX4#v=onepage&q&f=false. Accessed 11 Mar 2025

Bohunicky B, Mousa SA (2010) Biosensors: the new wave in cancer diagnosis. Nanotechnol Sci Appl 4:1. https://doi.org/10.2147/NSA.S13465

Bossé Y, Dasgupta A, Abadier M, Guthrie V, Song F, Saavedra Armero V, Gaudreault N, Orain M, Lamaze FC, Melton C et al (2024) Prognostic implication of methylation-based circulating tumor DNA detection prior to surgery in stage I non-small cell lung cancer. Cancer Lett 594:216984. https://doi.org/10.1016/J.CANLET.2024.216984

Cancer screening tests | Cancer | CDC. Available online: https://www.cdc.gov/cancer/prevention/screening.html. Accessed 11 Mar 2025

Chen W, Wu S, Li G, Duan X, Sun X, Li S, Zhao Y, Gu D, Zeng G, Liu H (2023) Accurate diagnosis of prostate cancer with CRISPR-based nucleic acid test strip by simultaneously identifying PCA3 and KLK3 genes. Biosens Bioelectron 220. https://doi.org/10.1016/J.BIOS.2022.114854

Chen Y, Ye Z, Ma M, Wu Y, Yang J, Ma P, Zhang Z, Song D (2025) Electrochemiluminescence resonance energy transfer biosensor based on BNCs@Zn-PTC for ultrasensitive and low-potential detection of CA125 in pancreatic cancer diagnostics. Sensors Actuators B Chem 427:137136. https://doi.org/10.1016/J.SNB.2024.137136

Connal S, Cameron JM, Sala A, Brennan PM, Palmer DS, Palmer JD, Perlow H, Baker MJ (2023) Liquid biopsies: the future of cancer early detection. J Transl Med 21:1–18. https://doi.org/10.1186/S12967-023-03960-8/FIGURES/7

Crosby D, Bhatia S, Brindle KM, Coussens LM, Dive C, Emberton M, Esener S, Fitzgerald RC, Gambhir SS, Kuhn P et al (2022) Early detection of cancer. Science (80-) 375. https://doi.org/10.1126/SCIENCE.AAY9040/ASSET/1D6DF757-2AD3-41DA-A919-79A20A65C881/ASSETS/IMAGES/LARGE/SCIENCE.AAY9040-FA.JPG

Das S, Devireddy R, Gartia MR (2023) Surface plasmon resonance (SPR) sensor for cancer biomarker detection. Biosensors 13:396. https://doi.org/10.3390/BIOS13030396

Driussi A, Lamaze FC, Kordahi M, Armero VS, Goudreault N, Orain M, Enlow W, Abbosh C, Hodgson D, Dasgupta A et al (2025) Clinicopathological predictors of the presence of blood circulating tumor DNA in early-stage non-small cell lung cancers. Mod Pathol:100744. https://doi.org/10.1016/J.MODPAT.2025.100744

Engel R, Kudura K, Antwi K, Denhaerynck K, Steinemann D, Wullschleger S, Müller B, Bolli M, von Strauss und Torney M (2024) Diagnostic accuracy and treatment benefit of PET/CT in staging of colorectal cancer compared to conventional imaging. Surg Oncol 57:102151. https://doi.org/10.1016/J.SURONC.2024.102151

Feng B, Wang J, Zhang RY, Wei AY, Zhao C, Yen YT, Ji YR, Kim H, Ju Y, Smalley M et al (2024) Click chemistry-mediated enrichment of circulating tumor cells and tumor-derived extracellular vesicles for dual liquid biopsy in differentiated thyroid cancer. Nano Today 58:102431. https://doi.org/10.1016/J.NANTOD.2024.102431

Fishman DA, Cohen L, Blank SV, Shulman L, Singh D, Bozorgi K, Tamura R, Timor-Tritsch I, Schwartz PE (2005) The role of ultrasound evaluation in the detection of early-stage epithelial ovarian cancer. Am J Obstet Gynecol 192:1214–1221. https://doi.org/10.1016/J.AJOG.2005.01.041

Fortuna A, Luz P, Cordeiro M, Gosalbez B, Campoa ER, Claudino M, Alves P, Costa JG, Fernandes AS, Pinto C (2024) Exploring the feasibility and implications of cranioencephalic computed tomography in HER2-positive breast cancer: a pilot study. Heliyon 10:e33886. https://doi.org/10.1016/J.HELIYON.2024.E33886

Frangioni JV (2008) New technologies for human cancer imaging. J Clin Oncol 26:4012. https://doi.org/10.1200/JCO.2007.14.3065

Frumovitz M, Morani AC, Aziz A, Jhingran A, Ramalingam P, Gonzales NR, Salvo G, Sun J, Bhosale P (2023) PET/CT scan improves detection of metastatic disease compared with CT scan alone in women with high-grade neuroendocrine cervical cancer: a NeCTuR study. Int J Gynecol Cancer 33:1690–1694. https://doi.org/10.1136/IJGC-2023-004907

Fu L, Karimi-Maleh H, Professor A (2024) Leveraging electrochemical sensors to improve efficiency of cancer detection. World J Clin Oncol 15:360. https://doi.org/10.5306/WJCO.V15.I3.360

Galeş LN, Păun MA, Anghel RM, Trifănescu OG (2024) Cancer screening: present recommendations, the development of multi-cancer early development tests, and the prospect of universal cancer screening. Cancers (Basel) 16:1191. https://doi.org/10.3390/CANCERS16061191

Ganesh S, Premachandran S, Venkatakrishnan K, Tan B (2024) Enhancing the cancer metastasis diagnosis: ultrasensitive nano sensors exploiting cancer stem cell associated DNA methylation as a liquid biopsy marker. Sensors Actuators B Chem 403:135206. https://doi.org/10.1016/J.SNB.2023.135206

García-Hernández LA, Martínez-Martínez E, Pazos-Solís D, Aguado-Preciado J, Dutt A, Chávez-Ramírez AU, Korgel B, Sharma A, Oza G (2023) Optical detection of cancer cells using lab-on-a-chip. Biosensors 13:439. https://doi.org/10.3390/BIOS13040439

Goetz L, Seedat N, Vandersluis R, van der Schaar M (2024) Generalization—a key challenge for responsible AI in patient-facing clinical applications. NPJ Digit Med 7:126. https://doi.org/10.1038/S41746-024-01127-3

Gong S, Zhang S, Lu F, Pan W, Li N, Tang B (2021) CRISPR/Cas-based in vitro diagnostic platforms for cancer biomarker detection. Anal Chem 93:11899–11909. https://doi.org/10.1021/ACS.ANALCHEM.1C02533/ASSET/IMAGES/LARGE/AC1C02533_0003.JPEG

Gong C, Wu Y, Zhang G, Liu X, Zhu X, Cai N, Li J (2025) Computer-assisted diagnosis for axillary lymph node metastasis of early breast cancer based on transformer with dual-modal adaptive mid-term fusion using ultrasound elastography. Comput Med Imaging Graph 119:102472. https://doi.org/10.1016/J.COMPMEDIMAG.2024.102472

Griffeth LK (2005) Use of PET/CT scanning in cancer patients: technical and practical considerations. Proc (Bayl Univ Med Cent) 18:321. https://doi.org/10.1080/08998280.2005.11928089

Gu Y, Cao D, Mao Y, Ge S, Li Z, Gu Y, Sun Y, Li L, Cao X (2022) A SERS microfluidic chip based on HpDNA-functioned Au-Ag nanobowl array for efficient simultaneous detection of non-small cell lung cancer-related microRNAs. Microchem J 182:107836. https://doi.org/10.1016/J.MICROC.2022.107836

Guo X, Peng Y, Song Q, Wei J, Wang X, Ru Y, Xu S, Cheng X, Li X, Wu D et al (2023) A liquid biopsy signature for the early detection of gastric cancer in patients. Gastroenterology 165:402–413.e13. https://doi.org/10.1053/J.GASTRO.2023.02.044

Hofman MS, Kasivisvanathan V, Link E, Buteau J, Roberts MJ, Francis RJ, Tang C, Vela I, Thomas P, Rutherford N et al (2024) Baseline nodal status on 68Ga PSMA-11 positron emission tomography/computed tomography in men with intermediate- to high-risk prostate cancer is prognostic for treatment failure: follow-up of the ProPSMA trial. Eur Urol Oncol. https://doi.org/10.1016/J.EUO.2024.11.006

Hofste LSM, Geerlings MJ, von Rhein D, Rütten H, Westenberg AH, Weiss MM, Gilissen C, Hofste T, van der Post RS, Klarenbeek BR et al (2023) Circulating tumor DNA detection after neoadjuvant treatment and surgery predicts recurrence in patients with early-stage and locally advanced rectal cancer. Eur J Surg Oncol 49:1283–1290. https://doi.org/10.1016/J.EJSO.2023.01.026

Huang CH, Lee KC, Doudna JA (2018) Applications of CRISPR-Cas enzymes in cancer therapeutics and detection. Trends Cancer 4:499. https://doi.org/10.1016/J.TRECAN.2018.05.006

Hussain S, Mubeen I, Ullah N, Shah SSUD, Khan BA, Zahoor M, Ullah R, Khan FA, Sultan MA (2022) Modern diagnostic imaging technique applications and risk factors in the medical field: a review. Biomed Res Int 2022:5164970. https://doi.org/10.1155/2022/5164970

Ibrahimi KM, Kumar R, Pakhira W (2023) A graphene/Au/TiO2 coated dual-core PCF SPR biosensor with improved design and performance for early cancer cell detection of with high sensitivity. Optik 288. https://doi.org/10.1016/J.IJLEO.2023.171186

Iranmakani S, Mortezazadeh T, Sajadian F, Ghaziani MF, Ghafari A, Khezerloo D, Musa AE (2020) A review of various modalities in breast imaging: technical aspects and clinical outcomes. Egypt J Radiol Nucl Med 51:1–22. https://doi.org/10.1186/S43055-020-00175-5/FIGURES/26

Jalalvand AR, Karami MM (2025) Roles of nanotechnology in electrochemical sensors for medical diagnostic purposes: a review. Sens Bio-Sensing Res 47:100733. https://doi.org/10.1016/J.SBSR.2024.100733

Jiao J, Yin M, Wang Z, Hu B, Chi J, Lu L, Dai F, Xue L, Wang T, Wang X et al (2025) An oriented self-assembly biosensor with built-in error-checking for precise midkine detection in cancer diagnosis and prognosis evaluation. Biosens Bioelectron 268:116905. https://doi.org/10.1016/J.BIOS.2024.116905

Ke H, Kao S, van Zandwijk N, Rasko JEJ, Yeo D (2024) Circulating tumor cell detection may offer earlier diagnosis in patients suspected of asbestos-related lung cancer. Lung Cancer 192. https://doi.org/10.1016/J.LUNGCAN.2024.107829

Korucu Ş, Kose A, Fellah MF (2024) Biosensor for the early diagnosis of lung cancer: a DFT study on the applicability of metal-doped graphene structures. Sensors Actuators A Phys 376:115637. https://doi.org/10.1016/J.SNA.2024.115637

Kotwal AA, Walter LC (2020) Cancer screening in older adults: individualized decision-making and communication strategies. Med Clin North Am 104:989. https://doi.org/10.1016/J.MCNA.2020.08.002

Lawrence R, Watters M, Davies CR, Pantel K, Lu YJ (2023) Circulating tumour cells for early detection of clinically relevant cancer. Nat Rev Clin Oncol 20:1. https://doi.org/10.1038/S41571-023-00781-Y

Li SY, Cheng QX, Liu JK, Nie XQ, Zhao GP, Wang J (2018) CRISPR-Cas12a has both cis- and trans-cleavage activities on single-stranded DNA. Cell Res 28(4):491–493. https://doi.org/10.1038/s41422-018-0022-x

Lian S, Wang Q, Liu Y, Lu Y, Huang L, Deng H, Xie X (2024a) Multi-targeted nanoarrays for early broad-spectrum detection of lung cancer based on blood biopsy of tumor exosomes. Talanta 276:126270. https://doi.org/10.1016/J.TALANTA.2024.126270

Lian S, Lu C, Li F, Yu X, Ai L, Wu B, Gong X, Zhou W, Xie Y, Du Y et al (2024b) Circulating DNA genome-wide fragmentation in early detection and disease monitoring of hepatocellular carcinoma. iScience 27:109701. https://doi.org/10.1016/j.isci.2024.109701

Liquid Biopsy Consortium | Division of Cancer Prevention. Available online: https://prevention.cancer.gov/major-programs/liquid-biopsy-consortium. Accessed 12 Mar 2025

Liu X, Zhang M, Shao C, Sun H, Zhang B, Guo Z, Sun J, Qi F, Zhang Y, Niu H et al (2023) Blood- and urine-based liquid biopsy for early-stage cancer investigation: taken clear renal cell carcinoma as a model. Mol Cell Proteomics 22:100603. https://doi.org/10.1016/J.MCPRO.2023.100603

Liu Z, Zhou Y, Lu J, Gong T, Ibáñez E, Cifuentes A, Lu W (2024) Microfluidic biosensors for biomarker detection in body fluids: a key approach for early cancer diagnosis. Biomark Res 12:153. https://doi.org/10.1186/S40364-024-00697-4

Liu R, Li Y, Liu Y, Wang Y, Si Q, Yakoba Agyapong DA, Feng J, Fang R, Tang L, Cao F et al (2025) A highly sensitive and reusable magnetic nano-electrochemical biosensor for the detection of the liver cancer biomarker heat shock protein 70. Chem Eng J 505:159860. https://doi.org/10.1016/J.CEJ.2025.159860

Loud JT, Murphy J (2017) Cancer screening and early detection in the 21st century. Semin Oncol Nurs 33:121. https://doi.org/10.1016/J.SONCN.2017.02.002

Loureiro A, Da Silva GJ (2019) CRISPR-Cas: converting a bacterial defence mechanism into a state-of-the-art genetic manipulation tool. Antibiotics 8:18. https://doi.org/10.3390/ANTIBIOTICS8010018

Martin TK, Dinerman A, Sudhaman S, Budde G, Palsuledesai CC, Krainock M, Liu MC, Smith E, Tapias L, Podgaetz E et al (2024) Early real-world experience monitoring circulating tumor DNA in resected early-stage non–small cell lung cancer. J Thorac Cardiovasc Surg 168:1349–1359.e2. https://doi.org/10.1016/J.JTCVS.2024.01.017

Mehta P, Antonelli M, Ahmed HU, Emberton M, Punwani S, Ourselin S (2021) Computer-aided diagnosis of prostate cancer using multiparametric MRI and clinical features: a patient-level classification framework. Med Image Anal 73:102153. https://doi.org/10.1016/J.MEDIA.2021.102153

Mengstie MA, Wondimu BZ (2021) Mechanism and applications of CRISPR/Cas-9-mediated genome editing. Biologics 15:353. https://doi.org/10.2147/BTT.S326422

Ming Y, Wu N, Qian T, Li X, Wan DQ, Li C, Li Y, Wu Z, Wang X, Liu J et al (2020) Progress and future trends in PET/CT and PET/MRI molecular imaging approaches for breast cancer. Front Oncol 10:507927. https://doi.org/10.3389/FONC.2020.01301/PDF

Moleyar-Narayana P, Leslie SW, Ranganathan S (2024) Cancer screening. StatPearls

Mun B, Jeong H, Kim R, Gu B, Kim J, Son HY, Rho HW, Lim EK, Haam S (2024) 3D-nanostructured microfluidic device arranged in a herringbone pattern for the highly effective capture of HER2-positive cancer-derived exosomes in urine. Chem Eng J 482:148851. https://doi.org/10.1016/J.CEJ.2024.148851

Ogi H (2013) Wireless-electrodeless quartz-crystal-microbalance biosensors for studying interactions among biomolecules: a review. Proc Jpn Acad Ser B Phys Biol Sci 89:401. https://doi.org/10.2183/PJAB.89.401

Parisi F, De Luca G, Mosconi M, Lastraioli S, Dellepiane C, Rossi G, Puglisi S, Bennicelli E, Barletta G, Zullo L et al (2024) Front-line liquid biopsy for early molecular assessment and treatment of hospitalized lung cancer patients. Cancer Treat Res Commun 41. https://doi.org/10.1016/J.CTARC.2024.100839

Pei J, Li L, Li C, Li Z, Wu Y, Kuang H, Ma P, Huang L, Liu J, Tian G (2025) Dumbbell probe-bridged CRISPR/Cas13a and nicking-mediated DNA cascade reaction for highly sensitive detection of colorectal cancer-related microRNAs. Biosens Bioelectron 273. https://doi.org/10.1016/J.BIOS.2025.117190

Peng J, Liu T, Guan L, Xu Z, Xiong T, Zhang Y, Song J, Liu X, Yang Y, Hao X (2024) A highly sensitive lock-Cas12a biosensor for detection and imaging of MiRNA-21 in breast cancer cells. Talanta 273. https://doi.org/10.1016/J.TALANTA.2024.125938

Prasanth BK, Alkhowaiter S, Sawarkar G, Dharshini BD, Baskaran AR (2023) Unlocking early cancer detection: exploring biomarkers, circulating DNA, and innovative technological approaches. Cureus 15:e51090. https://doi.org/10.7759/CUREUS.51090

PSMA PET-CT Accurately detects prostate cancer spread – NCI. Available online: https://www.cancer.gov/news-events/cancer-currents-blog/2020/prostate-cancer-psma pet-ct-metastasis. Accessed 12 Mar 2025

Pulumati A, Pulumati A, Dwarakanath BS, Verma A, Papineni RVL (2023) Technological advancements in cancer diagnostics: improvements and limitations. Cancer Rep 6:e1764. https://doi.org/10.1002/CNR2.1764

Qiu SF, Zhang QZ, Wu ZY, Liu MZ, Ding Q, Sun FM, Wang Y, Yang HX, Zheng L, Chen X et al (2024) Establishment and validation of circulating cell-free DNA signatures for nasopharyngeal carcinoma detection. EBioMedicine 108:105321. https://doi.org/10.1016/j.ebiom.2024.105321

Rahimi S, Balusamy SR, Perumalsamy H, Ståhlberg A, Mijakovic I (2024) CRISPR-Cas target recognition for sensing viral and cancer biomarkers. Nucleic Acids Res 52:10040–10067. https://doi.org/10.1093/NAR/GKAE736

Ren D, Wei H, Li N, Fu W, Huang Z, Yang L, Mu S (2024) Colorimetric detection of circulating tumor cells in breast cancer based on ladder-branch hybridization chain reaction and DFs/AuNCs nanozyme. Talanta 274. https://doi.org/10.1016/J.TALANTA.2024.125921

Safaeian M, Solomon D, Castle PE (2007) Cervical cancer prevention – cervical screening: science in evolution. Obstet Gynecol Clin N Am 34:739. https://doi.org/10.1016/J.OGC.2007.09.004

Saini A, Dilbaghi N, Yadav N (2025) CRISPR integrated biosensors: a new paradigm for cancer detection. Clin Chim Acta 569:120179. https://doi.org/10.1016/J.CCA.2025.120179

Salehjahromi M, Karpinets TV, Sujit SJ, Qayati M, Chen P, Aminu M, Saad MB, Bandyopadhyay R, Hong L, Sheshadri A et al (2024) Synthetic PET from CT improves diagnosis and prognosis for lung cancer: proof of concept. Cell Rep Med 5. https://doi.org/10.1016/J.XCRM.2024.101463/ATTACHMENT/9F0C7E27-D2DC-4F4F-A2E8-2FFAF59B6A73/MMC2.PDF

Sarkar S, Hazra S, Patra S, Gogoi M (2024) Biosensors for cancer detection: a review. TrAC Trends Anal Chem 180:117978. https://doi.org/10.1016/J.TRAC.2024.117978

Schiffman JD, Fisher PG, Gibbs P (2015) Early detection of cancer: past, present, and future. Am Soc Clin Oncol Educ Book:57–65. https://doi.org/10.14694/EDBOOK_AM.2015.35.57

Słomka A, Wang B, Mocan T, Horhat A, Willms AG, Schmidt-Wolf IGH, Strassburg CP, Gonzalez-Carmona MA, Lukacs-Kornek V, Kornek MT (2022) Extracellular vesicles and circulating tumour cells – complementary liquid biopsies or standalone concepts? Theranostics 12:5836. https://doi.org/10.7150/THNO.73400

Sornambikai S, Divya KP, Vasanth S, Viswanathan C, Ponpandian N (2023) CRISPR based biosensing: an ultrasensitive theranostic tool for the detection of early breast cancer biomarkers – a mini review. Biosens Bioelectron X 14:100367. https://doi.org/10.1016/J.BIOSX.2023.100367

Stewart GD, Godoy A, Farquhar F, Kitt J, Cartledge J, Kimuli M, Rossi SH, Shinkins B, Burbidge S, Burge SW et al (2024) Abdominal noncontrast computed tomography scanning to screen for kidney cancer and other abdominal pathology within community-based computed tomography screening for lung cancer: results of the Yorkshire Kidney Screening Trial. Eur Urol. https://doi.org/10.1016/J.EURURO.2024.08.029

Tran HT, Heeke S, Sujit S, Vokes N, Zhang J, Aminu M, Lam VK, Vaporciyan A, Swisher SG, Godoy MCB et al (2024) Circulating tumor DNA and radiological tumor volume identify patients at risk for relapse with resected, early-stage non-small-cell lung cancer. Ann Oncol 35:183–189. https://doi.org/10.1016/J.ANNONC.2023.11.008

Wahab MRA, Palaniyandi T, Thamada S, Viswanathan S, Baskar G, Surendran H, Baraneedharan P, Kannan J, Ravi M, Rajinikanth S et al (2024) Assessment of genome mutation analysis for tumor-informed detection of circulating tumor DNA in patients with breast cancer. Clin Chim Acta 561:119818. https://doi.org/10.1016/J.CCA.2024.119818

Wang X, Oldani MJ, Zhao X, Huang X, Qian D (2014) A review of cancer risk prediction models with genetic variants. Cancer Inform 13:19. https://doi.org/10.4137/CIN.S13788

Wang X, Song J, Fan X, Shi C, Zeng B, Xiao Y, Sun F, Hu X (2023) Universal and highly accurate detection of circulating tumor DNA mutation in non-small cell lung cancer based on CRISPR/Cas12a system. Sensors Actuators B Chem 383. https://doi.org/10.1016/J.SNB.2023.133493

Wang R, Wang B, Zhang H, Liao X, Shi B, Zhou Y, Zhou C, Yan Y, Zhang W, Wang K et al (2024a) Early evaluation of circulating tumor DNA as marker of therapeutic efficacy and prognosis in breast cancer patients during primary systemic therapy. Breast 76:103738. https://doi.org/10.1016/J.BREAST.2024.103738

Wang CH, Shao YS, Hsu KF, Lee GB (2024b) detection of dual-methylated BRCA1/BRCA2 cell-free DNA for ovarian cancer on an aptamer-based integrated microfluidic system. Chem Eng J 495:153478. https://doi.org/10.1016/J.CEJ.2024.153478

Wang Y, Long W, Wang Y, Han Y, Zeng F, Li J, He B, Song Y, Gao Y (2025) A portable microfluidic platform for ultra-sensitive detection of ovarian cancer biomarkers via cascade signal amplification. Chem Eng J 503:158289. https://doi.org/10.1016/J.CEJ.2024.158289

Wasilewski T, Kamysz W, Gębicki J (2024) AI-assisted detection of biomarkers by sensors and biosensors for early diagnosis and monitoring. Biosensors 14:356. https://doi.org/10.3390/BIOS14070356

National Cancer Institute (2025) Screening tests. National Institutes of Health. https://www.cancer.gov/about-cancer/screening/screening-tests

Yang G, Ye Q, Xia J (2022) Unbox the black-box for the medical explainable AI via multi-modal and multi-centre data fusion: a mini-review, two showcases and beyond. Inf Fusion 77:29. https://doi.org/10.1016/J.INFFUS.2021.07.016

Zamri AZM, Mustafa MK, Awang NA, Zalkepali NUHH, Mahmud NNHEN, Muhammad NAM (2024) Fiber-laser based on D-shaped fiber biosensor for prostate cancer biomarker detection. Mater Today Proc. https://doi.org/10.1016/J.MATPR.2024.04.071

Zhang Z, Nagrath S (2013) Microfluidics and cancer: are we there yet? Biomed Microdevices 15(4):595–609. https://doi.org/10.1007/S10544-012-9734-8

Zhang Y, Qi J, Li J, Jia S, Wang Y, Sun Q, Kang Y, Liu Y, Cao Y, Yu J (2020) Utility of circulating tumor cells for detection of early-stage luminal a breast cancer. Am J Med Sci 360:543–551. https://doi.org/10.1016/J.AMJMS.2020.01.020

Zhang B, Shi H, Wang H (2023) Machine learning and AI in cancer prognosis, prediction, and treatment selection: a critical approach. J Multidiscip Healthc 16:1779–1791. https://doi.org/10.2147/JMDH.S410301

Zhang A, Gao Q, Tian C, Chen W, Pan C, Wang L, Huang J, Zhang J (2024a) Liquid biopsy in lung cancer: nano-flow cytometry detection of non-small cell lung cancer in blood. Lab Investig 104. https://doi.org/10.1016/J.LABINV.2024.102151

Zhang B, Nie Q, Yan X, Jiang Q, Ren J, Xu P, Lu D, You R, Lu Y, Li L (2024b) Machine learning-based SERS label-free detection of plasma and exosome binding in early-stage lung cancer. Microchem J 205:111306. https://doi.org/10.1016/J.MICROC.2024.111306

Zhu W, Qian H, Cao S, Xia W, Wang X, Jin J, Wang X, Zhang H, Liu D, Chen Y (2025) A new platform of electrowetting-on-dielectric digital microfluidics for rapid detection of early-stage hepatocellular carcinoma (HCC) specific biomarker. Anal Chim Acta 1336:343533. https://doi.org/10.1016/J.ACA.2024.343533

Next-Generation Biosensing Devices and the Use of AI/ML

13

Fatemeh Sharifi, Sasha Cai Lesher Perez, Alev Erdi, and Volkan Cecen

Abstract

Biosensing systems have evolved from basic laboratory devices to advanced platforms that measure specific biological molecules. These devices offer benefits like low cost, speed, and portability, making them useful for health monitoring and environmental applications. The integration of machine learning (ML) and artificial intelligence (AI) enhances the functionality of biosensors, improving data analysis and decision-making. This technology aids in real-time monitoring of diseases and supports personalized healthcare by analyzing data from various biofluids. Additionally, connecting biosensors to smartphones has expanded their accessibility, especially in rural areas. Despite the advancements, further research is needed to overcome challenges and commercialize smarter biosensors for broader applications. Overall, AI enhances the accuracy and effectiveness of biosensing, allowing for better health diagnostics and environmental monitoring. We have examined the progress and challenges in developing biosensing systems, along with the significant impact of AI and machine learning. In conclusion, when proper precautions and safe conditions are maintained, biosensing systems can effectively measure concentrations of specific biological molecules. Moreover, advancements in nanotechnology and AI have greatly enhanced the functionality and applications of these systems.

F. Sharifi · S. C. L. Perez
Department of Chemical Engineering, University of Michigan, Ann Arbor, MI, USA

A. Erdi · V. Cecen (✉)
Department of Biomedical Engineering, Newark College of Engineering, New Jersey Institute of Technology, Newark, NJ, USA

V. Patel et al. (eds.), *Biosensor Technology in Translating Novel Materials into Practical Devices*, https://doi.org/10.1007/978-981-95-5519-2_13

Keywords
Healthcare monitoring · Artificial intelligence · Machine learning · Personalized medicine · In silico models

13.1 Introduction

Biosensing systems were initially electrochemical laboratory devices designed to measure the concentration of specific substances containing targeted biological molecules. Various biosensing devices have been developed through advances in nanotechnology, biomedical sciences, and manufacturing, in response to the increasing need for measuring different analytes (Mohan et al. 2017; Sharifi et al. 2020; Yunus et al. 2023). Such platforms offer advantages such as low cost, scalability, rapidity, simplicity, high throughput, high specificity, versatility, and portability. They have become rapidly widespread with multiple applications, including real-time monitoring of health parameters and disease diagnosis, which can be applied in various clinical applications (Sharifi et al. 2020; Yunus et al. 2023), point of care, and personalized health care devices, food safety (Bao et al. 2024), and environmental observations (Islam et al. 2023; Pouyanfar et al. 2022; Zevallos-Aliaga et al. 2024).

Biosensing devices are designed to measure specific metabolites using biomarkers obtained from the body's biofluids, such as urine, sweat, saliva, tears, exhaled breath, interstitial fluid, and blood, aiming to diagnose and monitor multiple diseases (Giarola et al. 2024; He et al. 2023).

ML, deep learning, and computer programming can ameliorate the proficiency of biosensors and make them innovative to help physicians better monitor and forecast the status of diseases. The great competence of ML models in processing data obtained from biosensors is inevitable (Bhaiyya et al. 2024; Dave et al. 2022). It can be applied in various stages, such as data cleaning and classification, data pattern recognition, enhancing device performance, and facilitating the output of results and decision-making. The innovative biosensors empowered by AI utilize ML methods to enhance outputs obtained from signal processing and image analysis (Bhatia et al. 2024; Haghayegh et al. 2024).

Combining biosensors with smartphones will lead to the widespread adoption of smart bio-sensing devices, which can provide detection systems for areas with limited access to medical facilities, such as farms and rural regions. A similar procedure happened for the automatic detection of COVID-19, where paper-based biosensors were developed, which benefited from using smartphones and augmented reality to identify the fluorimetric and colorimetric changes using the smartphone cameras, and developed mobile software (Gowri et al. 2021; Xu et al. 2021).

(Wu et al. 2024). In this regard, neural network-based systems have been applied to acceleration and strain sensors for the detection and automatic prediction of some physical performances, like gesture recognition and activity of the sensors (Qureshi et al. 2023). These advanced machine-learning methods enable real-time measurement and assessment of metabolite concentrations.

Although the integration of AI algorithms is inevitable in creating intelligent biosensors, further research and innovation must be done to overcome the challenges mentioned above, so that smarter biosensors with various applications become commercialized and available for different sensory applications (Chen et al. 2024; Flynn and Chang 2024).

The latest advancement in AI in the past decades has resulted in a rapid shift in the prevalent mathematical methods for data analysis. AI has also effectively found optimized solutions and predictions for systems with complicated and uncertain behavior (Turan et al. 2018). ML is a known part of AI, composed of computational algorithms that can learn from previous datasets and adapt to new circumstances (Kalmady et al. 2017). Such methods have been applied to analyze the data, detect trends and patterns, find inefficiencies, and make decisions based on the outcome of the analysis (Patcha and Park 2007).

Different approaches exist for the learning process of ML algorithms: unsupervised, semi-supervised, supervised, and reinforcement types of learning (Heo et al. 2017; Kadian et al. 2021, 2022). In a supervised algorithm, the machine is trained based on the related mapping methods (i.e., neural networks, support vector machines, Bayesian classifiers, etc.) to notice specific patterns, such as detecting specific colors in a biosensor's graph, while in unsupervised learning approaches, the computer algorithm processes the variables without considering any feedback from previous experiences. Therefore, the input for the supervised algorithms includes a set of predefined labels and the primary datasets. In contrast, for unsupervised methods, the first inputs are the data sets, and no pre-defined labels are given to the algorithms initially. Based on the input, the algorithm will find the initial meaningful features and parameters to predict the aforementioned labels and make the procedure more accurate. Semi-supervised learning is a method used to distinguish between supervised and unsupervised learning (Kadian et al. 2021). A reinforcement learning procedure is developed to optimize the reinforcement signals by mapping the situations to actions (Kadian et al. 2022).

Incorporation of AI into the electrochemical biosensing platforms will be beneficial since the innovative biosensors will have higher sensitivity, selectivity, and accuracy by providing more robust capabilities in data processing and analyzing, and real-time monitoring of patients' specific biomarkers (Yunus et al. 2023). The progress in advanced AI algorithms, especially in long-term real-time monitoring, will result in ameliorating signal processing, detecting trends, observing rapid changes, extracting data, and better decision-making, which will improve the sensitivity, accuracy, and selectivity of electrochemical biosensors (Zhang et al. 2023). Such excellent capabilities are valuable in the real-time monitoring of analytes with applications like monitoring biological analytes for medical diagnostics or observing the concentration of chemical compounds for environmental applications. Moreover, such advanced systems can provide versatile multimodal sensing devices where a couple of complex analytes will be monitored simultaneously, and their interactions or influence can be analyzed. ML algorithms continuously improve by learning from fresh data collected with the biosensors, resulting in an intelligent biosensing platform whose resilience and reliability improve over time (Turan et al. 2018).

ML algorithms will also increase the precision and reliability of the data obtained from medical imaging by providing an intelligent, in-depth data analysis (Chaulagain et al. 2022). Moreover, ML methods in applications like personalized therapy can provide long-term monitoring and massive analysis of specific patient data to create personalized patient pathological and physiological health profiles (Nittala et al. 2020).

Incorporating biosensors and IoT can also facilitate detecting and comprehending physiological and biochemical signals (Turan et al. 2018). Improvements in computer technologies, such as accelerated AI and edge computing, make this integration possible, allowing for faster data processing and decision-making at the device level.

13.2 Biosensing Devices

The general physics behind the Biosensing devices' performance is that they transfer biochemical interactions between specific antibodies previously coated over the biosensor surface and the targeted antigens inside the solution into the electrical, optical, or mechanical/piezoelectric signals, and with the help of some correlations, the output signal relates to the initial analyte concentration in the solution. Biosensors can fall into various categories based on the signal transduction they use and the nature of bio-recognition elements employed (Qureshi et al. 2023). Biosensing devices can be categorized into electrochemical, AI/ML, optical, piezoelectric, and thermometric biosensors based on the type of signal transduction. Biosensing platforms can also be classified based on their bio-recognition elements, such as enzyme-based, affinity-based, DNA, cell-based, tissue-based, and microbial biosensors (Mishra et al. 2020).

Electrochemical biosensors are considered the primary category of biosensing devices, where their detection is primarily based on converting a biological reaction into an electrical signal. Electrochemical biosensors are categorized into amperometric, potentiometric, voltammetric, and conductometric biosensors based on their detection mechanisms. Amperometric AI/ML biosensors work based on the current induced by the oxidation or reduction of the electroactive species (Borgmann et al. 2011). Glucose-level monitoring devices are a good example of this category. The physics of potentiometric biosensors is based on measuring the potential differences in the electrochemical environments (Pullano et al. 2022). PH sensors are a good example of potentiometric biosensors widely used in various applications, such as health monitoring, food and water quality assurance, and environmental analysis (Manjakkal et al. 2020). Voltammetric AI/ML biosensors are analytical devices that combine a biological recognition element with an electrochemical transducer. By applying a variable voltage and measuring the resulting current, these AI/ML biosensors can provide highly sensitive and selective detection of biomolecules, such as glucose, DNA, and proteins, in various sample matrices (Perumal and Hashim

2014). Their ability to offer rapid, real-time analysis with minimal sample preparation makes them valuable tools in medical diagnostics, environmental monitoring, and food safety applications (Dincer et al. 2019).

The general principle behind conductometric AI/ML biosensors is based on the alteration of conductivity in a solution by changing the ion concentration through the production or consumption of ion species. Conductometric biosensors have several advantages, including the ability to work without reference electrodes, light sensitivity, operation at low amplitude voltage, and ease of miniaturized fabrication compared to their counterparts. Electrochemical AI/ML biosensors offer significant advantages, including high sensitivity and selectivity, ease of miniaturization, and the potential for real-time analyte monitoring (Heo et al. 2017).

Microfluidic platforms are generally used to manipulate and analyze small volumes of fluids with high precision, enabling the development of lab-on-a-chip systems that revolutionize biochemical analyses and diagnostics. Integrating AI with these platforms is poised to enhance their capabilities, opening new avenues for automation, data analysis, and decision-making. AI algorithms can efficiently process complex datasets generated by microfluidic devices, allowing for real-time monitoring and optimization of experiments. By leveraging ML and other AI techniques, these integrated systems can potentially predict outcomes, adapt to changing conditions, and improve the accuracy of diagnostics and analytical measurements, thus fostering advancements in personalized medicine and other scientific fields (Rehan 2024).

Huang et al. developed a label-free microfluidic-based blood cell counting device where they used cell images and analyzed them with convolutional neural network techniques named single-frame super-resolution method, which could improve low-resolution cell images, providing a lensless microfluidic cell counting platform, which can be employed in point-of-care applications (Heo et al. 2017). In another study, T-cells and B-cells were differentiated using a microfluidic device comprising parallel pillars. Cell counting was done via a Support Vector Machine (SVM) classifier to distinguish the cells from the background. Then, algorithms like the histogram of oriented gradients and radial basis function-kernel SVM were employed to identify color and distinguish T-cells from B-cells (Kadian et al. 2022).

The integration of microfluidic platforms with AI holds great promise for developing intelligent continuous monitoring of biomarkers and analytes, and they can ameliorate the detection, characterization, and prediction of species. Commercialized microfluidic devices have been developed to detect chemical compounds like volatile organic compounds and CO_2 for environmental and food safety (Kadian et al. 2021). Similarly, paper-based microfluidic devices have been developed to classify bacterial species using supervised machine-learning techniques. The human tongue inspired the microfluidic design, which used fewer peptides as less specific receptors. The inclusion of supervised ML-enabled bacterial classification without the necessity of particular receptors. The AI/ML biosensors had four parallel channels accessing the loading zone spontaneously. The smartphone was taken video from the flow inside the channels, and the data were evaluated and supervised using an ML algorithm (Chaulagain et al. 2022).

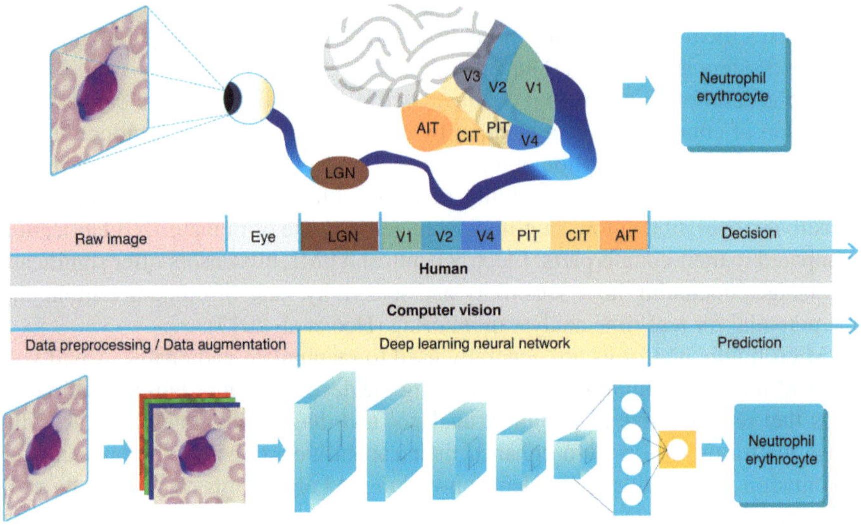

Fig. 13.1 Cell recognition through human eyes, brain, and computer vision. (Zhou et al. 2023)

Dou et al. devised a portable three-in-one biosensor to detect the SARS-CoV-2 viral RNA, antigen, and antibody. This AI/ML biosensor, coupled with a smartphone, can intelligently identify infected individuals (Mishra et al. 2020).

Computer vision constitutes a branch of artificial intelligence that employs algorithms to replicate how the human visual system acquires, processes, analyzes, and synthesizes visual information. The human visual cortex comprises over 140 million neurons and possesses unparalleled visual perception capabilities, achieved through the segmentation and integration of visual data transmitted from the retina, as well as through the instantaneous recognition of objects and patterns (Fig. 13.1). This advanced method showed higher throughput and was easier to use, especially in the initial sample preparation required for flow cytometry analysis (Zhou et al. 2023). Similarly, optical microfluidic channels and sensors are used to detect cells. The cells are circulated inside the microchannel and detected using laser-scattered light microscopy. The microfluidic chamber is a portable point-of-care detection platform in advanced optical flow cytometry. Various ML algorithms were employed to analyze the images for cell classification. In research conducted by Hoe et al., a convolutional neural network algorithm was applied to identify 21-by-21-pixel single-cell image datasets. Their results indicated that their device could accurately differentiate the label-free cells in a large-volume sample (Nittala et al. 2020).

13.3 Role of AI/ML in Biosensing

Choosing an appropriate intelligent model for a biosensing device is essential for enhancing data processing and its applications, as various AI and ML models can help analyze measurements, information, and images from biosensing platforms

(Wang et al. 2020). These intelligent AI-powered biosensing devices can constantly collect physiological data and monitor various patient biomarkers. Machine learning algorithms then analyze this data to identify patterns. These algorithms improve over time as more data is gathered, and any changes in signal patterns are carefully reviewed (Dhillon and Verma 2020).

ML models can be applied in various fields, including data collection, data analysis and classification, signal processing, understanding current trends, predicting outcomes, monitoring variations, image analysis, image recognition, and dimension reduction (Wang et al. 2020; Dhillon and Verma 2020) Selecting appropriate ML models for biosensing devices depends on the application and data types, as these models directly impact raw data collection and logical data processing. Such smart models will enable the development of advanced biosensors across various fields, including diagnostics, screening, personalized medicine, point-of-care devices, food safety, and environmental monitoring (Ramprasad et al. 2017).

Several machine learning tools have been developed, such as artificial neural networks (ANN), response surface methodology (RSM), and genetic algorithms (GA). Artificial neural networks are computational models inspired by the human nervous system and are commonly used to analyze complex empirical data from multisensory arrays (MSA) and multisensor systems (MSS), especially in pharmaceutical applications. A smart electrochemical method for monitoring glucose and insulin levels in diabetic patients has been developed. The results showed promising accuracy in forecasting concentrations based on the data sets (Shukla et al. 2023).

RSM employs various statistical methods to analyze how different factors interact and how these interactions influence the specific outcome (Janiesch et al. 2021). GA is an AI-based computational method incorporated with the results of ANN to provide an optimized final output. The logic of the GA is based on the process of natural selection through biological evolution, and therefore, the GA methodology benefits from genetic operators such as crossover, selection, and mutation. Such characteristics make the GA the ideal candidate to optimize the data in the biological process (Kumari and Toshniwal 2020).

ML and AI approaches have been applied to analyze various disease biomarkers and symptoms to facilitate disease detection, monitoring, and planning an optimized treatment. In this regard, the integrative technique was developed to quantify the interaction of virus–host interaction, where, with the help of bioinformatics, the drug-induced gene profiles were predicted (Dissanayake et al. 2019).

13.4 Applications in Regenerative Medicine, Personalized Medicine

The field of tissue engineering and regenerative medicine has shown great promise in future healthcare procedures to restore patients' cells and regenerate damaged tissues and organs, opening new opportunities for a wide range of diseases (Kumari and Toshniwal 2020). However, this field also faces several challenges and obstacles due to the complex nature of the organs within the body and the limited knowledge and medical facilities available for regenerating specific tissues and organs. AI appears highly beneficial in overcoming some of these barriers in this field. Its main role is to analyze the patient's data precisely and identify patterns and correlations between trends that human clinicians might overlook. The results of such analysis can be used, based on patients' personalized data, to find the best treatment plans and procedures, relying on informed predictions obtained from various resources such as real-time patient data, genetic information, medical history, disease specifics, and previous experiences with similar treatments (Zevallos-Aliaga et al. 2024). Researchers at the Cedars-Sinai Medical Center developed an AI algorithm to select specific stem cell therapies based on patients' genetics and medical histories. Their findings show that AI improved the success rate of stem cell treatments, reduced adverse reactions, and provided the most effective treatment options that cannot be achieved through conventional methods (Kumari and Toshniwal 2020). It is worth noting that such treatment protocols are continually enhanced by the flexible nature of ML algorithms, which boost the AI's ability to learn, improve predictive models, and refine input data, ensuring that treatment plans stay innovative and highly effective. Machine learning and AI algorithms can also integrate with tissue engineering to develop more efficient and intelligent methods for creating complex tissues. Since tissues have intricate structures, AI can assist in replicating these detailed architectures by developing new techniques, such as designing complex tissue scaffolds with variable configurations and mechanical properties. This enables more precise culturing methods, resulting in tissues that resemble their natural counterparts (Paleyes et al. 2022; Ristoski and Paulheim 2016).

The innovative technologies, with their extraordinary capabilities in processing complex data like genetic information and medical images, can also be applied in personalized medicine, where patients' genetics and medical history, as well as real-time monitoring of biomarkers, can be fed into these algorithms as input, and based on the result of these patient-specific analysis, the treatment strategies can be tailored and optimized (Shu and Ye 2023).

Moreover, ML and AI can also play a crucial role in drug discovery and development, where vast amounts of data can be processed to identify potential compounds, resulting in faster and more accurate drug molecules compared to conventional drug discovery processes. For example, Silico Medicine is a biotechnological company that uses AI to analyze numerous chemical candidates and predict their potential biological effects. ML and AI algorithms bring new ways to accelerate drug discovery and find better patient therapies. Generative AI is emerging as a pivotal tool in designing new molecules for regenerative therapies, providing advantages that traditional methods lack. Generative AI, through models like variational autoencoders (VAEs), generative adversarial networks (GANs), and retrieval-augmented generation (RAG), significantly accelerates this process by efficiently exploring vast molecular spaces and generating novel candidates for therapeutic use (Oliveira Jr and Oliveira 2022). These AI models contribute by identifying complex patterns within large datasets, predicting the efficacy of potential molecules, and optimizing them for specific regenerative applications. This computational power enables researchers to design more precise and efficient molecules than traditional methods.

AI algorithms can also predict patient responses to these molecules, facilitating personalized therapy plans tailored to individual patient needs (Nittala et al. 2020). This personalization is critical in regenerative medicine, where patient-specific treatments can significantly enhance outcomes.

Furthermore, integrating AI in regenerative medicine extends to enhancing diagnostic precision and improving patient outcomes by analyzing complex biological data. AI tools are instrumental in deciphering these data patterns, allowing for better decision-making in therapy design (Wang et al. 2022). This advanced data analysis capability, combined with the ability to rapidly generate and test new molecules, positions AI as a transformative force in regenerative medicine. The advantages of using AI in molecule design for regenerative therapies are multifold. AI-driven approaches reduce the time and cost associated with drug discovery and development, offer the potential for higher success rates by predicting biological activity and toxicity early in the process, and ensure the molecules are tailored to address specific regenerative needs (Paleyes et al. 2022; Ristoski and Paulheim 2016; Shu and Ye 2023; Oliveira Jr and Oliveira 2022). This technological synergy is poised to address numerous current challenges in regenerative medicine, paving the way for innovative treatments and enhanced patient care.

Biotechnology, particularly cell culture, has played a crucial role in drug development and regenerative medicine. ML techniques have increased real-time cell growth and tissue engineering monitoring accuracy and efficiency. This has become more prominent, with AI integrated with advanced robotic or automated 3D printing or culturing methods, leading to an advanced, validated, reproducible cellular patterning and screening, which can revolutionize the in vitro culturing systems in crucial applications like biomanufacturing, regenerative medicine, and drug discovery and development (Fig. 13.2) (Filippi et al. 2024). These advanced systems minimize manual work in the lab through automated cell culture processes, offering complete control over each step, which leads to more reliable and consistent results by reducing contamination and human error (Mahboob et al. 2024; Nguyen et al. 2023). Through these smart systems, 24/7 monitoring of cellular growth, viability, morphology, genetic stability, and behavior of sophisticated spheroids and organoids will become feasible (Kumari and Toshniwal 2020). Moreover, integrating ML in cell culture monitoring is also beneficial in analyzing cellular behavior and its related datasets, leading to enhanced accuracy and reliable, reproducible outcomes. Since these innovative platforms can handle large data sets, such integrated methods will enable the scaling of complex cell culture processes. In AI-driven systems, cell culture and image analysis workflows run continuously, reducing the need for manual intervention and minimizing the potential for human error. This capability enables more consistent and reproducible experimental results, which are essential for progressing regenerative medicine research (Xu et al. 2021).

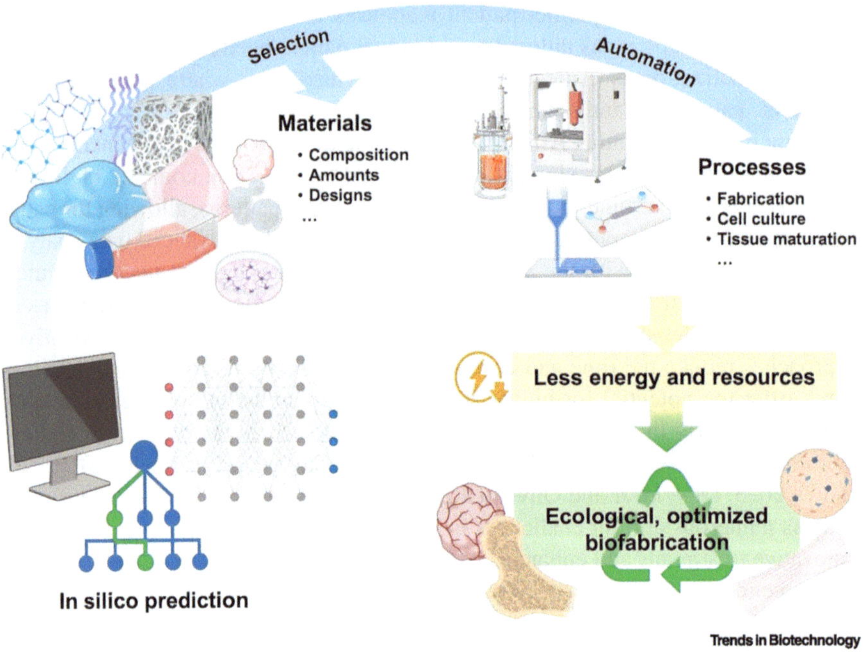

Fig. 13.2 Computational methods, such as holistic or hypothesis-driven methods, and materials with the highest specific performance scores enable more automation for tissue fabrication, culture, and development in vitro. (Filippi et al. 2024)

13.5 Challenges and Future Directions

The ML algorithm plays a crucial role in the analysis results. Therefore, choosing the ML algorithm and its design directly impacts the computational learning processes, adaptation, and data analysis. The performance of these ML algorithms also relies on data quality, meaning the availability of clean and diverse datasets, which significantly affects the outcomes evaluated. Additionally, ethical obligations require data privacy and security (Singh and Singh 2020).

The demand for smart biosensing devices drives researchers toward AI-powered biosensors that can monitor various biomarkers in real-time to enhance data accuracy, reliability, and security for personalized and clinical applications (Pouyanfar et al. 2022). These advanced biosensors integrate sophisticated machine learning algorithms and data analytics to interpret complex biological signals, enabling adaptive calibration and enhanced detection of subtle changes in biomarker levels. By delivering precise and personalized diagnostic insights, AI-enhanced biosensors have the potential to revolutionize patient care, enhance clinical decision-making, and support the development of targeted therapeutic strategies (Kalmady et al. 2017). Integrating AI into regenerative medicine presents several challenges and ethical concerns that require careful consideration. One of the main obstacles is managing the large volume of patient data while ensuring privacy and security (Yaqoob et al. 2022). AI algorithms must process extensive datasets to identify patterns and predict patient responses to treatments. Ensuring the confidentiality of this sensitive information requires robust data encryption, strict access controls, and compliance with privacy regulations (Sargiotis 2024).

The accuracy of AI predictions also presents challenges. ML algorithms used in drug discovery must be carefully trained and validated to ensure their predictions of drug efficacy, toxicity, and interactions are dependable. Mistakes in this area can cause significant delays in development and potentially harm patients (Donaldson et al. 2000; Leape et al. 1991). Collaboration between AI researchers and pharmaceutical scientists is essential to tackle these challenges. Strong partnerships can help bridge the gap between AI capabilities and real-world medical applications, ensuring the technology reaches its full potential (Nayyar et al. 2021).

Additionally, ethical issues such as bias in AI algorithms require attention. AI systems can unintentionally reinforce existing biases in healthcare, leading to unequal treatment outcomes. Regular testing and ongoing monitoring are essential to reduce these risks and ensure fairness (Kadian et al. 2022).

13.6 Discussion

Despite the recent advances in biosensor devices, they still face significant challenges related to fabrication, sensory components, detection, and analysis. These limitations slow down the widespread adoption of these powerful platforms in various commercial applications. The main concerns with biosensors, especially point-of-care devices, include issues such as poor sensitivity, high signal noise, accuracy, stability, and selectivity (Qureshi et al. 2023; Nittala et al. 2020; Wang et al. 2022; Wang et al. 2023). These limitations will affect the reliability of detection for these biosensing platforms, which in turn hinders their practical use in further medical and diagnostic applications. To address the limitations mentioned earlier, some researchers used multiple sensors, called sensor arrays, to enhance overall detection performance (Nittala et al. 2020). Recent advances in conducting polymers and metal oxide-based electronic noses have resulted in a range of sensing platforms with significant potential for biological applications. These sensor-array devices employ multiple sensors that have partial specificity. A key challenge with these parallel platforms is interpreting the data, as they produce complex, high-dimensional datasets. Consequently, analyzing and translating this data into clear, practical insights remains a major obstacle to the widespread commercialization of these platforms (Wang et al. 2023). ML techniques can assist in analyzing complex, high-dimensional data using various approaches, leading to better understanding, interpretation, and analysis of data, which results in improved sensors with higher detection and data prediction capabilities (Fig. 13.3).

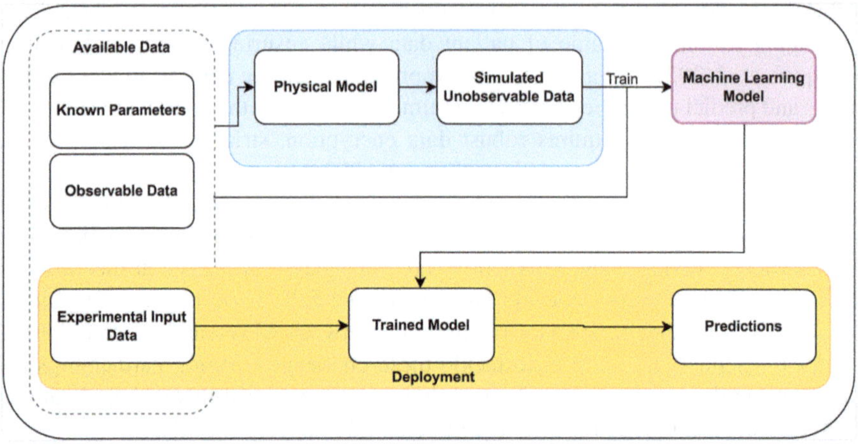

Fig. 13.3 The hybrid model employs physics-based modeling, which maps observable parameters to unobservable parameters and then feeds this information into the ML algorithm. (Wu et al. 2024)

13.7 Conclusion

The promise of AI-enhanced biosensing devices lies in their ability to transform personalized patient care and clinical decision-making, as well as their potential to revolutionize many sectors. For example, in personalized medicine, AI-enabled devices can continuously monitor biomarker levels, customize treatments to individual patient profiles, improve therapeutic outcomes, and minimize adverse effects. In environmental monitoring and food safety, these devices are crucial for detecting chemical compounds or biological organisms with unmatched accuracy and speed. However, the journey to fully unlock the potential of these technologies is filled with challenges that require careful attention.

Significant technical challenges include integrating AI/ML algorithms with hardware components to ensure seamless, real-time data processing and analysis. The complexity of these systems requires robust computational infrastructures capable of handling large datasets while maintaining efficiency and reliability. Similarly, ethical concerns such as data privacy, patient consent, and biases in AI models are pressing issues that must be addressed to prevent potential misuse or unintended consequences of these technologies. Protecting the confidentiality and security of sensitive patient information, along with ensuring fair and equitable outcomes from AI algorithms, will demand strict adherence to data protection regulations and ongoing oversight.

The potential breakthroughs in integrating AI/ML with biosensors are promising despite these challenges. Researchers and industry stakeholders need to collaborate to overcome current obstacles, leveraging AI to turn these innovations into practical uses. Through focused research, cross-disciplinary teamwork, and strict ethical review, the full potential of AI-powered biosensing technologies can be achieved, ensuring their responsible and effective use in both clinical and non-clinical settings, ultimately helping many communities worldwide.

References

Bao F et al (2024) Toward intelligent food packaging of biosensor and film substrate for monitoring foodborne microorganisms: a review of recent advancements. Crit Rev Food Sci Nutr 64(12):3920–3931

Bhaiyya M et al (2024) Role of machine learning assisted biosensors in point-of-care-testing for clinical decisions. ACS Sens 9(9):4495–4519

Bhatia D et al (2024) Biosensors and their widespread impact on human health. Sens Int 5:100257

Borgmann S et al (2011) Amperometric biosensors. Adv Electrochem Sci Eng 13:1–83

Chaulagain N et al (2022) Synergistic enhancement of the photoelectrochemical performance of TiO2 nanorod arrays through embedded plasmon and surface carbon nitride co-sensitization. ACS Appl Mater Interfaces 14(21):24309–24320

Chen Y et al (2024) Intelligent biosensors promise smarter solutions in food safety 4.0. Foods 13(2):235

Dave S et al (2022) Biosensors for healthcare: an artificial intelligence approach. In: Biosensors for emerging and re-emerging infectious diseases, pp 365–383

Dhillon A, Verma GK (2020) Convolutional neural network: a review of models, methodologies and applications to object detection. Prog Artif Intell 9(2):85–112

Dincer C et al (2019) Disposable sensors in diagnostics, food, and environmental monitoring. Adv Mater 31(30):1806739

Dissanayake T et al (2019) An ensemble learning approach for electrocardiogram sensor based human emotion recognition. Sensors 19(20):4495

Donaldson MS, Corrigan JM, Kohn LT (2000) To err is human: building a safer health system. National Academies Press (US), Washington (DC)

Filippi M, Mekkattu M, Katzschmann RK (2024) Sustainable biofabrication: from bioprinting to AI-driven predictive methods. Trends Biotechnol 43(2):290–303

Flynn CD, Chang D (2024) Artificial intelligence in point-of-care biosensing: challenges and opportunities. Diagnostics 14(11):1100

Giarola JF et al (2024) Validation of a plasmonic-based serology biosensor for veterinary diagnosis of COVID-19 in domestic animals. Talanta 271:125685

Gowri A, Kumar NA, Anand BS (2021) Recent advances in nanomaterials based biosensors for point of care (PoC) diagnosis of COVID-19–a minireview. TrAC Trends Anal Chem 137:116205

Haghayegh F et al (2024) Revolutionary point-of-care wearable diagnostics for early disease detection and biomarker discovery through intelligent technologies. Adv Sci 11(36):2400595

He L et al (2023) Smart chemical sensor and biosensor networks for healthcare 4.0. Sensors 23(12):5754

Heo YJ et al (2017) Real-time image processing for microscopy-based label-free imaging flow cytometry in a microfluidic chip. Sci Rep 7(1):11651

Islam MS et al (2023) Electrochemical biosensor for evaluation of environmental pollutants toxicity. Environments 10(4):63

Janiesch C, Zschech P, Heinrich K (2021) Machine learning and deep learning. Electron Mark 31(3):685–695

Kadian S et al (2021) Effect of sulfur-doped graphene quantum dots incorporation on morphological, optical and electron transport properties of CH3NH3PbBr3 perovskite thin films. J Mater Sci Mater Electron 32(13):17406–17417

Kadian S, Singh M, Manik G (2022) Graphene based hybrid nanocomposites for solar cells. In: Applications of nanomaterials in energy storage and electronics. Bentham Science Publishers, pp 61–77

Kalmady KS et al (2017) Improved transfer learning through shallow network embedding for classification of leukemia cells. In: 2017 ninth international conference on advances in pattern recognition (ICAPR). IEEE

Kumari P, Toshniwal D (2020) Impact of lockdown on air quality over major cities across the globe during COVID-19 pandemic. Urban Clim 34:100719

Leape LL et al (1991) The nature of adverse events in hospitalized patients: results of the Harvard medical practice study II. N Engl J Med 324(6):377–384

Mahboob K et al (2024) Integrating Apriori algorithm with data mining classification techniques for enhanced primary tumor prediction. In: Intelligent Data Analytics for Bioinformatics and Biomedical Systems, pp 213–234

Manjakkal L, Dervin S, Dahiya R (2020) Flexible potentiometric pH sensors for wearable systems. RSC Adv 10(15):8594–8617

Mishra RK et al (2020) Continuous opioid monitoring along with nerve agents on a wearable microneedle sensor array. J Am Chem Soc 142(13):5991–5995

Mohan AV et al (2017) Continuous minimally-invasive alcohol monitoring using microneedle sensor arrays. Biosens Bioelectron 91:574–579

Nayyar A, Gadhavi L, Zaman N (2021) Machine learning in healthcare: review, opportunities and challenges. In: Machine learning and the internet of medical things in healthcare, pp 23–45

Nguyen M, Roman GW, Soibam B (2023) Drosophila genotypes can be predicted from their exploration locomotive trajectories using supervised machine learning. Behav Process 212:104944

Nittala AS et al (2020) PhysioSkin: rapid fabrication of skin-conformal physiological interfaces. In: Proceedings of the 2020 CHI conference on human factors in computing systems

Oliveira ON Jr, Oliveira MCF (2022) Materials discovery with machine learning and knowledge discovery. Front Chem 10:930369

Paleyes A, Urma R-G, Lawrence ND (2022) Challenges in deploying machine learning: a survey of case studies. ACM Comput Surv 55(6):1–29

Patcha A, Park J-M (2007) An overview of anomaly detection techniques: existing solutions and latest technological trends. Comput Netw 51(12):3448–3470

Perumal V, Hashim U (2014) Advances in biosensors: principle, architecture and applications. J Appl Biomed 12(1):1–15

Pouyanfar N et al (2022) Artificial intelligence-based microfluidic platforms for the sensitive detection of environmental pollutants: recent advances and prospects. Trends Environ Anal Chem 34:e00160

Pullano SA et al (2022) Glucose biosensors in clinical practice: principles, limits and perspectives of currently used devices. Theranostics 12(2):493

Qureshi R et al (2023) Artificial intelligence and biosensors in healthcare and its clinical relevance: a review. IEEE Access 11:61600–61620

Ramprasad R et al (2017) Machine learning in materials informatics: recent applications and prospects. npj Comput Mater 3(1):54

Rehan H (2024) Advancing cancer treatment with AI-driven personalized medicine and cloud-based data integration. J Mach Learn Pharm Res 4(2):1–40

Ristoski P, Paulheim H (2016) Semantic web in data mining and knowledge discovery: a comprehensive survey. J Web Semant 36:1–22

Sargiotis D (2024) Data security and privacy: protecting sensitive information. In: Data governance: a guide. Springer, pp 217–245

Sharifi F, Sedighi A, Rehman M (2020) Design and simulation of a point-of-care microfluidic device for acoustic blood cell separation. Eng Proc 2(1):76

Shu X, Ye Y (2023) Knowledge discovery: methods from data mining and machine learning. Soc Sci Res 110:102817

Shukla S et al (2023) Computational approaches to delivery of anticancer drugs with multidimensional nanomaterials. Comput Struct Biotechnol J 21:4149–4158

Singh D, Singh B (2020) Investigating the impact of data normalization on classification performance. Appl Soft Comput 97:105524

Turan B et al (2018) A pillar-based microfluidic chip for T-cells and B-cells isolation and detection with machine learning algorithm. ROBOMECH J 5:1–9

Wang M et al (2020) Gesture recognition using a bioinspired learning architecture that integrates visual data with somatosensory data from stretchable sensors. Nat Electron 3(9):563–570

Wang M et al (2022) A wearable electrochemical biosensor for the monitoring of metabolites and nutrients. Nat Biomed Eng 6(11):1225–1235

Wang B et al (2023) Smartphone-based platforms implementing microfluidic detection with image-based artificial intelligence. Nat Commun 14(1):1–18

Wu Y, Sicard B, Gadsden SA (2024) Physics-informed machine learning: a comprehensive review on applications in anomaly detection and condition monitoring. Expert Syst Appl 255:124678

Xu W et al (2021) Rapid, label-free, and sensitive point-of-care testing of anti-SARS-CoV-2 IgM/IgG using all-fiber Fresnel reflection microfluidic biosensor. Microchim Acta 188(8):261

Yaqoob I et al (2022) Blockchain for healthcare data management: opportunities, challenges, and future recommendations. Neural Comput & Applic 34:11475–11490

Yunus G et al (2023) Electrochemical biosensors in healthcare services: bibliometric analysis and recent developments. PeerJ 11:e15566

Zevallos-Aliaga D et al (2024) Highly sensitive whole-cell mercury biosensors for environmental monitoring. Biosensors 14(5):246

Zhang Y et al (2023) Wearable artificial intelligence biosensor networks. Biosens Bioelectron 219:114825

Zhou S et al (2023) Computer vision meets microfluidics: a label-free method for high-throughput cell analysis. Microsyst Nanoeng 9(1):116

On-Chip Sensors Commercialized for Medical Diagnostics Applications

14

Vikas Kumar Shukla and Tanushri

Abstract

On-chip sensors have emerged as a transformative device in medical diagnostics, facilitating rapid, sensitive, and cost-effective detection of multiple biomarkers in complex biological fluids. Their advancement has been significantly influenced by interdisciplinary developments in materials science, microfabrication, and the integration of machine learning. This chapter provides an in-depth exploration of various fabrication methodologies for on-chip sensors, including screen printing, laser-induced graphene production, and nanocomposite functionalization. It further evaluates these methods in terms of scalability, in contrast with high-precision yet costly techniques such as lithography and 3D printing. A particular focus is directed toward the evolution of electrochemical, optical, and mechanical transduction systems, which have progressed from conventional silicon-based devices to innovative platforms enhanced by nanomaterials and driven by machine learning, featuring multiplexing capabilities. The chapter highlights significant real-world applications, including the monitoring of conditions such as myocardial infarction, sepsis, diabetes, and cancer, alongside the development of emerging non-invasive wearable devices designed for the analysis of sweat and tears. The discourse also critically examines pathways to commercialization, addressing key challenges such as sensitivity to low-abundance biomarkers, data standardization, regulatory compliance, and the enhancement of user accessibility in resource-limited environments. Case studies, including

V. K. Shukla (✉)
Department of Chemistry and Biochemistry, Worcester Polytechnic Institute, Worcester, MA, USA
e-mail: vshukla@wpi.edu

Tanushri
Department of Mathematics and Computing Technology, National Institute of Technology Patna, Patna, India

V. Patel et al. (eds.), *Biosensor Technology in Translating Novel Materials into Practical Devices*, https://doi.org/10.1007/978-981-95-5519-2_14

the Dexcom G7 continuous glucose monitor and Ellume's COVID-19 test, effectively illustrate both the challenges and triumphs encountered during the process of market translation. Moreover, the chapter discusses the role of machine learning methodologies, particularly fuzzy logic frameworks, in improving data interpretation, mitigating sensor drift, and enhancing clinical decision-making processes. The socioeconomic implications of on-chip sensors are also contemplated, underscoring their potential to alleviate healthcare burdens, strengthen disease surveillance systems, and foster equitable access to diagnostic tools. The on-chip sensors exhibited high accuracy with real patient samples. In conclusion, the chapter emphasizes the future promise of CRISPR-based sensing technologies, advanced nanomaterials, AI integration, and sustainable manufacturing approaches in addressing current limitations. Consequently, these advancements position on-chip sensors as fundamental components of precision medicine and global healthcare innovation.

Keywords

On-chip sensors · Fabrication · Invasive and Non-invasive · Machine Learning · Fuzzy logic

14.1 Introduction

The on-chip sensors have significantly made a paradigm shift in medical diagnostics due to fundamental alterations in routine medical diagnostics and early detection (Papamatthaiou et al. 2025). The on-chip sensors, often referred to as Lab-on-a-chip sensors (LOCs), integrated with a variety of sensing devices (electrochemical, lateral flow assay, and optical), microfluidics, and a data analysis processing unit, facilitate the robust, early, highly sensitive, and cost-effective medical diagnostics (Dkhar et al. 2023). An on-chip sensor is a small portable device that consists of pretreatment, separation, dilution, and a chemical reaction chamber, and requires a reduced sample volume (Arfin 2021). The on-chip sensors significantly reduce human interference, which improves the efficacy and efficiency of medical diagnosis. The reduced volume sample for on-chip sensors is essential in the medical discipline due to the scarcity of large volume biofluid samples. Moreover, miniaturization of these devices requires less reagent consumption, which reduces the cost of each diagnostic test (Bahnemann and Grünberger 2022). The on-chip sensors integrate the laboratory functionality, paving the way to overcome the gap between clinical laboratory and real-time patient healthcare due to their portability and point-of-care testing (Squires and Quake 2005). These devices have the potential to reach out to underdeveloped regions with limited medical facilities and improve medical care (Sorger 2008).

The conventional method used for the detection of protein biomarkers is enzyme-linked immunosorbent assay (ELISA). However, ELISA is a multiple-step process including the requirement of rigorous washing steps, which makes it time-consuming and also requires comparatively more sample volume. ELISA has a high sensitivity in the detection of protein biomarkers and is also known as a gold standard technique for protein quantification (Hnasko et al. 2011; Liu and Lei 2021). ELISA can monitor infectious pathogens such as the dengue virus (Nascimento et al. 2018), the Zika virus (Nurtop et al. 2018), and the influenza virus (Rajendran et al. 2017). Although ELISA has a better detection limit, it requires trained personnel, and non-portability decreases its reach to the underdeveloped regions. The contemporary microfluidic on-chip sensors, combined with other techniques, achieve better detection results. Mass spectrometry combined with microfluidic on-chip sensors can improve the currently used tools by clinicians in terms of early detection, diagnosis, monitoring, and treatment of malignant diseases such as cancer, heart disease, stroke, and diabetes (Nilsson et al. 2010). The surface plasmon resonance method has a high accuracy and sensitivity for detecting cancer biomarkers and virus detection at an affordable cost (Azzouz et al. 2022; Moznuzzaman et al. 2021). These microfluidic devices, with inclusive techniques, can detect blood biomarkers with high accuracy (Lin et al. 2020; Lim et al. 2019). Moreover, the incorporation of the lateral flow assay with microfluidics is also used as a point-of-care (POC) diagnostic (Koczula and Gallotta 2016). A commonly used lateral flow assay is a pregnancy kit, used in urine by a sandwich-based immunoassay for detecting human chorionic gonadotropin by a change in color. The lateral flow integrated bar chip was used to analyze multiple biomarkers in whole blood (Wang et al. 2010). The inclusivity of these techniques with on-chip sensors increases the reach of medical diagnosis by enhancing the device's portability.

On-chip sensors are miniaturized chips, fabricated at the micro- and nanoscales using different fabrication techniques (Bhagoria et al. 2020; Qamar and Shamsi 2020; Ho et al. 2015). These developed sensors need further development to be used in a medical diagnosis using invasive and non-invasive biofluids to detect metabolites and proteins in the physiological range (De Castro et al. 2019). On-chip sensors have been developed using a variety of different transduction approaches, such as electrochemical (Khan et al. 2019), optical (Hengoju et al. 2022), acoustic (Zhang et al. 2018), mechanical, and many more (Parihar et al. 2020). Each modality exhibits different physical mechanisms for the identification of biomarkers for health monitoring. The on-chip sensors work in parallel with invasive and non-invasive samples that provide access to analytical measures of the biomarkers. Still, invasive biofluids require trained medical personnel to collect samples such as blood and serum. On the other hand, non-invasive samples do not require trained personnel to collect samples such as saliva, urine, and sweat. This provides the edge to the on-chip sensors to become a home-friendly personalized medical diagnostic kit. The commercially available implantable sensors are Dexcom G7(Garg et al. 2022) and Freestyle Libre (Yaron et al. 2019) for continuously monitoring glucose levels.

Applying on-chip sensors with the incorporation of machine learning (ML) models increases the ability to observe the subtle changes in biomarkers at physiological levels and improves the diagnosis. To use ML models before that, we need to do exploratory data analysis and understand the recorded data, for which data preprocessing, such as correction in baseline and data standardization, is required (Ha et al. 2020; Kiani et al. 2016). The preprocessing of signals is essential to remove the signal drift from the signal, which improves the sensor response. The ML models are artificial neural networks (ANN) (Shahid et al. 2019), Recurrent Neural Network (RNN) (Ordóñez and Roggen 2016), Convolution Neural Network (CNN) (Saric et al. 2019), Support Vector Machine (SVM), Decision Trees (DT), Linear discriminant analysis (LDA), Principal Component Analysis (PCA), and Random Forest (RF) (Mahmud et al. 2018; Nakhleh et al. 2017). However, integrating machine learning with fuzzy logic provides enhanced accuracy and medical diagnosis (Nambison et al. 2024).

The on-chip sensors have immense potential to attract more users in the future. The global point-of-care medical diagnosis market size is estimated at $64.08 billion in 2025 and is expected to reach around $82.78 billion by 2034, expanding with a compound annual growth rate (CAGR) of 2.89% (https://www.precedenceresearch.com/). The tremendous growth in the commercial sector clearly indicates the need for on-chip sensors for medical prognosis and diagnosis.

The scope of this chapter is focused on the evolution of on-chip sensors, highlighting advances in different fabrication techniques, and material innovations. It also examines the transduction mechanisms that enable effective data acquisition from these on-chip sensors. In addition to this, we will also emphasize the integration and role of machine learning using a multitude of ML-based models to enhance the accuracy of diagnosis in complex biological fluids. Moreover, we will see the advancement in the commercialization of on-chip sensors from the laboratory to the market, and the transformative impact on the socioeconomic and decentralization of health care.

14.2 Evolution of On-Chip Sensors for Medical Diagnostics

The development of on-chip sensors for medical diagnostics showed a significant leap in medical care due to the integration of innovative research in microfabrication, nanotechnology, electrical engineering, chemistry, and biotechnology. These sensors are small and compact in size, like a coin, and provide robust and cost-effective monitoring of biomarkers. This is a big transformation from the clinical laboratory to personalized care. As we know, initially it was developed as a sensing device, and further it evolved into a lab-on-chip sensor fulfilling the needs of healthcare in the rural and urban areas where medical facilities are not reachable. In this section, we learn about the historical background, technological development, and keep our emphasis on the innovations of on-chip sensors, as shown in Fig. 14.1.

The miniaturization of microelectromechanical systems (MEMS) electronic components led to the development of a micro gas analysis system in the 1970s by Stanford University. The system was made up of silicon and glass using photolithography and chemical etching technology (Terry et al. 1979). The initial on-chip sensors were used for industrial and environmental applications. However, the silicon-based microfabricated transducers are used for temperature and pressure sensing. This paves the way for the application of pressure and temperature sensors to be used in the medical discipline for the measurement of physiological parameters

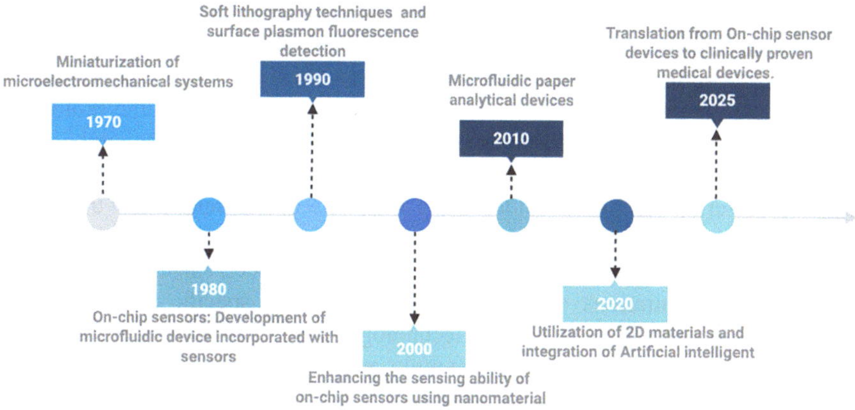

Fig. 14.1 A schematics of on-chip sensors from miniaturization to the translation of medical devices

such as blood pressure and glucose levels. Bergveld *et.al*; developed the ion-sensitive field effect transistors (ISFETs) in 1970(Bergveld 1970). The ISFETs are also used for measuring the ions in the solution, which paved the way to measure the pH of the solution using silicon-based substrates. Due to its ability, it can be used for the measurement of biomarkers. But due to a lack of sensitivity and specificity, it was difficult to use it in biological fluids for medical diagnostic applications. The microfluidic channel was developed around the 1980s with the incorporation of sensors for the use of small volumes from pico-litres to micro-litres (Manz et al. 1990). These advancements helped to lay the foundation of microfluidic sensors, but there was an external data processing unit.

In the 1990s, there was a significant development in sensor technology because of developments in material science and biotechnology. The chip-based sensors' specificity, sensitivity, and limit of detection were improved due to functionalization of recognition elements such as antibodies, proteins, enzymes, and nucleic acid sequences. The detection of glucose, lactate using electrochemical techniques such as amperometric and potentiometric gave fame to the sensors (Turner 2013). For example, the detection of glucose using enzyme-incorporated glucose electrochemical sensors became commercially viable for the treatment of diabetes. This decade has observed a significant enhancement in the on-chip sensors. The multiplex detection of analytes is made possible by a combination of a signal processing unit and microfluidic channels. Soft Lithography techniques were invented by George Whitesides. Using this lithography, we can use PDMS, a biocompatible, cost-effective, and easy-to-manage material during microfluidic channel fabrication (Whitesides et al. 2025). This development facilitates the use of portable diagnostic devices. In the case of optical sensors around the 1990s, the surface plasmon phenomena and fluorescence-based detection techniques were used to increase sensitivity (Homola 2008). The developed optical sensors were utilized for the detection of biomolecules such as proteins and DNA, which is crucial for the diagnosis of genetic and viral diseases. However, the expensive manufacturing cost limited the commercial scalability of the sensors.

In the 2000s, the incorporation of conductive nanomaterials into on-chip sensors tremendously increased the sensitivity and specificity and reduced the biofouling effects. The conductive material used such as graphene, carbon nanotubes, and nanoparticles. For example, the early detection of diseases is possible by attomolar limit of detection for biomolecules using nanowire-based field effect transistors (FETs) (Patolsky and Lieber 2005). These advancements have had a significant impact on the diagnosis of malignant diseases such as cancer, since it is possible to detect low concentrations of analytes such as prostate-specific antigen (PSA). Further, the application of multi-array technology is used for the detection of multiplex analytes in complex biofluids. The multi-array on-chip sensors provided high-throughput screening, which was crucial for the medical diagnosis (Schena 1996). For example, protein microarrays enabled proteomic research for the identification of disease biomarkers, while DNA microarrays enabled genetic profiling for customized therapy. Companies like Abbott and Roche brought portable diagnostic devices, which made the commercialized on-chip sensors available for personalized healthcare. Abbott's i-STAT system is a perfect example of on-chip sensors, as it quickly analyzes the blood for electrolytes, gases, and cardiac indicators for the treatment (Abbott Point of Care (2020), i-STAT System, https://www.pointofcare.abbott). To ensure the reproducibility between the sensors, they have used microfabrication techniques such as photolithography and thin-film deposition.

The easy-to-use, affordable, home-testing point of care increased the demand for these on-chip sensors in the 2010s. Another advancement in microfluidic devices was paper-based microfluidic sensors, also known as microfluidic paper analytical devices (μPADs) (Martinez et al. 2007). This development brought the cost of device fabrication very low, almost inexpensive in terms of scalability. In the microfluidic device, the flow of fluids by capillary action does not require the use of pumps like other microfluidic devices. In developing nations, HIV and malaria, the infectious diseases monitored using these devices.

In a similar vein, the wearable on-chip sensors were developed using a flexible substrate and controlled printing of electronic circuits on it. These wearable flexible sensors provide the real-time vital physiological parameters for personalized healthcare. These flexible sensors are easier to work with in the presence of non-invasive biological samples such as sweat, saliva, or interstitial fluids. And the biomarker is detected by sensors built into patches or wristbands (Gao et al. 2016). For example, continuous glucose monitoring using non-invasive methods was made feasible for diabetic care.

Further, the development was carried out from a data transmission perspective. The on-chip sensors were developed with wireless transmission of data and processing. Remote analysis of data and storage of healthcare data were made possible with the integration of on-chip sensors by cellphones and cloud-based systems (Liang et al. 2019). For example, the availability of diagnostic results at remote locations was enhanced using smartphone-based readers for lateral flow assays. Additionally, diagnostic accuracy and prediction were enhanced by the integration of machine learning, especially for malignant diseases such as cancer and neurological disorders. On-chip sensors have been developed with more complexity by integration of Internet-of-things (IoT) and artificial intelligence (AI) in 2020s. The prognosis and diagnosis of diseases in real time are made possible with AI algorithms and sensor data. AI-powered on-chip sensors help early diagnosis of Alzheimer's and heart diseases based on the minute trends in the biomarker profiles (Topol 2019). However, the addition of deep learning models and fuzzy logics decreases the false positive results in the complex biological samples and enhances the specificity of sensors.

The use of 2D materials such as quantum dots and MoS_2 is able to enhance the sensitivity of sensors in electrochemical and optical applications, and identify a single biomarker in complicated diseases for early detection of diseases (Nisar et al. 2024). Furthermore, the testing platform, such as an organ-on-chip, developed for the replication of physiological conditions, has improved the diagnostic sensors' accuracy (Huh et al. 2010). The application of on-chip sensors for rapid and robust diagnosis of the COVID-19 epidemic. The test result was available in a minute due to high-throughput data using microfluidic-based RT-PCR and incorporated antigen tests onto on-chip sensors (Nguyen et al. 2022). These developed sensors showed that they can be scalable and cost-effective compared to available techniques.

The interdisciplinary effort that has enabled the development of on-chip sensors throughout the years has facilitated the development of medical diagnostics. The on-chips sensors have changed the medical diagnostics from the first silicon-based transducers to nanomaterial functionalized ML-driven systems. They are robust, rapid, and affordable, which has improved the patients' healthcare across the globe. However, the challenges are still there, such as the sensitivity of low-abundance biomarkers, regulatory compliance, new developments in materials, and integration of advanced ML-based models. The on-chip sensors should be able to increase personalized healthcare monitoring and early detection of malignant diseases.

14.3 Materials and Promising Fabrication Techniques for Development of On-Chip Sensors

The fabrication of on-chip sensor devices is critical for advancing clinical diagnostics and improving patient personalized outcomes. This process involves selecting appropriate materials, designing based on specific medical requirements, and employing suitable fabrication methodologies. Key materials in lab-on-a-chip (LOC) development include silicon and glass, known for their structural integrity, alongside polymers like photoresists and elastomers such as polydimethylsiloxane (PDMS) (Nielsen et al. 2020). While silicon is often chosen for its surface functionalization capabilities, the high costs and hazardous production processes associated with silicon and glass limit their application in certain clinical contexts, particularly for continuous monitoring that requires gas permeation or extended cell culturing (Fuchs et al. 2021; Ren et al. 2013). In clinical applications, selecting materials that are cost-effective, biocompatible, and optically transparent is essential. Polymers, including thermoplastics like poly(methyl methacrylate) (PMMA) and polyethylene terephthalate (PET), have gained traction in clinical settings due to their versatility, despite their gas permeability limitations (Awaja et al. 2018; Xu et al. 2019). PDMS remains a popular material for microfluidic devices utilized in diagnostics due to its favorable characteristics, including ease of fabrication, non-cytotoxicity, and compatibility with biological samples. We integrate sensors into microfluidic channels made of polydimethylsiloxane (PDMS).

The photolithography (Moreira et al. 2015) process, while sophisticated and costly, is frequently employed in the manufacture of high-resolution sensors for clinical use. This multi-step procedure begins with the application of a photoresist onto a wafer, followed by UV exposure to create specific designs. After developing the patterns, metal deposition occurs, typically involving titanium (Ti) and gold layers, tailored to enhance sensor performance (Qamar and Shamsi 2020). The integration of insulating materials like SU-8 allows for the definition of electroactive areas, which is crucial for accurate biosensing applications (Whitesides et al. 2025; Fruncillo et al. 2021). Alternative fabrication techniques, such as screen printing (Lorestani et al. 2025), laser-induced printing, 3D printing, such as Inkjet printing (Carota et al. 2024), and paper-based microfluidic devices (Magro et al. 2017). These fabrication techniques are increasingly being explored for their potential in clinical diagnostics due to their cost-effectiveness and scalability. For example, *Uroš* et al. demonstrated the application of photolithography to develop multi-array electrochemical sensors for clinical analyte detection, enhancing the ability to diagnose conditions through precise and rapid measurement (Zupančič et al. 2021). *Ye* et al. further exemplified innovation in clinical sensor design by creating an inkjet-printed wearable sensor patch using a PET substrate. This patch, treated with oxygen plasma to increase hydrophilicity, incorporated a variety of electrodes for multimodal sensing, facilitating real-time patient monitoring (Ye et al. 2024). Such developments using photolithography and Ink-jet printing of clinical on-chip sensors for medical diagnosis illustrate the significant impact in clinical applications, providing tools for enhanced diagnostics and personalized healthcare.

However, screen printing is a promising, cost-effective, and relatively straightforward technique utilized in the development of clinical sensors, as shown in Fig. 14.2B. This method employs a mesh screen to transfer specific designs using a variety of inks, including gold, silver, and metal-based options. The resolution attained during screen printing spans from micrometres to millimetres, making it suitable for intricate sensor applications (Crapnell et al. 2022). Recent studies highlight the effectiveness of screen-printed gold electrodes in clinical diagnostics. For instance, Andreea-Cristina Mirica Ion et al. demonstrated the capability of these electrodes to detect cisplatin concentrations ranging from 0.0006 to 43.2 mg/mL and bleomycin levels between 0.23 and 7.56 μg/mL in serum samples, showcasing their potential for monitoring therapeutic drug levels (Mirica et al. 2024). Moreover, Lorestani et al. introduced an innovative wearable microfluidic on-chip system featuring enzymatic gold-graphene nanocomposite-modified laser-induced graphene (LIG) electrodes, coupled with a LIG-based pH sensor. This setup facilitates accurate and continuous monitoring of lactate levels in sweat, which is valuable for assessing metabolic conditions during physical activity (Lorestani et al. 2025).

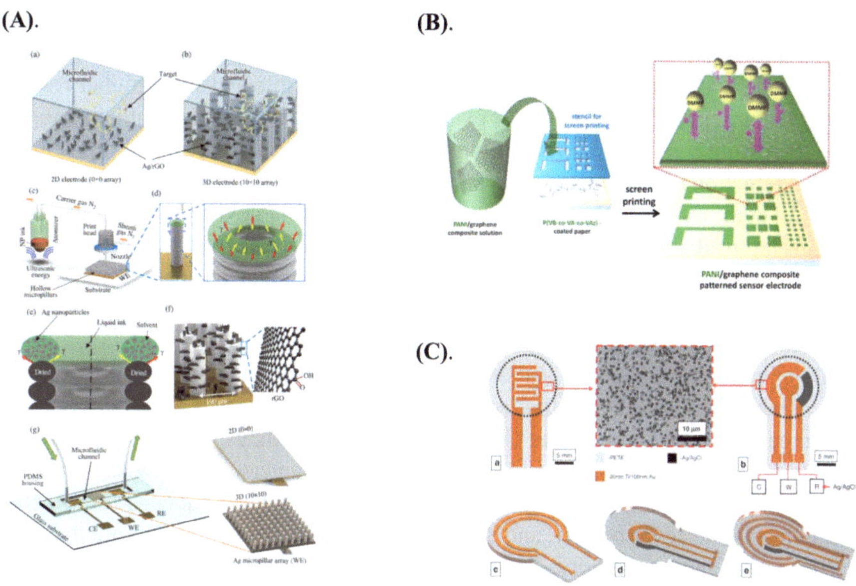

Fig. 14.2 Fabrication methodologies for on-chip multiarray electrode sensors (**A**). 3D printed micropillar array electrodes using Aerosol Jet nanoparticle for molecular sensing. (a, b) Schematic representations of random motion of molecules around electrodes. (c) Instrumentation of 3D printer with an atomizer and a print head. (d) The hollow-micropillar formation with concentric toroid-shaped rings of metal nanoparticle (NP) ink printed. (e) Cross-sectional view. (d). (f) A schematic showing the rGO flakes attached to the silver micropillars. (g) Schematic of the dopamine microfluidic sensing device (Ali et al. 2021). (**B**) Stencil-based screen printing of poly(aniline) (PANI)/graphene composite sensor electrodes (Yáñez-Sedeño et al. 2020). (**C**). (a, b) Fabrication of (a) interdigitated electrodes (IDEs) and (b) circular electrodes on PETE membranes. (c–e) Schematics of the (c) concentric IDEs on the top side (d) CV electrodes on the bottom side of the membrane, and (e) integration of both impedance and CV electrodes on one membrane (Ramiah Rajasekaran et al. 2020)

Zhou et al. focused on enhancing the reliability of DNA-based sensors by employing screen-printed gold leaf electrodes. They implemented a poly(vinyl alcohol) (PVA) hydrogel-based coating, which significantly improved the sensors' stability at ambient temperature. This advancement addresses the common stability issues faced by aptamer sensors, allowing them to maintain functionality for at least 2 months and endure temperatures up to 65 °C without affecting the biological assay (Zhou et al. 2025). These developments highlight the transformative potential of screen printing in the realm of clinical sensor technology.

In recent years, three-dimensional (3D) printing has been used quite frequently for the development of on-chip sensors. This is layer-by-layer printing of on-chip sensors using CAD software for pre-designed sensors (Mirica et al. 2024). In this technique, the required materials should be photopolymer resins (Lorestani et al. 2025; Bagheri and Jin 2019). Currently, there is a variety of 3D printing technologies, such as stereolithography (SLA), two-photon polymerization, fused deposition modelling (FDM), and bioprinting (Ho et al. 2015). Moreover, from a commercialization perspective, the inkjet is most cost-effective for the development of on-chip sensors. An inkjet printer does not require any mesh screen printing masks. The inkjet printer on-chip sensors are reproducible and show higher resolution (Qamar and Shamsi 2020). For example, Ali et al. used an aerosol jet nanoparticle 3D printing process shown in Fig. 14.2A, for the micropillar on-chip sensors for the detection of dopamine in the attomolar range (Ali et al. 2021). In addition to this, Liu et al. used a 3D printed microneedle biosensing device for the continuous monitoring of diabetes (Liu et al. 2021). Moreover, Rajasekaran et Al. developed a 3D printed, shown in Fig. 14.2C, modular, electrochemical sensor-integrated transwell system for monitoring cellular and molecular events in situ (Ramiah Rajasekaran et al. 2020).

Despite the advantages of screen printing, it is important to note that its resolution is inherently lower than that achievable by microfabricated electrodes. Within the screen printing process, the choice of ink material plays a decisive role in the quality of the final product. Several ink material parameters, such as viscosity, density, solid percentage, electrical resistivity, curing temperature, squeegee durometer, cleanup solvents, cytotoxicity, and storage time, are pivotal in determining the ink's performance and printability. These factors not only influence the manufacturing process but also the reliability and effectiveness of the diagnostic devices produced. Interestingly, when considering the transition to inkjet printing, there is an opportunity to optimize these parameters further. Inkjet printing provides a controlled printing process that allows for higher resolution than screen printing, albeit still lower than traditional microfabrication methods (Paimard et al. 2023).

The optimization of fabrication methods for cost-effective clinical diagnostics is essential in advancing medical technology. Among the various techniques, screen printing and laser-induced graphene (LIG) electrodes stand out due to their cost efficiency and promising potential for scalable integration with clinical devices. These methods present a viable option for developing medical on-chip sensors, allowing for the production of devices that can be mass-produced at a lower cost. In contrast, while methods such as 3D printing offer a highly controlled fabrication environment, they fall short in terms of scalability and production speed due to longer fabrication times. This limitation makes them less competitive compared to screen printing, particularly in scenarios where rapid deployment and affordability are critical. Moreover, the lithography process, while capable of achieving high precision, is burdened by exorbitant costs and the impractical maintenance of cleanroom environments, which are not always feasible for cost-efficient on-chip sensor applications.

Given these factors, it is crucial to evaluate the trade-offs associated with each fabrication technique in the context of cost-effective clinical diagnostics. As we delve deeper into this analysis, we will present a comparative Table 14.1 summarizing the advantages and limitations of these techniques. Furthermore, we will discuss several key studies in which researchers have elaborated on their respective fabrication processes, shedding light on best practices and innovations in the field. Ultimately, the focus remains on identifying the most suitable fabrication method

Table 14.1 Comparative table for the fabrication of electrodes and their commercialization feasibility

Fabrication technique	Number of steps	Material selection	Advantages/disadvantages
Microfabrication (Fruncillo et al. 2021)	Involves photolithography, etching, and thin film deposition	Metals (Au, Ag, Cu) Semiconductors (Si,), Dielectrics (SiO_2) Substrate: Si, glass, quartz wafers	Advantage: High precision and performance. Disadvantage: Costly due to complex processes, not easy to commercialization
Screen Printing (Paimard et al. 2023)	Mesh screen for deposition of conductive ink	Carbon (graphite, carbon nanotubes), metals (Au, Ag, Pt), Ag/AgCl Substrate: Plastics (PET, polyimide), ceramics, paper (Whatman chromatography paper) Binders and solvents (ethylene glycol, cellulose acetate)	Advantage: Cost-effective, scalable, and *high potential of commercialization* Disadvantage: Lower resolution of fabrication
Inkjet printing (Carota et al. 2024)	Drop-on-demand deposition of functional inks	Inks: Metal nanoparticle (Ag, Au, Cu). Conductive polymers (PEDOT:PSS, polyaniline), carbon-based (graphene, CNTs). Substrate: PET, polyimide, paper, glass. Inks with lower viscosity (<20 mPa.s) and surface tension (<80 mN.m^{-1})	Advantage: High resolution, scalable, low material waste, compatible with digital prototyping, and *limited commercialization capability* Disadvantage: Slower printing speed, and trained personnel to operate
Roll-to-roll (R2R) printing	Continuous printing on flexible substrate using gravure, flexography	Similar to screen printing inks	Advantage: *Suitable for mass production*. Disadvantage: Complex setup, high initial costs, and only for flexible sensors
Laser-induced graphene (LIG) (Lorestani et al. 2025)	Use of laser to convert carbon-rich substrate into porous graphene. Maskless method	Substrate: Polyimide, paper. No use of inks, a mix of nanoparticles for the enhancement of the material preferred.	Advantage: Low cost, *high potential for scalability*. Disadvantage: Limited substrate choice
3D printing (Bagheri and Jin 2019)	Layer-by-layer deposition of conductive materials using extrusion, binder jetting, and stereolithography	Conductive filaments (carbon, graphene, metal-filled polymers), conductive resins.	Advantage: Controlled fabrication, high resolution, high reproducibility Disadvantage: Small-scale production, slower printing speeds, material costs, and mass resolution

that balances cost efficiency, scalability, and performance, ensuring that advancements in clinical diagnostics are accessible and effective for improving health outcomes.

14.4 Innovation in Multi-array On-Chip Sensors for Biomarker Detection

In the previous section, we delved into the diverse fabrication techniques employed in the development of sensors, highlighting the significant promise of screen printing technology. This segment focuses on applying these variously fabricated sensors for the detection, early monitoring, and diagnosis of diseases across a range of medical contexts. Initially, we will explore the critical role of multi-array sensors in medical diagnostics and point-of-care testing, emphasizing their ability to provide swift and accurate results that are crucial for timely medical intervention. Furthermore, the discussion will extend to wearable devices, which represent a groundbreaking advancement in personalized healthcare. These devices enable continuous health monitoring and deliver real-time updates, empowering individuals to take charge of their health and stay informed about their physiological status.

In the context of these innovations, it is essential to consider how on-chip sensors compare to traditional sensors in terms of medical diagnostics. The following Table 14.2 will illustrate the key differences between these two approaches, examining factors such as sensitivity, portability, cost-effectiveness, and integration with digital health technologies. Through this comparison, we can better understand the transformative impact that on-chip sensors can have on the future of medical diagnostics and personalized patient care.

The utilization of on-chip sensors for disease diagnosis has gained attention due to their potential to facilitate rapid and minimally invasive assessment. Traditionally, these sensors have relied on a single analyte biomarker for detecting various diseases. However, this method proves to be problematic as it can lead to unreliable diagnoses, particularly due to interference from other diseases. For example, in the case of bladder and oral cancers, the level of hydrogen peroxide is known to fluctuate in both conditions, thereby complicating the interpretation of results when assessed through a singular biomarker (Kishi et al. 2024; Ursini et al. 2016). This limitation underscores the necessity for a more robust diagnostic approach that employs multiplex biomarker strategies for both diagnosis and prognosis. By analyzing multiple biomarkers simultaneously, multiplex-based diagnostic methods can provide a more comprehensive view of a patient's health status, increasing the specificity and sensitivity of the detection process (Li et al. 2025). Such an approach is particularly advantageous in clinical settings where a definitive diagnosis is critical for effective treatment planning and patient management.

Furthermore, multiplex on-chip sensors leverage the advantages of cross-reactivity and partial selectivity, which are essential for overcoming the challenges posed by complex biological samples, such as blood or other biofluids. These challenges include biofouling, the gradual accumulation of unwanted substances onto

Table 14.2 A comparative study of traditional versus on-chip sensors for medical diagnosis

Criteria	Traditional sensors	On-chip sensors
Size and portability	Bench-top or bulky instruments	Miniaturized, portable, and usually handheld
Requirement of sample volume	Need for a comparatively large sample volume (mL)	Small sample volume (μL)
Result time	A longer time, usually more than few hours or a day	Rapid or real-time diagnosis
Sensitivity and specificity	Good, but needs amplification in the signal	Enhanced due to micro−/nano-scale effects, higher surface-to-volume ratio
Integration of the system	Usually, all devices are separate for sample preparation, reaction, and detection	Integrated combined platforms on on-chip sensors
Throughput	Usually low to medium	High throughput, parallel processing possible
User	Need for trained personnel to operate the instrument and LAN infrastructure	User-friendly and point-of-care testing
Cost per test	Expensive	Lower cost per test and cost-efficient for scalable use
Maintenance	Timely calibration and servicing	One-time use chips or minimal maintenance
Biofouling and contamination	More prone due to large use of sample volume.	Lower
Data integration	Usually off-line analysis	Integrate with electronics, cloud storage and smartphone-based readouts
Examples	ELISA plates, benchtop electrochemical potentiostat, and spectrophotometers	Glucose test strips, pregnancy tests, electrochemical on-chip sensors, and organ-on-chip systems

the sensor surfaces, which leads to an associated increase in signal drift over time, and the potential interference from various biomolecules present in the sample. As these issues can significantly affect sensor performance and the reliability of results, addressing them is crucial for ensuring the clinical viability of these technologies. To facilitate real-world adoption of multiplex on-chip sensors, it is imperative to engage in rigorous validation processes that reflect typical clinical environments. This includes conducting large-scale, multicenter studies to assess the performance of these sensors across diverse populations and disease states. Real-world validation not only enhances the credibility of the diagnostic tools but also provides insights into the practical challenges that may arise during implementation in clinical practice (Tibaduiza et al. 2024).

In conclusion, the advancement of multiplex on-chip sensors represents a significant leap forward in the diagnosis and prognosis of diseases. By prioritizing clinical adoption through real-world validation and addressing the inherent problems associated with single-biomarker detection, these technologies stand to improve patient outcomes and transform the landscape of medical diagnostics. Continued research and collaboration between academia, industry, and healthcare providers will be essential for overcoming existing barriers and ensuring the successful integration of these innovative diagnostic tools into everyday clinical use. Lee et al. fabricated micrometer-thick and porous nanocomposite coating for the electrochemical sensors. The nozzle printed antifouling layer is used to create a micrometer-thick conducting coating using cross-linked albumin, interconnected pores, and gold nanowires. The sensitivity of developed multianalyte sensors is 3.75 to 17-fold enhanced with high specificity. They used the developed system for the multi-analyte testing, such as CRISPR, antigen (Ag), and antibody (Ab), as shown in Fig. 14.3A (Lee et al. 2024). Timlsina *et.al* developed a multi-array sensor on a chip. On-chip fabricated with four electrodes and one counter electrode. Using this on-chip sensor, they detected four clinically relevant biomarkers of myocardial infarction (MI) and traumatic brain injury (TBI), cTnlTC, S100, NT pro-BNP, and GFAP in whole blood by modifying the electrode surface with antifouling conductive nanomaterials (Timilsina et al. 2022). In addition to this, there is another similar multiplex analyte on-chip graphene sensor used for the detection of sepsis biomarkers. The biomarkers were procalcitonin (PCT), C-reactive protein (CRP), phosphorylcholine (PC), and pathogen-associated molecular patterns (PAMPs) in whole blood samples (Zupančič et al. 2021). In both the above-mentioned articles, the author used the same strategy of modifying the electrode surface with bovine serum albumin (BSA) incorporated with conductive materials such as reduced graphene flakes, and then used glutaraldehyde for the crosslinking, which facilitates the open porous structure and enhances the conductivity of the deposited film. Later, they have used the specific assay of antibody horseperoxidase-poly-HRP streptavidin and then used 3,3′,5.5′-tetramethylbenzimide (TMB) substrate that facilitates the signal transduction. This device costs approximately $0.08, which is economical, suitable for on-site testing, and has the potential to be commercialized. Rosella *et.al* reported an easy-to-use array sensor for the detection of human salivary stress biomarkers such as cortisol, adrenaline, and dopamine. They have used 18 different fluorescent organic dyes to develop a biomimetic (tongue-mimic) multi-array sensor, shown in Fig. 14.3B, associated with an optical physicochemical transducer (Santonocito et al. 2025).

The multiplex on-chip sensor paves the way for the wearable sensing platform. After this, we are trying to make wearable devices, but unfortunately, we are facing some shortcomings, such as the need for flexible on-chip sensors, as a rigid substrate would not be efficient. Therefore, the researchers have taken advantage of Inkjet printing and made wearable devices. Ye *et.al* developed a personalized wearable patch sensor as explained in the previous section of this chapter. They have modified the thiol-based aptamer onto the gold and MXene printed electrode, and another working electrode with gold only. They used electrodeposition of polyaniline pH sensing membrane onto a gold electrode. The multiplexing wearable patch sensor used for non-invasive female oestradiol hormone, which is crucial for female fertility and women's health (Ye et al. 2024). Silva et al. presented a 3D printed immuno and geno-electrochemical sensor shown in the Fig. 14.3C for the quantitative detection of protein A29 and the DNA of monkeypox virus (Silva et al. 2024).

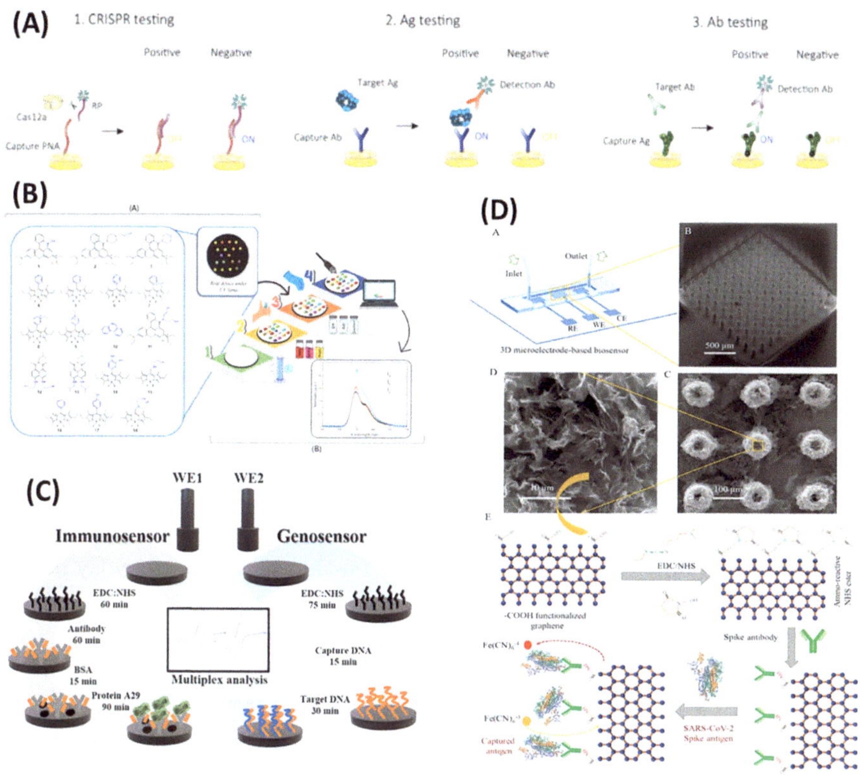

Fig. 14.3 Mechanism of on-chip multi-biomarkers medical diagnosis sensors (**A**). Antifouling functionalization for sensors (a). Schematics of multi-analyte enzymatic detection of SARS-CoV-2 RNA, antigen, and host antibody using antifouling coating sensors (Lee et al. 2024). (**B**) Schematic representation of the multiarray sensor using a fluorescent probe for the detection of stress biomarker by a portable spectrophotometer (Santonocito et al. 2025). (**C**). Specific electrochemical multiplex sensors by functionalization of (a). antibody (WE1—immunosensor) for label-free detection of the specific MKPV antigen and (WE2—genosensor) by anchoring the capture DNA and its hybridization with MKPV target DNA (Silva et al. 2024). (**D**). 3D printed electrochemical sensor for detection of SARS-CoV-2 VOCs. (A) Schematic presentation of a 3D printed gold nanoparticle sensor. (B) SEM image of micropillar electrode array. (C, D) SEM images of a gold microelectrode modified by graphene. (E) Surface functionalization by SARS-CoV-2 spike S1 antibodies on rGO-Au electrode to capture the antigens, which leads to hindering the electron transfer of Ferro/Ferricyanide molecules (Ali et al. 2024)

Lorestani et al. developed on-chip wearable sensors for the detection of lactate and pH in sweat samples. They have integrated the sweat collection system using a circular microfluidic channel with lactate oxidase (LOx) conductive nanocomposite functionalized laser-induced graphene (LIG) electrode and on-chip pH for on-body detection and monitoring of lactate levels from sweat samples (Lorestani et al. 2025). Ali et al. reported the advanced healthcare platform using an aerosol jet 3D printer, shown in Fig. 14.3D, the 3D microelectrode array modified by graphene and later antibodies specific to severe acute respiratory syndrome coronavirus-2 (SARS-CoV-2) spike antigens (Ali et al. 2024).

The advancement of on-chip sensors represents a significant innovation in medical diagnostics, enabling heightened accuracy in disease diagnosis and prognosis through multiplexing capabilities. These sensors utilize various materials and technologies, such as nanocomposite coatings and graphene, to enhance sensitivity and specificity in detecting multiple biomarkers simultaneously. Recent studies have demonstrated the successful application of on-chip sensors for monitoring conditions such as myocardial infarction, traumatic brain injury, and sepsis through the analysis of whole blood samples. Researchers are also exploring non-invasive methods, such as wearable devices, to track crucial health metrics like hormone levels and lactate in sweat. The integration of advanced manufacturing techniques, including inkjet printing and 3D printing, is paving the way for the development of flexible, user-friendly diagnostic tools. These innovations not only improve patient outcomes but also aim to streamline clinical workflows and enable on-site testing. Overall, ongoing research and collaboration among various sectors, such as the collaboration between industry and academia, are essential for overcoming existing challenges and fully realizing the potential of on-chip sensors in everyday healthcare settings.

14.5 Integration of Machine Learning with On-Chip Sensors for Medical Diagnosis

On-chip sensors have transformed medical diagnostics by enabling rapid, portable, and cost-effective point-of-care (PoC) testing. These systems process pico to microliter fluid volumes to detect biomarkers, cells, or molecules. The integration of Machine Learning with the on-chip sensors brought a paradigm shift in medical diagnosis due to enhanced accuracy and better prediction of diseases (Sakib et al. 2025). The compound annual growth rate is expected to increase 40% globally from $811 million due to the use of artificial intelligence in medical healthcare (Shahid et al. 2019). The recorded signals using on-chip sensors generally consist of noisy signals and do not follow a linear trend, such as an increase in concentration of analyte will not give you increase in peak current. The non-linear trend is mainly observed due to biological complexity, sensor limitations, low metabolite concentration in the physiological range in the biofluid, such as saliva, urine, blood, and sweat samples, using different transduction such as electrochemical and optical (Lee et al. 2024; Khondakar et al. 2025). Besides this, the biological fluids are very complex, made up of many proteins, enzymes, and other substances. These unwanted substances (matrix effect) cause biofouling on chip-on sensors, resulting in a decrease in the ability of sensors to detect the analyte of interest (Sabaté Del Río et al. 2019). Many researchers have tried to modify the electrode surface with different polymers crosslinked with a variety of linkers, zwitterion coating (Saxena et al. 2024), molecularly imprinted polymers (MIP) (Cetinkaya et al. 2025), and also polymer incorporated with conducting materials such as gold nanowires, MXenes, and graphene oxide (Pandey et al. 2023). This development definitely increases the ability and lifetime of on-chip sensors, but for a limited duration, and these additional antifouling strategies make the fabrication of on-chip sensors complicated. To overcome this challenge, machine learning plays a crucial role and enhances the ability of on-chip sensors.

However, the recorded electrochemical/optical noisy signal from biofluids can be useful for the machine learning models to find the trend in the dataset for medical diagnosis (Allegrini and Olivieri 2016). There are many ML models available, such as artificial neural network (ANN), random forest, gradient boosting methods, and many more. These models try to extract the features using recorded signals via principal component analysis (PCA). The features could be the area under the curve, peak potentials, peak current, shift in the signals, and change in noise level with variation of samples (Chen et al. 2023). After feature extraction, the model can be trained, validated, and tested using cross-validation on available datasets.

However, Machine learning models are highly dependent on high-dimensional data; the performance of ML-based models improves with more data. Machine learning is about learning from data and making predictions or classifications. Whereas Fuzzy logic is less dependent on large datasets, relies more on expert knowledge, and uses rule-based systems, Fuzzy logic is more about handling uncertainty and making decisions based on imprecise information. The modelling of imprecise data through membership functions with values between 0 and 1 offers a robust framework for handling uncertainty. A fuzzy logic system involves fuzzification, converting crisp sensor data (e.g., biomarker concentrations) into fuzzy sets (e.g., "low," "medium," "high"), a knowledge base with if-then rules, an inference engine mapping inputs to outputs, and defuzzification, yielding actionable diagnostic results. This approach excels in managing uncertainties from biological samples or low-power wireless body area network (WBAN) constraints, enhancing diagnostic accuracy (Nalbant 2024).

Key Functions of Fuzzy Logic

(i) *Handling Uncertainty*: On-chip sensors, such as electrochemical or optical biosensors, often produce noisy or incomplete data due to low analyte concentrations or interference from complex biological samples (e.g., blood, saliva). Fuzzy logic mitigates these issues by assigning partial memberships, enabling reliable classification of health states (e.g., "normal," "at-risk," "critical").

(ii) *Nonlinear Data Processing:* Biological systems exhibit nonlinear relationships, which fuzzy logic captures without requiring precise mathematical models, unlike traditional algorithms (Shahid et al. 2019). This is critical for interpreting multivariate sensor data, such as combining glucose, pH, and temperature readings.

(iii) *Decision Support:* Fuzzy inference systems (FIS) integrate multiple sensor inputs to provide nuanced diagnostic outputs, supporting clinicians in decision-making (Ieracitano et al. 2022). For instance, fuzzy logic can classify a patient's condition based on ambiguous biomarker levels, improving diagnostic accuracy.

(iv) *Adaptability*: Fuzzy systems are easily tuned by adjusting membership functions or rules, making them versatile for diverse diagnostic applications (Zadeh 1965).

Applications in Medical Diagnostics Fuzzy logic enhances several commercialized on-chip sensor applications in medical diagnostics, addressing challenges in data interpretation and decision-making. For example, in cardiovascular diagnostics, the QuidelOrtho Triage System uses fluorescence immunoassays with the Triage MeterPro to measure cardiac biomarkers, including troponin I, creatine kinase-MB, myoglobin, and B-type natriuretic peptide (BNP), in EDTA-anticoagulated whole blood or plasma, delivering results in 15–20 min to diagnose myocardial infarction or heart failure (https://www.quidelortho.com/global/en). Fuzzy logic can enhance interpretation by classifying biomarker levels as "normal," "elevated," or "critical," using rules like "IF troponin I is high AND BNP is elevated, THEN risk is critical," accounting for noise or patient-specific factors like age.

In diabetes management, Abbott's FreeStyle Libre 3 employs an electrochemical sensor to measure interstitial fluid glucose, providing readings every minute for up to 14 days. Fuzzy logic categorizes glucose levels as "low," "normal," or "high," addressing sensor drift or temperature variability with rules like "IF glucose is low AND trend is decreasing, THEN alert for hypoglycemia". Recent advancements have further enhanced non-invasive glucose testing by combining a fuzzy logic-based calibration mechanism with an infrared (IR) sensor and Arduino controller, utilizing mid-infrared (MIR) absorbance in fingertips and human tears. This calibration technique achieves high accuracy and reliability, with an error rate of less than 3% according to the Error Grid Analysis (EGA), where 97.5% of 360 measurements fell into zone A, 2.2% into zone B, and 0.3% into zone C of the Clarke Error Grid, demonstrating robust performance for PoC diabetes monitoring (Nazha et al. 2023).

For infectious diseases like influenza, combining neural networks and fuzzy c-means (FCM) clustering achieved efficient detection of higher-risk influenza patients with $SpO2 < 96\%$ within 10 s (Sun et al. 2015). Fuzzy logic also enhances chronic disease and cancer diagnostics. Microfluidic aptamer-based sensors detect biomarkers like glycated hemoglobin (HbA1c) for diabetes or chronic kidney disease, improving accuracy in PoC settings (Moznuzzaman et al. 2021). Adaptive neuro-fuzzy inference systems (ANFIS) enhance cancer detection, such as glioma brain tumors, by classifying biosensor-derived MRI data in low-power WBAN systems, reducing errors from noisy signals (Selvapandian and Manivannan 2018). In cancer diagnostics, plasmonic metamaterial sensors detect biomarkers like circulating tumor cells at high sensitivity, where fuzzy logic integrates multiple signals to classify cancer risk despite data ambiguity.

Fuzzy logic enhances accuracy by handling low-concentration analytes and noisy signals, classifying results as "positive," "probable," or "negative" through integrated inputs like viral load and temperature, as seen in smartphone-based reverse transcription loop-mediated isothermal amplification (RT-LAMP) platforms (Kumar et al. 2024; Khalil and Rahman 2023).

The incorporation of machine learning, particularly through fuzzy logic frameworks, significantly enhances the clinical adoption and real-world validation of on-chip sensors utilized in medical diagnostics. This synergy improves data interpretation and decision-making processes, thus elevating the accuracy and reliability of diagnostic tools employed in diverse clinical settings, including cardiovascular assessment, diabetes monitoring, and oncological detection. Machine learning algorithms adeptly classify biomarker levels while accounting for patient-specific variables, environmental influences, and sensor noise, thereby addressing prevalent challenges such as sensor drift and data ambiguity. Such capabilities not only facilitate timely and personalized patient care but also ensure that emerging diagnostic technologies undergo robust validation processes. This promotes heightened confidence among healthcare practitioners and patients in the application of these innovative solutions across a range of medical scenarios, ultimately contributing to the advancement of precision medicine.

14.6 Clinical Validation of On-Chip Sensors with Real Patient Samples

Clinical validation using real patient specimens is crucial for establishing the reliability and diagnostic application of the on-chip sensor. For example, a silicon photonic microring resonator immunosensor designed to detect MCP-1, a key inflammatory biomarker, demonstrated outstanding analytical performance when tested with spiked human serum samples. It achieved a limit of detection (LOD) as low as approximately 0.5 pg/mL and exhibited a linear detection range that spans nearly two orders of magnitude (from 84 to 1582 pg/mL). Additionally, the sensor showed excellent dynamic range and specificity, successfully meeting clinically relevant thresholds for conditions such as fibromyalgia and ovarian cancer (Valera et al. 2016). The other cost-effective on-chip-based clinical validation case studies are Laksanasopin T. et al., who reported a smartphone dongle for diagnosis of HIV and syphilis using the mChip platform for \$1 to \$1.50 for 96 patients. The result time is only 15 min. The triplex assay has 92–100% sensitivity and 79–100% specificity versus the gold standard of the lab (Laksanasopin et al. 2015). Ganguli A. et al. reported a 3D portable rapid isothermal amplification microfluidic detection system for SARS-CoV-2. They demonstrated the 20 unidentified clinical samples with 100% agreement, and the detection limit is 50 RNA copies/μL in 30–40 min (Ganguli et al. 2020). Recent studies have provided interesting evidence for the clinical validation of cost-effective on-chip sensors utilizing real patient samples, establishing their diagnostic reliability compared to traditional laboratory methods. These findings suggest that on-chip platforms are adequately prepared for routine application in clinical settings.

14.7 Decentralization and Socioeconomic Impact of On-Chip Sensors

On-chip sensors represent a significant advancement in healthcare technology, potentially transforming socioeconomic outcomes by alleviating the pressures existing healthcare systems face. These devices provide rapid, low-cost, point-of-care diagnostics, reducing the reliance on centralized laboratories and hospitals. This structural shift leads to a noticeable decrease in healthcare expenditures for patients and providers. Additionally, detecting diseases early with these sensors helps prevent costly medical complications. Decentralized diagnostic testing improves access to healthcare services in rural and underserved areas, ultimately addressing disparities in healthcare delivery. On-chip sensors can seamlessly integrate with hospital infrastructure and existing healthcare systems. They can be connected to electronic health record (EHR) systems, allowing automatic data entry and real-time updates. This integration enables healthcare providers to quickly access and analyze patient data, leading to more informed clinical decisions. Furthermore, these sensors can be incorporated into telemedicine platforms, enhancing remote patient monitoring and supporting healthcare providers in managing patients outside traditional clinical settings. By lowering out-of-pocket costs and enabling extensive screening initiatives, these technologies improve operational efficiency and alleviate overcrowding in healthcare facilities, promoting more strategic resource allocation (Ordóñez and Roggen 2016; Saric et al. 2019).

Beyond the immediate economic implications, deploying on-chip sensors strengthens public health resilience through real-time disease monitoring and surveillance, crucial during epidemiological outbreaks and pandemics. Furthermore, these sensors empower patients by providing self-monitoring capabilities, encouraging healthier lifestyle choices, and enabling seamless integration with digital health platforms. This integration accelerates clinical decision-making processes. On a macroeconomic level, adopting on-chip sensor technology catalyzes innovation, generates employment opportunities, and enhances national competitiveness in biomedical markets. Collectively, these factors help alleviate systemic burdens, improve health equity, and produce sustainable economic and social benefits (Mahmud et al. 2018; Nakhleh et al. 2017).

14.8 Challenges and Future Directions

14.8.1 Challenges of the On-Chip Sensors

Some challenges still obstruct the widespread adoption and performance of on-chip sensors. The challenges are in the technical, regulatory, and commercial domains; we need a solution to enhance the efficacy and accessibility of on-chip sensors. As we understand in the previous section of this chapter, the sensors' sensitivity and specificity are challenged in the complex biofluid matrices. The electrochemical and optical on-chip sensors must detect low concentration analytes, such as prostate-specific antigen for cancer, in the presence of interfering species in biofluids like blood or saliva (Malik et al. 2023). Non-specific binding and cross-reactivity can lead to false-positive results that decrease the reliability of the diagnosis. For example, electrochemical sensors suffer greatly due to biofouling (Meng et al. 2023). However, in the case of optical sensors, they need a signal amplification technique to overcome the limitation of low analyte detection (Homola 2008). To address these challenges, we need to advance in surface chemistry, such as antifouling coating, specific bioreceptors (Chen et al. 2024), and the design of sensors (Lee et al. 2024). The scalability of On-chip sensors is a significant hurdle due to their reproducibility (Yager et al. 2006; Scott and Ali 2021). However, paper-based microfluidic devices are affordable, but their sensitivity and reproducibility are often lower than the silicon-based devices (Aryal and Henry 2024). Facilitating the affordable On-chips sensors is essential for the global adoption that enhances personalized medical diagnostics (Balsam et al. 2013).

The combination of the existing healthcare system with the on-chip sensors poses challenges in terms of compatibility and standardization of data. As we know, on-chip sensors generate a variety of data sets that must be integrated with electronic health records and workflows (Hosain et al. 2024). Lack of standardization of data collection protocols may hinder interoperability and acceptance in hospitals (Bukowski et al. 2020). In addition to this, multiplexed diagnosis using multiple sensors can cause complexity in the design, data set, and power requirements (Sattar et al. 2023). Regulatory approval for on-chip sensors is a significant barrier due to strict requirements from agencies like the US Food and Drug Administration (FDA) and the European Medicines Agency (EMA) for ensuring the safety of humans. The developed device must be able to demonstrate clinical accuracy of more than 90%, be safe to use, and undergo multiple extensive validation studies, which are non-economical and time-consuming (Center for Devices and Radiological Health 2025). For example, Dexcom G7 needs to do thorough testing for continuous glucose monitoring across diverse patient populations and conditions (Avari et al. 2023). The inefficient standard protocols for novel sensor types, such as the utilization of nanomaterials, further complicate regulatory approvals (Fischer 2008). These obstacles delay the product entry to the market and increase the costs.

The point-of-care devices require user training to ensure proper operation and interpretation of results. For non-invasive biofluids, without proper guidance, the sample collection and preparation can be error-prone (Hosseinzadeh Fakhr et al. 2024). In limited resource settings, user-friendly designs and clear guidelines are crucial but challenging to implement without compromising device complexity (Nayak et al. 2019). However, providing access to everyone will be challenging due to costs and a lack of infrastructure (Patel et al. 2024).

14.8.2 Future Directions

The future of On-chip sensors for medical diagnosis is due to more complex designs and miniaturization of devices such as ingestible electronic capsules capable of sensing different gases and H_2S in the gut (Kalantar-Zadeh et al. 2018; Stine et al. 2024). The advancement in novel materials, digitization, and sustainable manufacturing each contributes to enhanced performance and accessibility.

To overcome the limitation of sensitivity and specificity by using the CRISPR-based detection on on-chip sensors. The CRISPR-modified on-chip sensors facilitate high specificity for nucleic acid detection, which increases the sensitivity. For the detection of RNA or DNA mutations, an on-chip CRISPR-Cas 12 and Cas 13 platform is used, and the sensitivity is comparable to that of PCR. This enables the rapid diagnosis of infectious diseases and genetic disorders (Hu et al. 2024). A microfluidic chip with a potential for commercialization in portable diagnosis of SARS-CoV-2 with an attomolar detection limit using CRISPR-cas (Robin et al. 2023). However, the 2D materials such as graphene, molybdenum disulfide, and quantum dots have the potential to increase the sensitivity, durability, and reduce the biofouling of on-chip sensors. These 2D materials enable single-molecule detection, facilitating ultra-early disease diagnosis (Barbosa et al. 2021). For example, in cancer and neurodegenerative disease, a graphene-based field effect transistor has detected the low-abundance biomarker (Krishnan et al. 2023). Besides this, antifouling nanomaterials such as zwitterionic coatings can reduce the biofouling effect and decrease the signal drift in complex biofluids (Amoako et al. 2025). These advancements will improve specificity, sensitivity, and address the signal challenges.

Implantable on-chip sensors are an advanced, continuous health monitoring device. These devices get power from biocompatible energy harvesting methods such as piezoelectric or thermoelectric systems, and can measure biomolecules such as glucose and lactate within the human body (Liu et al. 2023). For example, implantable electrochemical sensors provide real-time feedback about diabetes management by wireless transmission (Ameen et al. 2025). Wearable flexible sensors, such as sweat-based patches, will address non-invasive metabolite monitoring (Gao et al. 2023).

Machine learning is more familiar with biosensors due to their wide application. However, the integration of artificial intelligence and machine learning into on-chip sensors will enhance quick data analysis, diagnostic accuracy, and reproducible results. Machine algorithms use models such as artificial neural networks and random forests to analyze the subtle changes in the biomarker patterns, increasing reliability and reducing false positives in the multiplexed diagnosis (Wasilewski et al. 2024). For example, the detection of Alzheimer's disease by analyzing the protein profile in cerebrospinal fluid using AI-on-chip sensors (Hou et al. 2025). For improving the interoperability and supporting telehealth, real-time data processing and integration with EHRs using a cloud platform is suitable (Ehrenstein et al. 2019). The advancements integrating fuzzy logic with artificial intelligence (AI) and the Internet of Things (IoT), as seen in recent studies, promise smarter diagnostics, particularly for chronic diseases and viral detection using biodegradable or smartphone-integrated LoC systems. Fuzzy logic's robustness and flexibility make it integral to systems like the Triage System, FreeStyle Libre, and Check4, driving innovation in precise, reliable PoC testing (Ieracitano et al. 2022; Sun et al. 2015).

Sustainability in the on-chip sensors can be addressed by using biodegradable and eco-friendly materials for fabrication. Biodegradable polymers and paper-based on-chip microfluidic sensors can reduce the impact while ensuring the enhancement in medical diagnostics (Macdonald et al. 2017). Use of 3D printing will lower the fabrication costs and scalable production of customized sensors (Zhang et al. 2025). This will enable low-cost device production and promote global health equity.

Integration of Digital Health The integration of on-chip sensor data with the patient's health records provides a platform for clinicians to tailor treatments to individual needs (Shahid et al. 2019). For example, to optimize diabetes management strategies, the combination of glucose sensor data with lifestyle and genetic data is essential (Ordóñez and Roggen 2016). IoT sensors facilitate real-time monitoring and data sharing with healthcare providers and improve patient outcomes in acute disease management (Saric et al. 2019).

Regulatory and Standardization Advances To develop a standard validation protocol for on-chip sensors and streamline the regulatory approval process. The product to get market fit needs collaborative efforts of manufacturers, regulatory agencies, and academic institutions to speed up product market entry and ensure safety and efficacy (Mahmud et al. 2018). For example, the standard testing protocol for nanomaterial-based sensors could drastically reduce the validation costs (Nakhleh et al. 2017).

The on-chip sensors for commercialization faced multiple challenging hurdles, such as sensitivity and specificity limitations, high production costs, regulatory hurdles, and standard operating procedures. However, in the future, the incorporation of CRISPR-based on-chip sensors can overcome the sensitivity and specificity, advance material integration, inclusion of fuzzy with AI, and digitization of patient data for personalized healthcare, suggesting promising solutions. These advancements will enhance on-chip sensor performance for medical diagnostics and enhance personalized healthcare.

14.9 Conclusion

The commercialization of on-chip sensors for medical diagnostics showed a significant leap in personalized healthcare monitoring, detection, and management. The miniaturized, integrated with microfluidics, compact-sized device has exploited point-of-care diagnostics by the combinatorial effect of sensing and data processing with accurate results in complex biofluids. This conclusion will focus on the key advancement in terms of on-chip sensor development, emphasizing the pivotal role in advancing personalized medicine, improving accessibility to global health, and pressing healthcare needs.

On-chip sensors are fabricated using different techniques, but only a few affordable fabrication techniques, such as screen printing, are available for scalability. These devices are preferred due to their excellent working ability in complex biofluids and are also capable of multiplexing biomarker analysis for the diagnosis of diseases (Xu et al. 2019; Carota et al. 2024). The diverse application of sensors from disease diagnosis to continuous monitoring plays an essential role in the personalized health sector (Garg et al. 2022; Seshadri et al. 2019; Krutkyte et al. 2025). Commercial examples such as Dexcom G7(Garg et al. 2022) and Abbott FreeStyle Libre for continuous glucose monitoring, and Ellume's COVID-19 home test based on antigen detection, have demonstrated the practical and significant impact of on-chip sensors, which are making life better. The integration of cloud-based systems and real-time processing of data in mobile phones enables on-time diagnosis updates using a user-friendly interface (Yager et al. 2006).

The importance of on-chip sensors is their ability to address critical healthcare challenges. Their portability and small sample volumes make them suitable for POC testing, essentially in resource-limited settings where access to laboratory infrastructure is limited (Yetisen et al. 2013). For example, paper-based microfluidic sensors have affordable diagnostic tools for malaria and HIV diseases in developing regions (Lehnert and Gijs 2024). Wearable electrochemical sensors are used as continuous monitoring devices that empower patients with acute or chronic conditions to manage their health proactively, improving results such as A1C levels and time in range for diabetes (Martens et al. 2021). The rapid and robust response of on-chip sensors, exemplified by their role in high-throughput COVID-19 testing, has proven invaluable during public health crises and favors timely interventions (Richens et al. 2020). Besides this, the inclusion of machine learning models such as ANN and RF with fuzzy logics has enhanced the diagnostic and prognosis accuracy by complex matrices of biofluids, such as lung cancer (Shabu et al. 2024), breast cancer (Algehyne et al. 2022), and Alzheimer's (Shahid et al. 2019).

Notwithstanding these developments, on-chip sensors still have several issues that need to be resolved if their full potential is to be achieved. Since non-specific binding and biofouling make it difficult to detect low-abundance biomarkers in complex biofluids, sensitivity and specificity continue to be significant obstacles (Carroll and Mendes 2023). Because high-precision fabrication methods like photolithography are expensive and restrict mass production, scalability is another issue (Fruncillo et al. 2021). Extensive validation is necessary for regulatory approval from organizations such as the FDA and EMA, which delays market launch and raises costs (https://www.fda.gov). Standardized data protocols are necessary for integration with current healthcare systems, such as electronic health records, in order to guarantee compatibility (Ehrenstein et al. 2019). Accessibility presents additional difficulties since infrastructure constraints and user training may prevent adoption in environments with limited resources (Anawade et al. 2024). These difficulties highlight the necessity of ongoing innovation to improve affordability and performance.

By allowing people to conduct tests at home and communicate the results with doctors through cloud platforms, its integration with smartphones has democratized diagnostics (Ates et al. 2022). This has made telehealth and remote monitoring easier, which has increased patient involvement and the effectiveness of healthcare. Global health equity has been aided by the expansion of diagnostic capacities to low-income areas due to the cost of instruments such as paper-based lateral flow assays (Budd et al. 2023). On-chip sensors are valuable in evidence-based medicine, as clinical trials show that they improve patient outcomes, including lower hospitalization rates for diabetes complications (Glennie et al. 2022).

On-chip sensors have significant social and economic ramifications. These devices enhance access and reduce healthcare costs, especially in poor places, by reducing reliance on centralized laboratories (Bhatia et al. 2024). Their contribution to early disease diagnosis lessens the strain on healthcare systems by promoting preventative care. These advantages can reach a large audience because to the scalability of smartphone-integrated systems, which take advantage of the 6.8 billion smartphones in use worldwide in 2025. But, especially in environments with limited resources, resolving differences in smartphone ownership and digital literacy is necessary to achieve fair access. Cooperation between producers, legislators, and healthcare providers will be crucial to guarantee that on-chip sensors realize their full potential in global healthcare (Hernández-Neuta et al. 2019).

In conclusion, the key component of on-chip sensors are point-of-care (POC) diagnostics, enabling both patients and physicians through their integration of sophisticated sensing, microfluidics, and smartphone connectivity. Even if issues like sensitivity, scalability, and regulatory restrictions still exist, new developments in CRISPR, nanotechnology, artificial intelligence, and sustainable manufacturing hold out the possibility of overcoming these obstacles. Devices like the Dexcom G7 and Ellume's COVID-19 test have demonstrated their practical influence through their commercial success, and they have enormous potential to promote personalized treatment and global health equity. On-chip sensors will be essential in determining the direction of healthcare in the future, providing accurate diagnosis, enhancing patient outcomes, and promoting a more just and effective global health ecosystem as they develop further.

References

Algehyne EA, Jibril ML, Algehainy NA, Alamri OA, Alzahrani AK (2022) Fuzzy neural network expert system with an improved gini index random forest-based feature importance measure algorithm for early diagnosis of breast cancer in Saudi Arabia. Big Data Cogn Comput 6(1):1. https://doi.org/10.3390/bdcc6010013

Ali MA et al (2021) Breaking the barrier to biomolecule limit-of-detection via 3D printed multi-length-scale graphene-coated electrodes. Nat Commun 12(1):7077. https://doi.org/10.1038/s41467-021-27361-x

Ali MA, Zhang GF, Hu C, Yuan B, Gao S-J, Panat R (2024) An advanced healthcare sensing platform for direct detection of viral proteins in seconds at Femtomolar concentrations via aerosol jet 3D-printed Nano and Biomaterials. Adv Mater Interfaces 11(14):2400005. https://doi.org/10.1002/admi.202400005

Allegrini F, Olivieri AC (2016) Sensitivity, prediction uncertainty, and detection limit for artificial neural network calibrations. Anal Chem 88(15):7807–7812. https://doi.org/10.1021/acs.analchem.6b01857

Ameen SSM, Omer KM, Mansour FR, Bedair A, Hamed M (2025) Non-invasive wearable electrochemical sensors for continuous glucose monitoring. Electrochem Commun 173:107894. https://doi.org/10.1016/j.elecom.2025.107894

Amoako K, Ukita R, Cook KE (2025) Antifouling Zwitterionic polymer coatings for blood-bearing medical devices. Langmuir 41(5):2994–3006. https://doi.org/10.1021/acs.langmuir.4c04532

Anawade PA, Sharma D, Gahane S (2024) A comprehensive review on exploring the impact of telemedicine on healthcare accessibility. Cureus 16(3):e55996. https://doi.org/10.7759/cureus.55996

Arfin T (2021) Emerging trends in lab-on-a-chip for biosensing applications. In: Functionalized nanomaterials based devices for environmental applications. Elsevier, pp 199–218. https://doi.org/10.1016/b978-0-12-822245-4.00008-8

Aryal P, Henry CS (2024) Advancements and challenges in microfluidic paper-based analytical devices: design, manufacturing, sustainability, and field applications. Front. Lab Chip Technol 3. https://doi.org/10.3389/frlct.2024.1467423

Ates HC et al (2022) End-to-end design of wearable sensors. Nat Rev Mater 7(11):887–907. https://doi.org/10.1038/s41578-022-00460-x

Avari P et al (2023) The accuracy of continuous glucose sensors in people with diabetes undergoing hemodialysis (ALPHA Study). Diabetes Technol Ther 25(7):447–456. https://doi.org/10.1089/dia.2023.0013

Awaja F, Wong T, Arhatari B (2018) Lab-on-a-chip device made by autohesion-bonded polymers. Biomed Microdevices 20(1). https://doi.org/10.1007/s10544-017-0250-8

Azzouz A et al (2022) Advances in surface plasmon resonance–based biosensor technologies for cancer biomarker detection. Biosens Bioelectron 197:113767. https://doi.org/10.1016/j.bios.2021.113767

Bagheri A, Jin J (2019) Photopolymerization in 3D printing. ACS Appl Polym Mater 1(4):593–611. https://doi.org/10.1021/acsapm.8b00165

Bahnemann J, Grünberger A (eds) (2022) Microfluidics in biotechnology, In advances in biochemical engineering/biotechnology. Springer, Cham. https://doi.org/10.1007/978-3-031-04188-4

Balsam J, Ossandon M, Bruck HA, Lubensky I, Rasooly A (2013) Low-cost technologies for medical diagnostics in low-resource settings. Expert Opin Med Diagn 7(3):243–255. https://doi.org/10.1517/17530059.2013.767796

Barbosa AI, Rebelo R, Reis RL, Bhattacharya M, Correlo VM (2021) Current nanotechnology advances in diagnostic biosensors. Med Devices Sens 4(1):e10156. https://doi.org/10.1002/mds3.10156

Bergveld P (1970) Development of an ion-sensitive solid-state device for neurophysiological measurements. IEEE Trans Biomed Eng BME-17(1):70–71. https://doi.org/10.1109/tbme.1970.4502688

Bhagoria P, Mathew Sebastian E, Kumar Jain S, Purohit J, Purohit R (2020) Nanolithography and its alternate techniques. Mater Today Proc 26:3048–3053. https://doi.org/10.1016/j.matpr.2020.02.633

Bhatia D, Paul S, Acharjee T, Ramachairy SS (2024) Biosensors and their widespread impact on human health. Sens Int 5:100257. https://doi.org/10.1016/j.sintl.2023.100257

Budd J et al (2023) Lateral flow test engineering and lessons learned from COVID-19. Nat Rev Bioeng 1(1):13–31. https://doi.org/10.1038/s44222-022-00007-3

Bukowski M et al (2020) Implementation of eHealth and AI integrated diagnostics with multidisciplinary digitized data: are we ready from an international perspective? Eur Radiol 30(10):5510–5524. https://doi.org/10.1007/s00330-020-06874-x

Carota AG et al (2024) Low-cost inkjet-printed nanostructured biosensor based on CRISPR/Cas12a system for pathogen detection. Biosens Bioelectron 258:116340. https://doi.org/10.1016/j.bios.2024.116340

Carroll DP, Mendes PM (2023) Recent advances in surface modification and antifouling strategies for electrochemical sensing in complex biofluids. Curr Opin Electrochem 40:101319. https://doi.org/10.1016/j.coelec.2023.101319

Center for Devices and Radiological Health. Overview of device regulation. FDA. Accessed: July 23, 2025. [Online]. Available: https://www.fda.gov/medical-devices/device-advice-comprehensive-regulatory-assistance/overview-device-regulation

Cetinkaya A, Kaya SI, Ozkan SA (2025) A review of point-of-care (POC) and lab-on-chip (LOC) approaches in molecularly imprinted polymer-based electrochemical sensors for biomedical applications. Anal Chim Acta 1357:344080. https://doi.org/10.1016/j.aca.2025.344080

Chen H, Kätelhön E, Compton RG (2023) Machine learning in fundamental electrochemistry: recent advances and future opportunities. Curr Opin Electrochem 38:101214. https://doi.org/10.1016/j.coelec.2023.101214

Chen J, Ding X, Zhang D (2024) Challenges and strategies faced in the electrochemical biosensing analysis of neurochemicals in vivo: a review. Talanta 266:124933. https://doi.org/10.1016/j.talanta.2023.124933

Crapnell RD, Ferrari AG-M, Dempsey NC, Banks CE (2022) Electroanalytical overview: screen-printed electrochemical sensing platforms for the detection of vital cardiac, cancer and inflammatory biomarkers. Sens Diagn 1(3):405–428. https://doi.org/10.1039/D1SD00041A

De Castro LF, De Freitas SV, Duarte LC, De Souza JAC, Paixão TRLC, Coltro WKT (2019) Salivary diagnostics on paper microfluidic devices and their use as wearable sensors for glucose monitoring. Anal Bioanal Chem 411(19):4919–4928. https://doi.org/10.1007/s00216-019-01788-0

Dkhar DS, Kumari R, Malode SJ, Shetti NP, Chandra P (2023) Integrated lab-on-a-chip devices: fabrication methodologies, transduction system for sensing purposes. J Pharm Biomed Anal 223:115120. https://doi.org/10.1016/j.jpba.2022.115120

Ehrenstein V, Kharrazi H, Lehmann H, Taylor CO (2019) Obtaining data from electronic health records. In: Tools and technologies for registry interoperability, registries for evaluating patient outcomes: a user's guide, 3rd edition, Addendum 2 [Internet]. Agency for Healthcare Research and Quality (US). Accessed 22 July 2025. [Online]. Available: https://www.ncbi.nlm.nih.gov/books/NBK551878/

Fischer DB (2008) Nanotechnology—scientific and regulatory challenges. Vill Envtl L J 19:315. Available at: https://digitalcommons.law.villanova.edu/elj/vol19/iss2/2

Fruncillo S, Su X, Liu H, Wong LS (2021) Lithographic processes for the scalable fabrication of micro- and nanostructures for biochips and biosensors. ACS Sens 6(6):2002–2024. https://doi.org/10.1021/acssensors.0c02704

Fuchs S, Johansson S, Tjell AØ, Werr G, Mayr T, Tenje M (2021) In-line analysis of organ-on-chip systems with sensors: integration, fabrication, challenges, and potential. ACS Biomater Sci Eng 7(7):2926–2948. https://doi.org/10.1021/acsbiomaterials.0c01110

Ganguli A et al (2020) Rapid isothermal amplification and portable detection system for SARS-CoV-2. Proc Natl Acad Sci USA 117(37):22727–22735. https://doi.org/10.1073/pnas.2014739117

Gao W et al (2016) Fully integrated wearable sensor arrays for multiplexed in situ perspiration analysis. Nature 529(7587):509–514. https://doi.org/10.1038/nature16521

Gao F et al (2023) Wearable and flexible electrochemical sensors for sweat analysis: a review. Microsyst Nanoeng 9(1):1. https://doi.org/10.1038/s41378-022-00443-6

Garg SK et al (2022) Accuracy and safety of Dexcom G7 continuous glucose monitoring in adults with diabetes. Diabetes Technol Ther 24(6):373–380. https://doi.org/10.1089/dia.2022.0011

Glennie JL, Berard L, Levrat-Guillen F (2022) Sensor-based technology: bringing value to people with diabetes and the healthcare system in an evolving world. Clin Outcomes Res CEOR 14:75–90. https://doi.org/10.2147/CEOR.S346736

Ha N, Xu K, Ren G, Mitchell A, Ou JZ (2020) Machine learning-enabled smart sensor systems. Adv Intell Syst 2(9). https://doi.org/10.1002/aisy.202000063

Hengoju S, Shvydkiv O, Tovar M, Roth M, Rosenbaum MA (2022) Advantages of optical fibers for facile and enhanced detection in droplet microfluidics. Biosens Bioelectron 200:113910. https://doi.org/10.1016/j.bios.2021.113910

Hernández-Neuta I et al (2019) Smartphone-based clinical diagnostics: towards democratization of evidence-based health care. J Intern Med 285(1):19–39. https://doi.org/10.1111/joim.12820
Hnasko R, Lin A, McGarvey JA, Stanker LH (2011) A rapid method to improve protein detection by indirect ELISA. Biochem Biophys Res Commun 410(4):726–731. https://doi.org/10.1016/j.bbrc.2011.06.005
Ho CMB, Ng SH, Li KHH, Yoon Y-J (2015) 3D printed microfluidics for biological applications. Lab Chip 15(18):3627–3637. https://doi.org/10.1039/c5lc00685f
Homola J (2008) Surface Plasmon resonance sensors for detection of chemical and biological species. Chem Rev 108(2):462–493. https://doi.org/10.1021/cr068107d
Md Najmul Hosain, Yi-Sub Kwak, Jaeeun Lee, Hongseok Choi, Jungwon Park, Jongnam Kim IoT-enabled biosensors for real-time monitoring and early detection of chronic diseases. Phys Act Nutr, 2024 28(4):60-69. Accessed: July 23, 2025. [Online]. Available: https://e-pan.org/journal/view.php?doi=10.20463/pan.2024.0033
Hosseinzadeh Fakhr M et al (2024) Recent advances in wearable electrochemical biosensors towards technological and material aspects. Biosens Bioelectron X 19:100503. https://doi.org/10.1016/j.biosx.2024.100503
Hou X et al (2025) Machine-learning based strategy identifies a robust protein biomarker panel for Alzheimer's disease in cerebrospinal fluid. Alzheimers Res Ther 17:147. https://doi.org/10.1186/s13195-025-01789-5
Hu K et al (2024) CRISPR-based biosensors for medical diagnosis: readout from detector-dependence detection toward naked eye detection. Biosensors 14(8):8. https://doi.org/10.3390/bios14080367
Huh D, Matthews BD, Mammoto A, Montoya-Zavala M, Hsin HY, Ingber DE (2010) Reconstituting organ-level lung functions on a Chip. Science 328(5986):1662–1668. https://doi.org/10.1126/science.1188302
Ieracitano C et al (2022) A fuzzy-enhanced deep learning approach for early detection of Covid-19 pneumonia from portable chest X-ray images. Neurocomputing 481:202–215. https://doi.org/10.1016/j.neucom.2022.01.055
Kalantar-Zadeh K et al (2018) A human pilot trial of ingestible electronic capsules capable of sensing different gases in the gut. Nat. Electron. 1(1):79–87. https://doi.org/10.1038/s41928-017-0004-x
Khalil AA, Rahman MA (2023) Adaptive neuro-fuzzy inference system-based lightweight intrusion detection system for UAVs. IEEE
Khan MS et al (2019) Electrochemical-digital immunosensor with enhanced sensitivity for detecting human salivary glucocorticoid hormone. Analyst 144(4):1448–1457. https://doi.org/10.1039/c8an02085j
Khondakar KR, Mazumdar H, Das S, Kaushik A (2025) Machine learning (ML)-assisted surface-enhanced raman spectroscopy (SERS) technologies for sustainable health. Adv Colloid Interf Sci 344:103594. https://doi.org/10.1016/j.cis.2025.103594
Kiani S, Minaei S, Ghasemi-Varnamkhasti M (2016) A portable electronic nose as an expert system for aroma-based classification of saffron. Chemom Intell Lab Syst 156:148–156. https://doi.org/10.1016/j.chemolab.2016.05.013
Kishi S, Nagasu H, Kidokoro K, Kashihara N (2024) Oxidative stress and the role of redox signalling in chronic kidney disease. Nat Rev Nephrol 20(2):101–119. https://doi.org/10.1038/s41581-023-00775-0
Koczula KM, Gallotta A (2016) Lateral flow assays. Essays Biochem 60(1):111–120. https://doi.org/10.1042/ebc20150012
Krishnan SK, Nataraj N, Meyyappan M, Pal U (2023) Graphene-based field-effect transistors in biosensing and neural interfacing applications: recent advances and prospects. Anal Chem 95(5):2590–2622. https://doi.org/10.1021/acs.analchem.2c03399
Krutkyte G et al (2025) Performance of the DEXCOM G7 CGM system during and after major surgery. Diabetes Obes Metab 27(8):4586–4589. https://doi.org/10.1111/dom.16462
Kumar KN, Sai Santhosh VC, Mane A, Rahimunnisa K, Nirmal G, Vaghulade M (2024) Enhancing lung cancer detection and localization with a hybrid VGG-19 and Adaptive

Neuro-Fuzzy Inference System (ANFIS) approach on imaging data. In: 2024 systems and information engineering design symposium (SIEDS), pp 280–285. https://doi.org/10.1109/SIEDS61124.2024.10534680

Laksanasopin T et al (2015) A smartphone dongle for diagnosis of infectious diseases at the point of care. Sci Transl Med 7(273):273re1. https://doi.org/10.1126/scitranslmed.aaa0056

Lee J-C et al (2024) Micrometer-thick and porous nanocomposite coating for electrochemical sensors with exceptional antifouling and electroconducting properties. Nat Commun 15(1). https://doi.org/10.1038/s41467-024-44822-1

Lehnert T, Gijs MAM (2024) Microfluidic systems for infectious disease diagnostics. Lab Chip 24(5):1441–1493. https://doi.org/10.1039/D4LC00117F

Li Z, Guo M, Zhong W (2025) Multiplex detection of biomarkers empowered by nanomaterials. Precis Chem 3(6):297–318. https://doi.org/10.1021/prechem.4c00096

Liang C, Liu Y, Niu A, Liu C, Li J, Ning D (2019) Smartphone-app based point-of-care testing for myocardial infarction biomarker cTnI using an autonomous capillary microfluidic chip with self-aligned on-chip focusing (SOF) lenses. Lab Chip 19(10):1797–1807. https://doi.org/10.1039/c9lc00259f

Lim WY, Thevarajah TM, Goh BT, Khor SM (2019) Paper microfluidic device for early diagnosis and prognosis of acute myocardial infarction via quantitative multiplex cardiac biomarker detection. Biosens Bioelectron 128:176–185. https://doi.org/10.1016/j.bios.2018.12.049

Lin Q et al (2020) Microfluidic immunoassays for sensitive and simultaneous detection of IgG/IgM/antigen of SARS-CoV-2 within 15 min. Anal Chem 92(14):9454–9458. https://doi.org/10.1021/acs.analchem.0c01635

Liu H, Lei Y (2021) A critical review: recent advances in 'digital' biomolecule detection with single copy sensitivity. Biosens Bioelectron 177:112901. https://doi.org/10.1016/j.bios.2020.112901

Liu Y, Yu Q, Luo X, Yang L, Cui Y (2021) Continuous monitoring of diabetes with an integrated microneedle biosensing device through 3D printing. Microsyst Nanoeng 7(1). https://doi.org/10.1038/s41378-021-00302-w

Liu T, Wang Y, Hong M, Venezuela J, Shi W, Dargusch M (2023) Advances in biodegradable piezoelectrics for medical implants. Nano Today 52:101945. https://doi.org/10.1016/j.nantod.2023.101945

Lorestani F et al (2025) A granular hydrogel-enabled wearable electrochemical biosensing platform for continuous non-invasive sweat lactate detection. Small. https://doi.org/10.1002/smll.202502655

Macdonald NP, Cabot JM, Smejkal P, Guijt RM, Paull B, Breadmore MC (2017) Comparing microfluidic performance of three-dimensional (3D) printing platforms. Anal Chem 89(7):3858–3866. https://doi.org/10.1021/acs.analchem.7b00136

Magro L et al (2017) Paper microfluidics for nucleic acid amplification testing (NAAT) of infectious diseases. Lab Chip 17(14):2347–2371. https://doi.org/10.1039/c7lc00013h

Mahmud MS, Fang H, Wang H, Carreiro S, Boyer E (2018) Automatic detection of opioid intake using wearable biosensor. In: 2018 international conference on computing, networking and communications (ICNC). IEEE, Maui, pp 784–788. https://doi.org/10.1109/iccnc.2018.8390334

Malik S et al (2023) Nanomaterials-based biosensor and their applications: A review. Heliyon 9(9):e19929. https://doi.org/10.1016/j.heliyon.2023.e19929

Manz A, Graber N, Widmer HM (1990) Miniaturized total chemical analysis systems: a novel concept for chemical sensing. Sens Actuators B Chem 1(1–6):244–248. https://doi.org/10.1016/0925-4005(90)80209-i

Martens T et al (2021) Effect of continuous glucose monitoring on glycemic control in patients with type 2 diabetes treated with basal insulin. JAMA 325(22):1–11. https://doi.org/10.1001/jama.2021.7444

Martinez AW, Phillips ST, Butte MJ, Whitesides GM (2007) Patterned paper as a platform for inexpensive, low-volume, portable bioassays. Angew Chem Int Ed 46(8):1318–1320. https://doi.org/10.1002/anie.200603817

Meng X, O'Hare D, Ladame S (2023) Surface immobilization strategies for the development of electrochemical nucleic acid sensors. Biosens Bioelectron 237:115440. https://doi.org/10.1016/j.bios.2023.115440

Mirica A-C (Ion) et al. (2024) Screen-printed electrodes—a promising tool for antineoplastic drug detection (cisplatin and bleomycin) in biological samples. Int J Mol Sci, 25, 15, 15. https://doi.org/10.3390/ijms25158030

Moreira FTC, Guerreiro JRL, Brandão L, Sales MGF (2015) Synthesis of molecular biomimetics. In: Biomimetic Technologies. Elsevier, pp 3–31. https://doi.org/10.1016/b978-0-08-100249-0.00001-x

Moznuzzaman M, Khan I, Islam MR (2021) Nano-layered surface plasmon resonance-based highly sensitive biosensor for virus detection: a theoretical approach to detect SARS-CoV-2. AIP Adv 11(6). https://doi.org/10.1063/5.0046574

Nakhleh MK et al (2017) Diagnosis and classification of 17 diseases from 1404 subjects via pattern analysis of exhaled molecules. ACS Nano 11(1):112–125. https://doi.org/10.1021/acsnano.6b04930

Nalbant KG (2024) Chapter 31—The interaction of fuzzy logic with machine learning and artificial intelligence in decision-making models. In: Allahviranloo T, Pedrycz W, Seyyedabbasi A (eds) Decision-making models, Uncertainty, computational techniques, and decision intelligence. Academic, pp 563–571. https://doi.org/10.1016/B978-0-443-16147-6.00006-2

Nambison NK et al (2024) Pathology report interpretation and disease diagnosis using fuzzy logic embedded in an artificial intelligence framework: a new paradigm for digital technologies. Cureus. https://doi.org/10.7759/cureus.71148

Nascimento EJM et al (2018) Development of an anti-dengue NS1 IgG ELISA to evaluate exposure to dengue virus. J Virol Methods 257:48–57. https://doi.org/10.1016/j.jviromet.2018.03.007

Nayak S et al (2019) Integrating user behavior with engineering design of point-of-care diagnostic devices: Theoretical framework and empirical findings. Lab Chip 19(13):2241–2255. https://doi.org/10.1039/c9lc00188c

Nazha HM et al (2023) Portable infrared-based glucometer reinforced with fuzzy logic. Biosensors 13(11):11. https://doi.org/10.3390/bios13110991

Nguyen PQM et al (2022) Modular micro-PCR system for the onsite rapid diagnosis of COVID-19. Microsyst Nanoeng 8(1). https://doi.org/10.1038/s41378-022-00400-3

Nielsen JB, Hanson RL, Almughamsi HM, Pang C, Fish TR, Woolley AT (2020) Microfluidics: innovations in materials and their fabrication and functionalization. Anal Chem 92(1):150–168. https://doi.org/10.1021/acs.analchem.9b04986

Nilsson T, Mann M, Aebersold R, Yates JR, Bairoch A, Bergeron JJM (2010) Mass spectrometry in high-throughput proteomics: ready for the big time. Nat Methods 7(9):681–685. https://doi.org/10.1038/nmeth0910-681

Nisar S et al (2024) 2D materials in advanced electronic biosensors for point-of-care devices. Adv Sci 11(31). https://doi.org/10.1002/advs.202401386

Nurtop E et al (2018) Combination of ELISA screening and seroneutralisation tests to expedite Zika virus seroprevalence studies. Virol J 15(1). https://doi.org/10.1186/s12985-018-1105-5

Ordóñez F, Roggen D (2016) Deep convolutional and LSTM recurrent neural networks for multimodal wearable activity recognition. Sensors 16(1):115. https://doi.org/10.3390/s16010115

Paimard G, Ghasali E, Baeza M (2023) Screen-printed electrodes: fabrication, modification, and biosensing applications. Chemosensors 11(2):2. https://doi.org/10.3390/chemosensors11020113

Pandey R et al (2023) Electrochemical DNAzyme-based biosensors for disease diagnosis. Biosens Bioelectron 224:114983. https://doi.org/10.1016/j.bios.2022.114983

Papamatthaiou S, Menelaou P, El Achab Oussallam B, Moschou D (2025) Recent advances in bio-microsystem integration and lab-on-PCB technology. Microsyst Nanoeng 11(1). https://doi.org/10.1038/s41378-025-00940-4

Parihar A, Ranjan P, Sanghi SK, Srivastava AK, Khan R (2020) Point-of-care biosensor-based diagnosis of COVID-19 holds promise to combat current and future pandemics. ACS Appl Bio Mater 3(11):7326–7343. https://doi.org/10.1021/acsabm.0c01083

Patel J et al (2024) Reshaping the equitable and inclusive access to healthcare: a qualitative study. Clin Epidemiol Glob Health 26:None. https://doi.org/10.1016/j.cegh.2024.101544

Patolsky F, Lieber CM (2005) Nanowire nanosensors. Mater Today 8(4):20–28. https://doi.org/10.1016/s1369-7021(05)00791-1

Qamar AZ, Shamsi MH (2020) Desktop fabrication of lab-on-Chip devices on flexible substrates: a brief review. Micromachines 11(2):126. https://doi.org/10.3390/mi11020126

Rajendran M et al (2017) Analysis of anti-influenza virus neuraminidase antibodies in children, adults, and the elderly by ELISA and Enzyme inhibition: evidence for original antigenic sin. MBio 8(2). https://doi.org/10.1128/mbio.02281-16

Ramiah Rajasekaran P, Chapin AA, Quan DN, Herberholz J, Bentley WE, Ghodssi R (2020) 3D-printed electrochemical sensor-integrated transwell systems. Microsyst Nanoeng 6(1):100. https://doi.org/10.1038/s41378-020-00208-z

Ren K, Zhou J, Wu H (2013) Materials for microfluidic chip fabrication. Acc Chem Res 46(11):2396–2406. https://doi.org/10.1021/ar300314s

Richens JG, Lee CM, Johri S (2020) Improving the accuracy of medical diagnosis with causal machine learning. Nat Commun 11(1):3923. https://doi.org/10.1038/s41467-020-17419-7

Robin P et al (2023) A DNA biosensors-based microfluidic platform for attomolar real-time detection of unamplified SARS-CoV-2 virus. Biosens Bioelectron X 13:100302. https://doi.org/10.1016/j.biosx.2022.100302

Sabaté Del Río J, Henry OYF, Jolly P, Ingber DE (2019) An antifouling coating that enables affinity-based electrochemical biosensing in complex biological fluids. Nat Nanotechnol 14(12):1143–1149. https://doi.org/10.1038/s41565-019-0566-z

Sakib S et al (2025) Comparative analysis of machine learning algorithms used for translating aptamer-antigen binding kinetic profiles to diagnostic decisions. ACS Sens 10(2):907–920. https://doi.org/10.1021/acssensors.4c02682

Santonocito R et al (2025) Detection of human salivary stress biomarkers using an easy-to-use array sensor based on fluorescent organic molecules. Biosens Bioelectron 270:116986. https://doi.org/10.1016/j.bios.2024.116986

Saric M, Russo M, Stella M, Sikora M (June 2019) CNN-based method for lung cancer detection in whole slide histopathology images. In: 2019 4th international conference on smart and sustainable technologies (SpliTech). IEEE, Split, pp 1–4. https://doi.org/10.23919/splitech.2019.8783041

Sattar F, Puhan NB, Fazel-Rezai R (eds) (2023) Acoustic sensors and their applications. MDPI. https://doi.org/10.3390/books978-3-0365-9848-2

Saxena S, Lu Y, Zhang Z, Li Y, Soleymani L, Hoare T (2024) Zwitter-repel: an anti-fouling coating promoting electrochemical biosensing in biological fluids. Chem Eng J 495:153522. https://doi.org/10.1016/j.cej.2024.153522

Schena M (1996) Genome analysis with gene expression microarrays. BioEssays 18(5):427–431. https://doi.org/10.1002/bies.950180513

Scott SM, Ali Z (2021) Fabrication methods for microfluidic devices: an overview. Micromachines 12(3):319. https://doi.org/10.3390/mi12030319

Selvapandian A, Manivannan K (2018) Fusion based glioma brain tumor detection and segmentation using ANFIS classification. Comput Methods Prog Biomed 166:33–38. https://doi.org/10.1016/j.cmpb.2018.09.006

Seshadri DR et al (2019) Wearable sensors for monitoring the physiological and biochemical profile of the athlete. Npj Digit Med 2(1). https://doi.org/10.1038/s41746-019-0150-9

Shabu SLJ et al (2024) An improved adaptive neuro-fuzzy inference framework for lung cancer detection and prediction on internet of medical things platform. Int J Comput Intell Syst 17(1):228. https://doi.org/10.1007/s44196-024-00635-0

Shahid N, Rappon T, Berta W (2019) Applications of artificial neural networks in health care organizational decision-making: a scoping review. PLoS One 14(2):e0212356. https://doi.org/10.1371/journal.pone.0212356

Silva LRG et al (2024) Dual-target additively manufactured electrochemical sensor for the multiplexed detection of protein A29 and DNA of human Monkeypox virus. ACS Omega 9(30):33099–33110. https://doi.org/10.1021/acsomega.4c04460
Sorger PK (2008) Microfluidics closes in on point-of-care assays. Nat Biotechnol 26(12):1345–1346. https://doi.org/10.1038/nbt1208-1345
Squires TM, Quake SR (2005) Microfluidics: fluid physics at the nanoliter scale. Rev Mod Phys 77(3):977–1026. https://doi.org/10.1103/revmodphys.77.977
Stine JM et al (2024) Miniaturized capsule system toward real-time electrochemical detection of H2S in the gastrointestinal tract. Adv Healthc Mater 13(5):2302897. https://doi.org/10.1002/adhm.202302897
Sun G, Matsui T, Hakozaki Y, Abe S (2015) An infectious disease/fever screening radar system which stratifies higher-risk patients within ten seconds using a neural network and the fuzzy grouping method. J Infect 70(3):230–236. https://doi.org/10.1016/j.jinf.2014.12.007
Terry SC, Jerman JH, Angell JB (1979) A gas chromatographic air analyzer fabricated on a silicon wafer. IEEE Trans Electron Dev 26(12):1880–1886. https://doi.org/10.1109/t-ed.1979.19791
Tibaduiza D et al (2024) Electronic tongues and noses: a general overview. Biosensors 14(4):190. https://doi.org/10.3390/bios14040190
Timilsina SS, Durr N, Yafia M, Sallum H, Jolly P, Ingber DE (2022) Ultrarapid method for coating electrochemical sensors with antifouling conductive nanomaterials enables highly sensitive multiplexed detection in whole blood. Adv Healthc Mater 11(8). https://doi.org/10.1002/adhm.202102244
Topol EJ (2019) High-performance medicine: the convergence of human and artificial intelligence. Nat Med 25(1):44–56. https://doi.org/10.1038/s41591-018-0300-7
Turner APF (2013) Biosensors: sense and sensibility. Chem Soc Rev 42(8):3184. https://doi.org/10.1039/c3cs35528d
Ursini F, Maiorino M, Forman HJ (2016) Redox homeostasis: the golden mean of healthy living. Redox Biol 8:205–215. https://doi.org/10.1016/j.redox.2016.01.010
Valera E, Shia WW, Bailey RC (2016) Development and validation of an immunosensor for monocyte chemotactic protein 1 using a silicon photonic microring resonator biosensing platform. Clin Biochem 49(1):121–126. https://doi.org/10.1016/j.clinbiochem.2015.09.001
Wang J et al (2010) A self-powered, one-step chip for rapid, quantitative and multiplexed detection of proteins from pinpricks of whole blood. Lab Chip 10(22):3157. https://doi.org/10.1039/c0lc00132e
Wasilewski T, Kamysz W, Gębicki J (2024) AI-assisted detection of biomarkers by sensors and biosensors for early diagnosis and monitoring. Biosensors 14(7):356. https://doi.org/10.3390/bios14070356
Whitesides GM, Ostuni E, Jiang X, Ingber DE (2025) Soft lithography in biology and biochemistry. Annu Rev Biomed Eng 3:335–373
Xu M, Obodo D, Yadavalli VK (2019) The design, fabrication, and applications of flexible biosensing devices. Biosens Bioelectron 124–125:96–114. https://doi.org/10.1016/j.bios.2018.10.019
Yager P et al (2006) Microfluidic diagnostic technologies for global public health. Nature 442(7101):412–418. https://doi.org/10.1038/nature05064
Yáñez-Sedeño P, Campuzano S, Pingarrón JM (2020) Screen-printed electrodes: promising paper and wearable transducers for (bio)sensing. Biosensors 10(7):76. https://doi.org/10.3390/bios10070076
Yaron M et al (2019) Effect of flash glucose monitoring technology on glycemic control and treatment satisfaction in patients with type 2 diabetes. Diabetes Care 42(7):1178–1184. https://doi.org/10.2337/dc18-0166
Ye C et al (2024) A wearable aptamer nanobiosensor for non-invasive female hormone monitoring. Nat Nanotechnol 19(3):330–337. https://doi.org/10.1038/s41565-023-01513-0
Yetisen AK, Akram MS, Lowe CR (2013) Paper-based microfluidic point-of-care diagnostic devices. Lab Chip 13(12):2210. https://doi.org/10.1039/c3lc50169h
Zadeh LA (1965) Fuzzy sets. Inf Control 8(3):338–353. https://doi.org/10.1016/S0019-9958(65)90241-X

Zhang M, Huang J, Lu Y, Pang W, Zhang H, Duan X (2018) Solid-state microfluidics with integrated thin-film acoustic sensors. ACS Sens 3(8):1584–1591. https://doi.org/10.1021/acssensors.8b00412

Zhang N et al (2025) 3D printing of micro-nano devices and their applications. Microsyst Nanoeng 11(1):35. https://doi.org/10.1038/s41378-024-00812-3

Zhou X, Slaughter J, Riki S, Kuo CC, Furst A (2025) Polymer coating for the long-term storage of immobilized DNA. ACS Sens. https://doi.org/10.1021/acssensors.5c00937

Zupančič U, Jolly P, Estrela P, Moschou D, Ingber DE (2021) Graphene enabled low-noise surface chemistry for multiplexed sepsis biomarker detection in whole blood. Adv Funct Mater 31(16). https://doi.org/10.1002/adfm.202010638

Unlocking the Potential of PCB-Based Biosensors in Medical Diagnostics

15

Chandhana J P and T. G. Satheesh Babu

Abstract

Printed circuit board (PCB) technology, traditionally utilized in the manufacturing of electronic devices, has recently emerged as a cost-effective and scalable platform for the development of biosensors. Its widespread availability, standardized fabrication processes, and compatibility with modern microfabrication techniques make PCBs an attractive choice for integrating both sensing elements and electronic circuitry into compact, reliable, and low-cost biosensing systems. Also, PCBs offer key advantages, such as seamless integration with electronic components and microfluidic modules, which help reduce the overall device size and support compatibility with mass production. This chapter explores the fundamental principle of PCB technology, recent progress in the design and implementation of PCB-based biosensors, and provides insights into challenges and future direction in this field. In particular, the chapter highlights the transformative potential of PCB-based biosensors in medical diagnostics, including applications in point-of-care testing, real-time disease monitoring, and biomarker detection, emphasizing their role in enabling accessible, rapid, and accurate diagnostic solutions.

Chandhana J P
Department of Chemistry, Amrita School of Physical Sciences Coimbatore, Coimbatore, India

Biosensor Research Lab, Amrita School of Engineering Coimbatore, Coimbatore, India

T. G. Satheesh Babu (✉)
Department of Chemistry, Amrita School of Physical Sciences Coimbatore, Coimbatore, India

Biosensor Research Lab, Amrita School of Engineering Coimbatore, Coimbatore, India

Amrita Biomedical Engineering Centre, Amrita School of Engineering Coimbatore, Coimbatore, India
e-mail: tg_satheesh@cb.amrita.edu

V. Patel et al. (eds.), *Biosensor Technology in Translating Novel Materials into Practical Devices*, https://doi.org/10.1007/978-981-95-5519-2_15

Keywords

Printed circuit board · ENIG · biosensors · flexible PCB

15.1 Introduction

Despite the advancements in healthcare technology, delays in the diagnosis of diseases and challenges in providing affordable care, particularly in rural areas, remain a significant concern (Wang 2006). Traditional diagnostic methods involving blood tests require sophisticated clinical laboratory, skilled personnel to operate the instruments, time-consuming procedures and are expensive (da Silva et al. 2017). Electrochemical biosensors are game-changers, offering affordable, user-friendly devices that enable rapid, point-of-care testing, making healthcare more accessible and efficient (Kim et al. 2024).

The potential of electrochemical biosensors lies in simplifying routine health checks with real-time monitoring, though developing these sensors comes with its own set of challenges. Various fabrication techniques can be used to develop electrochemical sensors. Microfabrication techniques are commonly used to design metal electrodes and deposit membranes on substrates, but they can be costly and limited in terms of scalability (Anastasova et al. 2018; Mirzajani et al. 2022). Different fabrication techniques, including ink-jet printing, xurography, screen printing, sputtering, chemical vapour deposition, and photolithography, are used for sensor fabrication (Chandhana et al. 2023, 2024a, 2025; De Santana et al. 2012; Tortorich et al. 2018). However, these techniques can be expensive, often require specialized instruments, and are not easily scalable for mass production (Anastasova et al. 2018; Shamkhalichenar et al. 2020). Here, Printed PCB technology emerges as a promising solution as it provides excellent design flexibility, enabling customization for specific applications. The use of PCB technology in the biosensor field has recently emerged as an alternative to traditional photolithographic techniques for electrode array microfabrication (Sánchez et al. 2016).

The concept of PCBs originated in the early 1930s and has since evolved dramatically, becoming integral to nearly every sector of electronics and daily life. PCBs have played a crucial role in enabling modern technological advancements. Over the past 25 years, ongoing pressure to enhance PCB performance, reduce costs, and achieve miniaturization has driven continuous innovation in this field (Zupančič et al. 2021). Advancements in high-specification commercial PCB technology have enabled significant progress in sensors and diagnostics, particularly in developing biosensors for detecting biomolecules in clinical (Sánchez et al. 2016) and environmental settings (Dutta et al. 2019; Wang et al. 2020). Recently, the use of PCB technology has expanded to include a wide range of biosensors, notably for the detection and quantification of biomolecules (Alhans et al. 2018), bacteria (Ahuja et al. 2025), mRNA markers (Sánchez et al. 2016) and DNA (Gassmann et al. 2012).

This chapter presents an overview of PCB technology applications in the development of electrochemical sensing platforms for medical applications. The chapter first covers the essential principles and recent innovations in PCB technology, before highlighting the current trends and breakthroughs in electrochemical sensors and sensing platforms built on PCB and flexible PCB substrates.

15.2 Printed Circuit Boards

John Baynes developed the first technique for something similar to a double-sided PCB in 1888. Albert Hanson created the first printed circuit board by bonding flat foil conductors to an insulating board in 1903. After many years, Arthur Berry used etching for electro-thermal applications like heaters, making them some of the first integrated actuators on insulating substrates in 1913. Charles Ducas developed a panel with metalized lines and electroplated additional metal in 1925. Paul Eisner later developed a technique for fabricating stacked metal and insulating materials, closely resembling today's PCBs. Finally, Eugene W Hutters patented the "electrical component mounting device" using hole technology in 1955, while the solder mask composition was designed by Gabrick (Perdigones and Quero 2022). The timeline of the evolution of PCB over the years is shown in Fig. 15.1.

Flame retardant 4 (FR4), FR5 (FR4 High Tg), FR1, FR2, CEM3, CEM1, Polyimide, PTFE, and metal substrate are the most common names for PCB

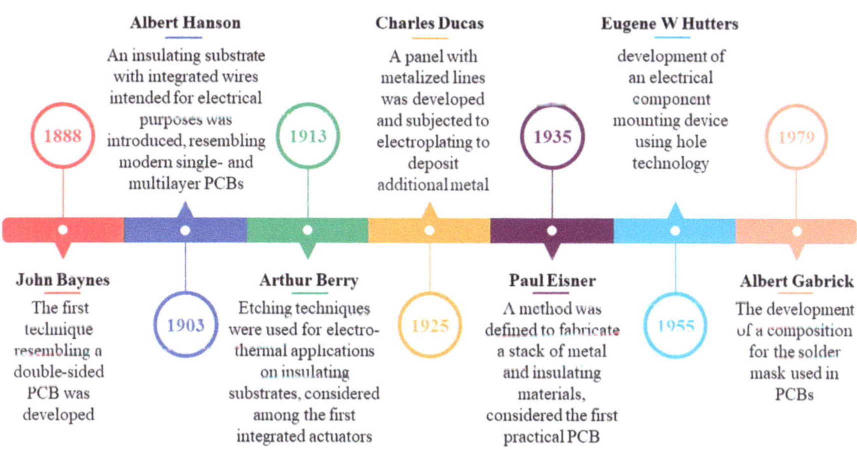

Fig. 15.1 Timeline flow chart illustrating the development of printed circuit boards (PCBs) from 1888 to 1979. Key milestones include: - 1888: Albert Hanson introduces an insulating substrate with integrated wires. - 1903: John Baynes develops a technique resembling a double-sided PCB. - 1913: Arthur Berry uses etching techniques for electro-thermal applications. - 1925: Charles Ducas develops a panel with metalized lines for electroplating. - 1935: Paul Eisner defines a method for fabricating a stack of materials, leading to the first practical PCB. - 1955: Eugene W. Hutter develops a mounting device using hole technology. - 1979: Albert Gabrick develops a composition for solder masks in PCBs. Each milestone is marked with a colored circle and corresponding text.

substrate classifications. FR4 is the most common substrate material used in PCBs due to its excellent electrical, mechanical, and thermal properties. It is made from woven glass cloth impregnated with epoxy resin binder, offering flame-resistant, excellent strength-to-weight ratio, near-zero water absorption rate, and excellent insulation (Ezema Ike-Eze et al. 2023).

Polyimide resin, reinforced with aramid fibres, is used for flexible and rigid-flex PCBs. It offers excellent thermal stability, a high glass transition temperature, a dielectric constant, and a good coefficient of thermal expansion. However, it has a high water absorption rate (up to 3% by weight) and is relatively expensive. The polyimide film thickness ranges from 12 to 125 μm, and its stiffness increases cubically with thickness. For example, doubling the thickness makes it eight times tougher but reduces flexibility by the same factor (Ezema Ike-Eze et al. 2023).

The design is created using computer-aided design (CAD), and the CAD file is checked for compatibility with the equipment before proceeding with production. A photographic image of the CAD design is transferred to the board using photosensitive film and ultraviolet light. After removing the film, excess copper is then etched, and an oxide layer is applied to the inner layers. These layers are stacked with prepreg for insulation and copper foil is added. The layers are laminated under high pressure and temperature, then drilled and cleaned. After cleaning, the board is treated with chemicals that deposit a layer of copper, with a thickness of 1.4 mil (35 μm), filling the drill holes and covering the top layer. The outer layers are coated with photoresist and plated with tin to protect the copper during etching. The panels are cleaned and prepared for a solder mask, after which ink epoxy and solder mask film are applied. The boards are exposed to ultraviolet light to define areas for removal, then baked to cure the solder mask (Fig. 15.2). Finally, the board is plated with gold using electroless nickel immersion gold (ENIG), silk-screened with labels, tested, and cut to the design specifications (LaDou 2006; Chan et al. n.d.).

Copper is commonly used for PCB traces and contacts, but is prone to oxidation, limiting its use in electrochemical sensors. To address this, inert metals like gold or

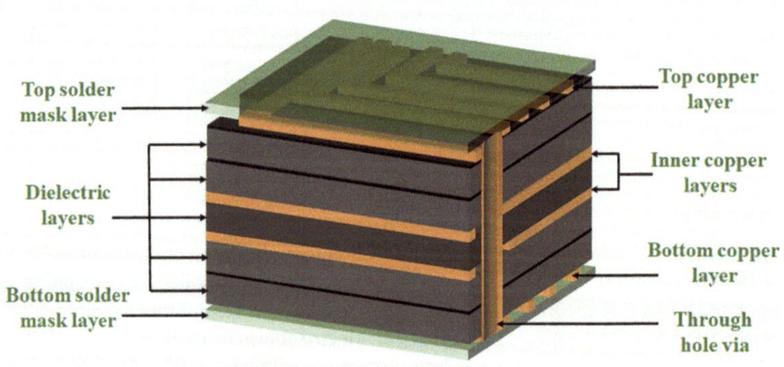

Fig. 15.2 A 3D sketch of a multilayer printed circuit board (PCB) showing its layered structure. The layers include a top solder mask layer, a top copper layer, multiple dielectric layers, inner copper layers, a bottom copper layer, and a bottom solder mask layer. A through-hole via is depicted, connecting the top and bottom copper layers. Each layer is labeled with arrows pointing to the respective sections

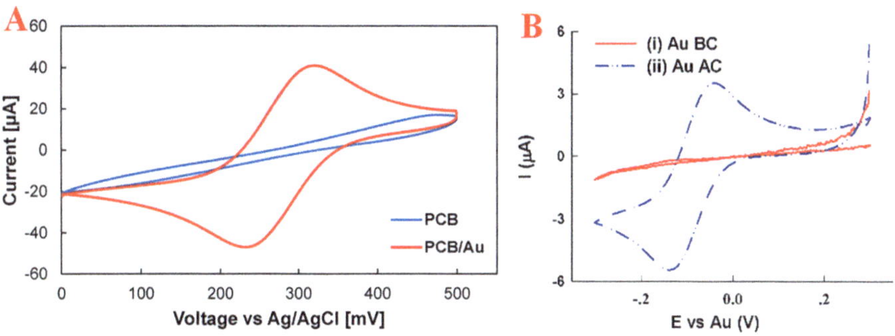

Fig. 15.3 (**A**) Comparison between cyclic voltammograms of PCB (blue line) and Au-plated PCB electrode (red line) recorded in 0.1 M KCl solution containing 5 mM $K_3Fe(CN)_6$ at a scan rate of 50 mV S^{-1}. Reproduced from (Shamkhalichenar et al. 2020), Creative Commons Attribution License (https://creativecommons.org/licenses/by/4.0/). (**B**) Comparison of cyclic voltammogram for Au-plated PCB electrode in PBS solution containing 4 mM $K_3Fe(CN)_6$ at a scan rate of 50 mV S^{-1} recorded before (red line - Au BC) and after cleaning (blue line - Au AC). Reproduced from (Dutta et al. 2018), Creative Commons Attribution License (https://creativecommons.org/licenses/by/4.0/)

platinum can be applied to PCB pads, improving he stability and performance. Various techniques, including electrodeposition, electroless, and sputtering techniques, are used for the deposition of gold. Electroless deposition is particularly efficient, offering good adhesion, uniform particle distribution, and cost-effectiveness without specialized equipment. Additionally, a thin layer of nickel is often electroplated to improve gold adhesion and act as a diffusion barrier, preventing copper from diffusing and forming an oxide layer (Mohammadzadeh and Haghighi 2021). ENIG coating is the most widely used finish for high-reliability electronic devices, in which a layer of nickel is applied on a copper surface to serve as the diffusion barrier, followed by a thin coating of immersion gold that protects the nickel from oxidation and ensures a solderable, corrosion-resistant finish (Shamkhalichenar et al. 2020).

A study demonstrated that a bare copper electrode shows a distorted cyclic voltammogram due to oxidation (Fig. 15.3a), a gold-plated electrode provides a stable and wide potential window suitable for electrochemical applications (Shamkhalichenar et al. 2020). Another study suggested cleaning PCB electrodes with acetone, ethanol, and water, followed by ultrasonication in a solution of ammonium hydroxide and hydrogen peroxide to remove surface contaminants and enhance their electrochemical activity (Fig. 15.3b) (Dutta et al. 2018).

15.3 Application of PCBs in Sensing

PCB technology has been widely employed in the development of various biosensors. The quantification of glucose plays a vital role in the diagnosis and management of diabetes mellitus. Recently, enzymatic glucose sensors have been reported using PCB-based sensors (Dutta et al. 2018). The glucose oxidase (GOx) enzyme is

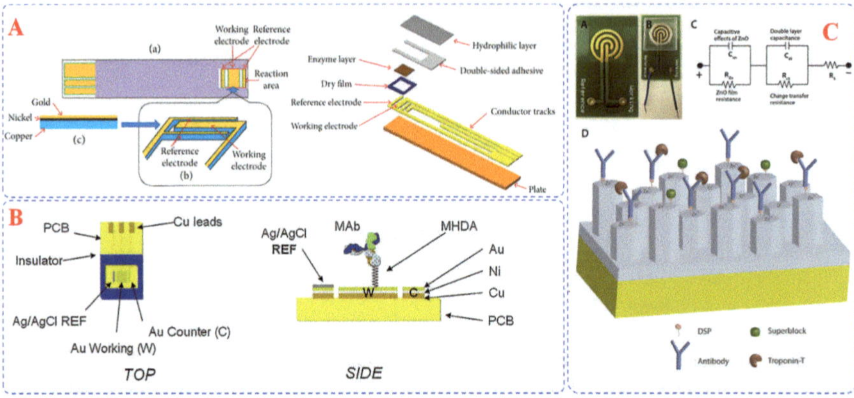

Fig. 15.4 (**A**) Schematic of the gold-coated blood glucose test strip, including the reaction zone electrode of the test strip, the corresponding circuit layout, and the layer-by-layer structure of the conducting material. Reproduced from (Kim et al. 2019), Creative Commons Attribution License (https://creativecommons.org/licenses/by/4.0/). (**B**) PCB-based sensing platform developed for electrochemical detection of Interleukin-12 (Top view and side view). Adapted with permission from (Bhavsar et al. 2009), Copyright 2009 Elsevier. (**C**) 3D representation of PCB-based sensing platform developed for electrochemical detection of Troponin-T biomarker, showing the PCB platform featuring electroplated gold electrodes and ZnO sputtered sensing site, the fully assembled sensor platform, the electrical circuit model of the sensor, and the schematic illustration of troponin-T immunoassay fabricated on the nano-columnar ZnO surface. Adapted with permission from (Jacobs et al. 2014), Copyright 2014 Elsevier

commonly used in the enzymatic sensing of glucose, and the immobilization of the enzyme plays a vital role in the sensor performance. Drop casting GOx onto a gold-coated PCB-based sensor strip has been reported for blood glucose measurement. For the fabrication of a PCB-based sensor strip, a negative film of the desired pattern was laminated onto a dry photoresist-coated copper layer on FR4 substrate. The substrate is then exposed to UV light, causing the photoresist under transparent regions to polymerize. The polymerized areas protect the copper during the etching process, allowing the formation of the desired pattern, including the working and reference electrodes. Then the exposed copper is electroplated with a nickel layer, followed by deposition of a gold layer via immersion plating. The GOx solution is drop cast onto a 2 × 2 mm reaction zone (Fig. 15.4A) containing both electrodes using a jet dispenser, then dried and coated with a hydrophobic layer (Kim et al. 2019). An amperometric sensor was developed by immobilizing GOx on an electropolymerized phenol red modified electrode. The PCB was fabricated on FR4 substrate with a low-cost ENIG finish. The layout included 8 circular working electrodes with 2 reference electrodes, each with 400 μm and 300 μm working area, along with a rectangular counter electrode (1900 × 500 μm). An excellent sensitivity of 3.13 μA mM^{-1} cm^{-2} was obtained with a detection range of 1–15 mM (Kassanos et al. 2018). In another work, GOx was modified on a pretreated PCB gold electrode employing EDC-NHS chemistry. A self-assembled monolayer was initially formed on PCB gold electrode using 3-mercaptopropionic acid, providing carboxylic groups. The carboxylic groups were then activated with EDC and NHS to covalently attach GOx to the electrode. The developed PCB-based sensor could detect a wide range of glucose, ranging from 0.5 to 20 mM, with a limit of detection of 500 μM (Dutta et al. 2018). Single-walled carbon nanotube (SWCNT) and multi-walled carbon nanotube (MWCNT) were drop-cast on the working area of PCB-based in order to facilitate immobilization GOx on gold-coated PCB electrodes. Both SWCNT/Au-PCB and MWCNT/Au-PCB-based sensors exhibited a wide detection range from 1–100 mM, with a limit of detection of 0.1 mM (Alhans et al. 2018). Minimally invasive self-powered glucose sensor based on an enzymatic fuel cell using a gold electrode on PCB. To enhance the surface area, the PCB electrode was modified with a nanoporous gold film. GOx with osmium redox polymer was used at the anode and bilirubin oxidase with a blocking agent at the cathode. The developed enzymatic fuel cell exhibited linear current response from 0.05 to 1 mM (sensitivity 14.13 μA mM^{-1} cm^{-2} in phosphate buffer saline and from 0.75 to 2 mM (sensitivity 21.5 μA mM^{-1} cm^{-2}) in saliva samples (Gonzalez-Solino et al. 2021).

Electrostatic interaction was utilized in another work to incorporate the enzyme on the PCB substrate for the detection of glucose and lactate in mouse serum. A positively charged chitosan/polyvinyl imidazole-Os/carbon nanotube composite was utilized for the immobilization of the enzyme where polyvinyl imidazole-Os act as a redox mediator, and carbon nanotube acts as a crosslinker. The positively charged chitosan electrostatically binds with negatively charged enzymes, enabling effective enzyme immobilization. The glucose sensor displayed a sensitivity of 2.44 μA mM^{-1} cm^{-2} with a detection range of 0–6 mM, whereas the lactate sensor showed a sensitivity of 25.46 μA mM^{-1} cm^{-2} over 0–0.6 mM (Li et al. 2013). Lactate plays a major role in energy metabolism under low O_2 levels and crucial biomarker for respiratory failure, sepsis, and acidosis. A solid-state electrode was fabricated on a PCB substrate for the detection of lactate. The sensor consists of a 3 mm diameter gold electrode as the working electrode, silver–silver chloride as the reference, and platinum wire as the counter electrode. Nickel oxide was electrodeposited using a mixture of nickel chloride, nickel acetate, and sodium sulphate and pretreated in 0.1 M sodium hydroxide to convert to nickel hydroxide or nickel oxyhydroxide. The electrocatalytic oxidation of lactate to pyruvate is facilitated by the conversion from Ni^{3+} to Ni^{2+} (Patel et al. 2023).

Cortisol and neuropeptides are key biomarkers associated with stress. An aptamer-based sensor for cortisol and neuropeptide was developed on a PCB substrate using Electrochemical Impedance Spectroscopy. The aptamer sensor platform was able to detect cortisol and neuropeptides in sweat samples with a detection range of 1–256 ng mL^{-1} and 1–256 pg mL^{-1}, respectively (Churcher et al. 2022). Troponin-T is a key biomarker found in the bloodstream of patients suffering from acute myocardial damage. A thin film of nanostructured zinc oxide (ZnO) was sputtered on an electroplated Au-PCB substrate. The immunoassay is fabricated by immobilizing a cross-linking molecule (dithiobissuccinimidylpropionate (DSP)) on the substrate, followed by adding antibodies (anti-troponin-T) and blocking unoccupied sites with superblock (Fig. 15.4C). The sensor revealed a detection limit of 10 fg mL^{-1} in PBS and 100 fg mL^{-1} in human serum samples (Jacobs et al. 2014).

The glycan-lectin interaction offers valuable insights into early cancer diagnosis, as biomarkers like MUC1, CEA, CA125, and PSA are highly glycosylated. A label-free glycan-lectin interaction was studied using impedance spectroscopy. Galactose-binding peanut agglutinin (PNA) and sialic acid-binding *sambucus nigra* agglutinin (SNA) are covalently bound on ENIG finish PCB substrate. This study highlights the label-free glycan-lectin interaction, showcasing its potential in cancer diagnostics, especially for identifying tumours associated with carbohydrate antigens (La Belle et al. 2007). Multiple sclerosis is an autoimmune disorder affecting the central nervous system and the overexpression of serum cytokine, often characterized by the overexpression of interleukin-12 (IL-12). A Label-free immunosensor was developed on PCB for the detection of IL-12 (Fig. 15.4B). To immobilize antibodies on the PCB electrode, 16-mercaptohexadecanoic acid was initially added, followed by EDC-NHS activation to facilitate antibody binding. After antibody immobilization, unreacted carboxylic acid groups were blocked with methanolamine. The developed sensor could detect IL-12 at a physiological level (Bhavsar et al. 2009). C-reactive protein (CRP) is produced in the liver in response to inflammation, and it is considered a key biomarker for monitoring inflammatory conditions. A ZnO-based immunosensor was developed on a PCB. A co-planar copper electrode was made on a FR4 substrate to fabricate an immunosensor. This work utilizes the development of an electrochemical equivalence circuit model (EEC) for a ZnO biosensor platform, designed to measure the varying CRP concentrations using impedance spectroscopy. The EEC, based on the Randles model, successfully correlated experimental and model data, quantifying charge modulations caused by CRP binding within the double layer at the ZnO–PBS interface. The developed impedimetric sensor could detect CRP within the concentration range of 1–10 ng mL^{-1} (Eveness et al. 2022).

PCB-based electrochemical sensors are also reported for virus and bacteria detection. An electrochemical immunosensor was developed on an ENIG finish PCB platform for SARS-CoV-2 detection. The cysteamine and glutaraldehyde were sequentially added to the gold working electrode to immobilize the SARS-CoV-2 spike protein antibody, with glutaraldehyde crosslinking cysteamine and binding to the amino group of the antibody. The polyclonal antibodies were immobilized on the surface, and BSA was used to block the vacant sites (Nandeshwar et al. 2021). A DNA-based electrochemical sensor was fabricated for the detection of SARS-CoV-2 amplicons employing methylene blue-DNA intercalation. The PCB electrode manufactured using the ENIG process is directly used as the sensing platform, without requiring additional modification steps. The change in current in voltammetric responses resulted from the adsorption of methylene blue-DNA complex on the electrode surface (Kumar et al. 2021). Tuberculosis (TB) is a contagious bacterial infection primarily affecting the lungs, caused by *Mycobacterium tuberculosis*. An amperometric PCB-based sensor was developed for cytokine detection using enzyme-linked immunosorbent assay (ELISA), providing an efficient method for TB diagnosis. The study employs an Au-coated PCB platform to immobilize the antibody via cysteine (thiol) linkage. A combination of colourimetric and electrochemical measurement was used to detect anti-interferon-gamma (IFNγ). The assays are performed using a modified ELISA protocol with TMB as the reporter molecule, enabling amperometric detection (Evans et al. 2017). A similar PCB-based microfluidics was developed for the detection for IFNγ. They improved the sensor range to 10–2048 pg mL^{-1} with a sensitivity of 40 pg mL^{-1} (Evans et al. 2018). An aptamer-based sensor was developed for *Salmonella enterica* serovar Typhimurium protein using an electroplated PCB gold electrode (la Belle et al. 2009). Tetracycline (Tet), ciprofloxacin (Cfx), and tobramycin (Tob) are antibiotics commonly used against a wide variety of bacterial infections. Thermally reduced graphene oxide was drop-cast to modify the PCB platform and incubated with 1-pyrene butanoic acid succinimidyl ester to facilitate the binding of antibodies (Mukherjee et al. 2025).

Another aptamer-based sensor was developed for *Salmonella Typhi* Hemolysin E protein using graphene oxide-chitosan modified PCB gold electrode. This label-free detection could detect 1.25–20 ng μL^{-1} with LOD 0.137 ng μL^{-1}. The aptamer-based sensor effectively detected in serum samples of *S. Typhi*-infected patients, with good correlation to commercial Typhidot assay (Awang et al. 2025). A cost-effective electrochemical sensor for viral nucleic acid detection was developed using PCB-based electrodes, showing a linear detection range from 10 pg μL^{-1} to 20 ng μL^{-1}. The electrodes were fabricated using the commercially available and affordable electroless nickel immersion gold technique, which provides extended shelf life without requiring special storage conditions (Ahuja et al. 2022).

A platform for nucleic acid detection on microarrays was developed, using gold electrode coated with SAM containing DNA probes. The unlabelled nucleic acid hybridizes with probe, while the signalling probe with ferrocene-modified nucleotide forms a sandwich complex. This system enables sequence-specific detection, single-nucleotide polymorphism discrimination, and gene expression monitoring (Umek et al. 2001). In another work, peptide nucleic acid (PNA) was utilized as a sequencing probe for genetic analysis. The gold-plated copper platform was functionalized with a thiolated PNA probe (Jolly et al. 2019).

Alzheimer's disease is a progressive and irreversible neurodegenerative disorder that primarily affects memory, thinking, and behaviour. Aβ40 and Aβ42 peptides are the key biomarkers associated with the disease (Ghasemi et al. 2018). PCB sensing electrodes electrodeposited with polypyrrole have been reported for the simultaneous detection of Aβ40 and Aβ42 (Supraja et al. 2021). The detection of Ubiquitin-carboxy terminal hydro-lase L1(UCHL1), a Traumatic Brain Injury (TBI) specific biomarker, using a PCB-based sensing platform has been developed. Polypyrrole (PPy)-functionalized multiwalled carbon nanotube composite synthesized by in-situ chemical oxidative polymerization was used to immobilize antibodies using glutaraldehyde as a crosslinker (Supraja et al. 2022). Using a similar approach, a PPy-MWCNT composite-based portable sensor was developed for UCHL1 and Glial Fibrillary Acidic protein (GFAP) (Supraja et al. 2023). A summary of electrode modification for PCB-based sensors, their target analytes, and sensor performance is presented in Table 15.1.

Table 15.1 Summary of PCB-based sensors

Platform	Electrode modification	Target analyte	Sensitivity	Analytical range	LOD	References
Electroplated Ni/Au	GOx	Glucose	–	50–250 mg dL^{-1}	–	Kim et al. (2019)
ENIG, Electroplated Au	Red phenol/CNT	Glucose	3.13 μA mM^{-1} cm^{-2}	1–15 mM	0.8 mg dL^{-1}	Kassanos et al. (2018)
Electroplated Au	GOx	Glucose	–	0.5–20 mM	500 μM	Dutta et al. (2018)
Au	CNT/GOx	Glucose	–	1–100 mM	0.1 mM	Alhans et al. (2018)
hPG/Au	Os/GOx	Glucose	21.50	0.05–1 mM	50 μM	Gonzalez-Solino et al. (2021)
PCB GE	NiO	Lactate	42.71 μA mg dL^{-1}	0.1–10 mg dL^{-1}	–	Patel et al. (2023)
Electroplated Au	ZnO/DSP	Troponin-T	–	0–100 pg mL^{-1}	100 fg mL^{-1}	Jacobs et al. (2014)
Electroplated Ni, Au	Ab	*Salmonella typhimurium*	–	–	10 pg mL^{-1}	La Belle et al. (2007)
Electroplated Ni, Au	Ab	Interleukin-12	–	0–25 pg mL^{-1}	–	Bhavsar et al. (2009)
ENIG	Ab/Cysteamine/Gluteraldehyde	SARS-CoV-2	–	0.1–500 ng mL^{-1}	0.1 ng mL^{-1}	Nandeshwar et al. (2021)
Electroplated Au	Ab	*Mycobacterium tuberculosis*	–	–	10 pg mL^{-1}	Evans et al. (2017)
Electroplated Au	Ab	IFNγ	–	16–2048 pg mL^{-1}	40 pg mL^{-1}	Evans et al. (2018)
Electroplated Au	DNA probe	DNA	–	–	–	Umek et al. (2001)

15.4 Application of Flexible Printed Circuit Boards in Sensing

Flexible printed circuit boards (FPCBs) are distinguished by their thin, lightweight, and flexible nature, setting them apart from conventional rigid PCBs. Their application in electronic devices has grown rapidly in recent years, fuelled by increasing demand for compact, portable, and wearable technologies (Yang and Yan 2021). In recent years, flexible PCB technology has attracted considerable interest in biosensing applications. Its widespread manufacturability, lightweight design, and mechanical flexibility make it an excellent choice for developing compact, thin, wearable measurement systems integrated with microfabricated biosensors (Shamkhalichenar et al. 2020).

A FPCB was developed using a polyimide substrate modified with graphene and AuNPs for GOx immobilization for glucose monitoring. The flexible sensor consists of a working electrode (1.2 × 0.2 mm) and a counter electrode (1.2 × 0.2 mm). A 5 μm gold layer was electrodeposited onto the electrode by depositing nickel on the copper layer, then replacing the nickel with gold through immersion in $KAu(CN)_2$ solution. The graphene layer was casted via inkjet printing, followed by gold nanoparticle electrodeposition to improve sensitivity. The GOx was then immobilized onto the working graphene AuNP layer by electropolymerization (Fig. 15.5A).

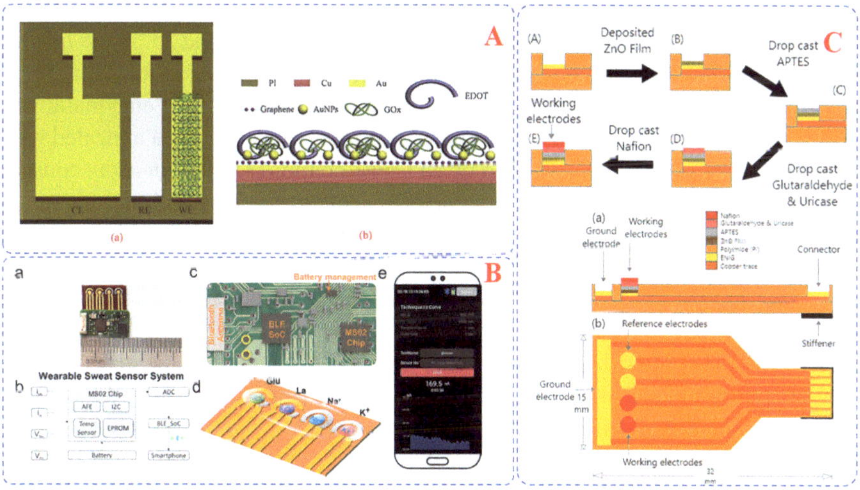

Fig. 15.5 (**A**) FPCB-based glucose sensor with a detailed view of the structure of the working electrode showing layers including PI, Cu, Au, graphene, AuNPs, GOx, and EDOT. Adapted with permission from (Pu et al. 2016), Copyright 2009 Elsevier. (**B**) FPCB-based sensing of glucose, lactate, Na^+, K^+, including an optical photograph of the integrated sweat sensor system, system-level block diagram of the wearable sensor, PCB responsible for biological signal processing, schematic of the electrochemical sensor array-integrated sensors and smartphone interface displaying data. Adapted with permission from (Wang et al. 2022), Copyright 2009 Elsevier. (**C**) FPCB-based uric acid sensor, illustrating fabrication of the working electrode along with cross-sectional and plan view representations. Reproduced from (Yang et al. 2023a), Creative Commons Attribution License (https://creativecommons.org/licenses/by/4.0/)

The FPCB-based glucose sensor could detect low glucose concentrations with a detection limit of 0.3 mg dL^{-1}, with a detection range of 0–40 mg dL^{-1} (Pu et al. 2016). Another work described the development of a glucose and lactate sensor by coating platinum black on the gold working electrode of a flexible. The platinum black enhanced the catalytic oxidation of hydrogen peroxide, which is produced during enzyme-catalysed reactions of glucose and lactate. The developed sensor can detect glucose up to 20 mM with a sensitivity of 41 nA mM^{-1} and lactate up to 0.8 mM with a sensitivity of 106.8 nA mM^{-1} (Kassanos et al. 2023).

An enzymatic glucose sensor was developed using a RuO_2 sputtered flexible PCB platform. The glucose sensor was fabricated on an FPCB composed of rolled annealed copper, electroless nickel gold, and polyimide. RuO_2 was modified on the substrate by radiofrequency sputtering and functionalized with (3-aminopropyl) triethoxy silane (APTES) and glutaraldehyde to immobilize the GOx enzyme. It detected glucose in the concentration range of 3–7 mM with a sensitivity of 44.42 mV/mM (Kuo et al. 2024). A similar platform was developed using a miniaturized MgO multi-sensor on an FPCB for simultaneous glucose and pH measurement. A thin layer of MgO was RF sputtered on ENIG modified FPCB. The glucose oxidase is immobilized on the modified substrate using glutaraldehyde and APTES for the fabrication of the glucose sensor. The potentiometric pH sensor involves the reaction of the MgO surface with H^+ ions, forming $MgOH^+$ and OH^- ions. As the pH changes, shifts in the ion concentrations alter the surface potential, which is measured as voltage differences for pH detection. The developed multi-sensor showcased excellent sensitivity, showing 6.78 mV/mM for glucose and 25.27 mV/pH for pH, respectively (Yang et al. 2025). A potentiometric uric acid sensor with a temperature correction unit was fabricated on an FPCB platform. The enzymatic uric acid sensor was fabricated on a polyimide substrate, with rolled and annealed copper applied on copper wire, followed by an ENIG coating. The sensor array consists of two working electrodes (2 mm diameter), a reference electrode, and a counter electrode with the working area modified with Nafion/uricase/APTES/zinc oxide structures (Fig. 15.5C). A thin ZnO layer was initially deposited using radiofrequency sputtering and functionalized with APTES. The uricase enzyme was then immobilized on the APTES layer using glutaraldehyde, and Nafion was added to prevent the enzyme leakage (Yang et al. 2023a). A similar sensor platform was developed for potentiometric dopamine detection using aluminium-doped zinc oxide. A thin layer of aluminium-doped zinc oxide (AZO) was deposited by radio frequency sputtering on a FPCB (ENIG) platform. The tyrosinase enzyme (Tyr) was immobilized on the AZO-modified electrode using APTES and glutaraldehyde. The AZO/ENIG/Cu/PI electrode exhibited superior performance compared to Tyr/AZO/ENIG/Cu/PI electrodes due to the excellent electrocatalytic activity of tyrosinase towards dopamine, resulting in an increased sensitivity from 33.68 to 71.66 mV dec^{-1} (Yang et al. 2023b).

A flexible electrochemical sensor array is integrated with a PCB to analyse multiple biomarkers in sweat during exercise. The electrodes were fabricated by screen printing technology on a flexible polyimide sheet and then modified for the selective detection of glucose, lactate, Na^+, and K^+ (Fig. 15.5B). A Prussian blue layer was electrodeposited on the working electrode as an electron transport mediator, followed by immobilization of the respective enzyme (GOx for glucose and lactate oxidase for lactate) using chitosan and carbon nanotubes. To fabricate Na^+ and K^+ sensor, poly(3–4)ethylenedioxythiophene: polystyrene sulphonate (PEDOT:PSS) was deposited on the electrode to reduce potential drift, and ion-selective membranes for Na^+ and K^+ ions were prepared and dropped on the respective electrodes. The Na^+ selective membrane mixture, containing sodium ionophore X, Na-TFPB, PVC, and DOS, was dissolved in THF, while the K^+ selective membrane mixture, including valinomycin, Na-TFPB, PVC, and DOS, was dissolved in cyclohexanone (Wang et al. 2022). In another work, a multi-ion sensor was developed on a PCB and a flexible PCB for potentiometric detection of pH, Na^+, and K^+. The developed sensor demonstrated sensitivity of 73.4 mV/log [H^+], 56.3 mV/log [Na^+], and 57.14 mV/log [K^+] (Anastasova et al. 2018). A non-enzymatic FPCB-based sensor was developed for ammonium ion detection in sweat samples, using a flexible electrolyte-gated carbon nanotube field effect transistor on polyimide. Carbon nanotubes were used as the active material with a nonactin ionophore-based ion-selective membrane for the selective detection of ammonium ions. The platform achieved a sensitivity of 4.516 $\mu A\ dec^{-1}$ with a detection range of 0.1–100 mM (Petrelli et al. 2023).

Label-free DNA sensor was fabricated on a flexible printed circuit for the detection of SARS-CoV-2. The electrodes were screen printed directly onto the FPCB, where graphene ink is used for printing the working electrode. The study used a two-step strategy involving the immobilization of a biotinylated complementary sequence on a streptavidin-modified surface, followed by hybridization with the target sequence. This graphene-based DNA sensor exhibited a linear range of detection from 100 fg mL^{-1} to 1 μg mL^{-1} with a 100 fg mL^{-1} limit of detection (Damiati et al. 2021). Graphene-based sensor arrays are fabricated on a flexible polyimide substrate for the detection of CRP in sweat. The study used laser-engraved graphene-based impedimetric immobilized with AuNP conjugated CRP capture antibodies for the immunosensor fabrication (Tu et al. 2023).

15.5 Conclusion

Throughout this chapter, key advancements in PCB based technology, from rigid to flexible platforms, have been discussed in the context of various medical applications. PCB-based biosensors are revolutionizing the field of medical diagnostics by offering a unique combination of scalability, cost-effectiveness, miniaturization, and rapid prototyping. In contrast to conventional microfabrication processes, which often rely on cleanroom facilities and specialized equipment, PCB-based sensor fabrication utilizes the mature and globally established electronics manufacturing infrastructure. Leveraging well-established PCB fabrication techniques, a wide spectrum of biosensor applications, including enzymatic, immunosensor, aptamer-based, and label-free systems, have been integrated on rigid and flexible PCBs. While traditional PCBs are constructed using copper, which presents limitations for direct electrochemical sensing, innovative modification techniques and alternative electrode finishes (e.g., Au, Ni, or carbon ink) have been developed to enable reliable biofunctionalization and signal transduction. Furthermore, the integration of novel materials such as carbon nanotubes, reduced graphene oxide, and metal or metal oxide nanoparticles can significantly enhance sensor sensitivity, selectivity, and stability.

The adaptability of PCB substrates for electrochemical sensing, combined with advancements in surface modification, nanomaterial integration, and microfabrication techniques, underscores their potential for point-of-care diagnostics. Moreover, FPCB-based platforms are proving to be critical in the development of next-generation wearable biosensors. These systems are capable of conforming to the body and monitoring physiological markers in real-time via non-invasive sampling of sweat, saliva, or interstitial fluid. This opens doors for applications in continuous health monitoring, early disease detection, and personalized medicine, especially in resource-limited or remote settings.

References

Ahuja S, Kumar MS, Nandeshwar R, Kondabagil K, Tallur S (2022) Longer amplicons provide better sensitivity for electrochemical sensing of viral nucleic acid in water samples using PCB electrodes. Sci Rep 12. https://doi.org/10.1038/s41598-022-12818-w

Ahuja S, Kulkarni A, Pandey R, Kondabagil K, Tallur S (2025) Practical considerations for DNA sensing using faradaic electrochemical impedance spectroscopy on ENIG PCB electrodes. Biosensors Bioelectronics: X 22. https://doi.org/10.1016/j.biosx.2024.100569

Alhans R, Singh A, Singhal C, Narang J, Wadhwa S, Mathur A (2018) Comparative analysis of single-walled and multi-walled carbon nanotubes for electrochemical sensing of glucose on gold printed circuit boards. Mater Sci Eng C 90:273–279. https://doi.org/10.1016/j.msec.2018.04.072

Anastasova S, Kassanos P, Yang GZ (2018) Multi-parametric rigid and flexible, low-cost, disposable sensing platforms for biomedical applications. Biosens Bioelectron 102:668–675. https://doi.org/10.1016/j.bios.2017.10.038

Awang MS, Zambry NS, Bustami Y, Ahmad Najib M, Khalid MF, Beh KK, Md Zawawi MA, Hamzah HH, Aziah I, Abd Manaf A (2025) A new Aptasensor to detect Salmonella Typhi Hemolysin E protein utilising a graphene oxide-chitosan modified printed circuit board gold electrode. Int J Biol Macromol 311. https://doi.org/10.1016/j.ijbiomac.2025.143534

Bhavsar K, Fairchild A, Alonas E, Bishop DK, La Belle JT, Sweeney J, Alford TL, Joshi L (2009) A cytokine immunosensor for multiple sclerosis detection based upon label-free electrochemical impedance spectroscopy using electroplated printed circuit board electrodes. Biosens Bioelectron 25:506–509. https://doi.org/10.1016/j.bios.2009.07.017

Chan CM, Tong KH, Leung SL, Wong PS, Yee KW, Bayes MW (n.d.) Development of novel immersion gold for Electroless nickel immersion gold process (ENIG) in PCB applications. IEEE

Chandhana JP, Punnakkal N, Vasu SP, Pradeep A, Nair BG, Babu TGS (2023) Zirconium copper oxide microflowers based non-enzymatic screen-printed electrochemical sensor for the detection of glucose in saliva, urine, and blood serum. Microchim Acta 190:390. https://doi.org/10.1007/s00604-023-05965-y

Chandhana JP, Punnakkal N, Vasu SP, Babu TGS (2024a) Development of a reagent-free electrochemical disposable sensor strip for the quantification of sweat chloride. Microchem J 208:112344. https://doi.org/10.1016/j.microc.2024.112344

Chandhana J P, Vasu SP, Pradeep A, G. SBT. (2025) Platinum copper oxide decorated niobium MXene graphene oxide nanocomposite for non-enzymatic glucose detection in saliva and urine. Electrochim Acta 535:146640. https://doi.org/10.1016/j.electacta.2025.146640

Churcher NKM, Greyling C, Upasham S, Lin KC, Rice P, Pali M, Spiro J, Prasad S (2022) AptaStrensor (aptamer-based sensor for stress monitoring): the interrelationship between NPY and cortisol towards chronic disease monitoring. Biosensors and Bioelectronics: X 10. https://doi.org/10.1016/j.biosx.2022.100145

da Silva ETSG, Souto DEP, Barragan JTC, Giarola J d F, de Moraes ACM, Kubota LT (2017) Electrochemical biosensors in point-of-care devices: recent advances and future trends. ChemElectroChem 4:778–794. https://doi.org/10.1002/celc.201600758

Damiati S, Sopstad S, Peacock M, Akhtar AS, Pinto I, Soares RRG, Russom A (2021) Flex printed circuit board implemented graphene-based DNA sensor for detection of SARS-CoV-2. IEEE Sensors J 21:13060–13067. https://doi.org/10.1109/JSEN.2021.3068922

De Santana PP, De Oliveira IMF, Piccin E (2012) Evaluation of using xurography as a new technique for the fabrication of disposable gold electrodes with highly reproducible areas. Electrochem Commun 16:96–99. https://doi.org/10.1016/j.elecom.2011.12.005

Dutta G, Regoutz A, Moschou D (2018) Commercially fabricated printed circuit board sensing electrodes for biomarker electrochemical detection: the importance of electrode surface characteristics in sensor performance. MDPI AG, p 741. https://doi.org/10.3390/proceedings2130741

Dutta G, Jallow AA, Paul D, Moschou D (2019) Label-free electrochemical detection of S. Mutans exploiting commercially fabricated printed circuit board sensing electrodes. Micromachines (Basel) 10:575. https://doi.org/10.3390/mi10090575

Evans D, Papadimitriou KI, Greathead L, Vasilakis N, Pantelidis P, Kelleher P, Morgan H, Prodromakis T (2017) An assay system for point-of-care diagnosis of tuberculosis using commercially manufactured PCB technology. Sci Rep 7. https://doi.org/10.1038/s41598-017-00783-8

Evans D, Papadimitriou KI, Vasilakis N, Pantelidis P, Kelleher P, Morgan H, Prodromakis T (2018) A novel microfluidic point-of-care biosensor system on printed circuit board for cytokine detection. Sensors (Switzerland) 18. https://doi.org/10.3390/s18114011

Eveness J, Cao L, Kiely J, Luxton R (2022) Equivalent circuit model of a non-faradaic impedimetric ZnO nano-crystal biosensor. J Electroanal Chem 906. https://doi.org/10.1016/j.jelechem.2021.116003

Ezema Ike Eze IC, Ucheji ON, Ubi PA, Oji EO, Aigbodion VS, Omah AD, Ogbuefi UC (2023) An overview of flame retardants in printed circuit boards for LEDs and other electronic devices. J Mater Environ Sci 14:410–420. http://www.jmaterenvironsci.com

Gassmann S, Gotze H, Hinze M, Mix M, Flechsig GU, Pagel L (2012) PCB based DNA detection chip. In: IECON proceedings (Industrial Electronics Conference), pp 3982–3986. https://doi.org/10.1109/IECON.2012.6389254

Ghasemi F, Reza Hormozi-Nezhad M, Mahmoudi M (2018) Label-free detection of β-amyloid peptides (Aβ40 and Aβ42): a colorimetric sensor array for plasma monitoring of Alzheimer's disease. Nanoscale 10:6361–6368. https://doi.org/10.1039/c8nr00195b

González-Solino C, Bernalte E, Bayona Royo C, Bennett R, Leech D, Di Lorenzo M (2021) Self-powered detection of glucose by enzymatic glucose/oxygen fuel cells on printed circuit boards. ACS Appl Mater Interfaces 13:26704–26711. https://doi.org/10.1021/acsami.1c02747

Chandhana JP, Roshith M, Punathil Vasu S, Kumar DVR, Satheesh SB (2024b) High aspect ratio copper nanowires modified screen-printed carbon electrode for interference-free non-enzymatic detection of serum creatinine in neutral medium. J Electroanal Chem 971:118605. https://doi.org/10.1016/j.jelechem.2024.118605

Jacobs M, Muthukumar S, Panneer Selvam A, Engel Craven J, Prasad S (2014) Ultra-sensitive electrical immunoassay biosensors using nanotextured zinc oxide thin films on printed circuit board platforms. Biosens Bioelectron 55:7–13. https://doi.org/10.1016/j.bios.2013.11.022

Jolly P, Rainbow J, Regoutz A, Estrela P, Moschou D (2019) A PNA-based lab-on-PCB diagnostic platform for rapid and high sensitivity DNA quantification. Biosens Bioelectron 123:244–250. https://doi.org/10.1016/j.bios.2018.09.006

Kassanos P, Anastasova S, Yang G-Z (2018) A low-cost Amperometric glucose sensor Basedon PCB technology. IEEE Sens:1–4

Kassanos P, Gowers S, Boutelle M (2023) Glucose and lactate Amperometric sensors on a flexible printed circuit for low-cost sensing applications. In: Proceedings of IEEE sensors. Institute of Electrical and Electronics Engineers Inc. https://doi.org/10.1109/SENSORS56945.2023.10325314

Kim KY, Chang H, Der Lee W, Cai YF, Chen YJ (2019) The influence of blood glucose meter resistance variation on the performance of a biosensor with a gold-coated circuit board. J Sens 2019. https://doi.org/10.1155/2019/5948182

Kim J, Jeong J, Ko SH (2024) Electrochemical biosensors for point-of-care testing. Biodes Manuf 7:548–565. https://doi.org/10.1007/s42242-024-00301-6

Kumar MS, Nandeshwar R, Lad SB, Megha K, Mangat M, Butterworth A, Knapp CW, Knapp M, Hoskisson PA, Corrigan DK, Ward AC, Kondabagil K, Tallur S (2021) Electrochemical sensing of SARS-CoV-2 amplicons with PCB electrodes. Sens Actuators B-Chem 343. https://doi.org/10.1016/j.snb.2021.130169

Kuo PY, Liao CH, Wang TH, Hsu MT (2024) Design and fabrication of enzymatic potentiometric biosensor based on flexible printed circuit board for glucose detection. IEEE Trans Nanobioscience 23:283–290. https://doi.org/10.1109/TNB.2023.3337381

La Belle JT, Gerlach JQ, Svarovsky S, Joshi L (2007) Label-free impedimetric detection of glycan-lectin interactions. Anal Chem 79:6959–6964. https://doi.org/10.1021/ac070651e

la Belle JT, Shah M, Reed J, Nandakumar V, Alford TL, Wilson JW, Nickerson CA, Joshi L (2009) Label-free and ultra-low level detection of salmonella enterica serovar typhimurium using electrochemical impedance spectroscopy. Electroanalysis 21:2267–2271. https://doi.org/10.1002/elan.200904666

LaDou J (2006) Printed circuit board industry. Int J Hyg Environ Health 209:211–219. https://doi.org/10.1016/j.ijheh.2006.02.001

Li X, Zang J, Liu Y, Lu Z, Li Q, Li CM (2013) Simultaneous detection of lactate and glucose by integrated printed circuit board based array sensing chip. Anal Chim Acta 771:102–107. https://doi.org/10.1016/j.aca.2013.02.011

Mirzajani H, Cheng C, Vafaie RH, Wu J, Chen J, Eda S, Aghdam EN, Ghavifekr HB (2022) Optimization of ACEK-enhanced, PCB-based biosensor for highly sensitive and rapid detection of bisphenol a in low resource settings. Biosens Bioelectron 196:113745. https://doi.org/10.1016/j.bios.2021.113745

Mohammadzadeh M, Haghighi B (2021) Fabrication and characterization of a low-cost microvolume electrochemical cell using PCB for electroanalytical applications. J Electrochem Soc 168:057517. https://doi.org/10.1149/1945-7111/ac0016

Mukherjee P, Sen S, Das A, Kundu S, RoyChaudhuri C (2025) Graphene FET biochip on PCB reinforced by machine learning for ultrasensitive parallel detection of multiple antibiotics in water. Biosens Bioelectron 271. https://doi.org/10.1016/j.bios.2024.117023

Nandeshwar R, Kumar MS, Kondabagil K, Tallur S (2021) Electrochemical Immunosensor platform using low-cost ENIG PCB finish electrodes: application for SARS-CoV-2 spike protein sensing. IEEE Access 9:154368–154377. https://doi.org/10.1109/ACCESS.2021.3128668

Patel V, Bhargava A, Puri A, Ghosh A, Srivastava R (2023) A pretreated electrodeposited nickel oxide film on gold PCB electrode for solid-state lactate sensing. In: 2023 IEEE BioSensors conference, BioSensors 2023 – proceedings. Institute of Electrical and Electronics Engineers Inc. https://doi.org/10.1109/BioSensors58001.2023.10281096

Perdigones F, Quero JM (2022) Printed circuit boards: the layers' functions for electronic and biomedical engineering. Micromachines (Basel) 13. https://doi.org/10.3390/mi13030460

Petrelli M, Golparvar A, Meimandi A, Shkodra B, Angeli MAC, Falco A, Lugli P, Petti L, Carrara S (2023) Flexible sensor and readout circuitry for continuous ion sensing in sweat. IEEE Sens Lett 7. https://doi.org/10.1109/LSENS.2023.3274682

Pu Z, Wang R, Wu J, Yu H, Xu K, Li D (2016) A flexible electrochemical glucose sensor with composite nanostructured surface of the working electrode. Sens Actuators B Chem 230:801–809. https://doi.org/10.1016/j.snb.2016.02.115

Sánchez JLA, Henry OYF, Joda H, Solnestam BW, Kvastad L, Johansson E, Akan P, Lundeberg J, Lladach N, Ramakrishnan D, Riley I, O'Sullivan CK (2016) Multiplex PCB-based electrochemical detection of cancer biomarkers using MLPA-barcode approach. Biosens Bioelectron 82:224–232. https://doi.org/10.1016/j.bios.2016.04.018

Shamkhalichenar H, Bueche CJ, Choi JW (2020) Printed circuit board (PCB) Technology for Electrochemical Sensors and Sensing Platforms. Biosensors (Basel) 10:159. https://doi.org/10.3390/bios10110159

Supraja P, Tripathy S, Singh R, Singh V, Chaudhury G, Singh SG (2021) Towards point-of-care diagnosis of Alzheimer's disease: multi-analyte based portable chemiresistive platform for simultaneous detection of β-amyloid (1–40) and (1–42) in plasma. Biosens Bioelectron 186. https://doi.org/10.1016/j.bios.2021.113294

Supraja P, Tripathy S, Krishna Vanjari SR, Singh SG (2022) Label-free, ultrasensitive and rapid detection of FDA-approved TBI specific UCHL1 biomarker in plasma using MWCNT-PPY nanocomposite as bio-electrical transducer: a step closer to point-of-care diagnosis of TBI. Biosens Bioelectron 216. https://doi.org/10.1016/j.bios.2022.114631

Supraja P, Tripathy S, Govind Singh S (2023) Smartphone-powered, ultrasensitive, and selective, portable and stable multi-analyte chemiresistive immunosensing platform with PPY/COOH-MWCNT as bioelectrical transducer: towards point-of-care TBI diagnosis. Bioelectrochemistry 151. https://doi.org/10.1016/j.bioelechem.2023.108391

Tortorich RP, Shamkhalichenar H, Choi JW (2018) Inkjet-printed and paper-based electrochemical sensors. Appl Sci (Switz) 8. https://doi.org/10.3390/app8020288

Tu J, Min J, Song Y, Xu C, Li J, Moore J, Hanson J, Hu E, Parimon T, Wang TY, Davoodi E, Chou TF, Chen P, Hsu JJ, Rossiter HB, Gao W (2023) A wireless patch for the monitoring of C-reactive protein in sweat. Nat Biomed Eng 7:1293–1306. https://doi.org/10.1038/s41551-023-01059-5

Umek RM, Lin SW, Vielmetter J, Terbrueggen RH, Irvine B, Yu CJ, Kayyem JF, Yowanto H, Blackburn GF, Farkas DH, Chen YP (2001) Electronic detection of nucleic acids: a versatile platform for molecular diagnostics. J Mol Diagn 3:74–84. https://doi.org/10.1016/S1525-1578(10)60655-1

Wang J (2006) Electrochemical biosensors: towards point-of-care cancer diagnostics. Biosens Bioelectron 21(10):1887–1892. https://doi.org/10.1016/j.bios.2005.10.027

Wang L, Xue L, Guo R, Zheng L, Wang S, Yao L, Huo X, Liu N, Liao M, Li Y, Lin J (2020) Combining impedance biosensor with immunomagnetic separation for rapid screening of salmonella in poultry supply chains. Poult Sci 99:1606–1614. https://doi.org/10.1016/j.psj.2019.12.007

Wang J, Wang L, Li G, Yan D, Liu C, Xu T, Zhang X (2022) Ultra-small wearable flexible biosensor for continuous sweat analysis. ACS Sens 7:3102–3107. https://doi.org/10.1021/acssensors.2c01533

Yang A, Yan F (2021) Flexible electrochemical biosensors for health monitoring. ACS Appl Electron Mater 3:53–67. https://doi.org/10.1021/acsaelm.0c00534

Yang PH, Chan CT, Chang YS (2023a) A flexible printed circuit board-based ZnO enzymatic uric acid potentiometric biosensor measurement and characterization. IEEE J Electron Devi Soc 11:114–121. https://doi.org/10.1109/JEDS.2023.3243056

Yang PH, Chang YS, Chan CT (2023b) Aluminum-doped zinc oxide enzymatic dopamine biosensor integrated with potentiometric readout circuit board. IEEE Sensors J 23:1809–1817. https://doi.org/10.1109/JSEN.2022.3231412

Yang PH, Huang JM, Chou JC, Lai CH, Kuo PY, Nien YH, Chen WS, Hsu MT, Liao CH (2025) A miniaturized MgO multi-sensor device based on a flexible printed circuit Board for Glucose and pH detection. IEEE Trans Nanobioscience. https://doi.org/10.1109/TNB.2025.3536456

Zupančič U, Rainbow J, Estrela P, Moschou D (2021) Utilising commercially fabricated printed circuit boards as an electrochemical biosensing platform. Micromachines (Basel) 12:793. https://doi.org/10.3390/mi12070793

MIX
Papier aus verantwortungsvollen Quellen
Paper from responsible sources
FSC® C105338

If you have any concerns about our products,
you can contact us on
ProductSafety@springernature.com

In case Publisher is established outside the EU,
the EU authorized representative is:
Springer Nature Customer Service Center GmbH
Europaplatz 3, 69115 Heidelberg, Germany

Printed by Libri Plureos GmbH
in Hamburg, Germany